ADVANCES IN THE BIOLOGY, IMAGING AND THERAPIES FOR GLIOBLASTOMA

Edited by **Clark C. Chen**

Advances in the Biology, Imaging and Therapies for Glioblastoma
Edited by Clark C. Chen

Published by InTech
Janeza Trdine 9, 51000 Rijeka, Croatia

Publishing Process Manager Petra Nenadic

Technical Editor Teodora Smiljanic

Cover Designer InTech Design Team

Additional hard copies can be obtained from orders@intechopen.com

Advances in the Biology, Imaging and Therapies for Glioblastoma,
Edited by Clark C. Chen
p. cm.
ISBN 978-953-307-284-5

Meet the editor

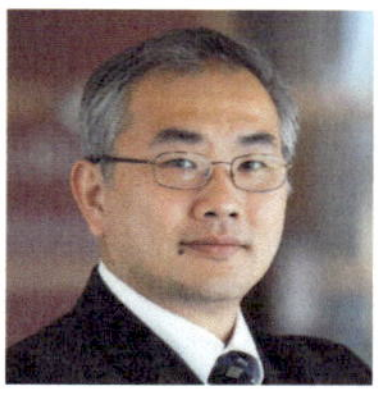

Dr. Clark C. Chen received his B.S. from Stanford University in 1992, M.S. from Columbia University in 1993, and his M.D.-Ph.D. from Harvard Medical School in 2001. He completed his neurosurgery training at the Massachusetts General Hospital and subsequently completed independent fellowships in stereotactic neurosurgery and radiosurgery. Dr. Chen previously served as the director of Clinical Neuro-Oncology at the Beth Israel Deaconess Medical Center before his current role as the Director of Stereotactic and Radiosurgery and Co-Director of Surgical Neuro-Oncology at the University of California, San Diego. Dr. Chen's research is directed at identifying alterations in DNA repair pathways as they relate to brain cancer therapy. Dr. Chen is the recipient of the Damon Runyon Fellowship Award, the James Kerr Award, American Brain Tumor Association Investigator Award, Paul Calabresi Scholar Award, Burroughs Wellcome Career Award, William Guy Forbeck Scholar Award, the Doris Duke Clinical Scientist Award and the Kimmel Scholar Award.

Contents

Preface

Glioblastoma remains one of the deadliest of human cancers, with almost uniform fatality of those afflicted. Any potential hope of improved clinical outcome would necessarily be grounded in advances in tumor imaging as it relates to biologic tenets and therapeutic strategies. It is in this context that this compendium is assembled. The selected articles are meant to highlight novel paradigms in hopes of stimulating thoughts that may ultimately contribute to meaningful improvement in clinical outcome. Emphasis was placed on key concepts as they relate to clinical translation. I hope that the work will contribute to the collective effort to ultimately cure the devastating disease of glioblastoma.

Clark C. Chen, M.D., Ph.D.
University of California,
San Diego
USA

Part 1

Biology of Malignant Gliomas

1

Radiobiology of Radioresistant Glioblastoma

Jerry R. Williams, Daila S. Gridley and James M. Slater
Radiation Research Laboratories,
Department of Radiation Medicine,
Loma Linda University and Medical Center,
Loma Linda, CA
USA

1. Introduction

Therapy of glioblastoma has been very problematic with disappointing results using multiple therapeutic approaches. In general, glioblastomas are considered radioresistant tumors with different radiation modalities failing to control them in the clinic. However a comprehensive and detailed analysis of the radiosensitivity of glioblastoma cells has not been performed. We now present such an analysis in this chapter seeking a better definition of patterns of radiosensitivity in glioblastomas compared to other tumor cells. These data show that some glioblastomas have unusual responses to radiation that may render them more resistant to some forms of radiotherapy but also render them amenable to exploitation by other forms of radiotherapy.

Multiple mechanisms have been proposed to be associated with radioresistance in human glioblastoma cells: Bao et al (1) have suggested increased DNA damage response. Karim et al (2) have proposed differential cyclo-oxygenase response in radioresistant glios. Brandani et al (3) have suggested HSP 70 elevation. Akuguka et al (4) have suggested increased rates in DNA double strand break rejoining association with micronuclei. Scmidberger et al (5) observed variation interferon-induced β associates with increased radiosensitivity in four out of five glioblastomas. Yao et al (6) suggest variation in cell cycle arrest, modulation of the expression of cyclin-dependent kinase inhibitors, and autophagy. Streffer et al (7) showed BCL- family proteins modulate radiosensitivity in human malignant glioma cells. Kraus et al (8) showed aberrant p21 regulation in radioresistant primary glioblastoma multiforme cells bearing wild-type p53. Haas-Kogan (9) et al showed p53 function influences the effect of fractionated radiotherapy on glioblastoma tumors. Hsiao et al (10) showed functional expression of human p21(WAF1/CIP1) gene in rat glioma cells suppresses tumor growth in vivo and induces radiosensitivity. Yount et al (11) showed cell cycle synchrony unmasks the influence of p53 function on radiosensitivity of human glioblastoma cells. Britten et al (12) showed differential level of DSB repair fidelity effected by nuclear protein extracts derived from radiosensitive and radioresistant human tumour cells. Guichard et al (13) suggest potentially lethal damage repair as a possible determinant of human tumour radiosensitivity including glioblastoma. Kal et al (14) have suggested rhabdomyosarcomas, similar to glioblastomas are sensitive to low dose-rate irradiation.

These studies used multiple types of glioblastoma cells, but they did not define glioblastoma cells based on essential cellular response mechanisms. We will identify classes of glioblastoma cells that exhibit distinct mechanisms of radiosensitivity in vitro and in vivo. In general there is an overall correlation between radiosensitivity of tumor cells in vivo, radiosensitivity of xenograft tumors as measured in the laboratory and radiosensitivity of tumors in the clinic, although it is clear more studies between these three forms of radiosensitivity is needed. One purpose of this article is to provide such data for radioresistant glioblastoma

Radiosensitivity as assayed by clonogenic inactivation is a precise and accurate endpoint measurable over a wide range of inactivation levels (circa 10^5) induced by a wide range of radiation doses (circa 10^3). Over this dynamic range, clonogenic inactivation can be measured with acceptable variation. Further, clonogenic inactivation is a dichotomous endpoint based on whether individual cells are either clonogenically inactivated or not. Mathematically, this enables the application of Poisson statistics to estimate the probability of inactivation for each increment of dose. Since 1956 when Puck and Marcus (15) published the first "survival curve" such patterns have been examined to discern underlying mechanisms that produce cellular inactivation. Although "hit-target" theory did not identify exact "hits" defined as patterns of ionizations or exact "targets" that once induced inactivates cell, these studies demonstrated a continuing concept that improves such estimates over specific dose-segments. The observation of a log-linear relationship over a specific dose-segment, e.g. logarithm of cells inactivated are a linear function of dose, indicates a constant rate of inactivation over that dose segment.

From these early data a common pattern of inactivation was usually observed for tumor cells: a low rate of cell inactivation below circa 2 to 3 Gray (Gy) followed by increased rates of inactivation at higher doses. Further the patterns of inactivation at higher doses could be approximated as a log-linear response and the slope of such a dose-segment could be calculated as a Poisson probability of inactivation, usually expressed as the parameter Do, the dose needed to inactivate a single cell.

Results from the huge empirical data base obtained in the clinic for the relative effect of different doses and protocols that induced both tumor regression and normal tissue toxicity, clearly demonstrated radiotherapy of some tumors was more successful when multiple doses below 3 Gy were used. Mathematical models were proposed to explain the rate of inactivation of tumors at lower doses circa 1 to 3 Gy and the most successful model was the "linear-quadratic (LQ) model" as proposed by Hendry (16) and by Fowler (17, 18). The LQ model was based on the concept that tumor cell inactivation was induced at a linear rate at lower doses (the alpha response) but reflected a quadratic component at higher doses determined by a coefficient beta times the square of the dose (the beta response). These efforts failed to identify specific targets or hits, which in retrospect, was partially due to the complex processes involved in cellular inactivation. However one basic observation from these analyses is useful: identification of a dose-segment over which inactivation is log-linear, is still valid in identifying the rate of inactivation over such a dose-segment, represented by a single Poisson coefficient.

The pioneering work of Joiner and his colleagues in identifying "low-dose hyper-radiosensitivity" (19) demonstrated that at lower doses (< 0.5 Gy) there were additional changes in rates of clonogenic inactivation that could not be well explained by the linear-quadratic model.

We have recently proposed that patterns of inactivation in tumor cells are expressed as two general responses, the alpha response and the omega (or quadratic) response, are in fact actually comprised of four distinct components induced sequentially at increasing doses (20). Three of these responses can be well fitted to a log-linear relationship and a Poisson coefficient could be calculated over each of these log-linear responses over distinct dose-segments that represented the rate of inactivation. We will discuss these results subsequently but our data suggested that radiosensitivity of any cell line can be described as coefficients that describe four sequentially induced responses in each cell line. Some glioblastoma cells, not others, show specific values for these four responses.

1.1 Concept of a "radiosensitivity phenotype"

Our studies suggest that radiosensitivity of tumor cells cannot be expressed as a single parameter or histological type, but should be analyzed on the basis of descriptors of multiple responses that are specific to human tumor cell lines. We argue that the radiosensitivity phenotype of each cell line should be defined by a set of coefficients including: 1) relative rates of inactivation over four distinct, sequentially-induced components that comprise radiosensitivity of each cell; 2) the general radiosensitivity group into which cell lines segregate non-randomly based on the values of exceptional coefficients; these groups associated with tumor cell genotype; 3) modulation of inactivation by reduced dose-rates; and 4) modulation of inactivation by the effect of ionization density of delivered radiations; and 5) modulation by in vivo mechanisms that are particular to genotype.
In the next several paragraphs we identify those coefficients that together define the "radiosensitivity phenotype" of human tumor cells. One overall goal is to equate radiosensitivity phenotypes of tumor cells to genetic or epigenetic properties.

1.2 Coefficients that describe four sequentially-induced responses in each human tumor cell

We have measured clonogenic inactivation in multiple cell lines over different dose-segments (20). These studies showed that response of tumor cells to radiation in vitro can be resolved into two general responses, termed the alpha response and omega response (or quadratic response) that represent the overall rate of inactivation over the dose-segment from 0 to circa 2 Gy (alpha response) and over doses greater than circa 3 Gy (omega response). These two general responses can be approximated by the linear and quadratic components of the linear-quadratic model. These two general responses vary not only between glioblastoma cell lines and other tumor types but also vary between different glioblastoma lines.
Our data show these two general responses are actually comprised of four more specific responses induced sequentially in each cell line. Thus one goal of this chapter is to measure coefficients that describe these four responses in tumor cells and to suggest their relative importance in clinical radiotherapy.
As stated above we have defined four sequentially-induced responses in ten tumor cell lines by increasing doses from 0.0 to 10.0 Gy. These responses are common to all tumor cells, induced at the same doses but vary in the rates of inactivation over these common dose-segments. These four responses are:
The hypersensitive (H) response is observed over the dose-segment from 0.0 to 0.10 Gy and is characterized by highest rates of clonogenic inactivation observed in tumor cells. This

response is related to low-dose radio-hypersensitivity as described by Joiner and his colleagues (19). In each cell line in which the H response is observed, it is expressed over the dose segment from 0.0 and 0.10 Gy with a very low threshold if any but ends at 0.10 Gy. The survival level at 0.10 Gy can be used to calculate the slope of the H response between 0.0 Gy and 0.10 Gy as α (SF.1). The H response varies strongly in different types of tumor cells with some genotypes not expressing this response. Thus each cell line can be classified as to whether the H response is induced and the slope of the rate of inactivation. Interestingly, some glioblastoma cells express the H response at a high rate but are very radioresistant at higher doses.

The resistant (R) response is observed over the dose-segment from 0.1 to 0.2 Gy and is characterized as increased resistance to clonogenic inactivation exhibited in each cell line that expresses the H response. The R response appears to be induced at circa 0.10 Gy in all cells and persists until it is terminated when the alpha* response is induced. The R response is coupled strongly to the H response. In our studies shown below the R response is not always expressed as a log-linear response across the dose-segment from 0.0 to 0.1 Gy and hence the change in rates of inactivation over the R response varies strongly with genotype. The expression of the H and R responses do not correlate with the expression of the alpha* and omega* responses.

The alpha* (repair) response is induced at 0.20 Gy in all cells and once induced extends to all higher doses. The alpha* response is a protective response preventing excessive loss of irradiated somatic cells. The rate of inactivation over the alpha response is more resistant than rates evidenced over the H response and also more resistant than increased sensitivity observed subsequently when the omega* response is induced. The alpha* response is characterized by transiently suppressed apoptosis, induction of repair responses and perturbation of cell cycle progression. We refer to this induced response specifically as the alpha* (α*) response and it is the only response determining inactivation between 0.2 and 2.0 Gy. The slope of the alpha* response is a correlate of the general alpha response observed between 0.0 and circa 3 Gy measured either by the slope of inactivation estimated between 0.0 and 2.0 Gy, α (SF2) or by linear component of the linear-quadratic model α (LQ). We will show examples of this relationship subsequently.

The omega* (triage) response is induced at circa 3.0 Gy in all cells and extends to all higher doses. We refer to this induced response as the omega* (ω*) response and consider it a triage response that results is increased inactivation of damaged cells. It can be approximated mathematically by the quadratic response of the linear-quadratic model. The omega response is determined by linear regression of data above circa 3.0 Gy and its slope designated as omega (ω). The omega response is the combined effect of the omega* response induced as circa 3 Gy and an extension of the alpha* response. The omega* response is characterized by increased rates of clonogenic inactivation and chromosomal aberrations but decreased rates of tumorigenesis, carcinogenesis and mutation. Thus the increased inactivation of cells at doses above 3 Gy preferentially removes cells more likely to express mutation or cancer and thus can be considered a triage process that preferentially eliminates cells by detecting radiation-induced properties and eliminating cells by post-repair apoptosis.

1.3 Coefficients that describe the rates of inactivation over the alpha and omega responses segregate human tumor cells into only four statistically-valid cellular radiosensitivity groups

In a broad survey of clonogenic inactivation in multiple tumor cells we observed that the rate of inactivation over the alpha response was the major determinant of overall cellular radiosensitivity Williams et al (21, 22). The values of the coefficients that describe the alpha response derived over doses from 0 to circa 2.5 Gy segregated all cell lines non-randomly into four distinct, statistically-valid radiosensitivity groups. Each radiosensitivity group is inactivated over the alpha response at different rates and the statistical variation is significant. While the alpha response, that is in reality the combined effects to the H, R and alpha* responses, is related to the omega response in the four radiosensitivity groups, measurements of the general alpha response as will be shown subsequently, correlates with the alpha* response as measured using the linear-quadratic model. Thus the radiosensitivity groups listed below are dependent on the values of the alpha* response. Our work showed these four radiosensitivity groups segregate with specific genotypes, one of which was a group of some glioblastoma cells that as stated earlier express what we refer to as the "glio" response.

All tumor types we examined segregated into only four cellular radiosensitivity groups:

A **VS (very sensitive) radiosensitivity group** was comprised of only a single hypersensitive tumor line that was mutated in the ataxia telangiectasia mutated (ATM) gene. This cell line is hypersensitive to radiation on the basis of clonogenic inactivation, expression of apoptosis, cell cycle progression and susceptibility to chromosomal aberrations.

An **S (sensitive) radiosensitivity group** was comprised of 17 cell lines all but one expressing wild type tumor protein 53 (wtTP53). The coefficients that describe the alpha response for these cell lines were intermediate between the VS cell line and other more resistant lines.

An **R (resistant) radiosensitivity group** was comprised predominantly of cell lines that expressed a mutant form of TP53 although the exact form of mutation that renders cells more resistant has not been defined. R cells are intermediate in their radiosensitivity between S and R cells.

A **VR (very radioresistant) radiosensitivity group** was identified that was comprised of only three human glioblastoma cells. For descriptive purposes, we will refer to the factor or gene that leads to this exceptional resistance as "glio". This is in contradistinction to the S and R groups that contain tumor cells that derive from multiple histological types.

1.4 Coefficients that describe radiosensitivity of tumor cells to low dose-rate irradiation

We also defined rates of clonogenic inactivation of glioblastoma cell lines to low dose-rates (0.25 Gy per hour) compared to high dose rate (circa 50 Gy per hour) and again find significant differences in some radioresistant glioblastoma cell lines 21, 22. Importantly, these data suggest that some glioblastoma cell lines are distinctly different in their response to low dose-rate irradiation compared to their resistance to radiation delivered at higher doses. We will show analysis of these data subsequently below, but they do demonstrate that some glioblastoma cell lines that are very resistant as measured over the alpha* responses have a unique response to low dose-rate radiation that perhaps can be exploited in the clinic. Therefore a broad assessment of the radiosensitivity phenotype of a human tumor cell should include response to protracted irradiation.

1.5 Coefficients that represent the susceptibility of radiosensitivity to differences in ionization-density

While we will publish data elsewhere on the effects of dose-rate and ionization density, here we can make the general statement here that these data show the H and R responses are generally not modified by either by dose-rate or ionization density. In contradistinction, the alpha* and omega* responses are highly susceptible to dose-rate and ionization density.

1.6 Coefficients that represent the modulation of in vivo radiosensitivity by genotype and dose

We demonstrated variation in the response of tumor xenografts to radiotherapy protocols based on genotype and dose-schedule. In these studies, Williams et al 21, we showed genotype of tumor cells influenced both in vitro radiosensitivity of tumor cells and also, by a different mechanism, influenced xenograft response in vivo. We attributed this effect, that was substantial in some cells, as an interaction between tumor genotype and the in vivo tumor microenvironment. Importantly one glioblastoma line that was in the VR cellular radiosensitivity group, expressed surprising sensitivity when irradiated as xenograft tumors in vivo.

2. Methods and materials

We have published in detail the exact protocols that we have used in these studies (21, 22, 23, 24).

2.1 Cell lines

We study 3 radioresistant glioblastoma cell lines (U251, T98G and U87) two other lines classified as glioblastoma but are more sensitive (GL-13, JW-1T). We compare them in detail with two human colorectal tumor cell lines (DLD-1 and 19S184), both cells expressing mutTP53 but 19S186 has been abrogated in CDKN1A (p21) and this abrogation while not effecting in vitro radiosensitivity causes increased radiosensitivity in xenograft tumors (Waldemann, 24).

2.2 Cell and culture techniques

The basic media for colon tumor cell lines was McCoy 5A, supplemented with 10% FBS, 1% penicillin and streptomycin, 1% L-glutamine; Human glioma cell lines were cultured in DMEM/F12 with 10% FBS, 1% L-glutamine and 1% Penicillin and streptomycin. All cells were sub-cultured twice a week to maintain exponential growth.

2.3 Cell survival assay

Cells were plated ~18 hours before irradiation. Surviving colonies were determined 10-14 days after irradiation depending on the cell line. Cells were stained with crystal violet and colonies counted (>50 cells/colony). Additional plates for each experiment were used as microcolony controls. Special care was taken in dispersing cell cultures to obtain single cell suspensions with high plating efficiencies.

2.4 Irradiation

Cells were irradiated in complete media in a Gammacell 40 (Nordion Ottawa ONT Canada) at approximately 0.7 Gy/min. Cells were plated 15 to 18 hours before irradiation with careful measurement of plating efficiency and multiplicity. After exposure, plates were incubated for 8-14 days depending on specific growth and colonies stained with crystal violet. Colonies with more than 50 cells were counted. For each cell line we performed controls to account for possible proliferation during the period between plating and irradiation. This control consisted of plating 10^5 cells in separate plates when replicates of cells were plated for colony formation. When irradiation was performed on the plates for colony formation, the microcolony plates were stained and the number of cells per colony measured. The average number of cells per colony was below 1.20 cells per microcolony for all cell lines and did not vary significantly between cell lines.

Low dose rate irradiation was carried out in a specially constructed Cs-137 irradiator with temperature control and the ability to irradiate cells with constant or exponentially-decreasing dose-rates.

2.5 Regrowth delay in xenograft tumors

Tumors were established by subcutaneous injection of 5 million cells suspended in PBS into the upper thigh of nude mice. Each cohort included 6 to 13 tumors. Tumor growth rate was determined by measuring three orthogonal diameters of each tumor twice a week and the tumor volume estimated as $\pi/6$ [D1 x D2 x D3], when individual tumor volumes reached ~0.1-0.3 cm^3, radiation treatment was initiated. Modal specific growth delay (mSGD) was measured for all cohorts in which a majority of tumors reached a volume four times the initial volume. Response was normalized to growth of unirradiated cells. We chose not to use the mean of specific regrowth delay patterns since a significant proportion of our cohorts included one or more tumors that did not regrow. Thus the mean became limited as a regrowth parameter. For cohorts for which some tumors did not regrow we estimated mSGD based on the regrowth pattern for the minority of tumors that did regrow. When we tested the sensitivity of modal to mean growth delay in selected cohorts in which all tumors regrew, the modal value always fell within one standard deviation of the mean. These methods share some characteristics of the methods described by Schwatchofer [25]. To provide an overview of the dichotomous response when some tumors regrow but some do not, we indicated such cohorts with an arrow showing this value, in terms of overall tumor response, was the common minimum response.

3. Analyses

3.1 Clonogenic inactivation of radioresistant glioblastoma cell lines

In our previous studies (21, 22) we identified three glioblastoma cell lines (U251, T98G, U-87) that were the most resistant of 39 cell lines examined as defined by comparison of clonogenic inactivation between circa 2 Gy and 10 Gy. These three radioresistant cell lines expressed two forms of TP53, with U251 and T98 expressing mutTP53 and U87 expressing wtTP53. For designation purposes we will refer to these three cell lines as expressing a VR radiosensitivity phenotype and expressing either a glio$^+$mutTP53 genotype (U251 and T98G) or a glio$^+$wtTP53 genotype. In figure 1 we compare clonogenic inactivation curves for these three VR (very radioresistant) glioblastoma cell lines compared to two colorectal cancer cell lines that fall into the R (radioresistant) radiosensitivity group wtTP53 (HCT116) and its subline abrogated in p21 (19S186) .

The data in figure 1 show relative radiosensitivity between the five cell lines but it is important in our interpretation of these data to show them in the context of overall radiosensitivity of human tumor cell lines. In figure 1 there are clear differences between the three glioblastoma cell lines and the two more sensitive colorectal tumors. These differences vary with the dose-segment over which the data are presented.

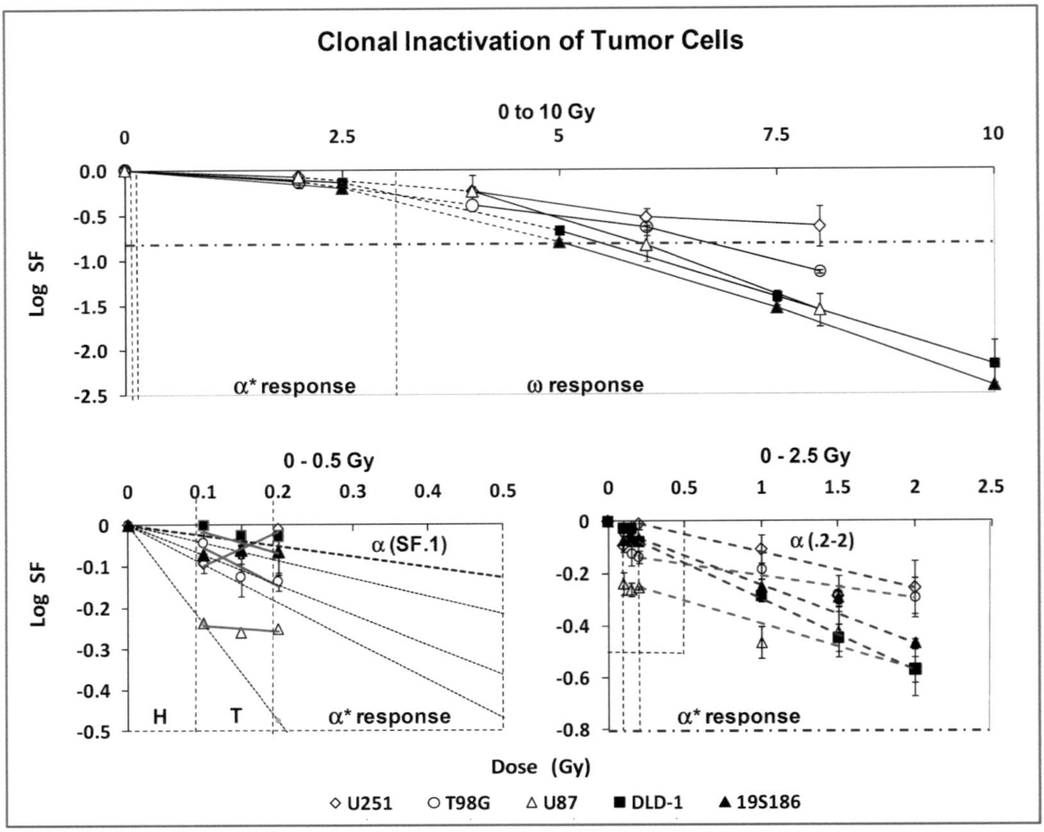

Fig. 1. Radiosensitivity curves (2 to 10 Gy) for five cell lines: three radioresistant human glioblastoma cell lines, U251, T98G, U87, and two human colorectal tumor cell lines, HCT116 and DLD-1. These data show standard survival measurements in the upper panel expressed as two general responses, the α response from 0.0 to circa 3.0 Gy and the ω response for doses greater than circa 3 Gy. The lower two panels show three components that together constitute the alpha response: the H response, the R response and the α* response.

In the top panel the overall responses are shown between 0 and 10 Gy for the five cell lines and these responses can be analyzed by measuring the slope of inactivation between 0.0 Gy and 2.0 Gy and defined as the alpha response. The values for the alpha response calculated in this manner are significantly higher for VR cells than R cells but these differences are difficult to visualize at the scale used in this panel so the dose-response patterns are expanded in the lower panels.

Similarly an omega response can be calculated for all five cell lines using linear regression of all data points above 4 Gy and the slopes of the five lines do not segregate between the two radiosensitivity groups, with two VR lines U251 and T98G showing a more resistant response than the third line U87. This dichotomy in response corresponds to the differences in these three lines in their expression of TP53. U251 and T98G express mutTP53 while U87 expresses wtTP53. These differences are shown more clearly subsequently.

In the bottom left panel the responses of all five cell lines are shown for their detailed responses over doses between 0.0 and 0.20 Gy. In this panel, the dashed lines are the slopes for each cell line defined by connecting 0.0 dose points to the points at 0.10 Gy, α (SF.1), extended to illustrate the strong variation in slope for the H responses.
All cell lines change in their rates of inactivation at 0.10 Gy that represents the induction of the R response. Note that the rates of inactivation over the R responses (0.1 to 0.2 Gy), varies between cell lines with U87 showing a marked increase compared to the other four lines. .
In the lower right panel, the rates of inactivation over the alpha* responses are shown. The rates for the slopes of the alpha* response are calculated by the slopes between 0.20 and 2.0 Gy indicated as α (.2-2.). The slopes of the For this dose-segment, all three VR cell lines are more resistant than the two R lines.
In a larger cohort of cells we have previously shown that the alpha responses of the three VR lines are distinctly more resistant (22). In our studies of multiple components (20) we showed that the alpha response is comprised of the "average" slope for the H, R and alpha* responses. This work also showed there is correlation between the alpha* response measured over the dose-segment from 0.2 Gy to 2.0 Gy an the general alpha response shown in the upper panel.

3.2 Coefficients that define the alpha and omega responses segregate human tumor cells into four radiosensitivity groups

In figure 2 we show a scatter diagram based on our data from Williams et al (21) expressed as values of the coefficients derived for the alpha and omega responses measured as shown in figure 1 and measured as the slope of the general alpha response and the omega response. This figure also specifically identifies the five cell lines that are the subject of our present analysis: U251, T98G, U87, DLD-1 and shows they are distinctly different in their radiosensitivity compared to the lines JW-1T and GL-13 purported also to be glioblastoma cells.
There are important implications of these data. First the values of the alpha response and omega response segregate all cell lines into four statistically distinct radiosensitivity groups: VS, S, R and VR. The alpha response is the predominant determinate of radiosensitivity group. Note that the five cell lines that we study in this chapter are distributed in two clusters: U-251 and T98G are clustered in cell lines that express extreme resistance based on their alpha and omega responses. Three cell lines cluster in patterns with the lowest values for both alpha and omega responses, but three cell lines, DLD-1, 19S186 and U-87 while showing resistance to lower doses (alpha response) have significantly larger values of the omega response are also determined as that are also resistant (alpha response) but show elevated values of their omega responses. Hence the three glioblastoma cells in the VR group share the smallest values for their alpha response but vary significantly in their omega responses. Two cell lines classified in the literature as glioblastoma GL-13 and JW-1T fall into distinctly different radiosensitivities segregating with the S radiosensitivity groups
The omega response for U87 cells is distinctly higher, reflecting, we hypothesize, the role of wtTP53 in "glio" cells. We hypothesize that over the alpha response, "glio" confers radioresistance beyond that characterized by expression of mutTP53. At higher doses, wtTP53 modulates radiosensitivity as shown for U87 cells. The data in this figure show three distinct clusters of glioblastoma cell lines.

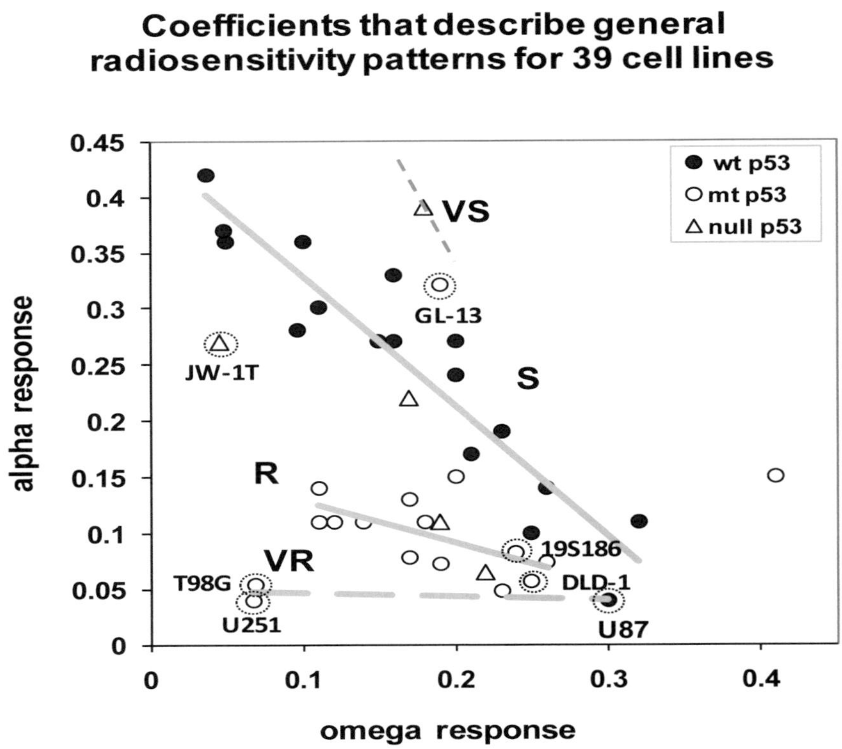

Fig. 2. Radiosensitivity of five glioblastoma cell lines in relationship to 34 other human tumor cell line data extracted from Williams et al 2008a. The ordinate is the coefficient that describes the slope of the alpha responses and the abscissa is the coefficient that describes the slope of omega responses as shown in figure 1. The diagonal lines are best fit estimates of regression and identify four distinct radiosensitivity groups (VS, S, R and VR). The "VR" (very resistant) group is comprised of only three radioresistant glioblastoma cell lines (U251, T98G, U87). In this figure we two cell lines that are also classified ad glioblastoma cell lines (JW-1T, GL-13) that do not segregate into the VR group. We also identify two R (resistant) cell lines DLD-1 and its subclone abrogated in p21, 19S186.

3.3 Radiosensitivity of radioresistant glioblastoma cell lines and human colorectal tumor cells to low dose-rate irradiation

We have previously measured the response of 27 human tumor lines to low dose-rate ionizing radiation (26) and in figure 3 we show the general responses of a VR cell line (U-251) and a less resistant colorectal tumor cell line (DLD-1).

These data show two important differences in these two cell lines. First the VR line is more resistant than the R line for both rates of radiation. Second, it is clear that within each line the differences between irradiation at HDR and LDR are markedly different for the two types of cells with the VR line showing a significant increase in inactivation by LDR.

These differences in rates of clonal inactivation between LDR and HDR are shown in more detail in the data in figure 4.

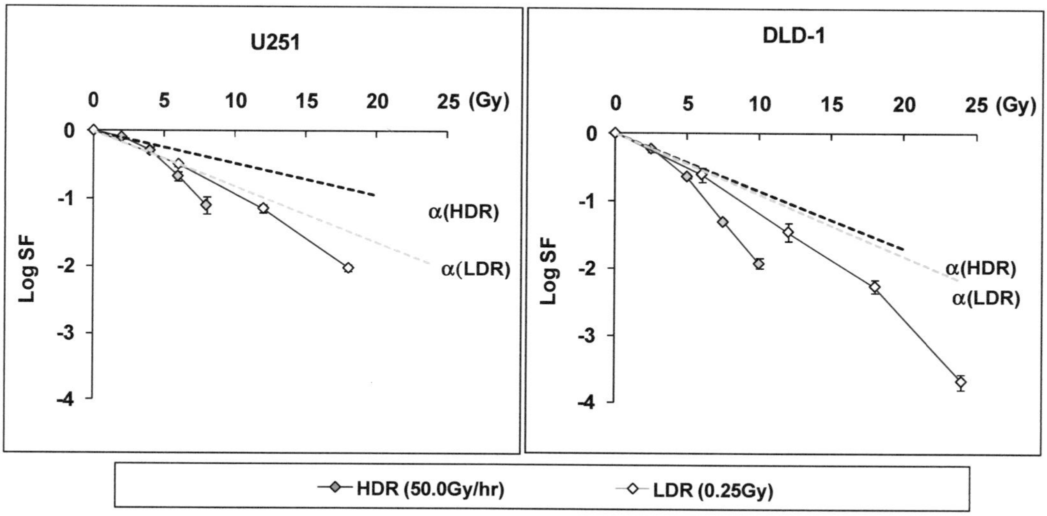

Fig. 3. Comparison of clonogenic inactivation induced by acute high dose-rate HDR (50 Gy/hr) and protracted irradiation LDR (0.25 Gy/hr). The dashed lines represent the extrapolation of the rate of inactivation at lower doses based on the slopes of inactivation by LDR and HDR.

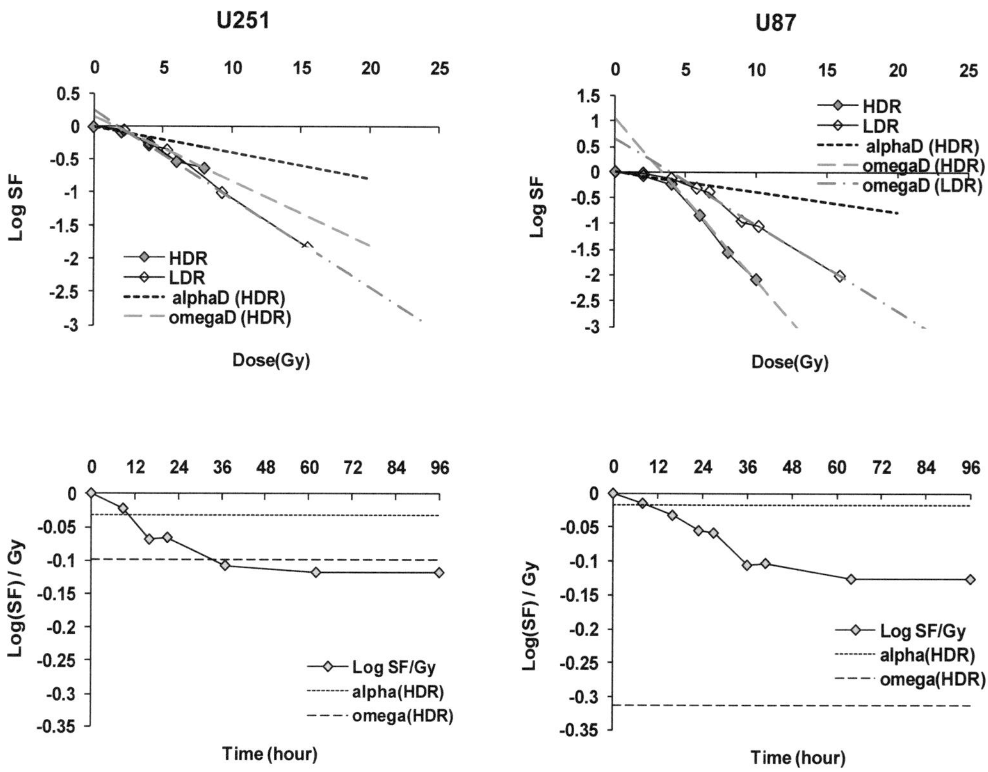

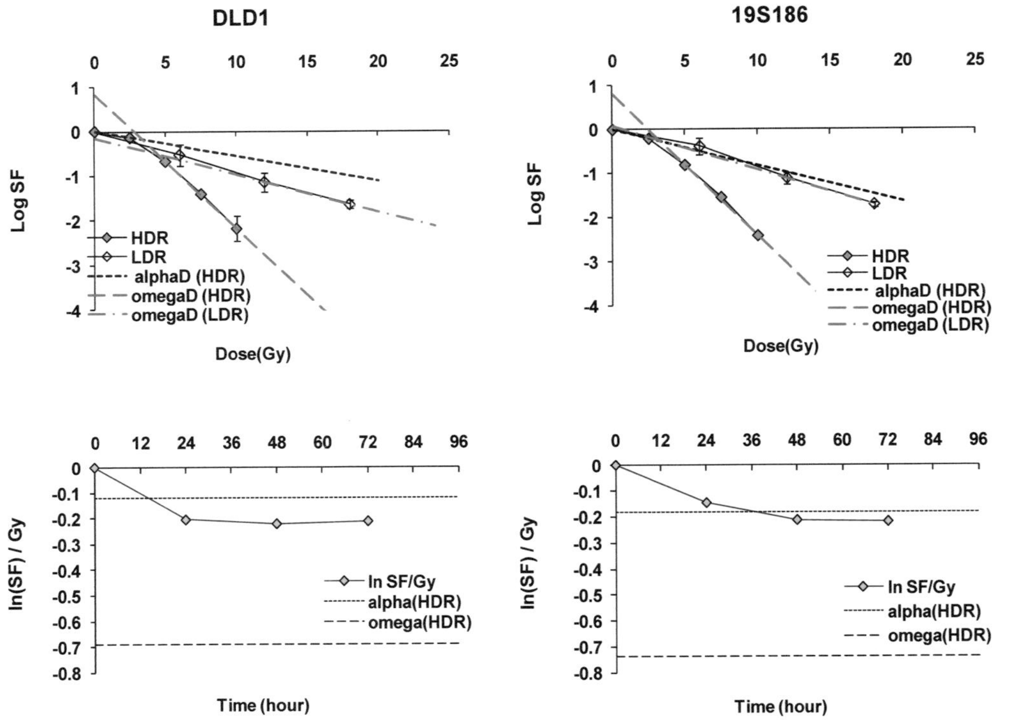

Fig. 4. Clonogenic survival patterns for two glioblastoma cell lines (U251, U87) and two colorectal tumor cell lines (HCT116 and DLD-1) irradiated with either HDR (50 Gy/hr) and LDR (0.25 Gy/hr). Data for each cell line are shown as two panels, the upper panel shows surviving fraction, lower panels show the rate of cell killing calculated as logs killed per Gy between sequential time points. The slopes of cell killing curves are represented by: α(HDR) which is measured from the slope of the line from 0.0 to surviving fraction at 2.0 Gy HDR; α (LDR) which is the slope of the line from 0.0 to 6.0 Gy LDR; the slope of the cell killing curve at doses greater than 4 Gy HDR determined by linear regression, ω (HDR); and the slope of cell killing at LDR doses greater than 6 Gy, ω (LDR). In the lower panels, the rate of cell killing by HDR is indicated by dotted, dashed lines.

These data show that both glioblastoma cell lines are inactivated by low dose-irradiation at approximately the same rates similar to rates for both colorectal tumor cells, showing a clear increase in rate that surpasses the levels of high dose-rate inactivation (omega response) of both cell types. This rate of LDR inactivation surpasses the rate of inactivation for the omega response for U-251 but the elevated level of U-87 cells for the omega response is not achieved.

These data suggest strongly that for radioresistant glioblastoma cells, the rate of inactivation by LDR irradiation can surpass the rate of inactivation for by multiple fractions that induce inactivation along the alpha response.

This in turn suggests using LDR radiotherapy for glioblastoma tumors and we synthesize our data to demonstrate the relative effect of different dose rates for induction of clonogenic inactivation. These data are shown in figure 5.

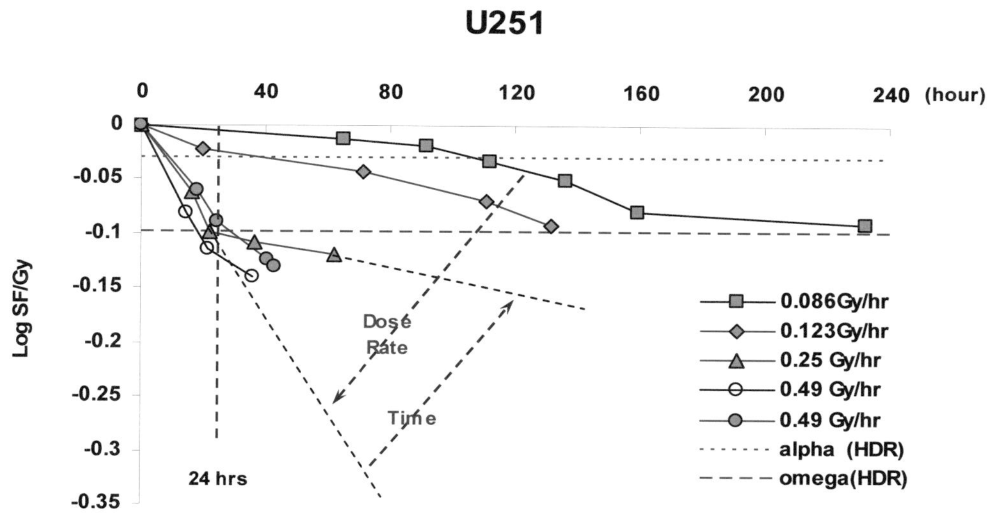

Fig. 5. Changes in the rate of cell killing expressed as Log10 of cells killed per Gy as a function of time of protracted irradiation in U251 cells irradiated with 4 different constant dose-rates and one that begins at 0.49 Gy/hr and decays with a half life of 2.7 days. The horizontal dotted and dashed lines represent the rate of cell killing for HDR irradiation at lower doses (alpha) and higher doses (omega).

These data show that increasing dose-rate increases the rate at which cells are inactivated until dose-rates reach approximately 0.12 Gy/hr when there is a relatively common response for higher dose-rates including our chosen LDR of 0.25 Gy/hr. The diagonal dashed lines in figure 5 are a general indication of the relative effects of dose-rate compared to the relative effects of duration of exposure (time). In our previous studies of LDR irradiation in multiple tumor cells we show that all cell lines change in their rates of inactivation at circa 20 to 24 hours, so duration of exposure and dose-rate are both factors in achieving changes in clonogenic inactivation.

The data in figure 5 suggests that dose rates in the range of 0.25 to 0.49 Gy/hr increase tumor cell inactivation to rates that exceed that can be achieved by the alpha response induced by HDR irradiation. Thus, these patterns of inactivation show that glioblastoma cells while resistant to radiotherapeutic protocols that use multiple fractions below circa 3 Gy, are more sensitive to protracted irradiation.

Together with J.A. Williams, we have shown that combining irradiation delivered by an implanted radioactive seed with concomitant external beam fractionated radiotherapy produces significant increases in tumor response (Williams JA et al 1998). This study established the feasibility of combining brachytherapy and external beam radiotherapy to achieve good responses in radioresistant glioblastoma cells.

3.4 Radiosensitivity of xenograft tumors comprised of two R cells compared to a radioresistant glioblastoma cell line

The response of xenograft tumors that differ in their susceptibility to clonogenic inactivation in vitro also vary in their radiosensitivity to different radiotherapy protocols delivered in vivo.

We performed a large set of experiments that compared the response of eight different cells that vary in their in vitro radiosensitivity to different radiotherapy protocols in vivo (Williams et al 2010). These studies showed a strong correlation between the total cells killed in vitro with tumor response but also showed a new in vivo effect that resulted from an in vivo interaction between tumor cell genotype and tumor microenvironment. Response of xenograft tumors comprised of two R cell lines, DLD-1 and 19S186 cells are compared to the very resistant VR line U-251 in figure 6.

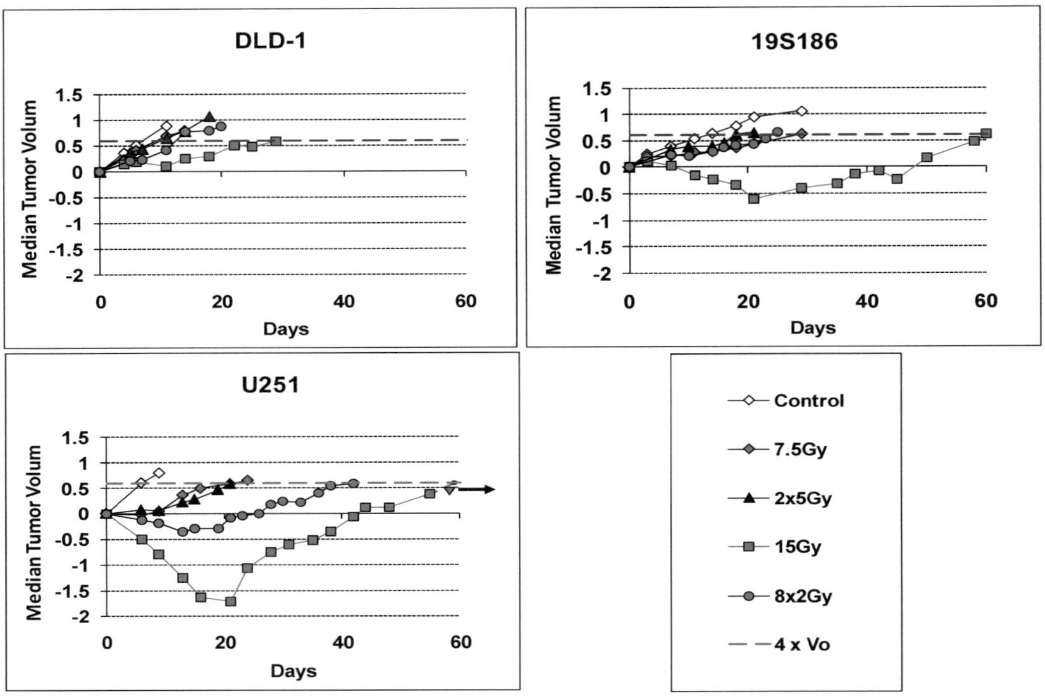

Fig. 6. Growth of cohorts of xenograft tumors comprised of DLD-1, 19S186 and U-251 glioblastoma cells to four radiation protocols: 8 x 2 Gy, 2 x 5Gy, 1 x 7.5 Gy and 1 x 15 Gy. The ordinate in these figures represent the median log V/Vo. Tumors that were irradiated at approximately 0.2 gm and their volumes measured with time. Tumor size is expressed as median tumor volume as a function of days after irradiation.

The data in figure 6 show an increase in tumor radiosensitivity compared to their in vitro radiosensitivity for glioblastoma cells.

In detailed analysis of 40 experiments similar to those shown in figure 6, we showed tumor response could be resolved into two independent sensitivity factors: **τ** and **ρ** (23). The factor τ is related to total cells inactivated in vitro by each protocol and is dependent on genotype, fraction-size ant total dose. The factor ρ is dependent on genotype, fraction-size and total dose, but is independent of τ. We showed that for each protocol and genotype tumor response was dependent on the product of τ and ρ.

The relationship between τ and ρ is a useful comparison for radiosensitivity of xenograft tumors induced in tumor that vary in genotype and treated with different protocols. These coefficients are shown in figure 7 for DLD-1, 19S186 and U-251 cells.

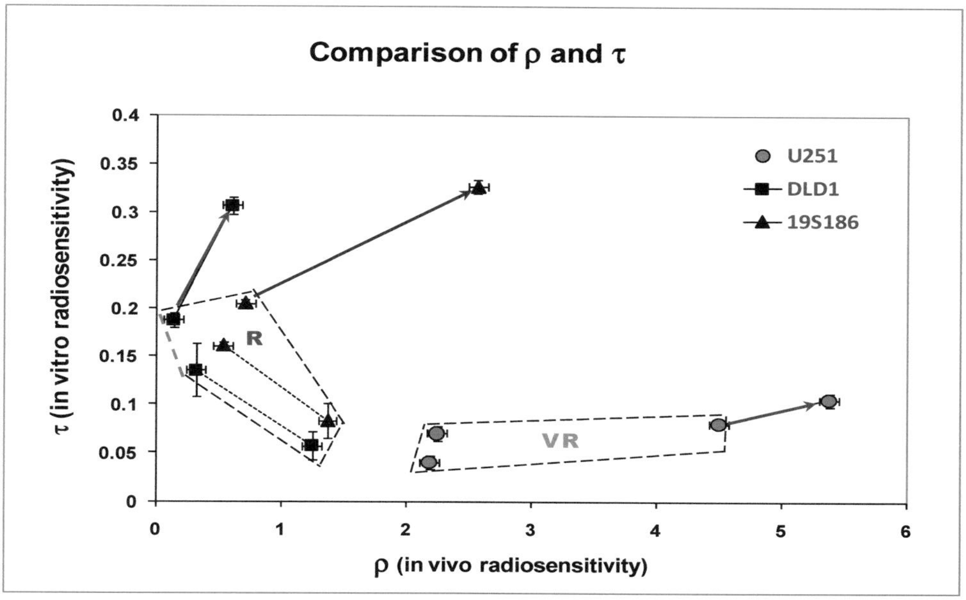

Fig. 7. Relative in vitro radiosensitivity (τ) and in vivo radiosensitivity (ρ) for two R cells, DLD-1 and 19S186 and a radioresistant glioblastoma cells U-251. Each data point represents tumor response of each cell line to one of four protocols. Data point representing the two fractionated protocols, 8 x 2 and 2 x 5, are connected by a dashed lines and these responses are very similar for U-251 cells but are markedly different for the two R cell lines. The response for each cell line to a single dose of 7.5 Gy is connected by an arrow to response of the same tumor to a single dose of 15 Gy. These increased responses are significant beyond the differences observed in fractionated protocols.

These data show important differences between the response of glioblastoma cell line and the two R cell lines. First, the contribution of in vivo radiosensitivity represented by ρ to responses of the glioblastoma line is remarkably greater than the contribution of this sensitivity in R cells. In contradistinction, the values for the in vitro component of tumor radiosensitivity in vitro, τ, are diminished, this diminution similar to differences predicted by in vitro clonogenic inactivation. The effects shown in this figure are large up to a factor of 50 to 100 in doses to induce equivalent regression or in doses needed to induce the same levels of regression.

4. Conclusions

4.1 Glioblastoma cells express a diverse radiosensitivity phenotype

Our studies show that cell lines designated as "glioblastoma" in the literature are diverse in their radiosensitivity phenotypes.

4.1.1 Some glioblastoma cell lines express a low rate of inactivation over the alpha* response

In our studies these reduced rates underlay the observation that such cell lines are refractory to doses over the alpha response. Specifically we hypothesized that these cell lines, express "glio", an unidentified genetic or epigenetic factor, that renders such glioblastoma cells resistant to radiation delivered at doses below circa 3 Gy. This in turn suggests that tumors comprised of cells that express glio and fall into the VR radiosensitivity group will be refractory to radiotherapy that is based on multi-fraction of cells when fractions are below 3.0 Gy.

4.1.2 The alpha* response can be uncoupled from the omega response in VR resistant glioblastoma cells

Our data show that while two radioresistant glioblastoma cell lines (U-251 and T98G) show resistance to inactivation at higher doses (omega response), one cell line (U-87) shows a more sensitive response. We hypothesize that this difference is associated with expression of TP53 in these cell lines, U-251and T98G express mutTP53 while U-87 expresses wtTP53. These differences are consistent with the ration between alpha and omega responses for cells that express mutTP53 versus wtTP53 as shown in figure 3 and are consistent with all VR cells expressing glio but susceptible to the effect of expression of TP53.

4.1.3 Glioblastoma cells that express VR radiosensitivity after high dose-rate irradiation show an unpredicted sensitivity to low dose-rate irradiation for dose-rates circa 0.25 to 0.49 Gy/hr

Glioblastoma cell lines that show VR radiosensitivity secondary to their expression of glio when irradiated with high dose-rate show a relatively more sensitive response to low dose-rate irradiation for dose-rates circa 0.25 to 0.49 Gy/hr. The data in figures 5 and 6 show that two VR lines, U-87 and U-251 show rates of inactivation when irradiated with lower dose-rates that are more sensitive than the rates of inactivation over the alpha response igh dose-rate irradiation, response to LDR irradiation by exhibiting a more sensitive response show elevated rates of inactivation.

4.1.4 Protocols that combine brachytherapy with external beam are highly effective in treating xenograft tumors of glioblastoma cells

Led by JA Williams (27) we have shown that xenograft tumors of U-251 glioblastoma cells are highly susceptible to the combined effects of brachytherapy using single seeds and external beam radiotherapy. These data shows that xenograft tumors that are resistant to lower fractions (2 and 5 Gy) and protracted radiation from implanted radioactive seeds are highly response to their response to protocols that combine these two modalities.

5.1 Implications for new approaches to radiotherapy of glioblastoma cell lines based on their radiosensitivity phenotype

Our data suggest relationships between the radiosensitivity phenotypes of glioblastoma cells and their predicted response to different radiotherapy protocols.

5.1.1 Cells that express the VR radiosensitivity phenotype will be refractory to protocols that use multiple fractions of doses lower than 3.0 Gy

Cells the express the VR radiosensitivity phenotype have low rates of inactivation by doses below 3 Gy (alpha response) and should not respond well to protocols that use smaller fraction sizes.

5.1.2 VR glioblastoma cells that express wtTP53 should be more responsive to protocols that use higher doses per fraction (> 3 Gy)

The data in figures 1, 2 and 3 show that U87 cells that express the VR phenotype but also express wtTP53 are more sensitive to doses that elicit the omega response (> 3 Gy) than the other two VR cells. This would suggest that tumors comprised of this form of VR cells would show significantly more inactivation than VR cells that express mut TP53 when doses are used that elicit the omega* response.

5.1.3 The VR cell line U 251 shows increased radiosensitivity of its xenograft tumors irradiated in vivo compared to other cell types

This increased response in vivo is observed for all protocols for glioblastoma cell line U-251 but is significantly elevated for protocols that use large fractions of 7.5 Gy and 15.0 Gy. This in turn suggests that some forms of VR glioblastoma cells will respond to hypofractionation with fractions circa 7.5 to 15.0 Gy.

6. Our observations suggest certain studies are needed to design protocols to exploit the VR radiosensitivity phenotype observed in some glioblastoma cell lines

Our research suggests several studies would improve selection of radiotherapy protocols that could improve therapeutic results from specific protocols.

6.1 Better markers are needed to define the VR radiosensitivity phenotype from tumor biopsies

Our studies overall suggest there is no single protocol that would be predicted to provide maximum improvement in tumor radiotherapy for all variations in the radiosensitivity phenotypes that we have observed in cells believed to be "glioblastoma" cells.

6.2 The data base on the VR radiosensitivity phenotype need to be extended to include more cells presumed to be glioblastoma cells

It seems clear from our work and that of others that a larger number of presumed glioblastoma cells need to be examined for their radiosensitivity phenotype including response to high dose-rate, to low dose-rate and their response as xenograft tumors to selected protocols.

6.3 The mechanisms that underlay increased in vivo response of tumors comprised of U-251 glioblastoma cells needs to be extended to other glioblastoma cells

Our data show this is a significant increase in radiosensitivity and the mechanisms that underlay it need to be studied in detail. The data we have presented offers a useful range of responses in different genotypes to study the role of genotype, fraction-size and total dose on this effect.

7. Overall conclusions

Radiosensitivity phenotypes of tumor cells are comprised of distinct, multiple responses to radiation. Glioblastoma cells exhibit responses that are both sensitive and resistant compared to other tumor cells. Specific protocols can be designed to exploit these differences in radiosensitivity.

8. References

[1] Bao S, Wu Q, McLendon RE, Hao Y, Shi Q, Hjelmeland AB, Dewhirst MW, Bigner DD, Rich JN. Glioma stem cells promote radioresistance by preferential activation of the DNA damage response. *Nature*. 2006 Dec 7;444(7120):756-60. Epub 2006 Oct 18.

[2] Karim A, McCarthy K, Jawahar A, Smith D, Willis B, Nanda A. Differential cyclooxygenase-2 enzyme expression in radiosensitive versus radioresistant glioblastoma multiforme cell lines. *Anticancer Res*. 2005 Jan-Feb;25(1B):675-9.

[3] Brondani Da Rocha A, Regner A, Grivicich I, Pretto Schunemann D, Diel C, Kovaleski G, Brunetto De Farias C, Mondadori E, Almeida L, Braga Filho A, Schwartsmann G. Radioresistance is associated to increased Hsp70 content in human glioblastoma cell lines. *Int J Oncol*. 2004 Sep;25(3):777-85.

[4] Akudugu JM, Theron T, Serafin AM, Böhm L. Influence of DNA double-strand break rejoining on clonogenic survival and micronucleus yield in human cell lines. *Int J Radiat Biol*. 2004 Feb;80(2):93-104.

[5] Schmidberger H, Rave-Fränk M, Lehmann J J, Weiss E, Gerl L, Dettmer N, Glomme S, Hess CF. Lack of interferon beta-induced radiosensitization in four out of five human glioblastoma cell lines.*Int J Radiat Oncol Biol Phys*. 2003 Apr 1;55(5):1348-57.

[6] Yao KC, Komata T, Kondo Y, Kanzawa T, Kondo S, Germano IM. Molecular response of human glioblastoma multiforme cells to ionizing radiation: cell cycle arrest, modulation of the expression of cyclin-dependent kinase inhibitors, and autophagy. *J Neurosurg*. 2003 Feb;98(2):378-84.

[7] Streffer JR, Rimner A, Rieger J, Naumann U, Rodemann HP, Weller M. BCL-2 family proteins modulate radiosensitivity in human malignant glioma cells.*J Neurooncol*. 2002 Jan;56(1):43-9.

[8] Kraus A, Gross MW, Knuechel R, Münkel K, Neff F, Schlegel J. Aberrant p21 regulation in radioresistant primary glioblastoma multiforme cells bearing wild-type p53. *J Neurosurg*. 2000 Nov;93(5):863-72.

[9] Haas-Kogan DA, Kogan SS, Yount G, Hsu J, Haas M, Deen DF, Israel MA. p53 function influences the effect of fractionated radiotherapy on glioblastoma tumors.*Int J Radiat Oncol Biol Phys*. 1999 Jan 15;43(2):399-403.

[10] Hsiao M, Tse V, Carmel J, Costanzi E, Strauss B, Haas M, Silverberg GD. Functional expression of human p21(WAF1/CIP1) gene in rat glioma cells suppresses tumor growth in vivo and induces radiosensitivity.*Biochem Biophys Res Commun*. 1997 Apr 17;233(2):329-35.

[11] Yount GL, Haas-Kogan DA, Vidair CA, Haas M, Dewey WC, Israel MA. Cell cycle synchrony unmasks the influence of p53 function on radiosensitivity of human glioblastoma cells.*Cancer Res*. 1996 Feb 1;56(3):500-6.

[12] Britten RA, Liu D, Kuny S, Allalunis-Turner MJ. Differential level of DSB repair fidelity effected by nuclear protein extracts derived from radiosensitive and radioresistant human tumour cells. *Br J Cancer*. 1997;76(11):1440-7.

[13] Guichard M, Weichselbaum RR, Little JB, Malaise EP. Potentially lethal damage repair as a possible determinant of human tumour radiosensitivity.*Radiother Oncol*. 1984 Jan;1(3):263-9.

[14] Kal HB, Barendsen BW, Bakker-van Haue R, Roeke H 1975. Increased radiosensitivity of rat rhabdomyosarcoma cells induced by protracted irradiation. Radiation Research 63, 521-530. (1975).

[15] Puck TT and Marcos PI. 1956 Action of x-rays on mammalian cells. J Exp Med 103: 653-666.

[16] Thames HD Jr, Withers HR, Peters LJ, Fletcher GH. 1982 Changes in early and late radiation responses with altered dose fractionation: Impliations for dose-survival relationships. International Journal of Radiation Oncology Biology and Physics. 8: 219-226.

[17] Fowler JF 1989 The linear-quadratic model and progress in fractionated radiotherapy. Br J Radiol 62:679-694 (1989).

[18] Fowler JF. 2009 Sensitivity analysis of parameters in linear-quadratic radiobiologic modeling.Int J Radiat Oncol Biol Phys. 73(5):1532-7.

[19] Joiner MC, Marples B, Lambin P, Short SC, Turesson I. 2001 Low-dose hypersensitivity: current status and possible mechanisms. Int J Radiat Biol Phys. Feb 1;49(2):379-89.

[20] Williams JR, Zhang Y, Zhou H, Gridley DS, Koch CJ, Slater JM, Dicello JF,Little JB.Sequentially-induced responses define tumour cell radiosensitivity.Int J Radiat Biol. 2011 Apr 18.

[21] Williams JR, Zhang Y, Russell J, Koch C, Little JB. Human tumor cells segregate into radiosensitivity groups that associate with ATM and TP53 status. *Acta Oncol*. 2007;46(5):628-38.

[22] Williams JR, Zhang Y, Zhou H, Gridley DS, Koch CJ, Russell J, Slater JS, Little JB. 2008b A quantitative overview of radiosensitivity of human tumor cells across histological type and TP53 status. Int J Radiat Biol. 84(4):253-64.

[23] Williams JR, Zhang Y, Zhou H, Russell J, Gridley DS, Koch CJ, Little JB. Genotype-dependent radiosensitivity: Clonogenic survival, apoptosis and cell-cycle redistribution. *Int J Radiat Biol*. 2008 Feb;84(2):151-64.

[24] Waldman, T., Zhang, Y., Dillehay, L., Yu, J., Kinzler, K., Vogelstein, B., Williams, J. Cell-cycle arrest versus cell death in cancer therapy. Nature Medicine 3(9):1034-1036, 1997.

[25] Schwachofer, JH, Hoogenhout J, Kal HB, Koedam J, van Wezel HP..Radiosensitivity of different human tumor lines grown as xenografts determined from growth delay and survival data. In Vivo 1990 4 (4): 253-7.

[26] Williams JR, Zhang Y, Russell J, Gridley DS, Koch CJ, Slater JS, and Little JB. 2008c Quantitative Overview of Human Tumor Cell Response to Low Dose-rate Irradiation. Int J Radiat Oncol Biol Phys;72(3):909-17. Review.

[27] Williams, J.A., Williams, J.R., Xuan, Y., and Dillehay, L.E. Protracted exposure radiosensitization of experimental human malignant glioma. Radiation Oncol. Invest., 6:255-263, 1998.

2

Impact of Metabolic and Therapeutic Stresses on Glioma Progression and Therapy

Kathryn J. Huber-Keener and Jin-Ming Yang
The Pennsylvania State University College of Medicine and
Penn State Hershey Cancer Institute
United States of America

1. Introduction

Glioma cells, both within solid tumors and during invasion, exist in surroundings that are subject to a variety of stresses, including metabolic and environmental stresses. Nonetheless, glioma cells survive and can even thrive under hostile conditions, such as hypoxia, nutrient deprivation, and therapeutic regimens. In order to survive, these tumor cells have to find a way to adapt to such an environment by activating certain growth factor and survival pathways while down-regulating cell death mechanisms. In fact, gliomas adapt so well that they not only survive but proliferate by creating a more hospitable environment through new blood vessel formation and dissemination, even as they endure additional stresses along the way. This chapter reviews the basic stresses that glioma cells encounter during the progression of tumor formation and therapeutic interventions.

2. Types of stress on glioma and their clinical implications

Internal stresses such as hypoxia, acidity, oxidative stress, and nutrient deprivation already exist within the cellular environment of tumors while external stressors like radiation treatment and genotoxic chemotherapy only worsen the internal factors. Encountering these stresses affects the process of carcinogenesis. Gliomas, especially GBM, are highly transformed tumors that react to stresses differently than less transformed cancers. Common markers of stress will be discussed along with their roles in induction of energy conservation and cell survival in glioma. Redistribution of energy resources towards survival pathways and away from energy-consuming processes is common.

Cellular stress can cause damage and mutations to numerous proteins, nucleic acid strands, and other macromolecules. The body has an innate reaction called the cellular stress response (CSR) to such damage. In the case of glioma and other cancers, the tumor is able to highjack the body's own machinery in order to help the cancerous cells survive usually by taking advantage of intrinsic or stress-related mutations. Thus, at times, stress may only further the growth and survival of tumor cells.

While the type of stress may vary, a common feature of many stresses is something referred to as the oxidative burst characterized by generation of oxidative stress and redox potential changes. Reactive oxygen species (ROSs) can be produced from activation of NADPH oxidase or other ceullar oxidases in the cell's various membranes. Stressor-specific responses, on the other hand, may be induced differentially depending on the type, severity, and duration of the stress. The following sections will cover these stresses and the resulting responses by normal cells and cancerous glioma cells.

2.1 Types of stress

Although gliomas can vary by type and stage, more advanced gliomas are characterized by high rates of mitosis, hypercellularity, evidence of angiogenesis, and areas of necrosis. Gliomas are known to have relatively high cellular heterogeneity, much of which may be caused by different areas of a tumor encountering different stresses and growing conditions. Thus, stress may be a driving factor in tumor heterogeneity. Although, medical professionals, along with patients, are able to control to a certain extent the extrinsic stresses put on patients' bodies and tumors such as treatments and environmental stressors (*e.g.* smoking), intrinsic stresses still naturally affect the tumor as it progresses.

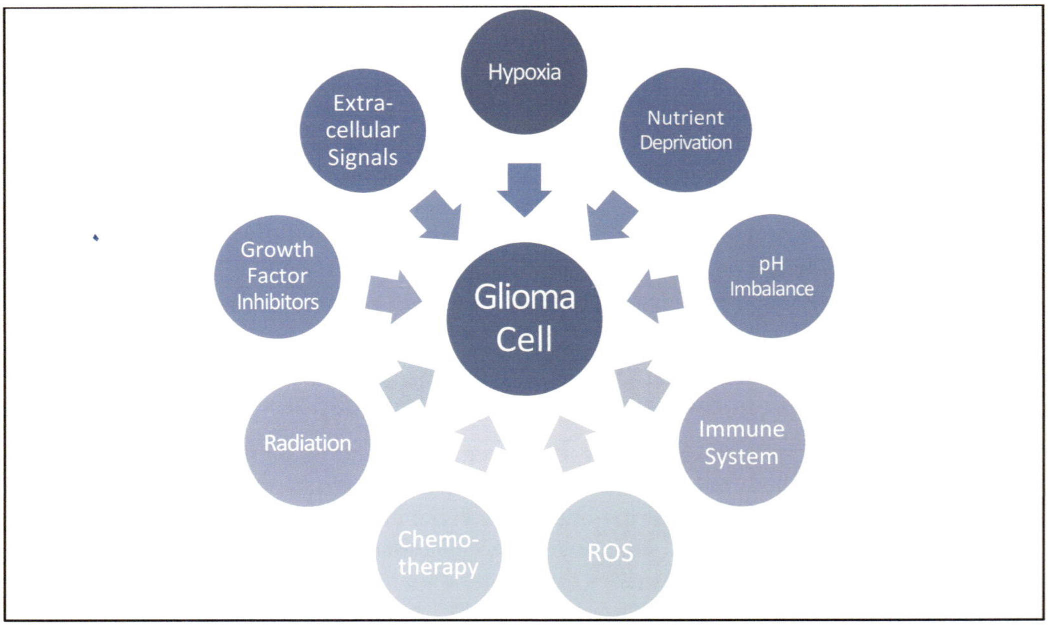

Fig. 1. Typical stresses encountered by glioma cells during tumor growth and progression.

2.1.1 Stresses during tumor development and progression

While research on glioma cells in laboratories is conducted primarily under nutrient-rich conditions, the micro-environments for cancer cells are actually quite hazardous. Rarely do tumor cells find themselves in conditions of perfect nutrient balance with necessary blood flow and comfortable living spaces. More often, glioma cells are constantly inundated with a barrage of stresses (Fig. 1). The internal stresses faced by glioma cells are not unique to brain tumors, but are actually shared by the majority of solid tumors types.

Environmental and metabolic stress occurs during tumor growth and progression. As cancer cells divide, they take up more space. Normal cells would stop growing through contact inhibition, but malignant cells overcome the signals to inhibit growth and continue to divide. As the tumor expands, it continually outgrows its blood supply. Tumors larger than 1 mm in diameter can no longer subsist on passive diffusion of nutrients (Gimbrone, 1973). The glioma cells, thus, go through periods of severe nutrient deprivation and hypoxia until enough tumor cells are able to signal new blood vessel formation or neoangiogenesis. Even after angiogenesis, cells are still subject to stress as the new vessels are prone to collapse due to their abnormal state and harsh surrounding conditions (Vajkoczy & Menger, 2004). During this time, cancer cells must adapt to survive in conditions and intermittent periods of limited amino acids, salts, and oxygen. Some researches indicate that this is when cancer cells start to rely on glycolysis, which continues even after oxygen is available, a phenomenon known as the Warburg effect. This contributes to the high metabolic demand of proliferating tumor cells and is a relatively inefficient method of producing energy (Warburg, 1956). Therefore, the cells are put under enormous stress just to keep up with energy production needs and are subjected to further metabolic stress when nutrients become unavailable.

The metabolic demands of the glioma cells are partially responsible for the increased acidity or pH imbalance found in many tumors. Human brain tumors measured with electrodes had a mean pH of 6.8, with measurements as low as 5.9; the normal pH for the human brain is ~7.1 (Vaupel et al., 1989). Such pH imbalance is even found in well vascularized areas of gliomas, thus indicating that tumor cells reside within a highly acidic environment even when oxygen is present. It was originally hypothesized that that hypoxia caused the acid buildup, but these new findings mean that hypoxia and acidity are not always linked. The increased energy metabolism of the glioma cells produce hydrogen ions and metabolites like lactic acid and carbonic acid. All these products are actively pumped out of the cell through proton exchangers and other transporters (Chiche et al., 2010). In cases with decreased perfusion, poor circulation contributes to the buildup of an acidic extracellular environment. As the tumor grows, the extracellular environment strives to slow down the progress of the cancer. Growth inhibition signals are sent that can either activate or deactivate cellular receptors depending on the need. Cancer cells survive by undergoing mutations in receptors like EGFR and PDGFR, changes that either stop the signaling cascades or rewire the signaling pathways to actually promote cancer cell growth. In this way, cellular proliferation is dissociated from nutrient availability by stress selection of surviving cells.

Hypoxia can play a major role in glioma development, with oxygen deprivation actually being necessary for tumor progression through alteration of gene expression, genomic instability, apoptotic dysregulation, and neoangiogenesis. In glioma, hypoxia is believed to be a key player due to the evidence of tumor necrosis in highly malignant forms like glioblastoma multiforme (GBM) (Brat & Meir, 2001). Brain tumors smaller than the previously stated 1 mm cutoff are found to be highly hypoxic and ill-perfused (Li et al. 2007). The oxygen deprivation is actually responsible for the growth of elaborate microvascular networks that indicate tumor progression in GBM. Even though larger GBM tumors are more vascularized, the blood vessels present are inefficient, and parts of the tumor environment remain hypoxic (Vajkoczy & Menger, 2004). Further transformation of the tumor cells occurs as reactive oxygen species (ROSs) increase during this time due to production by the mitochondria (Lui et al., 2008). Thus, hypoxia not only deprives cells of oxygen but leads to oxidative stress as well.

One of the hallmarks of a cancerous cell or tumor is its ability to invade through the basement membrane of one tissue into another type of tissue. The body has many stop guards in place to prevent this from happening, but somehow glioma cells overcome the challenge. Again, during this time, extracellular signals are sent to the cancer cells informing them to stop growing or to go through programmed cell death. Cell growth pathways are down-regulated by these signals causing severe stress to the cells. Without the normal nutrients or pathway activations, uncancerous cells would die, but glioma cells find a way to overcome the death signals. Cellular stress pathways that involve tumor suppressor p53 and metabolic stress pathways which activate the apoptotic protein Bim are often deregulated in human glioma (Tan et al.,2005). Therefore, the neoplastic cells are able to overcome invasion preventions.

The immune system is an added stress to cancer cells during all times of tumor progression, but is especially active during invasion and dissemination. While the immune system may ignore some cancer cells that stay in their own tissue, cells from different tissues are recognized by the markers or antigens they display. The innate immune system encounters the cancer cells first, with first-response cells like macrophages, granulocytes, and mast cells attacking foreign cells displaying unknown or altered markers. Even cancer cells that have managed to down-regulate these markers are subjected to hazardous surrounding environments due to the release of ROSs, metalloproteinases, chemokines, and cytokines created by the attack and death of neighboring cancer cells (Qian and Pollard, 2010). Dendritic cells transport the antigens from the neoplastic cells to the lymphoid organs in order to mount an adaptive response against the tumor. Yet somehow, in cases of cancer progression, tumor cells are able to survive these stresses and move to alternate locations. This is partially due to activated innate immune cells and paracrine signals from surrounding cells releasing soluble pro-survival molecules that initiated tumor cells can use to alter their levels of gene transcription, continuing the cell cycle and surviving (Egeblad et al., 2010). Even though the hazardous environment may kill some neoplastic cells, others may develop and thrive due to increased genomic instability from free radicals, creating additional, resistant cancer cells (Grivennikov et al., 2010). In fact, chronic inflammation has actually been linked to tumor development. Inflammatory cells can actually help in the angiogenesis and migration of glioma cells by promoting vasculature development and releases extracellular proteases that rebuild and mold the tumor environment (Colotta et al., 2009). The adaptive immune response eventually builds such that it can clear some of the neoplastic cells, but many of the cancer cells have further transformed so that they are not recognized by the cytotoxic T-cells. Even though the adaptive immune response may initially be helpful, as it continues it further promotes chronic inflammation and stress in the area, thereby contributing to cancer progression.

Those cells able to overcome the response of the immune system have a better chance of surviving invasion and migration into new tissues. Although very rare in glioma, occasionally cells do metastasize to other locations of the body, but more commonly disseminate to nearby areas of the brain. After breaking through the basement membrane, invasion may include entrance into nearby white matter tracks, and less frequently, blood vessels. By invading the white matter tracks, glioma cells are able to migrate along CNS developmental paths of the brain, taking up residence in new areas of ideal conditions, again through the process of invasion (Dai et al., 2001). In the uncommon case of hematogenous dissemination, the liver, lungs, pleura, lymph nodes and skeletal system are the most common sites of metastasis, although metastases outside of the brain are relatively rare due to the specificity of programming of glial cells (Pasquier et al., 1980). The cells that do survive are again subjected to the stresses of the immune system, new ECM signals, and lack of designated tumor blood vessels.

With the above intrinsic stresses attacking gliomas throughout their progression, it is a testament to cancer cell adaptability that any cancerous cells survive. By adapting to these stresses, gliomas have selected for the most stress resistant cells, making cancer therapy a challenge. However, while many therapies do produce the same types of stresses already present in the body, the treatments cause more effective and sustained stress, especially when combined.

2.1.2 Therapeutic stresses

Tumor cells have already found ways to survive the numerous internal stresses covered in the previous section, so it is of no surprise that glioma cells are often able to find ways around common therapies due to the similarity of the mechanisms of action of the interventions with the mechanism of the body's natural defenses. Table 1 lists some of the common and experimental therapies used to treat glioma in addition to the type of stress they cause. While the mechanisms of action are diverse, the treatments cause the same stresses already encountered by the glioma cells during the body's intrinsic response to aberrant cell growth.

Surgery is almost always used on patients who are surgical candidates. Debulking of the tumor not only allows for better brain function but also allows chemotherapies to be more effective by working on a smaller population. While surgery should be undertaken in situations where critical structures will not be disrupted, the act is extremely stressful on the brain. Small areas will be cut off from the blood supply creating a hypoxic and nutrient deprived environment leading to metabolic stress for unremoved cancer cells. The death of neighboring cells along with the immune response will cause an increase in oxidative stress and ROSs production.

Radiation is another first-line therapy against gliomas. While there are many variations of radiotherapy, ionizing radation (IR) tends to work through two basic mechanisms that ultimately damage the DNA by either charged particles or photons. In the case of photon radiation, like in intensity modulated radiation therapy (IMRT), this technique causes indirect damage that occurs after water is ionized producing free radicals. Double-stranded DNA breaks (DSBs) are the most significant cause of cell death. Photon radiotherapy requires well-oxygenated tumors to create the damaging free radicals, which requires adequate blood supply to all areas of the tumor. Because many areas of gliomas are hypoxic, this technique is often relatively unsuccessful long-term in many brain tumors (Harrison et al., 2002). Particle therapy, on the other hand, works by directly damaging the DNA by charged particles. Direct damage can occur through transfer of energy from charged particles like proton, carbon or boron ions that do not require oxygen. These particles can cause DBSB themselves. In either case, there are free radicals and ROSs produced by radiation; the ROSs are necessary for the efficacy of the treatment, further injuring cells (Dal-Pizzol et al., 2003). However, these reactive molecules are released during cell death causing increased stress to surviving cells. The body mounts an immune response to repair and clear damaged cells. Although many patients with gliomas take steroids to reduce the swelling and inflammation produced by radiotherapy, remaining neoplastic cells are still subjected to large amounts of stress, killing many while further transforming others into radioresistant tumor cells.

Therapy	Mechanism of Action	Form of Stress
Surgery	**Evacuation of tumor site**	**De-vascularization with subsequent hypoxia and nutrient deprivation, immune response**
Radiation External beam radiation Brachytherapy	Ionizing radiation	Oxidative stress, DNA damage
Genotoxic Chemotherapy Temozolomide, Procarbazine Carmustine (BCNU), Lomustine *Cis*-platinum, Carboplatin Vincristine Etoposide, Irinotecan	 Nonclassical alkylating agents Nitrosourea alkylating agents Platinum DNA crosslinkers Mitotic inhibitor Inhibits topoisomerase I or II	DNA and organelle damage due to interruption of replication, induces metabolic stress and ROSs
Monoclonal Antibodies Bevacizumab EGFR - Cetuximab, Nimotuzumab	 Anti-angiogenic Tyrosine kinase inhibitors	 Hypoxia Growth factor signaling inhibition leading to oxidative stress
Immunotherapies/Vaccines*	Immune system response	Oxidative stress, DNA damage, metabolic stress
Small Molecule Targeted Therapy* EGFR - Gefinitib, Erlotinib PDGFR - Imatinib mTOR - Everolimus	Tyrosine kinase inhibitors	Growth factor signaling inhibition leading to oxidative stress

Table 1. Common therapies and the stresses they cause. * Indicates experimental therapies

Chemotherapy is often used in conjunction with surgery and radiotherapy. Most of the common genotoxic chemotherapies for glioma produce their effects by disrupting the DNA strands. Alkylating agents like temozolomide (TMZ) and carmustine (BCNU) primarily work by alkylating the guanine base of DNA leading to cross-linking of the DNA strands which causes the strands to be unable to uncoil and separate. The platinum drugs, such as carboplatin and cis-platinum, work similarly by using the platinum ion to cross-link the guanine base pairs on the DNA strand. These therapies are more toxic to cells that replicate and proliferate faster, thus making cancer cells more sensitive than normal cells to genotoxic therapy. The stresses to the cell caused by chemotherapy are mostly due to interference of mitosis and induction of DNA repair mechanisms. When the cell is unable to unwind and repair its DNA, it causes apoptosis and metabolic stress. As apoptosis continues, ROSs are released into the ECM affecting nearby cells. Genotoxic stress through ROSs is dependent on activation of SAPK/JNK pathway (Benhar et al., 2001). Thus, chemotherapy stresses glioma cells through different mechanisms.

A general chemotherapy-induced stress response is seen in many types of cancer cells. This is a response to anti-neoplastic agents that can destroy many cancer cells but induce survival and resistance mechanisms in others. In yeast, stress changed the cell cycle and lead to increases in *de novo* protein synthesis, proliferation, HSP90 expression, and proton pump levels. The first line of defense in severe shock is *de novo* synthesis of protective proteins (Miligkos et al., 2000). Increasing key membrane component proteins can up- or down-regulate their efficacy to restore ionic balance. Changes in the heat shock protein (HSP) population of the cell due to chemotherapeutic stress also increase HSP27 and HSP70 in resistant cells; these cells are translocated to the nucleus in response to stress, increasing protein synthesis necessary for resistance (Nadin et al., 2003). Whole body response is also important as hormones production levels can change during the stress response; such hormones can affect the cell cycle or gene transcription. On a smaller scale, cell-to-cell interactions occur between transformed and non-transformed cells involving the transfer of survival signals, thus indicating that the extracellular environment is important. The stress response to chemotherapy-induced hyperthermia can even lead to induction of drug resistance through a general increase in MDR P-glycoprotein production (Benhar et al., 2001).

Anti-angiogenic therapies are becoming more common in glioma and are used to combat the tumor vasculature. Most of the inhibitors, like bevacizumab, are monoclonal antibodies that work by antagonistically binding vascular endothelial growth factors (VEGFs), the factors responsible for signaling growth of blood vessels. Contrary to other cancers, it is thought that anti-angiogenic drugs in glioma could work by transiently normalizing the tumor vasculature (Nagy et al., 2010). As discussed previously, tumor blood vessels are abnormal and unstable due to the mixture of pro- and anti-angiogenic factors. An angiogenesis inhibitor would override many of these signals. Although, this might decrease blood vessel formation, it might also stabilize the existing vasculature. By normalizing the vasculature, there could be improved delivery of chemotherapeutic agents. Either way, the neoplastic cells would be subject to stress caused either by hypoxia and nutrient deprivation or increased concentrations of anticancer drugs.

Progress in targeted therapies for glioma has been made in recent years. Numerous small molecule inhibitors are being tested in clinical trials to antagonize the commonly mutated or over-expressed growth factor pathways. These inhibitors, like erlotinib which works on EGFR and imatinib for PGDFR, work by intracellularly binding the tyrosine kinase receptors, interrupting the downstream PI3K and MAPK signaling cascades. Monoclonal antibodies like cetuximab and nimotuzumab (EGFR inhibitors) work similarly, except they bind extracellulary to the growth factor receptors. Most of the stress caused by these antagonists is through decreased growth factor signaling and the resulting metabolic stress.

All these therapies cause stresses already encountered by tumor formation, but the duration and severity of the stresses during therapy is more extreme. Prolonged exposure to these stresses can induce cell death programming more effectively than short, intermittent periods. However, in most cases, some cancer cells do survive. They evade the immune system and death signals, selected for by their unique mutations leading to therapy resistance. It is therefore important to determine accurate markers to identify these cells and to classify the mechanisms through which they survive.

2.2 Markers of stress

While glioma cells may be adept at surviving cellular stress, they do show indicators of the stresses they endure. These indicators or markers may eventually be exploited to determine what stresses the cancer cells are under, and thus what types of stress they may be more susceptible to if subjected further. This section will cover the most common markers of general cellular stress and the specific stresses mentioned previously.

When cells encounter stress, certain elements of the stress response are universal. There is a highly conserved minimal stress proteome that is shared among species. In a paper by Dieter Kültz, a list of the 41 proteins needed for the minimal stress proteome was compiled (Table 2).

While this table is not exhaustive for all proteins involved in the stress response, nor does it list the most reliable markers, it does indicate that cells all have a fundamental basic response to stress. The response is referred to as the conserved stress response (CSR). Various stresses may induce different proteins and markers, but certain responses are unchanged between stresses, even amongst species.

The general response of cells to stress originally focused on three types of proteins: heat shock proteins (HSPs), glucose-regulated proteins (GRPs) and ubiquitin-associated proteins, all of which are inter-related (Feder & Hofmann 1999). Of these three types of proteins, HSPs have been studied the most thoroughly. HSPs are induced during stress as a protective mechanism. While HSPs ordinarily play a more mundane role in the cell, folding proteins into their appropriate tertiary structures and facilitating steroid hormone binding, the subjection of cells to stress activates heat shock transcription factors (HSFs), allowing the transcription of stress-related HSPs like HSP27, HSP70 and HSP90 (Calderwood et al, 2006). In many gliomas and other cancers, binding of HSP90 to p53 mutants in the cytoplasm can further the damage caused by stress (Goetz et al., 2003). This is because p53 functions in the nucleus, and it leads to enhanced HSP70 transcription which allows for cancer cell growth (Ciocca & Calderwood, 2005). These HSPs, along with others, have been linked to cancer therapy resistance.

The unfolded protein response (UPR) has gained increasing coverage as a fundamental stress reaction caused by changes in the celluar redox potential, energy status, or Ca2+ levels leading to unfolded or misfolded proteins within the lumen of the endoplasmic reticulum (ER). This is also known as ER stress (Herr & Debatin, 2001). ER stress is closely linked to hypoxia and glucose depletion. Misfolded proteins can be a problem due to their propensity to aggregate together and cause harmful accumulations. The role of UPR is to stop protein translation, arrest the cell cycle, and to signal pathways that increase activation of protein folding chaperones, some of which are HSPs. Ultimately, UPR leads to cell death through apoptosis if translation is halted for a prolonged period. GPRs are related to UPR and are actually just specialized HSPs that are found in the ER of the cell. In fact, Grp78 is the protein responsible for chaperoning the misfolded proteins and signaling downstream activators of the UPR. Another GRP, grp94 or HSP90B1, is actually essential for immune responses as it is a chaperone that regulates both innate and adaptive immunity through secretory pathways (Maki et al., 1990). Upregulation of these proteins is often seen during stress, and thus could represent markers for stress induction.

Many stresses signal through the stress-activated protein kinase/c-Jun NH2-terminal kinase (SAPK/JNK) pathway, which is activated by numerous extracellular signals and stresses.

Minimal Stress Proteome		
Redox regulation	**DNA damage sensing/repair**	**Fatty acid/lipid metabolism**
Aldehyde reductase	MutS/MSH	Long-chain fatty acid ABC transporter
Glutathione reductase	MutL/MLH	Multifunctional beta oxidation protein
Thioredoxin	Topoisomerase I/III	Long-chain fatty acid CoA ligase
Peroxiredoxin	RecA/Rad51	
Superoxide dismutase		
MsrA/PMSR	**Molecular chaperones**	**Energy metabolism**
SelB	Petidyl-prolyl isomerase	Citrate synthase (Krebs cycle)
Proline oxidase	DnaJ/HSP40	Ca^{2+}/Mg^{2+}-transporting ATPase
Hydroxyacylglutathione hydrolase 6	GrpE (HSP70 cofactor)	Ribosomal RNA methyltransferase
NADP-dependent oxidoreductase YMN1	HSP60 chaperonin	Enolase (glycolysis)
Putative oxidoreductase YIM4	DnaK/HSP70	Phosphoglucomutase
Aldehyde dehydrogenase		
Isocitrate dehydrogenase	**Protein degradation**	**Other functions**
Succinate semialdehyde dehydrogenase	FtsH/proteasome-regulatory subunit	Inositol monophosphatase
Quinone oxidoreductase	Lon protease/protease La	Nucleoside diphosphate kinase
Glycerol-3-phosphate dehydrogenase	Serine protease	Hypothetical protein YKP1
2-hydroxyacid dehydrogenase	Protease II/prolyl endopetidase	
phosphogluconate dehydrogenase	Aromatic amino acid aminotransferase	
	Aminobutyrate aminotransferase	

Table 2. The minimal stress proteome as described by Kültz, 2005.

These kinases are part of the larger superfamily known as mitogen-activated protein kinases (MAPKs), which control many intracellular events. SAPK is activated by SEK1 or MKK4. The SAPK/JNK pathway is activated by stresses like hypoxia, radiation, drug therapy, ROSs, and inflammatory molecules (Benhar et al., 2001). They signal through a variety of receptors, including G-protein coupled receptors (GPCRs), cytokine receptors (TNFα), death receptors (Fas), and antigen receptors. SAPK/JNK pathways can control proliferation, apoptosis, transformation and differentiation along with migration. In response to many types of stress such as radiation and hypoxia, this pathway signals for mitochondrial-dependent apoptosis (Sanchez-Prieto et al., 2000). Thus, the SAPK/JNK signaling cascade is a protective mechanism for cells. However, any mutations or aberrant signaling could also lead to further glioma progression. Up-regulation of proteins involved in these pathways is a good indicator of cellular stress.

Additionally, other markers of general stress have also been found. The MDR1 (multi-drug resistance 1) gene, which encodes the P-glycoprotein responsible for reducing drug accumulation in cancer cells, is actually induced by stresses like acidity, drug treatment, and radiation (Szabo et al., 2000). Thus, cancer cells under stress have created multiple mechanisms to evade cell death. The original intent for non-transformed, normal cells was for them to be able to pump out toxins encountered in their environment for survival purposes. Transformed cancer cells have adapted those responses to their own needs.

Some indicators of specific stresses have also been revealed. An example of a marker for specific stress can be found in hypoxia. The transcription factor HIF-1 (hypoxia-inducting factor-1) is a major regulator of the cellular hypoxia response, which binds to hypoxia-responsive elements (HREs) leading to the transcription of genes involved in cell survival, metabolism, angiogenesis and invasion. It can increase expression of glycolysis genes and VEGF protein (Jiang et al., 1996). The expression of HIF-1 is increased in glioma usually through induction by EGFR signaling the PI3 kinase pathway and loss of the tumor suppressors p53 and PTEN. HIF-1 expression, and thus hypoxic stress, in tumors can be determined by immunohistochemical staining. Another indicator of stress linked to HIF-1 is NF-κB induction. NF-κB activation leads to the rapid transcription of important genes involved with the stress response. Because it is a transcription factor, it is often thought of as a first line of defense, especially against activators of the immune system (Garg & Aggarwal, 2002). NF-κB is able to regulate many proteins involved in proliferation and survival, including HIF-1. Another isoform, HIF-2α, appears to be a specific marker for pH imbalance as it is increased with exposure to acidic stress (Hjelmeland et al., 2010).

Overall, there are numerous markers of stress in glioma cells. Many are the result of a general response to stress, but as research continues, better markers for specific stress, like HIF-1 in the case of hypoxia, will be developed as our understanding continues to grow. These markers may eventually help clinicians to positively identify the stresses the tumor is under, which will inevitably lead to more effective glioma treatment.

2.3 Mitigation of metabolic and therapeutic stress by autophagy

Glioma cells are able to employ several ways to overcome stress and the resulting energy depletion. Autophagy, the catabolic recycling of the cell's own components, takes advantage of this idea as a survival mechanism. The autophagic process allows the tumor cells to reallocate amino acids, fatty acids and other macromolecules for energy and go into a hibernation-like state until the surrounding environment is more favorable. Glioma therapies, like temozolimide and etoposide, have been shown to induce autophagy as have various metabolic stresses. While autophagy is also viewed as a cell death mechanism, new research indicates that autophagy can actually be responsible for glioma cell survival and resistance to therapies and stresses. Molecules like beclin-1 and elongation factor-2 kinase (EF-2K) have been shown to play a critical role in the autophagic response in glioma.

2.3.1 Role of autophagy in stress response

Autophagy was first discovered as a Type II programmed cell death (PCD) mechanism with distinct differences from apoptosis in yeast. Most initial research was done in yeast, and later, it was found that many of the proteins involved are conserved in higher eukaryotes with human homologues. During autophagy, double membrane autophagosomes or autophagic vacuoles engulf cytoplasm along with long-lived proteins and damaged organelles through a process of self-digesting. The enveloped contents of the autophagosome are degraded by fusing with the lysosome. Their constituents of fatty acids and amino acids are recycled into new molecules or shunted into the synthesis of ATP to meet energy needs. If left unchecked, autophagy does indeed lead to cellular destruction and canabolitic cell death. Because autophagy occurs in many cells immediately preceding cell death, it was initially seen as a cell death mechanism (Levine & Yuan, 2005). However, cells can also utilize autophagy as a means to go into a cellular "hibernation" state where they have decreased energy needs as a strategy of survival (Kuma et al., 2004). Thus, autophagy can also be seen as a temporary protective response of cells.

Autophagy is known to occur in the brain during neurodegenerative processes such as Alzheimer, Parkinson, and Huntington disease. However, its role as a protector or cause of disease is debated (Nixon, 2006). As for its role in glioma, cancer cells were shown to have decreased levels of autophagy compared to non-malignant cells, while nutrient deprivation upregulated its autophagic activity in cancer cells (Wu et al., 2006). This could be due to the early stages of tumorigenesis needing increased protein synthesis and proliferation, where autophagy would impede the growth of the cells. Also, since autophagy removes damaged organelles, it can decrease the mutation rate of the cancer cells, leaving them at a disadvantage during early stages of the disease. Later stages of glioma progression see an increase in autophagy to protect against the numerous cellular stresses present at this stage like nutrient deficiency.

An important mechanism of regulation of autophagy is through the PI3K-Akt-mTOR pathway, which is activated in many cancers. Suppression of autophagy occurs through class 1 PI3K, while class III PI3K promotes autophagosome development (Lum et al., 2005). This is because class III PI3K binds to a molecule known as beclin-1 (BECN1). Beclin-1, the homologue of yeast Atg6, is part of an early-autophagy complex that participates in the autophagosome formation (Liang et al., 1999). It is also known to interact with the anti-apoptotic protein Bcl-2, binding the molecule and preventing cell death (Erlich et al., 2007). Bcl-2 may regulate the balance between autophagy and apoptosis, since it plays a role in both. Down-regulation of Bcl-2 or up-regulation of its binding protein, BNIP3, induces autophagy. Beclin-1 expression has been shown to be aberrant in cancers, including glioma (Liang et al., 2006). When beclin-1 binds class III PI3 kinase, the complex can activate autophagy. This complex is located in the cell cytoplasm and trans-Golgi network where it can sort the necessary autophagosome components. It, in turn, can be regulated through miRNA miR-30a which is able to down-regulate beclin-1 and thus regulate autophagy. miR-30a expression in glioma was initially implicated in a miRNA screen for differential expression during conditions that induce autophagy and was found to be decreased during autophagy. Further studies with the miRNA showed that expression of miR-30a in glioma cells decreased beclin-1 expression and decreased autophagy (Zhu et al., 2009). This was the first report of miRNA regulating autophagy, so it is certainly possible that other miRNA's may play a role in this process.

The formation of the autophagosome is mediated by a series of autophagy specific genes (ATGs) originally identified in yeast like Beclin-1. Other important human counterparts of regulators of autophagy have been found, such as LC3, a mammalian homologue of yeast gene Atg8, which is one of the primary markers of autophagy. It is a ubiquitin-like protein which cooperates with Atg4 protease (Mizushima, 2004). Other autophagy proteins include another system of an Atg12-Atg5-Atg16 complex in addition to gene products like Atg5, Atg7, and Atg10, which also play roles in activating autophagy.

Another regulator of autophagy is the protein synthesis inhibitor, elongation factor-2 kinase (EF-2K). EF-2K, a Ca^{2+}/calmodulin kinase, halts translation by phosphorylating elongation factor-2 (EF-2), a protein responsible for moving the peptide strand along the ribosome during elongation. It does so through hydrolyzing GTP to GDP, which provides the energy for elongation. Phosphorylation of EF-2 negatively reduces its affinity for the ribosome (Ryazanov et al., 1991). Regulating this energy-consuming step in translation is important to cell survival during periods of stress and reduced nutrients, so it is unsurprising that EF-2K protein and activity levels are found to be increased in glioma and other cancers.

The first link of EF-2K to cellular stress was found in hibernating squirrels. During hibernation, decreased respiration and blood flow along with abstinence from food intake, greatly reduces the amount of oxygen and nutrients that are available to cells. In tissues with high metabolic rate, both p-EF-2 and EF-2K levels were found to be increased(Chen et al., 2001). Further studies in cells and mouse models showed increases in EF-2K during nutrient deprivation, hypoxia, radiation exposure, and drug treatment. As EF-2K is a calmodulin kinase known to be activated by calcium flux, ER stress was also found to be dependent on EF-2K status (Py et al., 2009). Unsurprisingly, it was later discovered that EF-2K regulates autophagy. Down-regulation of EF-2K reduces autophagy and increases cell death during stress in glioma (Wu et al., 2006).

EF-2K is regulated through the PI3K/mTOR/S6 kinase pathway by nutrient and growth factor availability, which links together cellular stress and the autophagic response, as they are regulated by the same pathway (Hait et al., 2006). In fact, disruption of the PI3K/mTOR/S6K pathway is known to induce autophagy, probably through EF-2K activation (Fig. 2). Nutrients and growth factors activate mTOR that in turn activates S6 kinase. Both mTOR and S6 kinase negatively regulate EF-2K by phosphorylating it on Ser 78 and Ser366, respectively (Browne & Proud, 2004). This inhibits EF-2K activity and its induction of autophagy, since nutrients and cellular building blocks are plentiful. Nutrient deprivation not only inhibits mTOR signaling and regulation of EF-2K, but it also increases AMP kinase activity due to the depletion of ATP. AMP kinase can positively regulate EF-2K activity by phosphorylating it on a different site, Ser 398, leading to its activation and induction of autophagy, as measured by autophagic markers, like LC3 and acidic vacuole organelle staining (Browne et al., 2004).

It is through the mTOR/S6 kinase pathway that cellular stress can cause the induction of autophagy. Some stresses, dependent on severity and duration, can instantaneously cause both apoptosis and autophagy, while the same stress under different conditions make cause one or another. While it is not yet clear why one pathway is chosen over another, new studies into the induction of autophagy have helped to determine the conditions under which it is stimulated. Disruption of the PI3K/Akt pathway has been associated with autophagy induction as well as stimulation of the AMP kinase pathway. mTOR inhibits autophagy through activating one of its downstream targets, S6 kinase (Abeliovich, 2003).

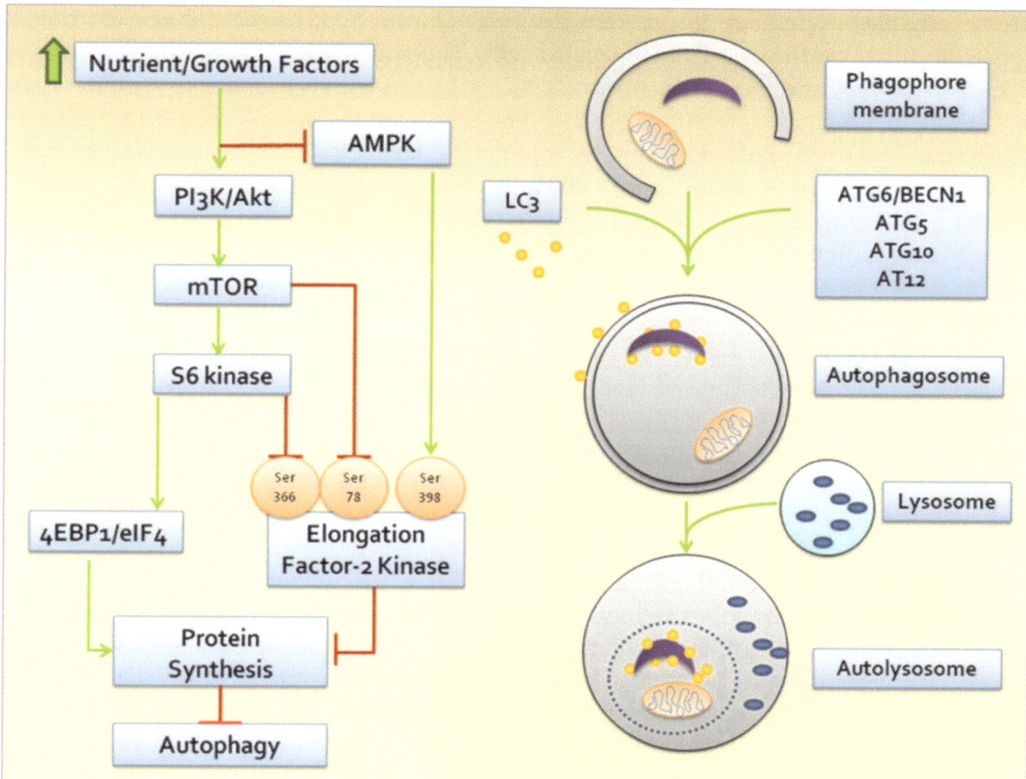

Fig. 2. Autophagy machinery and its regulation by EF-2K.

Many neoplastic cells, including glioma cells, survive metabolic stress through autophagy. Autophagy can originally act as a tumor suppressor due to the inactivation of apoptosis and subsequent immune reaction. In fact, autophagic markers localize *in vivo* to areas of tumors that are undergoing metabolic stress (White, 2007). Autophagy supports metabolic functions during periods of starvation by cannibalizing and recycling need elements, in short, providing alternative energy sources. Initially, autophagy in non-malignant cells can help prevent tumorigenesis through the removal of damaged organelles and defective proteins, since accumulation of these particulars can lead to oxidative stress. In fact, research shows that it even protects the genomic stability (White, 2007). However, as genetic mutations from other sources accumulate, autophagy allows compromised cells to survive. Defective autophagy can lead to cell death through apoptosis and necrosis, which further stresses neighboring cells through the recruitment of inflammatory molecules. Damage can occur to cellular DNA, creating further genomic instability. Increased mutation rate can further tumor progression at the expense of some cells.

Stresses known to induce autophagy include starvation, ER stress, mitochondrial damage, protein aggregation, radiation, hypoxia, and pathogens stimulation. Failure of autophagy has been reported to be the mechanism behind cell damage accumulation and aging.

Starvation is readily linked to autophagy through activation the mTOR pathway. Other stresses regulate autophagy in different manners. During hypoxia, autophagic clearing of damaged mitochondria is advantageous to cells. The source of pro-apoptotic signals and ROSs is removed, and thus the cancer cell is able to survive even under oxygen deprived conditions. Bcl-2 family protein, BNIP3, is known to induce autophagy during hypoxia, while others believe it induces apoptosis especially after the cellular environment becomes too acidic from hypoxia (Azad et al., 2008). Metabolic stress activates the p53 pathway, which can normally induce apoptosis through proteins like Puma and Noxa, but metabolic stress increases Bim instead, which signals through Bax and Bak (Vousden & Lane, 2007). Therefore, autophagy can suppress apoptosis during both hypoxia and metabolic stress in glioma.

In short, autophagy plays a critical role in glioma cell survival during various stresses. While autophagy can lead to cell death if not properly regulated, neoplastic cells can also use it as a protective mechanism. The autophagic response is activated by the typical hazards encountered by glioma cells during tumorigenesis, helping the cells to survive periods of limited oxygen and nutrients. Thus, exploiting autophagy as a therapeutic intervention is a subject that has been actively explored.

2.3.2 Glioma treatments and autophagy

Since autophagy can serve as a cell survival mechanism, it is unsurprising that cancer cells would adapt to use it to their advantage. Not only can neoplastic cells survive intrinsic stresses through autophagy, but they can use it to evade therapeutic interventions. Autophagy-associated therapy resistance is gaining recognition as a key resistance mechanism. Glioma cells tend to undergo autophagy rather than apoptosis, perhaps due to their advanced nature created by genomic instability. Autophagy has been shown to be induced in a wide range of glioma therapies.

Radiation was the first therapy shown to cause glioma cells to undergo autophagy. As stated previously, the main mechanism of damage caused by radiation is through DNA double-strand breaks (DBSs), which can lead to translocation, misrepair, and even loss of chromosomes. Gamma radiation is known to induce autophagy in human glioma cells, but there is some controversy as to whether it causes cell death or if it protects cells (Paglin et al., 2001). This could be due to autophagy playing different roles at different times, acting as a cell death mechanism during early stages and acting as a protective mechanism later in tumor development after the accumulation of more advantageous mutations. Autophagy itself is also regulated on many levels and at different stages of induction, producing differing effects in glioma cells. Inhibiting autophagy is sometimes protective and other times destructive, indicating that autophagy is a sensitive modulator of cell survival. Even with glioma cells using autophagy as a way of survival, prolonged radiation may eventually switch the autophagic program from cell survival to cell death as too many damaged proteins accumulate. Glioma cells treated with autophagic inhibitors were radiosensitized, and radiation was able to create more DBSs (Ito et al., 2005).

Many chemotherapies cause autophagy in glioma. Mainstay treatment, temozolomide (TMZ), is used for high-grade gliomas (late stage). It is a small, lipophilic agent that easily passes through the BBB. Although referred to as an alkylating agent, TMZ does not actually cause cross-linking but instead adds a methyl group to a guanine which gets mispaired with thymine instead of cytosine during the next cycle of DNA synthesis. Initial research into the mechanism of cell death by the drug indicated that TMZ causes cell death through autophagy not through apoptosis (Kanzawa et al., 2004). . However, not much cell death occurred, and it was eventually discovered that glioma cells were using autophagy initially as a protective mechanism as glioma cells were able to start proliferating again after a week of TMZ treatment. This could be due to the previously stated idea that inhibiting autophagy at different stages of induction leads to different outcomes. Before the recruitment of LC3, cells can be rescued from autophagy by treatment with 3-MA (inhibitor of PI3K) (Kanzawa et al., 2004). Bafilomycin A1, an inhibitor of lysosomal ATPase and atuophagy, in combination with TMZ induces apoptosis.

While TMZ induces autophagy and not apoptosis in glioma cell lines, another alkylating agent cisplatin induces both apoptosis and autophagy. Apoptosis is further activated if autophagic inhibitors were added to cisplatin-treated glioma cells due to the release of Bcl-2 from beclin-1. Thus, cisplatin also utlizes autophagy as a protective mechanism (Harhaji-Trajkovic, 2009). Additional studies were done on TMZ and etopside showing that autophagy clearly protects cells from the multimicronucleation and cell death normally associated with TMZ and etoposide treatment. This was discovered through the detection of a concomitant ATP-surge that occurred with treatment. The associated unsustained ATP surge was not through glycolysis but through a brief period of oxidative phosphorylation. This was due to an induction of autophagy that increased catabolic metabolism to increase ATP levels (Katayama et al., 2007). Many chemotherapeutic agents have also been shown to cause hyperthermia in areas of tumors due to increased inflammation and stress in glioma cells. Hyperthermia itself is also known to induce autophagy, adding another mechanism by which glioma chemotherapies are able to activate autophagic response (Sanchez-Prieto et al., 2000).

Growth factor inhibitors are in the experimental stage of glioma therapy development. Platelet-derived growth factor receptor (PDGFR) antagonists, such as imatinib, and epidermal growth factor receptor (EGFR) antagonists, like erlotinib, have been developed to inhibit the growth signals transmitted through these pathways. Autocrine signaling of growth factors can occur, with glioma cells over-expressing both the growth factor and its receptor together to signal through PI3K pathway. Inhibition of PDGF and EGF signaling induced autophagy but not apoptosis (Takeuchi et al., 2004). This result could be due to inhibitory effect of class I PI3K and/or stimulatory effect of class III PI3K. Downstream targets are also available for inhibition of growth factor pathways. Rapamycin, the inhibitor of mTOR, was able to induce autophagy along with suppressing proliferation. Since mTOR regulates both cell proliferation and autophagy, this could be a good target for future combined therapies. Combining rapamycin with an Akt or PI3K inhibitor increased glioma cell death, and future studies will look at the combination of rapamycin with growth factor inhibitors (Takeuchi et al., 2005).

Another category of experimental therapies, glycolytic inhibitors, work similarly to nutrient deprivation as they have preferential uptake by glioma cells that are normally dependent on high levels of glucose to satisfy their rapid glycolysis needs. 2-deoxy-D-glucose (2-DG) is a glycolytic inhibitor that blocks the effects of glucose on metabolic pathways. It had previously been shown to inhibit growth of cancer cells and enhance the efficacy of other glioma treatments. 2-DG causes oxidative stress in glioma cells which lead to the discovery of its induction of autophagy. The glycolytic inhibitor activated EF-2K and thus autophagy in a PTEN-independent manner. Inhibition of EF-2K blocked autophagy induction by 2-DG, thereby sensitizing the cells to 2-DG cell death through caspase-3 apoptosis. Cells under additional stress like hypoxia were further sensitized by concurrent treatment of 2-DG and EF-2K inhibition (Wu et al, 2009).

Thus, it appears that glioma cells have used autophagy to resist a wide range of current glioma therapies. Although originally thought to be a mechanism of cell death, autophagy obviously plays a major role in protecting glioma cells from therapeutic intervention. Studies do indicate, however, that inhibiting autophagy may re-sensitize cancer cells to currently used treatments, providing a way around tumor resistance.

2.4 Stress and glioma cancer stem cells

Neural stem cells (NSCs) are specific to the central nervous system and are multipotent able to generate neurons, astrocytes, and oligodendrocytes. Like other stem cells, they are self-renewing, proliferative, and quiescent until needed. NSCs are common during human embryonic development but are reduced in number and sequestered to specific regions of adult brains. These tiny subpopulations of cells can be recognized by their CD133+ status. In recent years, there has been a new consensus that gliomas contain a glioma cancer stem cell (GCSC) population in addition to other precursor and differentiated cancer cells. Thus, gliomas can express both neuronal and glial markers. There is accumulating evidence that NSCs are key players in tumor initiation and progression along with angiogenesis and dissemination. Thus, their presence is starting to redefine how therapy outcomes are determined and understanding their role in tumor progression and therapy resistance may be pivotal in improving patient prognoses.

For years it was thought that humans were born with all the brain cells that they were ever going to have and that mitosis of neural and glial cells only occurred during early development. While most cells in the CNS do exit the cell cycle as terminally differentiated cells early in life, it has come to light that neurogenesis continues throughout life in small areas of the brain including the subventricular zone (Lois & Alvarez, 1993) and the dentate gyrus (Kuhn et al., 1996). These locations are home to NSCs that exhibit the normal stem cell markers and are capable of migration and multipotency. The existence of these NSCs that are normally present in the brain provides precedence for the idea of mutipotent cells in the CNS and gliomas. As gliomas are known to be highly heterogeneous tumors with cells from multiple neural lineages, cancerous neural stem cells could explain this finding. Poor prognosis has been linked to glioma tumor heterogeneity (Pallini et al., 2008), which could be the result of GCSCs.

2.4.1 Stress-induced stem cell markers

Although, at present, there are no universally accepted markers of GCSCs, this section will cover known NSC markers along with frequently studied glioma stem cell markers (Fig. 3). Small side populations (SP) of glioma stem cells (0.01-5% of total cells) exist that rarely divide despite elevated proliferation potential (Hirschmann-Jax et al, 2004). These were first found through flow cytometry studies where a small SP of tumor cells could be sorted and differentiated from the rest of the population. These cells were shown to efflux the fluorescent nucleic acid-staining dye, Hoechst 33342 (Pattrawala et al, 2005). When isolated, this small percentage of cells was able to generate neurospheres and xenografts, which are key stem cell properties. The SPs were able to efflux both the dye and chemotherapeutic agents through up-regulation of an ATP-binding cassette (ABC) member, BCRP, which is involved in multi-drug resistance (Eramo et al., 2006). These SPs were the first indicator that there was probably a cancer stem cell population in gliomas.

The two most common markers of neural stem cells are CD133 and nestin. CD133, also known as prominin-1, is a cell membrane glycoprotein which is present on different types of stem cells and cancer cells while being down-regulated on differentiated cells (Uchida et al., 2000). CD133+ cells can be isolated from human brain tumors and are able to demonstrate stem cell properties *in vivo* like accelerated tumor growth and invasion (Singh et al., 2004). They pass the gold standard for determining stem cell properties, which is that cells must be able to initiate formation of tumor similar to the patient's and is able to undergo serial transplantations. These cells have increased levels of stem cell genes such as nestin, Msi-1, MELK, and CXCR4 (Lui et al., 2006). Recent studies indicate that CD133 expression may be linked to periods of angiogenesis or times of stress. In fact, hypoxia can induce a CD133+ brain tumor stem cell population. CD133+ cells are resistant to drug treatment and apoptosis with increased expression of several ABC transporters and DNA repair machinery (Eramo et al, 2006). These cells also show an increase in chemokine receptor CXCR4 that directs NSC migration and thus GSCS movement (Lui et al., 2006). Even though it appears that CD133+ status is indicative of a NSC, CD133- cells can still exhibit stem cell properties (Wang et al., 2008). Therefore, CD133 status is not the final determinant of stem cellness for glioma cells.

The another common marker, nestin, is an intermediate filament protein produced by NSCs that controls cellular morphology, proliferation, and adhesion. Differentiated cells down-regulate nestin and increase other neurofilaments involved in neurons and glial cells that have exited the cell cycle (Zimmerman et al., 1994). Nestin expression increases during stress like ischemia, traumatic brain injury, inflammation, and tumor progression (Holmin et al., 1997). As a glioma marker, it indicates an increased malignant potential in invasion and motility abilities associated with poor prognosis (Stronjnik et al., 2007). It was one of the first discovered NSC markers but is not ideal due to its cytoplasmic location. Thus, sorting methods like flow cytometry cannot be used to separate stem cells from non-stem cells according to nestin status.

Other stem cell markers may be more useful due to their location on the cell surface. A2B5 is cell surface marker of neural progenitor cells. It is a ganglioside normally found in cells in the subventricular zones that host NSCs (Nunes et al., 2003). It has recently been reported that cells in GBM have been found that are A2B5+ and exhibit stem cell properties like tumor initiation. In fact, A2B5+/CD133- cells are also capable of initiating tumors and forming neurospheres (Tchoghandjian et al., 2009). Thus, A2B5 status is a potential useful marker for stem cells in gliomas and should be added to initial screenings. Stage-Specific Embryonic Antigen -1 (SSEA-1), which is also known as CD15 or Lewis-X Antigen, is another cell surface antigen. It is a carbohydrate moity that associates with glycoproteins and glycolipids. SSEA-1+ cells have increased stem cell gene expressions and properties. The majority of GBM tumors analyzed for the marker were SSEA-1+, and SSEA-1+ cells are highly tumorigenic while SSEA-1- cells are not (Son et al., 2009). Therefore, these two surface markers may play an important role in determining a GCSC population.

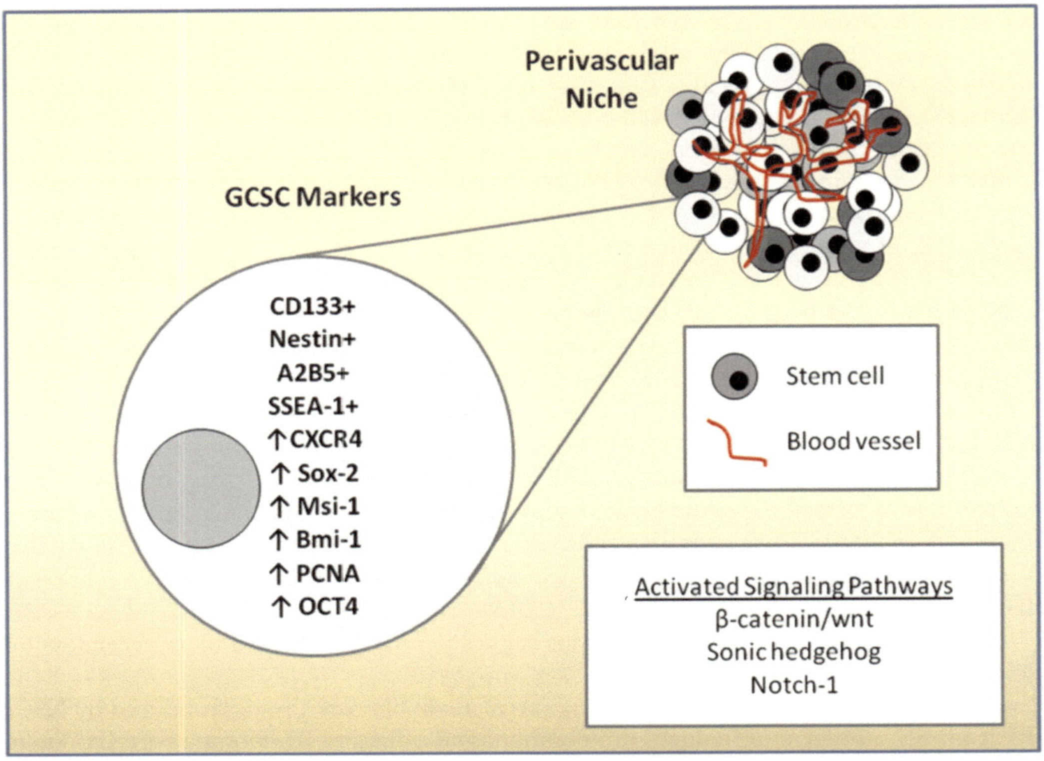

Fig. 3. Glioma cancer stem cell population in the perivascular niche. Common markers are listed.

Developmental pathways and other signaling pathways are also up-regulated in SPs, which later became indicators of stem cell activity (Hadnagy et al., 2006). The Wnt/β-catenin and the sonic hedgehog (SHH)/Gli1 pathways are both upregulated in GCSCs (Rich, 2007). Wnt signaling increases β-catenin activity. Over-expression of Gli1 and β-catenin have recently been shown to be correlated with poor prognosis (Pu et al., 2009), while EGFR and p53 were not predictive (Rossi et al., 2011). Some GCSCs have increased Notch-1 signaling, as do their healthy NSCs counterparts. Even PDGF status is linked to stem cells, as signaling of the growth factor is upregulated during oligodendrocyte proliferation and differentiation (Nait-Oumesmar et al., 1997).

Other stem cell pathways and molecules have been found in these populations. The Notch receptor pathway has also been implicated in GCSCs, as this signaling cascade mediates differentiation and proliferation (Koch and Radtke, 2007). Over-expression of Notch-1 leads to formation and proliferation of neurosphere-forming stem cells that are nestin-positive, while down-regulation leads to apoptosis (Hitoshi et al., 2002). Additional traditional stem cell markers such as Sox2, Bmi-1, PCNA, NANO, Msi-1, and OCT4 have all been found in these cells, indicating that gliomas do in fact have populations of cancerous cells that have stem-cell like properties and are probably GCSCs (Hemmati et al., 2003). This finding has a tremendous impact of glioma cell survival and important implications for new therapies regimens to treat patients with glioma.

2.4.2 Glioma cancer stem cells are obstacles to effective treatment

It remains a matter of debate whether GCSCs are derived from original NSCs or other progenitor cells. Some argue that cancer cells can actually transition from a differentiated cell back into an undifferentiated cell through epithelial-mesechymal transition (EMT) (Singh & Settleman, 2010). This would mean that signals that trigger EMT could also trigger cancer stem cell formation. Either way, it has been shown that stem cell pathways including Wnt/ β-catenin, SSH, and Bmi-1 can all be activated by common treatments used in glioma therapy, like ionizing radiation and TMZ, which may lead to resistance to radiation and chemotherapy (Bell & Miele, 2011).

Thus, regardless of the origins of the GCSCs, the presence of cancer stem cells would explain the seemingly inevitable recurrence of advanced gliomas. If cancer cells can either revert to a de-differentiated state or if original mutated stem cells from a tumor could survive a therapy, then the cancer could proliferate again. Stem cells are designed to survive assaults. They are a form of cellular dormancy that can wait until the cell encounters a more favorable environment, and then self-renew, proliferate, and create differentiated progeny that are suited to the present conditions (Hambardzumyan et al., 2008). GCSCs could shed light on why patients seem to have been cured of their cancer only to have it return months or even decades later after having undergone numerous surgeries, chemotherapies, and radiation treatments. Mounting evidence indicates that cancer stem cells are key to the survival or recurrence of glioma. In fact, current treatment regimens could worsen matters by putting the cancer cells under the exact stresses that actually select for GCSCs (Tetyana et al., 2010).

Stresses in different areas of a tumor could select for distinct subpopulations of normal tumor cells and CSCs. Since CSCs by definition are plastic, they are able to adapt to their current environment, at times lying dormant and at others, proliferating and differentiating cancer cells that have adapted through genomic instability that is inevitable with cancer progression. These cells are even able to create stromal support layers recruiting host cells to make some of the necessary growth factors and signals (Bao et al, 2006).

The GCSCs either migrate or produce their own local microenvironments or niches that created by cells and an ideal extracellular matrix (ECM) (Fig. 3). Niches shield the GCSCs from harsh environments present in the rest of the brain (Valshi et al., 2009). They support a specific mix of necessary growth factors, signaling molecules, and nutrients to sustain a stem cell population. Perivascular niches are also commonly home to healthy NSCs (Calabrese et al., 2007). In GBM, the niche is composed of vasculature that contacts the cells and allows secretion of factors that help to maintain stem cell quiescence. This increased density of microvessels is highly associated with GCSCs niches, which tightly regulates the availability of oxygen and nutrients while allowing the cells a means of migration to other areas if necessary. The stems cells continue to modulate this extracellular environment - they secrete VEGF and increase the number of endothelial cells, which in turn leads to increased GCSC and tumor growth (Gilbertson & Rich, 2007). Niches are abnormal in GCSCs because they cause the stem cells to renew and proliferate.

Protected by their ideal environment, GCSCs are easily able to resist common treatments. This is conceivable since even normal stem cells need to survive years of stress under normal circumstances. As mentioned previously, GCSCs express adenosine triphosphate

(ATP)-binding cassette transporters (ABC-transporters) such as MDR1 and breast cancer resistance protein (BCRP) that are able to efflux chemotherapeutic drugs. This allows stem cells to survive regardless of the type of chemotherapy delivered. Even when the cells cannot efflux all of the agent, GCSCs derived from patient tumors, when treated with common therapies, are able to show resistance within 48 hours with continued ability to proliferate (albeit at a lower rate) in the presence of the drugs (Eramo, 2006). Many of these cells also show increases in DNA-mismatch repair with over-expression of methyl guanine methyl transferase (MGMT) which is common in resistance to alkylating or alkylating-like agents (Jullierat-Jeanneret et al., 2008). Anti-apoptotic proteins like Bcl-2 and Bcl-XL were found to be over-expressed in the increased population of CD133+ cells GCSC treated with TMZ, carboplatin, or taxol, as were members of the inhibitor of apoptosis (IAP) family such as surviving (Lui et al., 2006). Numerous mechanisms and pathways have been associated with treatment resistance of GCSCs.

Not only are GCSCs able to survive therapeutic insults, but many interventions actually select for the cancer stem cells. Radiation has been shown to enrich for GCSC. These stem cells have increased survival advantages over their non-radiotreated counterparts. Radioresistant tumors showed increases in CD133+ status. Notch-1 signaling has also been shown to be activated upon radiation exposure (Scharpfenecker et al., 2009). All cells had the same amount of initial damage to DNA and organelles, but GCSCs were able to repair damage more quickly than matched non-stem cells (Bao et al., 2006). CD133+ cells are able to evade radiation damage by preferential activation of DNA damage checkpoints. Bao determined that the resistance to radiation can be partially circumvented by inhibiting cell cycle proteins, Chk1 and Chk2. Treatment with alkylating agents also increased GCSC populations, as determined by stem cell markers (Kang and Kang, 2007).

Due to the ability of gliomas to either induce stem cell dedifferentiation or to select for already present GCSC populations during treatment and stress, glioma cancer stem cells present a considerable problem for future therapeutic regimens. While common therapies can reduce the size of gliomas to microscopic levels, these small populations of stem cells remain within the tissues, resistant to therapies and selected due to their ability to survive. Recurring tumors will therefore be more malignant and progress more quickly than the original glioma. Therefore, focus on eliminating GCSCs should be pursued during brain cancer research treatment.

2.5 Targeting stress response as glioma therapy

The preceding sections have focused on how glioma cells manage to evade the deleterious effects of both intrinsic and extrinsic stressors. Future developments in glioma therapy should take into account these survival pathways. New treatment options should take advantage of the stress response and new survival mechanisms such as autophagy, while others could target GCSCs in order to completely, and hopefully, permanently eliminate glioma tumors. Novel treatments can be used to sensitize glioma cells to traditional therapies by exacerbating the stresses the cells are under (Table 3).

Most importantly, gliomas need to be characterized for the proteins that they express. This can then inform clinicians what therapies with which that particular tumor may be treated. For example, glioma cells or tumors that are shown to be deficient in autophagic proteins might be more susceptible to traditional apoptotic therapies or radiation. Tumors void of any stem cell markers might be less likely to recur, and those patients can be offered more simple treatment plans. The key is to make the most of the information available to personalize the therapies given to each patient. Therefore, a compilation of an assortment of markers and screening panels needs to be created to fit into the era of personalized medicine.

Category	Compound	Target
Autophagic Inhibitors	3-MA	Pre-autophagosomal structure inhibition
	Bafilomycin A1	Block autophagosome and lysosome fusion
	HCQ	Block autophagosome and lysosome fusion
	Monensin	Block autophagosome and lysosome fusion
	siRNA against BECN1,ATG5, ATG7, ATG10, etc.	Blocks translation of autophagic response
	NH125	Inhibits EF-2K
Autophagic Enhancers	Rapamycin	Inhibit mTOR pathway to increase stress
	Arsenic trioxide	Targets mitochondria for destruction to sensitize to autophagy inhibition
Agents Affecting Tumor Stem Cells	Bevacizumab	Anti-angiogenic to sensitize stem cell population to therapy
	Sodium Bicarbonate	Increase cellular pH to sensitize stem cell population to therapy
	siRNA against β-catenin/wnt, SSH, and Notch-1 pathways	Reduce stem cell signaling

Table 3. Proposed therapies for sensitization of gliomas to current treatments.

Since the majority of current glioma therapies induce autophagy in glioma cells, including radiation and chemotherapy, inhibition of autophagy would decrease the survival of these cells. Tumor cells may undergo apoptosis when autophagy is started and then disrupted. Adding the autophagy inhibitor bafilomycin A1 (H^+-APTase inhibitor) to TMZ lead to cell death via apoptosis through caspase-3 and mitochondrial permeabilization. Autophagy can be blocked at multiple levels, allowing for adjustment according to whether cells are using it as a protective or cell death mechanism. The P13K inhibitor, 3-methyladenine (3-MA), can be used to inhibit autophagy before formation of the autophagosome (Kanzawa et al., 2004). Other agents like bafilomycin A1 blocks the fusion of the autophagosome with the lysosome, as do several other drugs like hydroxychloroquine (HCQ) and the proton exchanger, monensin. The natural product arsenic trioxide targets mitochondria and induces autophagy in glioma cells, and when combined with bafilomycin A1, is able to eliminate all remaining tumor cells (Kanzawa et al., 2005). Drugs like rapamycin could be used to further the stress caused by nutrient starvation, activating autophagy, thereby leading to cell self-digestion. Synergistic killing of glioma cells has been shown with treatment of rapamycin and either Akt or PI3K inhibitors (Takeuchi et al., 2005). These are just a few examples of how therapies can be combined to sensitize and eliminate glioma cells through autophagic inhibition or enhancement.

In the future, genetic modification of cells will be more feasible, so eventually the autophagic response could also be targeted with small interfering RNA (siRNA) against autophagy proteins such as BECN1, ATG5, and ATG10 along with many others. EF-2K presents a novel target for inhibiting autophagy and sensitizing cells to other therapies. NH125 is the preclinical inhibitor of EF-2K and could be developed into a bioavailable agent for humans or an siRNA could be used against the kinase as well.

Glioma cancer stem cells are another cell type that could be targeted as glioma therapy for complete abolishment of the malignancy. Bmi-1 is an E3-ubiquitin ligase that is up-regulated in GCSCs and other cancer stem cells. GSCSs have low proteosome activity, which can be used to track stem cells through Bmi-1 degradation (Vlashi et al., 2009). Eliminating GCSCs by targeting Bmi-1 expressing cells was sufficient for causing regression of the solid glioma indicating that ridding the tumor of cancer stem cells may actually be curative.

Several possibilities exist for targeting stem cells. As mentioned previously, anti-VEGF treatments like bevacizumab might help to normalize the vasculature and allow for efficient delivery of chemotherapies (von Baumgarten et al., 2011). In xenotranpslants, bevacizumab synergizes with radio- and chemo-therapy to effectively kill glioma cells (Vredenburgh et al., 2007). Anti-angiogenic therapy could help reduce the stem cell niches. Bevacizumab blocked the GSCSs ability to induce the migration of endothelial cells necessary for neoangiogenesis and cell migration (Ailles & Weissman, 2007). Thus, anti-VEGF treatment might work in multiple ways.

GSCSs could be targeted by additional approaches. Treatment of tumors with sodium biocarbonate increased tumor pH and reduced invasion, while reducing stem cell markers in breast cancer (Robey et al., 2009). While not yet used in glioma, this could restore the non-acidic pH environment, targeting the tumor microenvironment. Also, developing agents against the stem cell signaling pathways will be important in eliminating tumors. The β-catenin/wnt and SHH pathways along with Notch-1 signaling are all good candidates for targeting. Markers, CD133 and nestin, could be used to identify potential responders.

Overall, new therapies should be used to take advantage of the stress that glioma cells already encounter, in addition to targeting their means of survival. Those gliomas that use autophagy as a protective mechanism could be treated with autophagic inhibitors to enhance efficacy of therapy. These therapies could be used to sensitize tumors to treatment with standard radiation and chemotherapies. Also, any gliomas that have markers indicative of cancer stem cells might be considered to be treated with agents that target stem cells to circumvent that avenue of cancer cell survival. Autophagy and GCSCs represent attractive, novel targets for future glioma therapy that can be combined with conventional therapy to fully eradicate glioma cells.

3. Conclusions/perspectives

The preceding chapter sought to introduce the concept that glioma cells are constantly under stress, a factor which needs to be taken into consideration during the treatment of brain cancers. Both intrinsic and extrinsic stresses impact the development and progression of glioma. Stresses like nutrient deficiency, hypoxia, acidity, and the immune response are present during normal tumor growth and throughout treatment. Tumor cells that survive these stresses are more adept at surviving hostile conditions and are more resistant to current therapies. Stress, therefore, shapes the tumor cell population. The autophagic response and glioma cancer stem cells are two of the prevalent survival and resistance mechanisms in glioma, and both can be induced by cellular stresses.

New treatment regimens should take advantage of various stresses and stress responses present in glioma. Stresses like hypoxia or acidity could be exacerbated and sustained with new agents, allowing traditional therapies, such as TMZ or radiation, to permanently eliminate the sensitized cells. Autophagy is a fragile state for cancer cells, and inhibition of the autophagic process at the level of EF2K, beclin-1, and other proteins may combat this glioma cell survival mechanism. Targeting the autophagy pathway has already been shown to render glioma cells and other types of cancers more susceptible to currently available treatments. Recognition of GCSC markers could lead to better diagnostic and prognostic tools in addition to targeted cancer stem cell therapy. Combining current therapy with inhibitors that interrupt the stress response of glioma cells is an attractive approach for future glioma treatment.

4. Acknowledgment

Research was supported by grants from the US Public Health Service and NCI with RO1CA135038.

5. References

Abeliovich H. (2003). Regulation of Autophagy by the Target of Rapamycin (Tor) Proteins, In: *Autophagy*. Daniel Klionsky, Landes Bioscience, ISBN: 1-58706-203-8, University of Michigan

Ailles LE, & Weissman IL. (2007). Cancer stem cells in solid tumors. *Curr Opin Biotechnol*, Vol. 18, No. 5, pp. 460-6.

Azad MB, Chen Y, Henson ES, Cizeau J, McMillan-Ward E, Israels SJ, & Gibson SB. (2008). Hypoxia induces autophagic cell death in apoptosis-competent cells through a mechanism involving BNIP3. *Autophagy*, Vol. 4, pp. 195–204.

Bao S, Wu Q, McLendon RE, Hao Y, Shi Q, Hjelmeland AB, Dewhirst MW, Bigner DD, & Rich JN. (2006). Glioma stem cells promote radioresistance by preferential activation of the DNA damage response. *Nature*, Vol. 444, pp. 756-60.

Bell D, & Miele L. (2011). A magnifying glass on glioblastoma stem cell signaling pathways. *Cancer Biology & Therapy*, Vol. 11, No. 8, (April 15, 2011), pp. 765-8.

Benhar M, Dalyot I, Engelberg D, & Levitzki A. (2001). Enhanced ROS production in oncogenically transformed cells potentiates c-Jun N-terminal kinase and p38 mitogen-activated protein kinase activation and sensitization to genotoxic stress. *Mol and Cell Bio*, Vol. 21, pp. 6913-26.

Brat DJ, & Van Meir EG. (2004). Vaso-occlusive and prothrombotic mechanisms associated with tumor hypoxia, necrosis, and accelerated growth in glioblastoma. *Lab Invest*, Vol. 84, pp. 397-405.

Browne GJ, Finn SG, & Proud CG. (2004). Stimulation of the AMP-activated protein kinase leads to activation of eukaryotic elongation factor 2 kinase and to its phosphorylation at a novel site, serine 398. *J Biol Chem,*Vol. 279., No. 13, (Mar 26, 2004), pp. 12220-31.

Browne GJ, & Proud CG. (2004). A novel mTOR-regulated phosphorylation site in elongation factor 2 kinase modulates the activity of the kinase and its binding to calmodulin. *Mol Cell Biol.* Vol. 24, No. 7. (Apr 24, 2004), pp. 2986-97.

Calabrese C, Poppleton H, Kocak M, Hogg TL, Fuller C, Hamner B, Oh EY, Gaber MW, Finkestein D, Allen M, Frank A, Kayazitov IT, Zakherenko SS, Gajjar A, Davidoff A, & Gilbertson RJ. (2007). A perivascular niche for brain tumor stem cells. *Cancer Cell,* Vol. 11, pp. 69-82.

Calderwood SK, Khaleque MA, Sawyer DB, & Ciocca DR. (2006). Heat shock proteins in cancer: chaperones of tumorigenesis. *Trends in Biochemical Sciences,* Vol. 31, pp. 164-72.

Chen Y, Matsushita M, Naim AC, Damuni Z, Cai D, Frerichs KU, & Hallenbeck JM. (2001). Mechanisms for increased levels of phosphorylation of elongation factor-2 during the hibernation in ground squirrels. *Biochemistry,* Vol. 140, pp. 11565-70.

Chiche J, Brahimi-Horn MC, & Pouyssegur J. (2010). Tumour hypoxia induces a metabolic shift causing acidosis: a common feature in cancer. *J Cell Mol Med.* Vol. 14, pp. 771-94.

Ciocca DR, & Calderwood SK. (2005). Heat shock proteins in cancer: diagnostic, prognostic, predictive, and treatment implications. *Cell Stress Chaperones,* Vol. 10, pp. 86-103.

Colotta F, Allavena P, Sica A, Garlanda C, & Mantovani A. (2009). Cancer-related inflammation, the seventh hallmark of cancer: links to genetic instability. *Carcinogenesis* Vol. 30, pp. 1073–81.

Dai C, Celestino JC, Okada Y, Louis DN, Fuller GN, & Holland EC. (2001) PDGF autocrine stimulation dedifferentiates cultured astrocytes and induces oligodendrogliomas and oligoastrocytomas from neural progenitors and astrocytes in vivo. *Genes Dev* Vol. 15, pp. 1913-25.

Dal-Pizzol F, Ritter C, Klamt F, Andrades M, da Frota Jr. MLC, Diel C, da Rocha A, de Lima C, Filho AB, Schwartsmann G, & Fonseca Moreira JC. (2003). Modulation of oxidative stress in response to gamma-radiation in human glioma cell lines. *Journal of Neuro-Oncology,* Vol. 61, pp. 89–94.

Egeblad M, Nakasone ES, Werb Z. (2010). Tumors as organs: complex tissues that interface with the entire organism. *Dev. Cell,* Vol. 18, pp. 884–901.

Eramo A, Ricci-Vitiani L, Zeuner A, Pallini R, Lotti F, Sette G, Pilozzi E, Larocca LM, Peschle C, & De Maria R. (2006). Chemotherapy resistance of glioblastoma stem cells. *Cell Death Differ,* Vol. 13, pp. 1238-41.

Erhrlich S Mizrachy L, Segev O, Lindenboim L, Zmira O, Adi-Harel S, Hirsch JA, Stein R, Pinkas-Kramarski R. (2007). Differential interactions between Beclin 1 and Bcl-2 family members. *Autophagy,* Vol. 3, pp. 561-8.

Feder M, & Hofmann GE. (1999) Heat shock proteins, molecular chaperones, and the stress response: evolutionary and ecological physiology. *Ann Rev of Phys,* Vol. 61, pp. 243-82.

Ferrara N. (2004). Vascular endothelial growth factor: basic science and clinical progress. *Endocr Rev.* Vol. 25, pp. 581-611.

Folkman J & Hochberg M. (1973) . Self-regulation of growth in three dimensions . *J. Exp . Med.* Vol. 138, pp. 745.

Garg A, & Aggarwal BB (2002). "Nuclear transcription factor-kappaB as a target for cancer drug development". *Leukemia,*Vol. 16, No. 6, (June 2002), pp. 1053–68.

Gilbertson RJ, & Rich JN. (2007). Making a tumour's bed: glioblastoma stem cells and the vascular niche. *Nat Rev Cancer* Vol. 7, No. 10, pp. 733-6.

Gimbrone, MA Jr ., Leapman S, Cotran RS , & Folkman J. (1973) . Tumor angiogenesis : iris neovascularization at a distance from experimental intraoculartumors . *J. Natl . Cancer Inst* . Vol. 50, pp. 219

Goetz MP, Toft DO, Ames MM, & Erlichmann C. (2003). The Hsp90 chaperone complex as a novel target for cancer therapy. *Annals of Oncology,* Vol. 14, pp. 1169-76.

Grivennikov SI, Greten FR, & Karin M. (2010). Immunity, inflammation, and cancer. *Cell,* Vol. 140, pp. 883–99.

Hadnagy A, Gaboury L, Beaulieu R, & Balicki D. (2006). SP analysis may be used to identify cancer stem cell populations. *Exp Cell Res,* Vol. 312, pp. 3701–10.

Hait WN, Wu H, Jin S, & Yang JM. (2006). Elongation factor-2 kinase: its role in protein synthesis and autophagy. *Autophagy,* Vol. 2, No.4 (Oct-Dec, 20060, pp. 294-6.

Hambardzumyan, D.; Becher, O.J.; & Holland, E.C. (2008). Cancer stem cells and survival pathways. *Cell Cycle,* Vol.7, No.10, (May 2008), pp. 1371-8.

Hanahan D, &Weinberg RA. (2011) Hallmarks of Cancer: The Next Generation. *Cell,* Vol. 144, (March 4, 2011), pp. 646-674.

Harhaji-Trajkovic L, Vilimanovich U, Kravic-Stevovic T, Bumbasirevic V, & Trajkovic V. (2009). AMPK-mediated autophagy inhibits apoptosis in cisplatin-treated tumor cells. *J Cell Mol Med,* Vol. Epub (Jan 16, 2009).

Harrison LB, Chadha M, Hill RJ, Hu K, & Shasha D. (2002). Impact of tumor hypoxia and anemia on radiation therapy outcomes. *Oncologist* Vol. 7, No. 6, pp. 492–508.

Hemmati HD, Nakano I, Lazareff JA, Masterman-Smith M, Geschwind DH, Bronner-Fraser M, & Kornblum HI. (2003). Cancerous stem cells can arise from pediatric brain tumors. *Proc Natl Acad Sci USA,* Vol. 100, pp. 15178–83.

Herr I, & Debatin KM. (2001). Cellular stress response and apoptosis in cancer therapy. *Blood* Vol. 98, pp. 2603-14.

Hirschmann-Jax C, Foster AE, Wulf GG, J. G. Nuchtern JG, Jax TW, Gobel U, Goodell MA, & Brenner MK, (2004). A distinct "side population" of cells with high drug efflux capacity in human tumor cells. *Proc Natl Acad Sci USA,* Vol. 101, pp. 14228–14233.

Hitoshi S, Alexson T, Tropepe V, Donoviel D, Elia AJ, Nye JS, Conlon RA, Mak TW, Bernstein A, and van der Kooy D. (2002). Notch pathway molecules are essential for the maintenance, but not the generation, of mammalian neural stem cells. *Genes Dev,* Vol. 16, pp. 846-58.

Hjelmeland AB, Wu Q, Heddleston JM, Choudhary GS, MacSwards J, Lathia JD, McLendon R, Lindner D, Sloan A, & Rich JN. (2010) Acidic stress promotes a glioma stem cell phenotype. *Cell Death and Differentiation,* Vol. 18. No. 5, pp. 1-12.

Holmin S, Almquist P, Lendahl U, & Mathiesen T. (1997). Adult nestin expressing subependymal cells differentiate to astrocytes in response to brain injury. *Eur J NeuroSci,* Vol. 9, pp. 65–75.

Ito H, Daido S, Kanzawa T, Kondo S, & Kondo Y. (2005). Radiation-induced autophagy is associated with LC3 and its inhibition sensitizes malignant glioma cells. *Int J Oncol,* Vol. 26, pp. 1401–10.

Jiang BH, Rue E, Wang GL, Roe R, & Semenza GL. (1996). Dimerization, DNA binding, and transactivation properties of hypoxia-inducible factor 1. *J Boil Chem,* Vol. 271, pp. 17771-8.

Juillerat-Jeanneret L, Bernasconi CC, Bricod C, Gros S, Trepey S, Benhattar J, & Janzer RC. (2008). Heterogeneity of human glioblastoma: glutathione-S-transferase and methylguanine-methyltransferase. *Cancer Invest,*Vol. 26, No. 6, pp. 597- 609.

Kang MK, & Kang SK. (2007). Tumorigenesis of chemotherapeutic drug-resistant cancer stem-like cells in brain glioma. *Stem Cells Dev,* Vol. 16, pp. 837–47.

Kanzawa T, Germano IM, Komata T, Ito H, Kondo Y & Kondo S. (2004) Role of autophagy in temozolomide-induced cytotoxicity for malignant glioma cells. *Cell Death Differ,* 11: 448–457.

Kanzawa T, Zhang L, Xiao L, Germano IM, Kondo Y, & Kondo S. (2005). Arsenic trioxide induces autophagic cell death in malignant glioma cells by upregulation of mitochondrial cell death protein BNIP3. *Oncogene,* Vol. 24, pp. 980–91.

Katayama M, Kawaguchi T, Berger MS, & Pieper RO. (2007). DNA damaging agent-induced autophagy produces a cytoprotective adenosine triphosphate surge in malignant glioma cells. *Cell Death and Differentiation,* Vol. 14, pp. 548–58.

Koch U, & Radtke F. (2007). Notch and cancer: A double-edged sword. *Cell Mol Life Sci,* Vol. 64, pp. 2746–62.

Kuhn, HG, Dickinson Anson H, Gage FH. (1996). Neurogenesis in the dentate gyrus of the adult rat: age-related decrease of neuronal progenitor proliferation. *J Neurosci,* Vol.16,pp. 2027-33.

Kültz D. (2005). Molecular and evolutionary basis of the cellular stress response. *Annu Rev Physiol,* Vol. 67, pp. 225-57.

Kuma A, Hatono M, Matsui M, Yamamoto A, Nakaya H, Yoshimori T, Ohsumi Y, Tokuhisa T, & Mizushima N. (2004). The role of autophagy during the early neonatal starvation period. *Nature,* Vol. 432, pp. 1032-6.

Levine B., & Yuan J. (2005).Autophagy in cell death: an innocent convict? *J Clin Invest,*Vol. 115, pp. 2679-88.

Liang C, Feng P, Ku B, Dotan I, Canaani D, Oh BH, & Jun JU. (2006). Autophagic and tumour suppressor activity of a novel Beclin-1 binding protein UVRAG. *Nat Cell,* Vol. 8, pp. 688-99.

Liang XH, Jacdson S, Seaman M, Brown K, Kempkes B, Hibshoosh H, & Levine B. (1999). Induction of autophagy and inhibition of tumorigenesis by beclin 1. *Nature,* Vol. 402, pp. 672-6.

Li JL, Sainson RC, Shi W, Leek R, Harrington LS, Preusser M, Biswas S, Turley H, Heikamp E, Hainfellner JA, Harris AL. (2007). Delta-like 4 Notch ligand regulates tumor angiogenesis, improves tumor vascular function, and promotes tumor growth in vivo. *Cancer Res,* Vol. 67, pp. 11244-53.

Liu G, Yuan X, Zeng Z, Tunici P, Ng H, Abdulkadir IR, Lu L, Irvin D, Black KL, & Yu JS. (2006). Analysis of gene expression and chemoresistance of CD133+ cancer stem cells in glioblastoma. *Mol Cancer,* Vol. 5, pp. 67–78.

Liu L, Wise DR, Diehl A, & Celeste Simon M. (2008). Hypoxc reactive oxygen species regulate the integrated stress response and cell survival. *J of Bio Chem* Vol. 283, No. 45, (Nov 7, 2008), pp. 31153-62.

Lois C, & Alvarez BA. (1993). Prolierating subventricular zone cells in the adult mammalian forebrain can differentiate into neurons and glia. *Proc Natl Acad Sci USA,* Vol. 90, pp. 2074-7.

Lum JJ, DeBerardinis RJ, & Thompson CB. (2005). Autophagy in metazoans: cell survival in the land of plenty. *Nat Rev Mol Cell Biol,* Vol. 6, pp. 439–48.

Maki RG, Old LJ, & Srivastava PK. (1990). Human homologue of murine tumor rejection antigen gp96: 5'-regulatory and coding regions and relationship to stress-induced proteins. *Proc. Natl. Acad. Sci. U.S.A.* Vol. 87, No. 15, (Aug 1990), pp. 5658–62.

Miligkos V, Tiligada E, Papmichael K, Ypsilantis E, & Delitheos A. (2000). Anticancer drugs as inducers of thermotolerance in yeast. *Folia Microbiologica,* Vol. 45, pp. 339-42.

Mizushima N. (2004). Methods for monitoring autophagy. *Int J Biochem Cell Biol,* Vol. 36,pp. 2491-502.

Nadin SB, Vargas-Roig LM, Cuello-Carrion FD, & Ciocca DR. (2003). Deoxyribonucleic acid damage induced by doxorubicin in peripheral blood mononuclear cells: possible roles for stress response and the deoxyribonucleic acid repair process. *Cell Stress Chaperones,* Vol. 8, pp. 361-72.

Nagy JA, Chang SH, Shih SC, Dvorak AM, & Dvorak HF. (2010). Heterogeneity of the tumorVasculature. *Semin Thromb Hemost,* Vol. 36, pp. 321–31.

Nait-Oumesmar B, Vignais L, & Baron-Van Evercooren A. (1997). Developmental expression of platelet-derived growth factor receptor in neurons and in glial cells of the mouse CNS. *J Neurosci* Vol. 17, pp. 125–39.

Nixon R. (2006). Autophagy in neurodegenerative disease: friend, foe or turncoat? *Trends in Neurosciences,* Vol. 29, No. 9, (Sept 2006), pp. 528-35.

Nunes MC, Roy NS, Keyoung HM, Goodman RR, McKhann G II, Jiang L, Kang J, Nedergaard M, & Goldman SA. (2003). Identification and isolation of multipotential neural progenitor cells from the subcortical white matter of the adult human brain. *Nat Med,* Vol. 9, pp. 439–47.

Paglin S, Hollister T, Delohery T, Hackett N, McMahill M, Sphicas E, Domingo D, & Yahalom J.(2001). A novel response of cancer cells to radiation involves autophagy and formation of acidic vesicles. *Cancer Res,* Vol. 61, pp. 439–44.

Pallini R, Ricci-Vitiani L, Banna GL, Signore M, Lombardi D, Todaro M, Stassi G, Martini M, Maira G, Larocca LM, & De Maria R. (2008). Cancer stem cell analysis and clinical outcome in patients with glioblastoma multiforme. *Clin Cancer Res,* Vol. 14, pp. 8205-12.

Pasquier B, Pasquier D, N'Golet A, Panh MH, & Couderc P. (1980) Extraneural metastases of astrocytomas and glioblastomas. Clinicopathological study of two cases and review of literature. *Cancer,* Vol. 45, pp. 112-25.

Pattrawala L, Calhoun T, Schneider-Broussard R, Zhou J, Claypool K, & Tang DG. (2005). Side population is enriched in tumorigenic, stem-like cancer cells, whereas ABCG2+ and ABCG2- cancer cells are similarly tumorigenic. *Cancer Res,* Vol. 65, (2005), pp. 6207-19.

Pu P, Zhang Z, Kang C, Jiang R, Jia Z, Wang G, & Jiang H. (2009).Downregulation of Wnt2 and β-catenin by siRNA suppresses malignant glioma cell growth. *Cancer Gene Ther,*Vol. 16, pp. 351-61.

Py BF, Boyce M, & Yuan J. (2009). A critical role of eEF-2K in mediating autophagy in response to multiple cellular stresses. *Autophagy,* Vol. 5, No. 3, (Apr 5, 2009), pp. 393-6.

Qian BZ, & Pollard JW. (2010). Macrophage diversity enhances tumor progression and metastasis. *Cell,* Vol. 141, pp. 39-51.

Rich JN. (2007). Cancer stem cells in radiation resistance. *Cancer Res,* Vol. 67, No. 19, pp. 8980–84.

Robey IF, Baggett BK, Kirkpatrick ND, Roe DJ, Dosescu J, Sloane BF, Hashim AI, Morse DL, Raghunand N, Gatenby RA, Gillies RJ. (2009). Bicarbonate increases tumor pH and inhibits spontaneous metastases. *Cancer Res.* Vol. 69, pp. 2260-8.

Rossi M, Magnoni L, Miracco C, Mori E, Tosi P, Pirtoli L, Tini P, Oliveri G, Cosci E, & Bakker A. (2011). Beta-catenin and Gli1 are prognostic markers in glioblastoma. *Cancer Biol Ther,* Vol. 11, pp. 742–50.

Ryazanov AG, Rudkin BB, & Spirin AS. (1991). Regulation of protein synthesis at the elongation stage. New insights into the control of gene expression in eukaryotes. *FEBS Lett,* Vol. 285, pp. 170-5.

Sanchez-Prieto R, Rojas JM, Taya Y, & Gutkind JS. (2000). A role for the p38 mitogen-activated protein kinase pathways in the transcriptional activation of p53 genotoxic stress by chemotherapeutic agents. *Cancer Res* Vol. 60, pp. 2264-72.

Scharpfenecker M, Kruse JJ, Sprong D, Russell NS, Ten Dijke P, & Stewart FA. (2009). Ionzing radiation shifts the PAI-1/ID-1 balance and activates notch signaling in endothelial cells. *Int J Radiat Oncol Biol Phys,* Vol. 73, pp. 506-13.

Singh SK, Hawkins C, Clarke ID, Squire JA, Bayani J, Hide T, Henkelman RM, Cusimano MD, & Dirks PB. (2004). Identification of human brain tumour initiating cells. *Nature,* Vol. 432, pp. 396-401.

Singh S, & Settleman J. (2010). EMT, cancer stem cells and drug resistance: an emerging axis of evil in the war on cancer. *Oncogene,* Vol. 29, pp. 4741-51.

Son MJ, Woolard K, Nam DH, Lee J, & Fine HA. (2009). SSEA-1 is an enrichment marker for tumor-initiating cells in human glioblastoma. *Cell Stem Cell,* Vol. 4, pp. 440–52.

Stronjnik T, Rosland GV, Sakariassen PO, Kavalar R, & Lah T. (2007) Neural stem cell markers, nestin and musashi proteins, in the progression of human glioma: correlation of nestin with prognosis of patient survival. *Surg Neurol,* Vol. 68, pp. 133-43.

Szabo D, Keyzer H, Kaiser HE, & Molnar J. (2000). Reversal of multi-drug resistance of tumor cells. *Anticancer Research,* Vol. 20, pp. 4261-74.

Takeuchi H, Kanzawa T, Kondo Y, & Kondo S. (2004). Inhibition of platelet-derived growth factor signalling induces autophagy in malignant glioma cells. *British Journal of Cancer,* Vol. 90, pp. 1069-75.

Takeuchi H, Kondo K, Fujiwara K, Kanzawa T, Aoki H, Mills GB, & Kondo S. (2005). Synergistic augmentation of rapamycin- induced autophagy in malignant glioma cells by phosphatidylinositol 3-kinase/protein kinase B inhibitors. *Cancer Res,* April 15, Vol. 65, (Apr 15, 2005), pp. 3336-46

Tan TT, Degenhardt K, Nelson DA, Beaudoin B, Nieves-Neira W, Bouillet P, Villunger A, Adams JM, & White E. (2005). Key roles of BIM-driven apoptosis in epithelial tumors and rational chemotherapy. *Cancer Cell,* Vol. 7, pp. 227–38.

Tchoghandjian A, Baeza N, Colin C, Cayre M, Metellus P, Beclin C, Ouafik L, & Figarella, Branger D. (2010). A2B5 cells from human glioblastoma have cancer stem cell properties. *Brain Pathol,* Vol. 20, No. 1, pp. 211-21.

Tetyana D, Gennero L, Roos MA, Melcarne A, Juenemann C, Faccani G, Morra I, Cavallo G, Reguzzi S, Pescarmona G, & Ponzetto A. (2010) Glioblastoma cancer stem cells: heterogeneity, microenvironment and related therapeutic strategies. *Cell Biochemistry and Function,* Vol. 28, (June 2010), pp. 343-351.

Uchida N, Buck DW, He D, Reitsma MJ, Masek M, Phan TV, Tsukamoto AS, Gage FH, & Weissman IL. (2000). Direct isolation of human central nervous system stem cells. *Proc Natl Acad Sci USA* Vol. 97, pp. 14720-25.

Vajkoczy P, & Menger MD. (2004). Vascular microenvironment in gliomas. *Cancer Treat Res,* Vol. 117, pp. 249-62.

Vaupel P, Kallinowski F, & Okunieff P. (1989). Blood flow, oxygen and nutrient supply, and metabolic microenvironment of human tumors: a review. *Cancer Res,* Vol. 49,pp. 6449-65.

Vlashi E, Kim K, Dealla Donna L, Lagadec C, McDonald T, Eghbali M, Sayre J, Stefani E, McBride W, & Pajonk F. (2009). In- vivo imaging, tracking, and targeting of cancer stem cells. *J Natl Cancer Inst,* Vol. 101, pp. 350-9.

Vousden KH, & Lane DP. (2007). p53 in health and disease. *Nat Rev Mol Cell Biol.* Vol. 8, pp. 275–83.

Von Baumgarten LD, von Baumgarten LD, Brucker D, Tirniceru AL, Kienast Y, Grau S, Burgold S, Herms J & Winkler F. (2011). "Bevacizumab has differential and dose-dependent effects on glioma blood vessels and tumor cells." *Clin Cancer Res,* (July 25, 2011) [epub ahead of print].

Vredenburgh JJ, Desjardins A, Herndon JE 2nd, Marcello J, Reardon DA, Quinn JA, Rich JN, Sathornsumetee S, Gururangan S, Sampson J, Wagner M, Bailey L, Bigner DD, Friedman AH, Friedman HS. (2007). Bevacizumab plus irinotecan in recurrent glioblastoma multiforme. *J Clin Oncol* Vol. 25, No. 30, pp. 4722-9.

Wang J, Sakariassen PO, Tsinkalovsky O, Immervoll H, Boe SO, Svendson A, Prestegarden L, Rosland G, Thorsen F, Stuhr L,

Molven A, Bjerkvig R, & Enger PO. (2008). CD133 negative glioma cells form tumors in nude rats and give rise to CD133 positive cells. *Int J Cancer,* Vol. 122, pp. 761-8.

Warburg, O. (1956). On Respiratory impairtment in cancer cells. *Science*, Vol. 124, pp. 269-70.

White E. (2007). Role of Metabolic Stress Responses of Apoptosis and Autophagy in Tumor Suppression. *Ernst Schering Found Symp Proc*, Vol. 4, pp. 23–34.

Wu H, Yang JM, Jin S, Zhang H, & Hait WN. (2006). Elongation factor-2 kinase regulates autophagy in human glioblastoma cells. *Cancer Res*. Vol. 66, No. 6, (Mar 15, 2006), pp. 3015-23.

Wu H, Zhu H, Liu DX, Niu T, Ren X, Patel R, Hait WN, &Yang JM. (2009) Silencing of elongation factor-2 kinase potentiates the effect of 2-deoxy-D-glucose against human glioma cells through blunting of autophagy. *Cancer Res*, Vol. 69, No. 6, pp. 2453-60.

Zimmerman L, Parr B, Lendahl U, Cunningham M, McKay R, Gavin B, Mann J, Vassileva G, & McMahon A. (1994). Independent regulatory elements in the nestin gene direct transgene expression to neural stem cells or muscle precursors. *Neuron*,Vol. 12, pp. 11–24.

Zhu H, Wu H, Liu X, Li B, Chen Y, Ren X, Liu CG, & Yang JM. (2009). Regulation of autophagy by a Beclin 1-targeted microRNA, miR-30a, in cancer cells. *Autophagy*, Vol. 5, No. 6, (Aug 16, 2009), pp. 816-23.

3

Key Principles in Glioblastoma Therapy

Bartek Jiri Jr.[1], Kimberly Ng[2], Bartek Jiri Sr.[3], Santosh Kesari[4], Bob Carter[5] and Clark C. Chen[1,6]
[1]*Department of Neurosurgery, Karolinska University Hospital, Stockholm*
[2]*Department of Radiation Oncology, Dana-Farber Cancer Institute, Boston, MA*
[3]*Institute of Cancer Biology and Centre for Genotoxic Stress Research*
Danish Cancer Society, Copenhagen
[4]*Department of Neurology, Moores Cancer Center, UCSD, San Diego, CA*
[5]*Center for Theoretical and Applied Neurosurgery, UCSD, San Diego, CA*
[6]*Division of Neurosurgery, Beth Israel Deaconess Medical Center, Boston, MA*
[1]*Sweden*
[2,4,5,6]*USA*
[3]*Denmark*

1. Introduction

Glioblastoma is the most common form of primary brain tumor. The incidence of this tumor is fairly low, with 2-3 cases per 100,000 people in Europe and North America [1]. It is one of the most aggressive forms of cancer [2]. Without treatment, the median survival is approximately 3 months [3]. The current standard of treatment involves maximal surgical resection followed by concurrent radiation therapy and chemotherapy with the DNA alkylating agent, temozolomide [4]. With this regimen, the median survival is approximately 14 months. For nearly all affected, the treatments available remain palliative.

The best available evidence suggests that glioblastomas originate from cells that give rise to glial cells[5, 6]. These glial derived tumors are graded by the World Health Organization (WHO) into 4 categories, termed WHO grade 1 to grade 4. The higher grade denotes histologic features of increased malignancy. WHO 4 glioma is essentially synonymous with glioblastoma[7].

Studies carried out over the past three decades suggest that glioblastomas, like other cancers, arise secondary to the accumulation of genetic alterations. These alterations can take the form of epigenetic modifications, point mutations, translocations, amplifications or deletions and modify gene function in ways that deregulate cellular signaling pathways leading to the cancer phenotype [8]. The exact number and nature of genetic alterations and deregulated signaling pathways required for tumorigenesis remains an issue of debate[9], although it is now clear that CNS carcinogenesis requires multiple disruptions to the normal cellular circuitry. The genetic alteration results in either activation or inactivation of specific gene functions that contribute to the process of carcinogenesis [9]. Genes, that when activated, contribute to the carcinogenesis are generally termed proto-oncogenes. The mutated forms of these genes are referred to as oncogenes. Genes, that when inactivated, contribute to the carcinogenesis are generally termed tumor suppressor genes.

Despite some progress in the clinical management of glioblastoma, prognosis of patients suffering from this deadly tumor remains dismal, and design of new and more effective therapies for glioblastoma is highly desirable. Arguably the most promising route to discoveries of innovative treatment strategies is to obtain better mechanistic insights into glioblastoma pathogenesis and biology. Indeed, recent research in this area of experimental and clinical oncology has identified the key signaling pathways, critical regulatory nodes, genes and their protein products, as well as their mutual cross-talks, thereby providing a solid molecular basis for selection of candidate therapeutic targets and drug discovery programs. These lines of investigation complement the recent efforts to sequence entire genomes of a growing number of human tumors including glioblastoma, formulation of new concepts and principles in tumor cell biology, and potential exploitation of these major advances for personalized disease management in oncology. Collectively, such efforts have begun to provide exciting leads to conceptual framework that afford innovative therapeutic strategies. This review will aim to review these critical concepts and their relevance for glioblastoma therapeutic development.

2. Concept 1: Glioblastoma subtypes

There is an old adage that cancer is a hundred diseases masquerading in one. While this adage is based on clinical and pathologic observations, systemic genomic characterization of a large number of glioblastoma specimens (TCGA) confirms the notion that subtypes with distinct pathologic molecular events and therapeutic response.

The Cancer Genome Atlas (TCGA) is a major NIH initiative involving institutions spanning the continental U.S. with the goal of tumor specimen collection and molecular characterization [10]. Glioblastoma was one of the first tumor types characterized in this effort. This vast wealth of data is unprecedented, and despite the enormous challenge to process and analyze this incoming information, correlations of such emerging 'genetic and expression profiles' or 'tumor landscapes' with tumor biology and clinico-pathological features of the patients including therapeutic responses are beginning to impact oncology.

This profiling approach [11] has led to the understanding that glioblastoma is but an umbrella term that encapsulates subtypes characterized by distinct molecular properties. Based on global transcript profiling, glioblastoma can be divided into three to four distinct subtypes [11, 12]. Interestingly, each subtype harbor distinct genetic aberrations [12] and proteomic profiles [13]. The recognition that glioblastoma consists of subtypes varying in molecular circuitry and biologic behavior suggests that no therapy can be universally efficacious. The major importance of this concept of heterogeneity is that meaningful therapeutic gain can only be attained by customizing the therapy to the underlying molecular circuit.

One subtype (termed classical by the TCGA and proliferative by Philips et al) is characterized by frequent amplification or mutations in the Epidermal Growth Factor Receptor (EGFR) gene [10, 11]. In contrast, in another subtype, termed proneural by both groups, harbored frequent mutations in p53, Platelet Derived Growth Factor Receptor A (PDGFRA), and Isocitrate Dehydrogenase 1 (IDH1) [12]. A third type, termed mesenchymal by both groups, is characterized by frequent mutations in the Neurofibromatosis type 1 gene (NF-1). Of note, these subtypes differ in their clinical responses to therapy. Patients afflicted with the classical (proliferative) or mesenchymal subtypes benefit from radiation and temozolomide treatment [12]. Such benefit was not observed in patients afflicted with the proneural subtype.

3. Concept 2: Oncogene addiction

The term "oncogene addiction" was initially coined by Dr. Bernard Weinstein to describe the phenomenon that some tumors exhibit exquisite dependence on a single oncogenic protein (or pathway) for sustaining growth and proliferation [14]. Such dependence has been convincingly demonstrated in both tissue culture and transgenic mice systems for oncogenic versions of MYC [15-17] and RAS [18]. Application of this concept to the clinical setting has achieved variable success in various cancer types, including chronic myelogeneous leukemia (CML) harboring the BCR-ABL translocation, Erb2 over-expression breast cancer, and Non-Small Cell Lung Cancer harboring selected EGFR mutations [19, 20]. A simplistic application of this concept in glioblastoma would involve identification of the critical "addicted" oncogene followed by the inhibition of such oncogene(s). Unfortunately, the actual biology of glioblastoma is far more complex.

To understanding this complexity, a careful analysis of the fundamental notion of oncogenic addiction is needed. In some ways, the observation that tumors exhibit dependence on a particular oncogenic pathway at some point in its history is not surprising. However, taken in the context of the plethora of dynamic genetic changes that accumulated during cancer progression [21], it is somewhat anti-intuitive to suspect that any particular pathway would play a prominent role in maintaining cell viability. Moreover, inactivation of the normal counterpart of the addicted oncogenic protein is often tolerated in normal tissue. These observations suggest that the genetic circuitry of the cancer cell have been extensively re-programmed to result in this "addicted" state [14].

The molecular nature of this re-programming remains poorly understood. Several hypotheses have been put forward. One hypothesis involves the notion of "genetic streamlining", where genetic instability in cancer cells is thought to mutationally or epigenetically inactivate certain signaling pathways that are operational in a normal cell but not required for growth in the cancer cell. In this "streamlined" state, the tumor cell becomes hyper-dependent on the oncogene driven processes [22]. A more generalized form of this explanation involved the notion of synthetic lethality. Two genes are considered synthetically lethal if cells remain viable with inactivation of either gene. Simultaneous inactivation of both genes, on the other hand, results in cell death [23]. It is thought that the cancer cells have accumulated mutations that are synthetically lethal with the absence of critical oncogenes. The main difference between this hypothesis and the "streamline" hypothesis is that the mutation in the former can result in a gain or loss of function, whereas the later specifically proposes a loss of function. A third hypothesis suggests that oncogenes reprogrammed the tumor cell by both pro-survival and pro-apoptotic signaling [22]. With acute inactivation, the pro-survival signaling decayed faster than the pro-apoptotic signaling, resulting in tumor death.

The main reason for revisiting the framework of oncogene addiction is that mechanism by which the cells can evolve to avoid such addiction. For instance, in the context of synthetic lethality, EGFR inhibition may be cytotoxic to glioblastoma cells only in the appropriate genetic context. Indeed, therapeutic effects of EGFR inhibition were observed only in patients with tumors harboring an oncogenic form of EGFR and an intact PTEN tumor suppressor gene [24]. To complicate the matter, recent studies demonstrate that glioblastomas harbor activation of multiple oncogenic Receptor Tyrosine Kinases (RTKs), such that inactivation of any single oncogene merely diverts signaling through other active oncogenes [25]. In these contexts, it is evident that meaningful therapy will require simultaneous inhibition of multiple oncogenes or identification of the fitting genetic context.

4. Concept 3: Non-oncogene addiction

Emerging literature suggests an alternative strategy to the multi-target approach. These studies reveal that oncogene activation introduces secondary physiologic changes that stress cellular capacity for survival. Consequently, tumor cells become hyper-dependent on processes required to compensate for these stressful conditions [26, 27]. This phenomenon is termed "non-oncogene addiction" since the compensatory processes required for tumor survival do not directly contribute to the cancer formation. In other words, even genes that are not themselves targeted by tumorigenic mutations may well become essential for the tumor to survive the stressful environment and fuel the demanding process of tumor progression. Consequently, interference with the function of such genes can be rate-limiting to the particular mechanism in the tumor, but not as much in the normal counterpart cells. Importantly, such adaptively essential genes that underlie the 'non-oncogene addiction' [26, 27] of cancer cells can be therapeutically targeted if suitable drugs or other approaches are available.

There are several examples of such critical non-oncogenic pro-survival functions required for maintenance of the tumorigenic state in glioblastoma. EGFR is a critical proto-oncogene in glioblastoma pathogenesis [10, 28]. Our laboratory has demonstrated that EGFR hyperactivation results in increased accumulation of reactive oxygen species (ROS), which in turn cause cytotoxic DNA damage. To compensate for the deleterious effect of ROS, EGFR hyperactive glioblastomas exhibit increased reliance on DNA repair process that repair ROS related DNA damage [29]. Selective targeting of EGFR hyperactive glioblastomas can, thus, be achieved by inhibition of these repair process. Other groups have demonstrated that EGFR hyperactivation in glioblastoma cell lines heightens requirement for lipogenesis [30, 31]. Other examples of such critical non-oncogenic pro-survival functions required for maintenance of the tumorigenic state include dependency on mechanism for compensating mitotic and proteotoxic stress and interplay with the tumor microenvironment including the immune system [26]. While illustrative examples of strategies based on these "non-oncogene" addiction paradigms have been established in other cancers, the pertinence to glioblastoma awaits rigorous interrogation.

The principle of non-oncogene addiction suggests that there is a wider spectrum of therapeutic options than afforded under the paradigm of "oncogene addiction". In many cases, compensatory processes involved in "non-oncogene addiction" are the same as those that basic scientists have studied for years (for instance, DNA repair). Mechanistic investigations into these biologic processes by the basic scientists have yielded a rich database of inhibitors. Thus, identifying gene functions that compensate for oncogene induced cellular stress should afford opportunities to tap into this rich database and expand the denominator of drugs available for combinatorial therapy. Identifying genes that are synthetically lethal with oncogenes constitute an attractive means to this end.

It is important to note that effects of therapies designed based on the principles of "oncogene addiction" and of "non-oncogene addiction" are inherently antagonistic. For instance, EGFR inhibition leads to a reduction of ROS, obviating the need for DNA repair [29]. In this context, combination of DNA repair inhibition and EGFR inhibition would not be desirable. Rational strategies for synthesizing the two therapeutic paradigms remains a major intellectual challenge.

5. Concept 4: Tumor initiating cells

Another advance that may profoundly change our thinking about solid tumors including glioblastoma involves the concept of tumor initiating cells. The experimental observation is that within a total population of glioblastoma cells, there appears to be a small sub-population of cells that are highly tumorigenic (hence the term "tumor initiating cells" or "TICs") with tremendous capacity for self-renewal [32, 33]. To the extent that glioblastoma tumor initiating cells share many common properties when compared to neural stem cells, it is proposed that the TICs originated from stem cells. While there are some data supporting this hypothesis [5], the universality of this hypothesis remain controversial.

Protein markers to prospectively identify and isolate these putative TICs such as the transmembrane glycoprotein CD133 (prominin-1) in glioblastomas have been identified [5]. However, the value of CD133 as a single marker of glioblastoma TICs remains controversial, partly because also CD133-negative glioblastoma cells could give rise to tumors in an intracranial mouse xenograft model [34-36]. These uncertainties motivate an ongoing search for additional candidate TIC markers. Candidate cell surface molecules suggested in this context include the adhesion glycoprotein L1CAM [37], surface carbohydrate antigen CD15 (SSEA-1) [38], surface marker A2B5 [39], and integrin α6 [40]. Currently, there are no generally accepted cell surface markers for defining TIC. The definition of TICs remains a functional one as defined by the ability of a tumor cell to sustain self-renewal and initiate glioblastoma formation in immuno-compromised xenograft models.

Arguably, the most important aspect of the concept of TICs is that this population appeared particularly resistant to conventional radiation and chemotherapy [32]. In this context, TICs may be responsible for glioblastoma recurrence after conventional therapy. Given such properties, it is understandable that glioblastoma research has recently focused on identification and development of potential anti-TIC therapies. Two of these strategies, namely targeting the TICs as part of a vascular niche, and attempts to overcome their therapeutic resistance, will be discussed in the following sections on glioblastoma angiogenesis and the role of DNA damage response pathways, respectively. Here, we briefly consider strategies that are emerging as potentially fruitful approaches to treat glioblastoma through targeting TICs.

The first strategy reflects the efforts to identify suitable cell surface markers to reliably identify glioblastoma TICs - with the hope of conjugating the corresponding antibody to cytotoxic compounds as therapeutic agents. The second strategy is based on observations that some TICs, like neural stem cells, can be induced into a differentiated state whereby the self-renewal properties are lost. Among the suggested agents to induce such TIC differentiation, the bone morphogenetic proteins (BMPs) appear promising [41]. The third strategy involves modulating specific signaling pathways required for maintaining the TIC state. Pathways targeted include those mediated by EGFR, Wnt-beta catenin, STAT3, Sonic Hedgehog-Gli, and Notch pathways [42]. To the extent that these pathways are also regulated by miRNAs such as miR-21 [43], such miRNA constitute therapeutic targets in this strategy. Finally, normal neural stem cells have been shown to migrate toward and track TICs. Based on this principle, neural stem cells have been as delivery vehicles to increase local concentration of therapeutic agents in the vicinity of TICs [44].

6. Summary

In this chapter, we have discussed key principles underlying current development of glioblastoma therapeutics. Emphasis was placed on conceptual framework rather than specific drugs or targets. These frameworks should serve as the basis for translating fundamental biologic tenets into clinically useful therapeutic strategies.

7. References

[1] Jemal A, Siegel R, Xu J, Ward E. Cancer statistics, 2010. *CA Cancer J Clin.* Sep-Oct 2010;60(5):277-300.
[2] Wen PY, Kesari S. Malignant gliomas in adults. *N Engl J Med.* Jul 31 2008;359(5):492-507.
[3] Walker MD, Alexander E, Jr., Hunt WE, et al. Evaluation of BCNU and/or radiotherapy in the treatment of anaplastic gliomas. A cooperative clinical trial. *J Neurosurg.* Sep 1978;49(3):333-343.
[4] Stupp R, Mason WP, van den Bent MJ, et al. Radiotherapy plus concomitant and adjuvant temozolomide for glioblastoma. *N Engl J Med.* Mar 10 2005;352(10):987-996.
[5] Alcantara Llaguno S, Chen J, Kwon CH, et al. Malignant astrocytomas originate from neural stem/progenitor cells in a somatic tumor suppressor mouse model. *Cancer Cell.* Jan 6 2009;15(1):45-56.
[6] Ignatova TN, Kukekov VG, Laywell ED, Suslov ON, Vrionis FD, Steindler DA. Human cortical glial tumors contain neural stem-like cells expressing astroglial and neuronal markers in vitro. *Glia.* Sep 2002;39(3):193-206.
[7] Louis DN, Ohgaki H, Wiestler OD, et al. The 2007 WHO classification of tumours of the central nervous system. *Acta Neuropathol.* Aug 2007;114(2):97-109.
[8] Hanahan D, Weinberg RA. The hallmarks of cancer. *Cell.* Jan 7 2000;100(1):57-70.
[9] Stratton MR, Campbell PJ, Futreal PA. The cancer genome. *Nature.* Apr 9 2009;458(7239):719-724.
[10] TCGA. Comprehensive genomic characterization defines human glioblastoma genes and core pathways. *Nature.* Oct 23 2008;455(7216):1061-1068.
[11] Phillips HS, Kharbanda S, Chen R, et al. Molecular subclasses of high-grade glioma predict prognosis, delineate a pattern of disease progression, and resemble stages in neurogenesis. *Cancer Cell.* Mar 2006;9(3):157-173.
[12] Verhaak RGW, Hoadley KA, Purdom E, et al. Integrated genomic analysis identifies clinically relevant subtypes of glioblastoma characterized by abnormalities in PDGFRA, IDH1, EGFR, and NF1. *Cancer Cell.* Jan 19 2010;17(1):98-110.
[13] Brennan C, Momota H, Hambardzumyan D, et al. Glioblastoma subclasses can be defined by activity among signal transduction pathways and associated genomic alterations. *PLoS One.* 2009;4(11):e7752.
[14] Weinstein IB. Cancer. Addiction to oncogenes--the Achilles heal of cancer. *Science.* Jul 5 2002;297(5578):63-64.
[15] Felsher DW, Bishop JM. Reversible tumorigenesis by MYC in hematopoietic lineages. *Mol Cell.* Aug 1999;4(2):199-207.
[16] Felsher DW, Bishop JM. Transient excess of MYC activity can elicit genomic instability and tumorigenesis. *Proc Natl Acad Sci U S A.* Mar 30 1999;96(7):3940-3944.
[17] Yokoyama K, Imamoto F. Transcriptional control of the endogenous MYC protooncogene by antisense RNA. *Proc Natl Acad Sci U S A.* Nov 1987;84(21):7363-7367.
[18] Chin L, Tam A, Pomerantz J, et al. Essential role for oncogenic Ras in tumour maintenance. *Nature.* Jul 29 1999;400(6743):468-472.
[19] Druker BJ. Inhibition of the Bcr-Abl tyrosine kinase as a therapeutic strategy for CML. *Oncogene.* Dec 9 2002;21(56):8541-8546.
[20] Roberts PJ, Der CJ. Targeting the Raf-MEK-ERK mitogen-activated protein kinase cascade for the treatment of cancer. *Oncogene.* May 14 2007;26(22):3291-3310.

[21] Greenman C, Stephens P, Smith R, et al. Patterns of somatic mutation in human cancer genomes. *Nature.* Mar 8 2007;446(7132):153-158.
[22] Sharma SV, Settleman J. Oncogene addiction: setting the stage for molecularly targeted cancer therapy. *Genes Dev.* Dec 15 2007;21(24):3214-3231.
[23] Kaelin WG, Jr. The concept of synthetic lethality in the context of anticancer therapy. *Nat Rev Cancer.* Sep 2005;5(9):689-698.
[24] Mellinghoff IK, Wang MY, Vivanco I, et al. Molecular determinants of the response of glioblastomas to EGFR kinase inhibitors.[see comment][erratum appears in N Engl J Med. 2006 Feb 23;354(8):884]. *New England Journal of Medicine.* 2005;353(19):2012-2024.
[25] Stommel JM, Kimmelman AC, Ying H, et al. Coactivation of receptor tyrosine kinases affects the response of tumor cells to targeted therapies. *Science.* 2007;318(5848):287-290.
[26] Luo J, Solimini NL, Elledge SJ. Principles of cancer therapy: oncogene and non-oncogene addiction.[erratum appears in Cell. 2009 Aug 21;138(4):807]. *Cell.* 2009;136(5):823-837.
[27] Luo J, Emanuele MJ, Li D, et al. A genome-wide RNAi screen identifies multiple synthetic lethal interactions with the Ras oncogene. *Cell.* 2009;137(5):835-848.
[28] Parsons DW, Jones S, Zhang X, et al. An integrated genomic analysis of human glioblastoma multiforme. *Science.* Sep 26 2008;321(5897):1807-1812.
[29] Nitta M, Kozono D, Kennedy R, et al. Targeting EGFR induced oxidative stress by PARP1 inhibition in glioblastoma therapy. *PLoS One.* 2010;5(5):e10767.
[30] Guo D, Hildebrandt IJ, Prins RM, et al. The AMPK agonist AICAR inhibits the growth of EGFRvIII-expressing glioblastomas by inhibiting lipogenesis. *Proc Natl Acad Sci U S A.* Aug 4 2009;106(31):12932-12937.
[31] Guo D, Prins RM, Dang J, et al. EGFR signaling through an Akt-SREBP-1-dependent, rapamycin-resistant pathway sensitizes glioblastomas to antilipogenic therapy. *Sci Signal.* 2009;2(101):ra82.
[32] Bao S, Wu Q, McLendon RE, et al. Glioma stem cells promote radioresistance by preferential activation of the DNA damage response. *Nature.* Dec 7 2006;444(7120):756-760.
[33] Singh SK, Hawkins C, Clarke ID, et al. Identification of human brain tumour initiating cells. *Nature.* Nov 18 2004;432(7015):396-401.
[34] Chen R, Nishimura MC, Bumbaca SM, et al. A hierarchy of self-renewing tumor-initiating cell types in glioblastoma. *Cancer Cell.* Apr 13 2010;17(4):362-375.
[35] Sun Y, Kong W, Falk A, et al. CD133 (Prominin) negative human neural stem cells are clonogenic and tripotent. *PLoS One.* 2009;4(5):e5498.
[36] Wang J, Sakariassen PO, Tsinkalovsky O, et al. CD133 negative glioma cells form tumors in nude rats and give rise to CD133 positive cells. *Int J Cancer.* Feb 15 2008;122(4):761-768.
[37] Bao S, Wu Q, Li Z, et al. Targeting cancer stem cells through L1CAM suppresses glioma growth. *Cancer Res.* Aug 1 2008;68(15):6043-6048.
[38] Son MJ, Woolard K, Nam DH, Lee J, Fine HA. SSEA-1 is an enrichment marker for tumor-initiating cells in human glioblastoma. *Cell Stem Cell.* May 8 2009;4(5):440-452.

[39] Ogden AT, Waziri AE, Lochhead RA, et al. Identification of A2B5+CD133- tumor-initiating cells in adult human gliomas. *Neurosurgery.* Feb 2008;62(2):505-514; discussion 514-505.
[40] Lathia JD, Gallagher J, Heddleston JM, et al. Integrin alpha 6 regulates glioblastoma stem cells. *Cell Stem Cell.* May 7 2010;6(5):421-432.
[41] Lee J, Son MJ, Woolard K, et al. Epigenetic-mediated dysfunction of the bone morphogenetic protein pathway inhibits differentiation of glioblastoma-initiating cells. *Cancer Cell.* Jan 2008;13(1):69-80.
[42] Ebben JD, Treisman DM, Zorniak M, Kutty RG, Clark PA, Kuo JS. The cancer stem cell paradigm: a new understanding of tumor development and treatment. *Expert Opin Ther Targets.* Jun 2010;14(6):621-632.
[43] Krichevsky AM, Gabriely G. miR-21: a small multi-faceted RNA. *J Cell Mol Med.* Jan 2009;13(1):39-53.
[44] Frank RT, Najbauer J, Aboody KS. Concise review: stem cells as an emerging platform for antibody therapy of cancer. *Stem Cells.* Nov 2010;28(11):2084-2087.

4

Biological Responses of Glioma Cell to Chemotherapeutic Agents

Yuichi Hirose and Shigeo Ohba
Department of Neurosurgery, Fujita Health University, Toyoake
Department of Neurosurgery, Ashikaga Red Cross Hospital, Ashikaga
Japan

1. Introduction

Because gliomas are not curable surgically, development of effective adjuvant therapies is warranted. A chemotherapeutic agent temozolimide (TMZ) has been widely used not only because it is well tolerated and easily administrated orally but because various clinical trials had revealed that high grade gliomas could show objective response or stable disease to this compound (Stupp et al., 2005). The action of TMZ had been extensively studied primarily in leukemia and lymphoma cells. TMZ spontaneously decomposes in aqueous solution to form the cytotoxic methylating agent, and the cytotoxicity of TMZ appears to be mediated mainly through adduction of a methyl group to O^6 position of guanine (G) in genomic DNA. The methyl group can be removed from O^6-methylguanine by O^6-methylguanine-DNA methyltransferase (MGMT). If MGMT is deficient in the cell, however, O^6-methylguanine is not repaired, and incorporation of a thymine (T) rather than a cytosine opposite the O^6-methylguanine during the next cycle of DNA replication leads to the formation of GT mismatches in DNA. This triggers the DNA mismatch repair (MMR) system which removes the T, only to have the T reinserted during repair synthesis. Futile cycles of MMR triggered by GT mismatches can lead to a variety of outcomes in TMZ-treated cells (Figure 1).

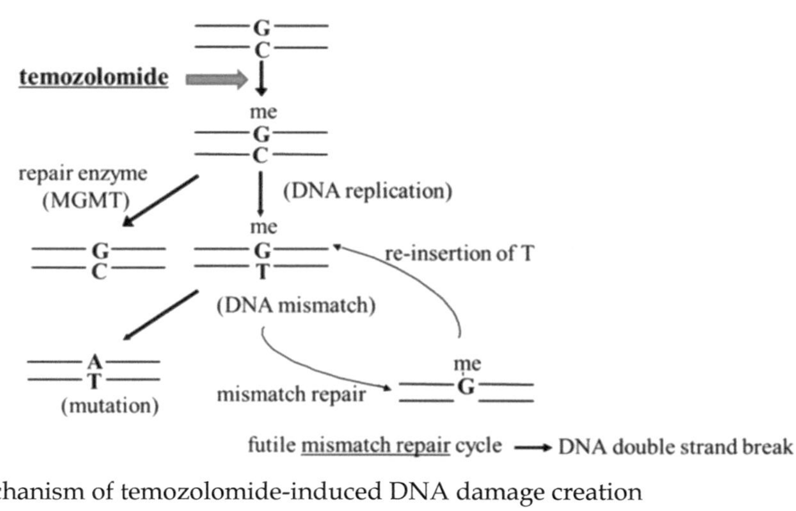

Fig. 1. Mechanism of temozolomide-induced DNA damage creation

Since MGMT has been considered as a key factor in the resistance of gliomas to TMZ, several clinical trials have been conducted. However, TMZ treatment in combination with MGMT-depleting compound did not show remarkable therapeutic affect for malignant gliomas, and recent clinical studies suggest that MGMT is just a prognostic marker for malignant gliomas treated with genotoxic agents including radiation and chemotherapy, and that MGMT is not the only factor that induces TMZ-resistance, and that further biological investigation on glioma cells is needed. In this chapter we review our studies on glioma biology in regard its cellular responses to DNA-damaging compounds, especially TMZ, which could provide a clue to develop safe and effective methods to potentiate anti-tumor activity of the drug.

2. Cell cycle arrest of glioma cells in response to temozolomide

Most of DNA-damaging chemotherapeutic agents induce cell cycle arrest, and so does TMZ (Hirose et al., 2001a). When MGMT-negative and p53 wildtype U87MG human glioblastoma cells were treated with TMZ at the concentration based on the published data of the plasma concentration of the drug in patients involved in its clinical trials (100 microM for 3 hours), FACS analysis revealed no significant difference in the percentage of cells in each phase of the cell cycle between untreated U87MG cells and the cells harvested at 1 day after TMZ treatment. However, cells began to accumulate at the G2/M boundary (4n DNA content) 2 days after TMZ treatment. This G2/M arrest (here defined as a greater percentage of cells in G2/M than G1) was sustained for at least 10 days after TMZ treatment, and was associated with the gradual appearance of hyperploid (>4n DNA content) cells and the gradual loss of cells with 2n DNA content (G1 cells). Although TMZ-treated cells underwent cell cycle arrest, the sub-G1 population, which represents apoptotic cells, was small and did not significantly increase throughout the 10 days following TMZ treatment. Consistent with the G2/M arrest data, p53 and $p21^{Waf1/Cip1}$ levels were increased approximately 2-4 fold at 2 days after TMZ treatment with the accumulation persisting at least 10 days after the treatment. On the other hand, genetically modified U87MG-E6 cells which have low levels of p53 because of transfection of human papilloma viral oncoprotein E6 mediating ubiquitination and destruction of p53 showed shorter G2/M after TMZ treatment. That is, the proportion of U87MG cells at G2/M began decreasing by 3 days after TMZ treatment and was considerably lessened by 10 days after treatment. The reduction in G2/M arrest in these cells was also associated with a gradual increase in cells with a sub-G1 (less than 2n). Because U87MG and U87MG-E6 cells share a common genetic background except for expression of E6, comparison of the responses of these cells provides more useful information than the comparison of responses of cells with completely different genetic backgrounds. These results support the idea that p53 (and $p21^{Waf1/Cip1}$), while not important for initiation of TMZ-induced G2/M arrest, do play a role in sustaining the arrest (Figure 2). Colony formation efficiency assay revealed that U87MG cells showed a dose-dependent decrease in clonogenicity, and, on the other hand, U87MG-E6 cells formed far less colonies. As well as being associated with the duration of TMZ-induced arrest in glioma cells, the p53 status of cells was also associated with the ultimate fate of the cells. p53-wildtype cells underwent a prolonged G2/M arrest which left the majority of cells viable yet non-proliferative showing the features of ascent cells. In contrast, p53-deficient cells underwent a more transient arrest, and lost viability in a manner consistent with mitotic catastrophy. Therefore while both p53-wt and p53-deficient cells became non-proliferative in response to

TMZ, the means by which this was accomplished differed in a manner consistent with p53 status.

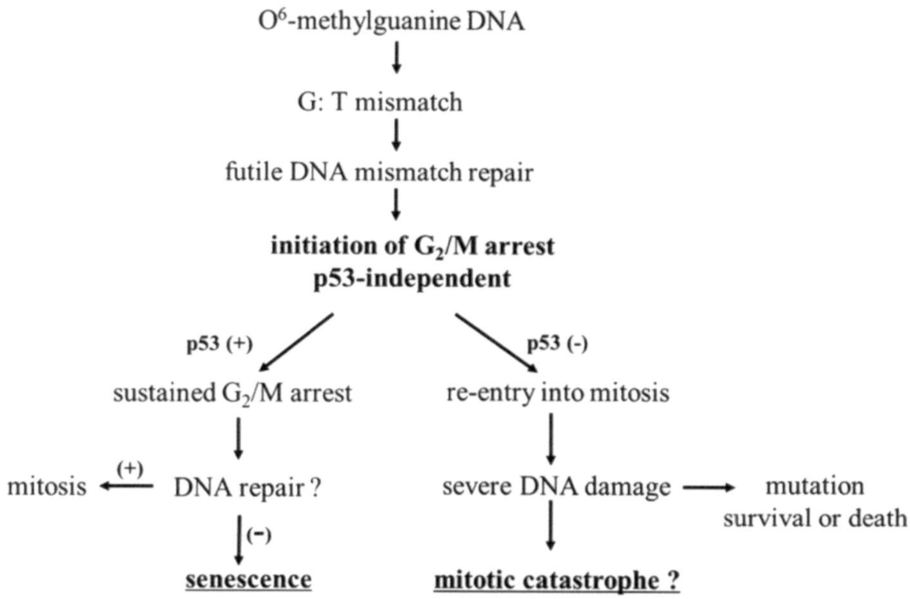

Fig. 2. TMZ-induced cell cycle arrest and the fate of the cells.

3. DNA checkpoint

While both p53-wt and p53-deficient cells initiate G2/M arrest and become non-proliferative in response to TMZ, p53-wt cells which undergo prolonged G2/M arrest are less sensitive than p53-deficient cells to the cytotoxic actions of TMZ. One possible explanation for this effect is that the prolonged G2/M arrest noted in p53-wt cells allows more time for reversal of the cytotoxic effects of the drug prior to entry into mitosis and death by mitotic catastrophe. G2/M arrest in response to TMZ may therefore represent a defense mechanism against the cytotoxic actions of TMZ.

While the linkage between TMZ-induced DNA damage and G2/M arrest has not been fully explored, the linkage between irradiation-induced DNA damage and G2/M arrest has been shown to involve a pathway controlling the cyclin-dependent kinase cdc2. Various types of DNA damage activate Chk1 kinase which phophorylates cdc25C phosphatase at serine-216 which enhances the binding of 14-3-3 proteins and the export of the cdc25C/14-3-3 complex to the cytoplasm. The cytoplasmic sequestration of phosphorylated cdc25C in turn eliminates the potential cdc25C-mediated dephosphorylation of cdc2. Cdc2 therefore remains bound to cyclin B in an inactive, phosphorylated state. The end result of DNA damage-induced Chk1 activation therefore is the phosphorylation of cdc2, and the arrest of cells with damaged DNA at the G2/M boundary. The ability of TMZ to induce DNA damage suggested that, like other DNA damaging agents, TMZ might initiate G2/M arrest via a Chk1-dependent pathway.

If Chk1 activation is critical in activation of G2/M arrest in TMZ-treated cells, and if G2/M arrest provides the opportunity for cells to avoid TMZ-induced cytotoxicity, inhibition of cdc2-dependent G2 arrest should sensitize cells to TMZ. A variety of small molecule inhibitors have recently been developed, and we analyzed the effect of UCN-01, a staurosporin derivative Chk1 inhibitor, as a pharmacologic tool to assess the linkage between TMZ exposure and G2/M arrest, to determine if G2/M arrest protects cells from TMZ-induced cytotoxicity, and to determine if Chk1 inhibitors might represent a way to sensitize cells to TMZ (Hirose et al., 2001b).

To better define how TMZ induces G2/M arrest, we analyzed alterations in levels of G2-checkpoint-associated proteins in TMZ-treated cells. The protein levels of Chk1 increased in a transient manner, rising at 1-2 days after TMZ exposure and returning to sub-control levels by 10 days after TMZ exposure. While total levels of cdc2 were unchanged or only slightly increased after TMZ, levels of phosphorylated cdc2 were transiently increased in both U87MG and U87MG-E6 cells in a timeframe and manner similar to that noted for induction of Chk1.

To more directly test the association between TMZ and alterations in G2 checkpoint proteins, U87MG and U87MG-E6 cells were treated with TMZ, and then exposed to UCN-01 for 3 days immediately following TMZ removal. Immunoblot analyses revealed that UCN-01 reduced the level of phosphorylated cdc2 in the cells and significantly inhibited TMZ-induced G2/M arrest of both U87MG and U87MG-E6 cells Furthermore, in agreement with the study described above, UCN-01 reduced TMZ-induced senescence-associated beta-galactosidase activity and enhances mitotic catastrophe. UCN-01 increases TMZ-induced cytotoxicity in both p53-wt and p53-deficient glioma cells (Figure 3).

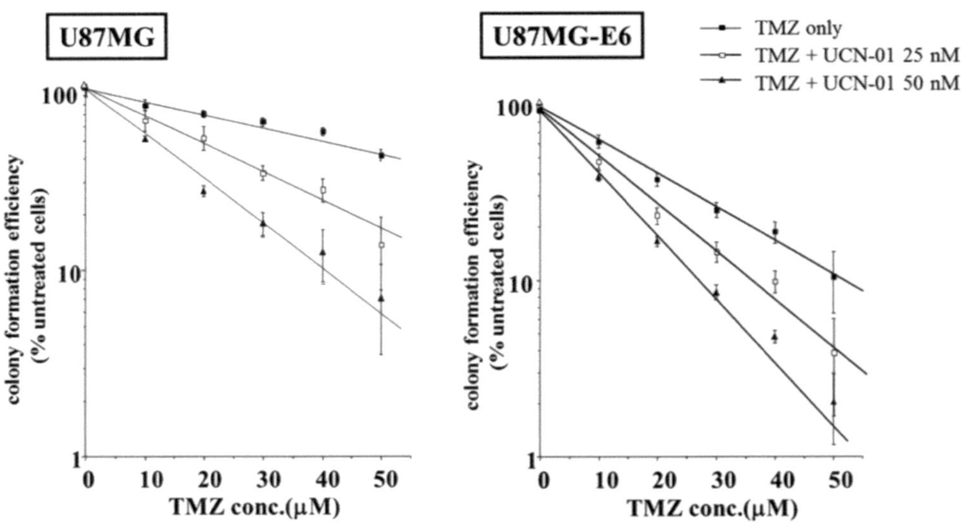

Fig. 3. p53-independent sensitization of glioma cells to TMZ by Chk1 inhibitor UCN-01.

Having established an association between TMZ-exposure, Chk1 activation, and TMZ-induced G2/M arrest, we examined the hypothesis that G2/M arrest is a protective response of cells to TMZ-induced cytotoxicity, and that elimination of the G2 checkpoint might sensitize cells (and in particular p53-wt cells) to TMZ. In p53 wt cells, which undergo a p53-associated prolonged G2/M arrest and senescence in response to TMZ, UCN-01 post-treatment greatly reduced the extent of G2/M arrest, reduced the percentage of cells undergoing TMZ-induced senescence, and increased the percentage of cells undergoing mitotic catastrophe. These results clearly suggested that in p53-proficient glioma cells, the G2 checkpoint serves a protective function, and that elimination of the checkpoint is associated with an increase in the number of cells that die by pre-mature entry into mitosis. UCN-01, however, not only sensitized p53-wt cells but also p53-deficient cells which underwent only a transient G2/M arrest in response to TMZ. This sensitization did not involve changes in TMZ-induced senescence (which was minimal in these cells) but rather was associated exclusively with increases in the number of cells undergoing mitotic catastrophe (Figure 4).

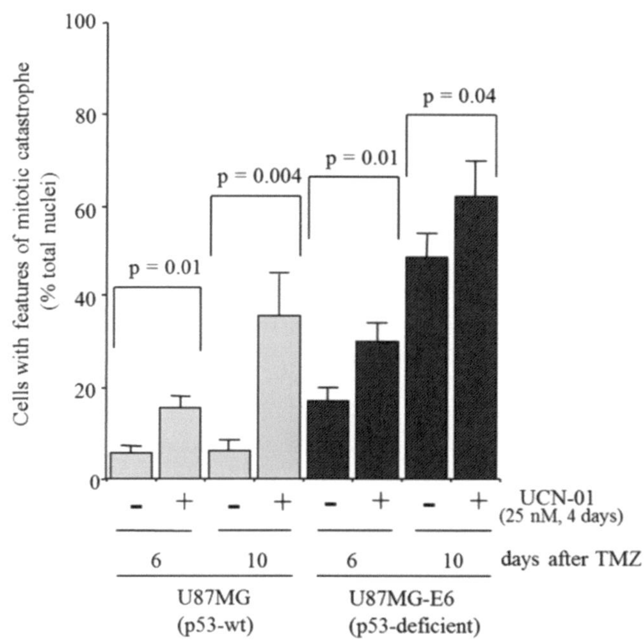

Fig. 4. Enhancement of TMZ-induced mitotic catastrophe by UCN-01.

While increased levels of MGMT and loss of MMR capacity can both confer TMZ resistance, very few gliomas over-express MGMT or are MMR deficient. It appears likely, therefore that at least some of the resistance of gliomas to TMZ involves events downstream of futile MMR activation. The ability of UCN-01 to prevent downstream events which may contribute to TMZ resistance may therefore prove useful in the treatment of TMZ-resistant as well as TMZ-sensitive tumors. As approximately two-thirds of gliomas have defects in the p53 pathway, the ability of UCN-01 to sensitize cells regardless of p53 status also increases the range of tumors for which this approach might be effective. While issues relating to duration of exposure, drug sequencing, and the events that link MMR to Chk1 activation remain to be examined, it has been suggested that the combinations of TMZ with G2 checkpoint inhibitors such as UCN-01 might be useful additions to existing therapies for brain tumors.

4. Stress-activated kinases

Stress-activated kinases (SAPKs) could be targeted in an effort to enhance the effect of chemotherapeutic agents because the tumor cells, which grow under various types of cellular stress including hypoxia and genetic instability, might survive in severe environment by modifying on stress-inducing events. We here discuss about two SAPKs, p38MAPK and c-Jun-N-terminal kinase (JNK).

4.1 p38 MAPK

While the cellular response to methylating agent exposure appeared highly dependent on DNA repair processes influenced by the G2 cell cycle checkpoint, the purpose of the cell cycle arrest remains unclear, although it has long been suggested that cell cycle arrest provides cells that have incurred DNA damage time in which to reverse the damage. Despite this suggestion has not been directly tested, it was clear that the prolonged G2 arrest noted in glioma cells exposed to cytotoxic methylating agents alters their response.

It has been appreciated for some time that cells lacking a functional MMR system undergo neither G2 arrest nor cytotoxicity in response to methylating agents, clearly suggesting a link between MMR and G2 arrest.

A potential signaling pathway that might help connect activation of the MMR system to G2 arrest is that controlled by the p38 MAPK family. The p38 family of stress kinases contains four members: α, β, γ, and δ. These MAP kinases are activated by the upstream kinases MKK3 and/or MKK6 in response to diverse stimuli including environmental stress and growth factors. p38 kinases in turn activate a variety of downstream targets including MAPKAP2, the C/EBP family of transcription factors, and various other transcription factors including p53. In this manner p38 is believed to play an important, although not well defined, role in co-ordinating a variety of cellular events including cell growth, cell differentiation, and cell death. At least two recent studies have suggested that the ability of the p38 pathway to co-ordinate cell growth and cell death might also extend to actions on cell cycle progression.

To begin to address the possible role of the p38 pathway in the response of cells to methylating agents, we exposed U87MG cells to TMZ, and the various p38 isoforms were then immunoprecipitated from the nuclear fractions, and equal amounts of the immunoprecipitated p38 isoforms from each time point were incubated with the p38 substrate ATF2 in the presence of ATP. TMZ exposure stimulated p38α kinase activity and p38β kinase activity was also modestly stimulated while the activity of p38γ and δ were not significantly affected (Hirose et al, 2003).

To investigate linkage between MMR and p38 activation, we first exposed MMR-deficient HCT116 human colorectal adenocarcinoma cells and paired MMR-proficient HCT116 cells containing a copy of *Mlh1*-containing chromosome 3 (HCT116 3-6 cells) to TMZ, after which the cells were collected and analyzed for levels of p38α phosphorylation/activation and extent of G2 arrest by Western blot and by FACS analysis, respectively. Neither HCT116 nor HCT116 3-6 cells exhibited p38 induction or G2 arrest in the first two days following TMZ exposure, consistent with previous studies showing that both these cell lines are MGMT-proficient and presumably repair TMZ-induced O^6-methylguanine before these lesions mispair with thymine and trigger downstream consequences. Following exposure to the highly specific MGMT depleting agent O^6-benzylguanine prior to and after TMZ exposure, however, the MMR-proficient HCT116 3-6 cells exhibited TMZ-induced p38α

activation in a manner similar to that noted in U87MG glioma cells, and underwent G2 arrest. O^6-benzylguanine-exposed, TMZ-treated MMR-deficient HCT116 cells, however, exhibited neither p38 activation nor G2 arrest. These results suggested in a preliminary manner that p38 activation in response to TMZ is dependent on O^6-methylguanine lesions and on the recognition and/or processing of these lesions by the DNA MMR system.
While studies in HCT cells suggested an association between the DNA MMR system and TMZ-induced G2 arrest, the MMR-corrected HCT116 3-6 cell line used was derived from a clone that contains a large portion of human chromosome three, and which therefore could differ from the MMR-proficient HCT116 cells in ways more dependent on clonal selection and multiple gene expression that on direct correction of the MMR defect. We therefore also examined TMZ-induced p38 activation and G2 arrest in MGMT-deficient, MMR-proficient human U87MG glioblastoma cells and in paired cells made MMR-deficient by expression of a retrovirally-encoded siRNA targeted to the MMR protein MLH1. Expression of the retrovirally encoded MLH1 siRNA blocked TMZ-induced G2 arrest such that cells expressing the MLH1 siRNA, but not cells expressing the blank vector, avoided TMZ-induced G2 arrest in a manner identical to that noted in HCT116 cells in which MLH1 was eliminated by mutation. More importantly, siRNA-mediated reduction of MLH1 levels also blocked the ability of the cells to activate the p38 pathway. These results, in connection with those derived from the studies with HCT cells, suggested that p38 activation was a common response of human cells to the methylating agent TMZ, that this activation is dependent on a functional MMR system, and that p38 activation is associated with methylating agent-induced G2 arrest.

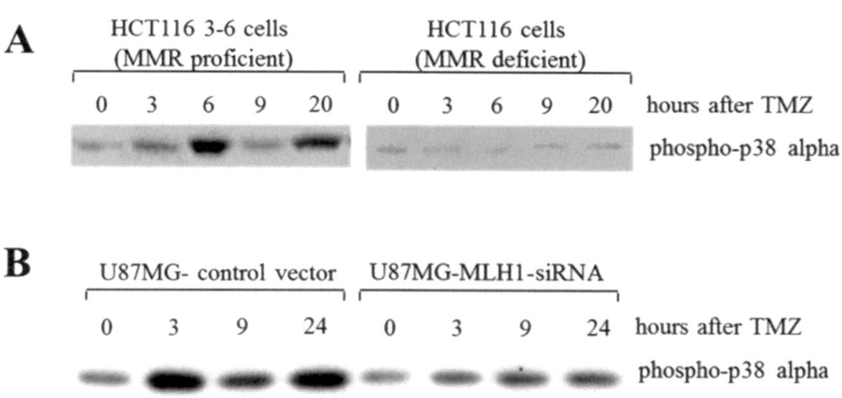

Fig. 5. TMZ-induced p38 activation in MMR-deficient colon carcinoma cells (A) and MMR-silenced glioma cells (B).

Having demonstrated the linkage between DNA MMR and p38 activation, we wished to more clearly define the potential linkage between p38 activation and G2 arrest. To do so we used both pharmacologic and genetic inhibitors of p38α, and monitored the effects of these inhibitors on G2 checkpoint proteins and on TMZ-induce G2 arrest. For pharmacologic inhibition studies, MGMT-deficient, MMR-proficient U87MG cells were exposed to the p38α/β selective inhibitors SB203580 or SB202190 prior to and following TMZ exposure, after which effects of p38 inhibition on TMZ-induced p38 activation, activation of the G2 checkpoint pathway, and activation of the G2 checkpoint itself were examined. Both compounds not only blocked TMZ-induced p38 activation but also dramatically inhibited the ability of U87 cells to undergo G2 arrest two days following TMZ exposure. Exposure of cells to SB203580 prior to and following TMZ exposure blocked the inactivation of both cdc25C and cdc2, consistent with the inability of SB compound-treated cells to undergo G2 arrest following TMZ exposure. SB203580 exposure, however, had no significant effect on TMZ-induced Chk1 or Chk2 activation. These results suggest that the p38 pathway, and p38α/β specifically, are linked not only to MMR but also to activation of the G2 checkpoint through Chk1/2-independent actions on cdc25C and/or cdc2.

We also employed genetic means to selectively inhibit p38α and to assess the consequences of p38α inhibition on the G2 arrest pathway. To do so, MGMT-deficient, MMR-proficient U87MG cells were transfected with a pool of siRNA targeting p38α, after which the cells were exposed to TMZ. Transfection of U87MG cells with p38α siRNA reduced basal levels of p38α, and blocked the TMZ-induced ability of immunoprecipitated p38α to phosphorylate the p38 substrate MAPKAP2 *in vitro*. Selective genetic inhibition of p38α blocked TMZ-induced G2 arrest in U87MG cells in manner identical to that mediated by pharmacologic inhibitors of p38α/β. Furthermore, as was noted in studies using pharmacological inhibitors, p38α siRNA blocked the phosphorylation/inactivation of both cdc25C and cdc2 without affecting TMZ-induced Chk1 or Chk2 activation (Figure 6). These results clearly show that p38α is activated by the DNA MMR system, and that this activation is in turn linked by Chk1- and Chk2-independent means to inactivation of cdc2, cdc25C, and ultimately to G2 arrest.

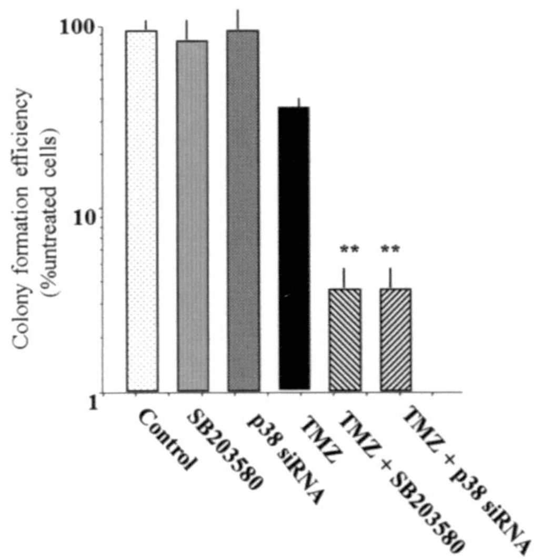

Fig. 6. p38 inhibition potentiated TMZ-induced cytotoxicity

Although pharmacologic or genetic inhibition of p38α did not alter clonagenicity, extent of senescence-associated beta-galactosidase expression, or extent of mitotic catastrophe, (data not shown), it did enhance the sensitivity of U87MG cells to TMZ-induced cytotoxicity, reducing the colony forming ability of these cells. p38 inhibition increased the percentage of TMZ-treated cells that died by mitotic catastrophe, consistent with the idea that cells incapable of undergoing G2 arrest enter mitosis with damaged DNA and die by mitotic catastrophe. These results suggest that p38α not only links MMR to the G2 checkpoint, but also influences the response of cells to cytotoxic methylating agents. It would be reasonable to suspect that tumors capable of activating the G2 checkpoint via the p38α pathway would be less sensitive than those incapable of doing so. Conversely, because inhibition of p38α sensitizes cells to TMZ, p38α might be a reasonable therapeutic target.

4.2 c-Jun N-terminal kinase

Since p38, a major component of mitogen-activated protein kinases (MAPKs), had been shown to be involved in TMZ-induced cellular responses, we were interested other MAPKS in terms they could be target for chemosensitization. MAPKs are components of a complex intracellular signaling network that regulates gene expression in response to extracellular stimuli, in turn regulating cell proliferation, differentiation, and cell death. The MAPK family includes components of three major pathways in humans: p38 kinase, c-Jun NH2-terminal kinase (JNK), and extracellular signal-regulated kinase. In the JNK pathway, specific stimuli activate various kinases leading to activation of JNK. Once activated, JNK is translocated to the nucleus, where it phosphorylates and activates transcriptional factors such as components of activator protein, including c-Jun, JunB, and JunD, as well as other factors including ATF-2 and STAT-3. As examples of the importance of JNK on cell signaling, JNK is associated with cell survival, oncogenesis, growth, differentiation, and cell death. The role of the JNK pathway in the mediation of cellular responses (including cellular transformation, cell growth, and cell death) to extracellular stimuli has been studied extensively. Interestingly, JNK can exert completely opposite effects depending on the cell type and stimuli. Since the question of whether JNK is associated with cell death or cell survival appeared to depend on the type of cellular stress, we investigated in the role of JNK in glioma cells treated with TMZ (Ohba et al., 2009).

We first investigated whether JNK was activated in response to TMZ and confirmed the activation of JNK in glioma cells treated with TMZ. Previous studies on gliomas had already shown that JNK was activated and played a pro-survival role in response to the DNA crosslinking agent CDDP, and that the inhibition of the JNK pathway sensitized glioma cells to CDDP. Sensitization to chemotherapeutic agents by the inhibition of the JNK pathway has also been reported either in other cancer cells although, on the other hand, the inhibition of JNK reportedly led to the suppression of chemotherapeutic agent-induced apoptosis in several studies. Therefore, we investigated the role of JNK in glioma cells treated with TMZ by utilizing the JNK inhibitor SP600125. As a result, we confirmed that SP600125 potentiated the TMZ-induced cytotoxicity in U87MG cells, and concluded that JNK activation played a cytoprotective role in glioma cells in response to TMZ-induced DNA damage (Figure 7A).

To clarify the mechanism responsible for the JNK inhibitor-induced potentiation of TMZ-induced cytotoxicity, the two main downstream proteins of JNK, c-Jun and ATF-2, were investigated, since these proteins are believed to be associated with chemoresistance. In our study, because SP600125 inhibited the phosphorylation of c-Jun but not of ATF-2 at the low concentration at which SP600125 induced chemosensitization to TMZ, c-Jun-related responses were considered to be more important in the JNK-mediated survival of glioma cells treated with TMZ than ATF-2-related pathways (Figure 7B).

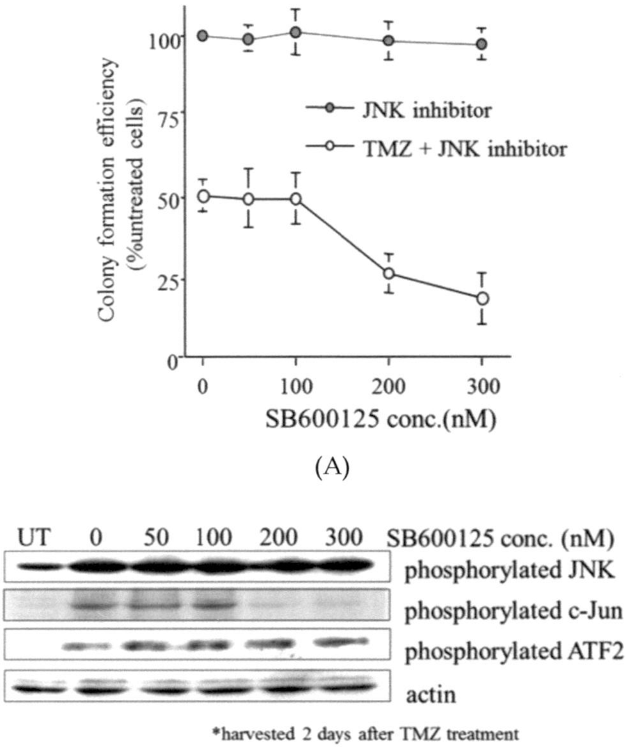

Fig. 7. Effect of JNK inhibitor SB600125 on TMZ-induced cytotoxicity (A) and phosphorylation of associated proteins (B).

As noted above, the inhibition of p38 increased the sensitivity of glioma cells to TMZ in association with the abrogation of G2 arrest, however, in contrast, JNK inhibitor did not affect the cell cycle distribution of TMZ-treated cells nor changed the protein level of phosphorylated cdc2. Thus, the SP600125-induced chemosensitization to TMZ in glioma cells was probably not a consequence of the abrogation of cell cycle arrest. Rather, JNK inhibition increased the percentage of senescence-like cells in U87MG cells and of mitotic catastrophe cells in U87MG-E6 cells after treatment with TMZ. These results suggest that the enhancement of TMZ toxicity by a JNK inhibitor in glioma cells was induced by the potentiation of cell death pathways induced by TMZ alone. These data might be in agreement with previous studies on gliomas which suggested involvement of the JNK pathway in DNA repair.. c-Jun-related responses could be key events in the JNK-mediated cytoprotection of glioma cells treated with TMZ, and further investigations of the involvement of c-Jun in the survival machinery of cells with DNA damage might promote the development of useful chemotherapeutic strategies against malignant gliomas.

5. Survival-promoting protein Akt

Survival promoting protein such as Akt, which is frequently activated in malignant gliomas, could be a target to enhance the effect of chemotherapeutic agents.

Whereas an extensive network of proteins are required to work together to initiate G2 arrest in response to DNA damage, a number of additional proteins have been reported to alter activation and maintenance of the G2 checkpoint. One of the most interesting of these is Akt, a member of the phosphatidylinositol-3 kinase family that is recruited to the cell membrane and activated in response to the generation of phospholipids by a variety of signaling pathways. Activated Akt in turn signals to a variety of key downstream molecules including mammalian target of rapamycin (mTOR), glycogen synthetase kinase 3, and S6 kinase, the sum of which is to suppress cell death and to promote cell survival. In addition to effects on apoptosis and cell metabolism, Akt activation has been reported to suppress activation of the G2 checkpoint in human colon carcinoma cells exposed to radiation. Whereas the mechanism by which Akt suppresses G2 arrest has not been defined, the observation that Akt influences the G2 checkpoint is of particular importance to the therapeutic application of TMZ whose cytotoxicity is influenced by the G2 checkpoint and which are frequently used in the treatment of PTEN-deficient, Akt overexpressing gliomas. Furthermore, because exposure of glioma cells to TMZ induces a senescence-like phenomenon and mitotic catastrophe, and because bypass of TMZ–induced G2 arrest by Chk1 inhibitors enhances, rather than suppresses, glioma cell death as described above, the consequences of potential Akt-mediated bypass of methylating agent–induced G2 arrest on cellular outcome remained uncertain.

To investigate the effect of Akt activation in biological responses of glioma cells to DNA-methylating compound, we created U87MD-derived cells of which Akt activity could be exogeneously controlled. U87MG human glioma cells were infected with a retroviral construct encoding a modified Akt (AktERM+) protein which, by virtue of deletion of the parathyroid hormone domain, fusion to a c-Src myristoylation signal, and fusion to a modified form of the mouse ER hormone binding domain, has been shown rapidly activated in response to 4-hydroxytamoxifen. The levels of AktER rose in response to exposures of 4-hydroxytamoxifen (Figure 8A).

Having created cells with inducible levels of activated Akt, we addressed the consequences of Akt pathway activation on TMZ-induced G2 arrest. In the absence of 4-hydroxytamoxifen, TMZ-treated U87MG-AktERM+ cells showed Cdc2 (Tyr15) phosphorylation/ inactivation, and G2 arrest 3 to 5 days following TMZ exposure. However, U87MG cells expressing the AktERM+ construct exhibited significant inhibition of TMZ-induced phosphorylation/ inactivation of Cdc2, and TMZ-induced G2 arrest (Figure 8B).

As described above, inhibition of TMZ-induced G2 arrest by Chk1 inhibitor forced cells into mitosis and enhances cell death by mitotic catastrophe in both p53-proficient and p53-deficient glioma cells. We therefore questioned whether bypass of TMZ-induced G2 arrest by Akt, a protein known to suppress apoptosis in response to radiation-induced DNA damage, would sensitize cells to TMZ or instead protect cells by suppressing pathways linked to senescence and/or mitotic catastrophe. As a result, AktERM+ activation protected rather than sensitized the p53-proficient U87MG cells to TMZ-induced cytotoxicity (Figure 8C). The cytoprotective effects of Akt overexpression were associated with a reduction in the percentage of cells expressing senescence-associated beta-galactosidase activity following TMZ exposure, suggesting that Akt overexpression not only reduced the percentage of cells undergoing TMZ-induced G2 arrest but also reduced the ability of p53-positive glioma cells to undergo a senescence-like phenomenon in response to TMZ. Furthermore, AktERM+

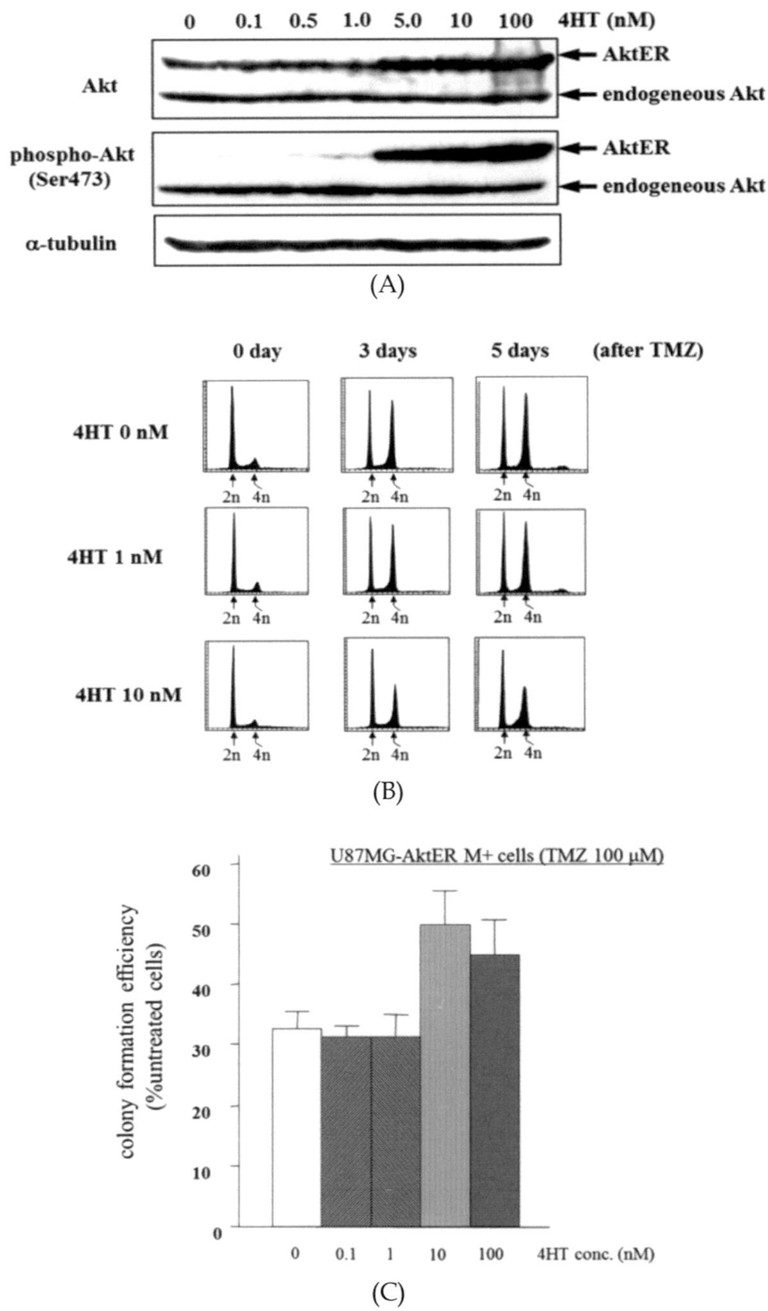

Fig. 8. Akt over-activation in U87MG-AktERM+ cells (A) and its effect on TMZ-induced cell cycle arrest (B) and cytotoxicity (C)

overexpression in U87MG-E6 cells suppressed not only TMZ-induced G2 arrest and loss of clonogenicity but also the percentage of cells undergoing death by mitotic catastrophe following TMZ exposure. These results suggest that Akt overexpression, whereas suppressing TMZ-induced G2 arrest, also protects cells from loss of clonogenicity caused by induction of senescence and mitotic catastrophe.

In summary, the results showed that Akt activation suppresses the G2 checkpoint by selectively altering activation of the DNA damage signal transducer Chk2 and the downstream effectors of the G2 checkpoint. The overriding effect of Akt activation, however, is suppression of TMZ-induced senescence and mitotic catastrophe in cells that avoid G2 arrest. The Akt pathway may therefore contribute to TMZ resistance in the clinical setting.

It is interesting to note that most high-grade human gliomas have high levels of Akt activation, which are believed to be a consequence of PTEN deletion. Given the role Akt plays in moving cells through the G2 checkpoint and in suppressing TMZ-induced cytotoxicity, it seems likely that an analysis of Akt pathway activation in gliomas before therapy may help identify those individuals for whom TMZ-based therapies are most likely to succeed. Similarly, strategies combining TMZ with inhibitors of the Akt pathway may enhance the likelihood of success. Because Akt overexpression has also been reported to increase the mutagenicity of agents that induce G2 arrest, presumably by promoting cell survival in the absence of genuine DNA repair, strategies designed to suppress Akt may contribute not only to improved tumor cell kill but also to suppression of unwanted mutagenic effects which might otherwise contribute to secondary malignancies.

6. Molecular chaperone 90kD heat shock protein

As reviewed above, several ways to potentiate the cytotoxicity of TMZ have been reported, and thus many pathways can be targeted in an effort to sensitize tumor cells to chemotherapeutic agents. A molecular chaperone, 90kD heat shock protein (hsp90) has recently attracted attention as a sensitizing agent because it is expressed at 2–10-fold higher levels in tumor tissue than in normal tissue, and is associated with many proteins (termed client proteins) involved in cell cycle regulation, cell survival and oncogenesis. Taken together, these studies indicated that many hsp90 client proteins are involved in cytoprotective mechanisms against cellular stressors such as DNA damage, suggesting that hsp90 might be important in the survival of tumor cells after exposure to DNA-damaging chemotherapeutic agents. Therefore we hypothesized that hsp90 inhibitors might act as antitumor agents against gliomas and might potentiate the cytotoxicity of DNA-damaging agents.

To investigate this hypothesis, we used 17-AAG, a geldanamycin derivative, as a pharmacological inhibitor of hsp90 and examined whether an hsp90-targeted strategy could be useful for chemosensitizing glioma cells to the DNA-damaging agents BCNU, cisplatin, and TMZ (Ohba et al., 2010).

The clonogenicity of cells treated with cisplatin, BCNU, or TMZ was depressed with 17-AAG. This 17-AAG–induced potentiation of the effects of these chemotherapeutic agents was recognized at a lower concentration than that needed to induce cytotoxicity with 17-AAG alone, and was more remarkable in the cisplatin- and BCNU-treated cells than in the

TMZ-treated cells. Isobologram analyses revealed that the interactions between 17-AAG and cisplatin or BCNU were synergistic, whereas the interaction between 17-AAG and TMZ was no more than additive (Figure 9).

The FACS analyses revealed that the population of cells with a sub-G1 DNA content was increased by combined treatment with 17-AAG and either cisplatin or BCNU; furthermore, the combined treatment remarkably increased the number of annexin V-positive and PI-negative cells. These results demonstrated that the 17-AAG- induced enhancement of the DNA crosslinking agents-induced cytotoxicity was either associated in part or entirely with an increase in apoptotic cell death.

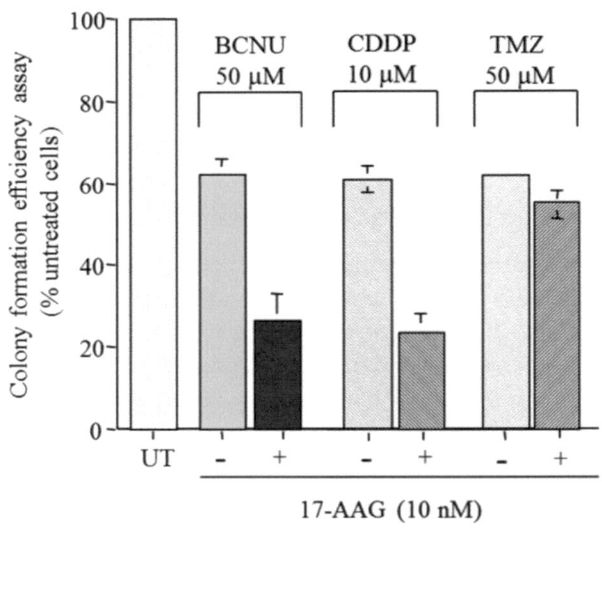

Fig. 9. Effect of Hsp90 inhibitor 17-AAG on cytotoxicity induced by various DNA damaging agents.

A reasonable concern is that hsp90 inhibitors may act not only on tumor cells, but also on normal cells; however, the authors of previous studies have shown that hsp90 is expressed at 2–10-fold higher levels in tumor than in normal tissue, and that hsp90 derived from

tumor cells has a 100-fold higher binding affinity for the hsp90 inhibitor 17-AAG than does hsp90 derived from normal cells. These data suggest that the effect of hsp90 inhibitors on normal cells may be much smaller than that on tumor cells and that an hsp90 inhibitor might therefore be useful for selectively killing tumor cells.
The mechanism of the 17-AAG–induced enhancement of the cytotoxicity of DNA-crosslinking agents has not yet been completely elucidated, and suppression of other survival-promoting factor(s) could be involved in enhancement of DNA-damaging agents, however.

7. Conclusion

We reviewed our studies focusing chemosensitization of gliomas. We propose that combination of conventional chemotherapy using DNA-damaging agents and molecular targeted therapy could be a potentially useful new antiglioma therapeutic strategy. However, enhancement of the effect of chemotherapeutic agents clearly depends on the mechanism by these compounds exhibit cytotoxicity. Therefore the development of a safe and effective therapeutic regimen will require further investigation

8. References

Hirose, Y., Berger, M. S. & Pieper, R. O. (2001a). p53 Effects Both the Duration of G2/M Arrest and the Fate of Temozolomide-treated Human Glioblastoma Cells. *Cancer Res*earch Vol. 61, No.5 (March 2001), pp1957-1963, ISSN 0008-5472

Hirose, Y., Berger, M. S. & Pieper, R. O. (2001b). Abrogation of the Chk1-mediated G2 Checkpoint Pathway Potentiates Temozolomide-induced Toxicity in a p53-independent manner in Human Glioblastoma Cells. *Cancer Res*earch Vol. 61, No.15 (August 2001), pp5843-6849, ISSN 0008-5472

Hirose, Y., Katayama, M., Stokoe, D., Haas-Kogan, D. A., Berger, M. S. & Pieper, R. O. (2003). The p38 Mitogen-activated Protein Kinase Pathway Links the DNA Mismatch Repair System to the G2 Checkpoint and to Resistance to Chemotherapeutic DNA-methylating Agents. *Molecular and Cellular Biology,* Vol.23, No.22 (November 2003), pp8306-8315, ISSN 0270-7306

Hirose, Y., Katayama, M., Mirzoeva, O. K., Berger, M. S. & Pieper, R. O. (2005). Akt Activation Suppresses Chk2-mediated, Methylating Agent-induced G2 Arrest and Protects from Temozolomide-induced Mitotic Catastrophe and Cellular Senescence. *Cancer Research* Vol.65, No.11 (June 2005), pp4861-4869, ISSN 0008-5472

Ohba. S., Hirose, Y., Kawase, T. & Sano, H. (2009). Inhibition of c-Jun N-terminal kinase enhances temozolomide-induced cytotoxicity in human glioma cells. *Journal of Neuro-oncology,* Vol.95, No.3 (December 2009), pp307-316, ISSN 0167-594X

Ohba, S., Hirose, Y., Yoshida, K., Yazaki, T. & Kawase, T. (2010). Inhibition of 90-kD heat shock protein potentiates the cytotoxicity of chemotherapeutic agents in human glioma cells. *Journal of Neurosurgery,* Vol.112, No.1 (January 2010), pp33-42, ISSN 0022-3085

Stupp, R., Mason, W. P., van den Bent, M. J., Weller, M., Fisher, B., Taphoorn, M. J., Belanger, K., Brandes, A. A., Marosi, C., Bogdahn, U., Curschmann, J., Janzer, R. C., Ludwin, S. K., Gorlia, T., Allgeier, A., Lacombe, D., Cairncross, J. G., Eisenhauer, E. & Mirimanoff, R. O. (2005). Radiotherapy Plus Concomitant and Adjuvant Temozolomide for Glioblastoma. *New England Journal of Medicine,* Vol.352, No.10 (March 2005), pp987-996, ISSN 0028-4793

5

Prognostic Significance of Immunohistochemical Markers in Glioma Patients

Tadej Strojnik
University Clinical Center Maribor
Slovenia

1. Introduction

Gliomas are the most common form of brain tumors, contributing to more than half of the incidence of brain tumors. They are derived from three basic types of glial cells: astrocytes, oligodendrocytes and ependymal cells. The most frequent are diffusely infiltrating astrocytomas, further classified into astroytomas (A), anaplastic astrocytomas (AA) and glioblastoma, equivalent to World Health Organization (WHO) grade II, II and IV, respectively (Kleihues & Cavenee, 2000). The term glioblastoma is used synonymously with glioblastoma multiforme (GBM), which suggests, the histopathology of this tumor is extremely variable (Kleihues & Cavenee, 2000). GBM is the most common and lethal type of astrocyte-derived tumor, corresponding to 50% of adult primary brain tumor cases, followed by anaplastic astrocytoma (30%) and astrocytoma (20%) (Greenberg, 2010). GBM may develop from astrocytoma or anaplastic astrocytoma (secondary GBM), but more frequently they manifest after a short clinical history *de novo*, without any evidence of a less malignant precursor lesion (primary GBM) (Farhadi & Rutka, 2008). Although primary brain tumors are relatively rare compared with carcinomas, they are characterized by higher mortality rates and increased disability. The overall annual incidence rate of primary malignant and benign brain tumors in developed countries is approximately 15 per 100,000 individuals, and for primary malignant brain tumors it is 7 per 100,000 (Minn et al., 2008). Brain tumor incidence and mortality have increased by up to 300% over the past 3 decades primarily in people aged over 75 years (Davis et al., 1996 as cited in Minn et al., 2008; Wrensch et al, 1993 as cited in Minn et al., 2008).

Malignant gliomas are among the most challenging of all cancers to treat successfully. The tumor cells vigorously invade surrounding tissue, which renders complete surgical resection difficult and contributes to the high incidence of the recurrence (Merzak et al., 1995). Invasion of glioma cells into adjacent brain tissue is dependent on their interaction with the extracellular matrix (ECM) and possible destruction of matrix barriers (Pilkington, 1994). Tumor cells at the invasive front have to detach from the primary tumor mass and re-attach to ECM components or to surrounding tissue elements. In general, invasiveness may result in deformation and destruction of the brain architecture which leads to the fatal outcome for the patient. Proteolytic modification of ECM components, such as laminin and fibronection, is believed to facilitate the invasive spread of tumor cells (Gladson, 1999; Goldbrunner et al., 1999). Lysosomal cysteine cathepsins have been implicated in tumor progression. Proteolytic enzymes, including cahtepsins (Cats), mediate the invasion process, either acting alone or participating in proteolytic cascades (Schmitt et al., 1992; Sloane et al., 1994). Increased activity of proteolytic enzymes is observed during brain tumor progression (Frosch & Sloane, 1998; Levičar et al., 2003). Cathepsins are responsible for intracellular protein turnover and are vitally important for normal cell and organ development. The activity of the cysteine cathepsins can be regulated at various levels, ultimately by their endogenous inhibitors (Lah & Kos, 1998; Calkins & Sloane, 1995). In brain tumors, down-regulation of the total inhibitory activity of cystatins has been observed, presumably contributing to tumor malignancy (Sivaparvathi et al., 1996a).

In addition, tumor growth is critically dependent on blood supply and the development of new capillaries. In the case of tumor cell-induced angiogenesis, endothelial cells invade surrounding tissue in a process similar to that observed for tumor cells (Paku, 1998).

Human GBM also contains a various amounts of brain tumor stem-like precursor cells (BTSC) (Singh et al., 2003), which indicates a hierarchical model of tumorigenesis. The BTSCs display self-renewal potential, ex vivo multipotency and, most importantly, the ability to establish and expand the tumor in vivo. Moreover, genetic analyses of the BTSC in various patients have revealed distinct patterns of up-regulated genes, including patient-specific genes expression (Galli et al., 2004).

Despite recent advances in neuro-imaging, neurosurgical resection techniques and the development of novel adjuvant therapies, the long-term survival of patients suffering from malignant glioma remains low. Although treatment with temozolomide and radiotherapy improved median survival after diagnosis of GBM from 12 months to 14 months (Kalkanis & Rosenblum, 2008), the survival rate still ranges from a few months to several years, which, together with the poor prognosis, points the need for new, independent prognostic factors that may enable individualized treatment modalities, including molecular based therapies, of patients with unfavourable prognosis. Our studies are aimed to reveal differential expression and compare the prognostic significance of potential biological markers in glioma patients.

2. Immunohistochemical investigation of human gliomas

High-grade gliomas often demonstrate immunoreactivity for various markers. Such biologic markers could be used to assess the patient prognosis and may thus provide the new information regarding the time of glioma recurrence. In recent years we investigated the possible prognostic significance of different biological markers. The particularity of present report is the fusion of author's clinical work with his own experimental studies on animal models.

2.1 The animal models for experimental studies of human malignant brain tumors

The objective of experimental neuro-oncology is to contribute to a better understanding of human malignant brain tumors (Wechsler et al., 1989). To this end, the development of several animal models has provided specific clues about the formation of gliomas (Pilkington et al., 1997). Such animal models are also beneficial for selective molecular and biochemical analyses of tumor markers (Brem & Sawaya, 2004).

Previously, either commercial cell lines derived from human GBM or multicellular tumor spheroids from human gliomas have been used as a model for the study of brain tumor invasion (Bjerkvig et al., 1990; Engebraaten et al., 1999). Since all these cell types can grow in vitro, the cultures must be characterized to ascertain the cell subpopulations which have been selected through the culture conditions. Morphological characterization is not sufficient and a panel of markers may be required to define the populations present. However, as the cells adapt to the tissue culture conditions, they may lose the ability to express one or more of these markers. The need for better and more relevant brain tumor models is generally acknowledged.

2.1.1 U87 human glioblastoma cell xenografts in rat brains and on the chicken chorioallantoic membrane

The objective of our experimental work was to develop a simple and cheap animal model, with high tumor take rate, for brain tumor progression studies (Strojnik et al., 2006; Strojnik et al., 2010). A tumorigenesis model was presented, originating from tumor spheroids prepared from U87 human glioblastoma cell line, in the brain of rats and on the chick chorioallantoic membrane (CAM). U87 cells are considered to be a rapidly proliferating cell line, which can be grown in culture as monolayers and tumor spheroids. The U87 cell suspension, or precultured U87 tumor spheroids, was inoculated into the brain of 4-week-old rats and on CAM on embryonic day seven.

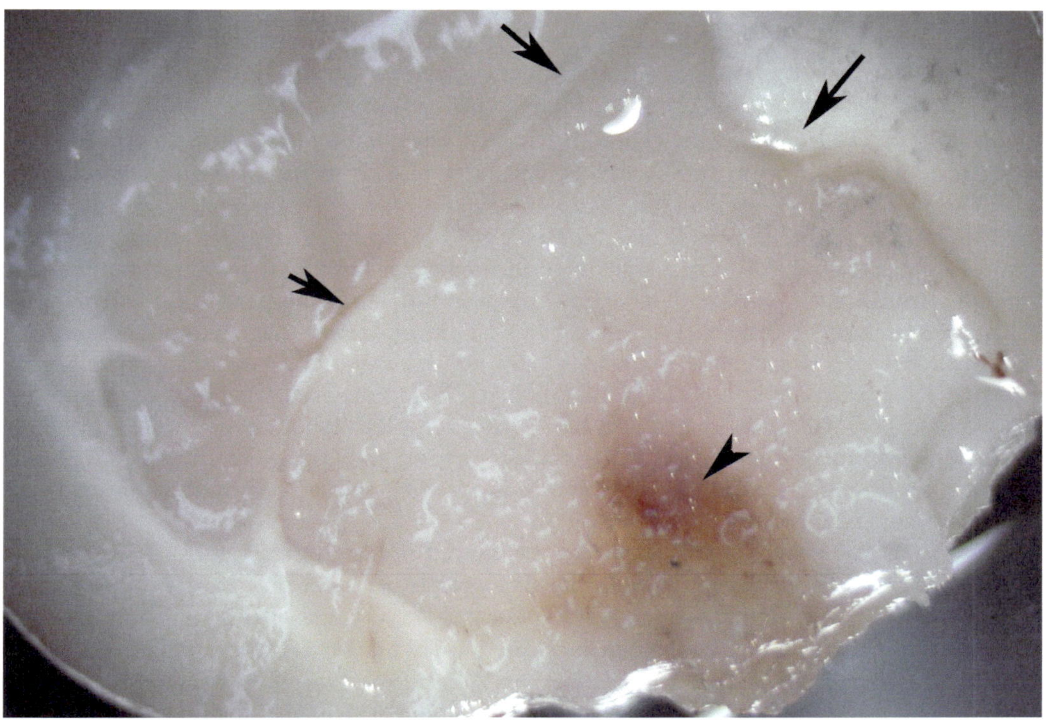

Fig. 1. Coronal rat brain tissue sections demonstrated solid, well demarcated, grayish tumor with an area of hemorrhage (arrow).

The resulting first generation tumors that were induced in rats were also transferred through serial transplantations from rat to rat, to obtain second and third generation tumors. The macroscopic tumor appearance, histopathology and immunohistochemistry of selected relevant tumor progression markers were monitored in U87 human glioblastoma cells xenografted into the brain of rats. In accordance with other reports, maximum progressive tumor growth was observed after 2 - 3 weeks (Wechsler et al., 1989). According to the WHO classification of human brain tumors (Kleihues & Cavenee, 2000), the transplantation tumors demonstrated features of anaplastic astrocytic tumor (WHO grade III), but become increasingly similar to glioblastomas (WHO grade IV) in the second and third generations. Parallel to this progression, increasing neovascularization and tumor necrosis was observed, both characteristic of glioblastoma. The benefits of inoculation of pre-cultured small tumor spheroids have been well described (Bjerkvig et al., 1990; Engebraaten et al., 1999). However, it should be stressed that spheroids from a biopsy specimen consist of heterogeneous cell populations, e.g. vascular elements (endothelial cells, pericytes), other mesenchyme-derived cells (fibroblasts) and microglia (a type of differentiated tissue macrophage) (Bressler et al, 1985; Badie & Schartner, 2001), requiring more careful characterization of the cellular composition of the inoculated spheroids when interpreting the resulting tumor behavior. In contrast, U87 cell-inoculated tumors have a relatively isomorphos cellular composition, due to their clonal origin, and further tumor development can be followed during subsequent generations, with respect to dedifferentiation of the tumor cells and induced recruitment of stromal cells from the tumor microenvironment (Mueller & Fusenig, 2004). The panel of marker protein expressions were followed in the first, second and third generations of tumors.

Anyway, the rodent models are somewhat limited by costs, experimental duration, variability and major ethical concerns, as well as by the difficulty of obtaining morphological data during tumor progression, resulting in large numbers of animals required to obtain conclusive results (Hagedorn et al., 2000). Another system consists of a human tumor grown in a xenogeneic host, the chick embryo. Consequently, we developed a tumorigenesis model, originating from the U87 human glioblastoma cell line, on the CAM, a densely vascularised extra-embryonic tissue (Strojnik et al., 2010). A few studies in chick embryos have been undertaken by others, but the primary focus was to demonstrate metastatic potential and not local invasiveness (Chambers et al., 1990; Ossowski & Reich, 1980). Our study aimed to compare the expression of various immunohistochemical markers of U87 cells and spheroids in culture and in rat brain with those grown on the CAM membrane. The macroscopic tumor appearance, histopathology and immunohistochemistry of selected relevant tumor progression markers were monitored in U87 human glioblastoma cells xenografted on the chick embryo CAM. In accordance with other reports, tumor growth was observed and well established tumors were seen after seven days in the CAM model.

There were few differences in histological appearance between tumor models. In both tumor models, the full range of cytological features of human glioblastomas were observed, including astrocytes, small anaplastic cells, spindle cells and giant cells. In rats, tumors were more sharply demarcated from the surrounding brain, while on CAM, tumor nodules grew, with smaller groups of tumor cells growing apart from the gross tumor mass. These cells were usually within the connective tissue with some also attached to the vessel walls. This might be the result of how the tumor cells initially seeded upon inoculation; however, it may possibly mean that this model is more suitable for studying tumor invasiveness.

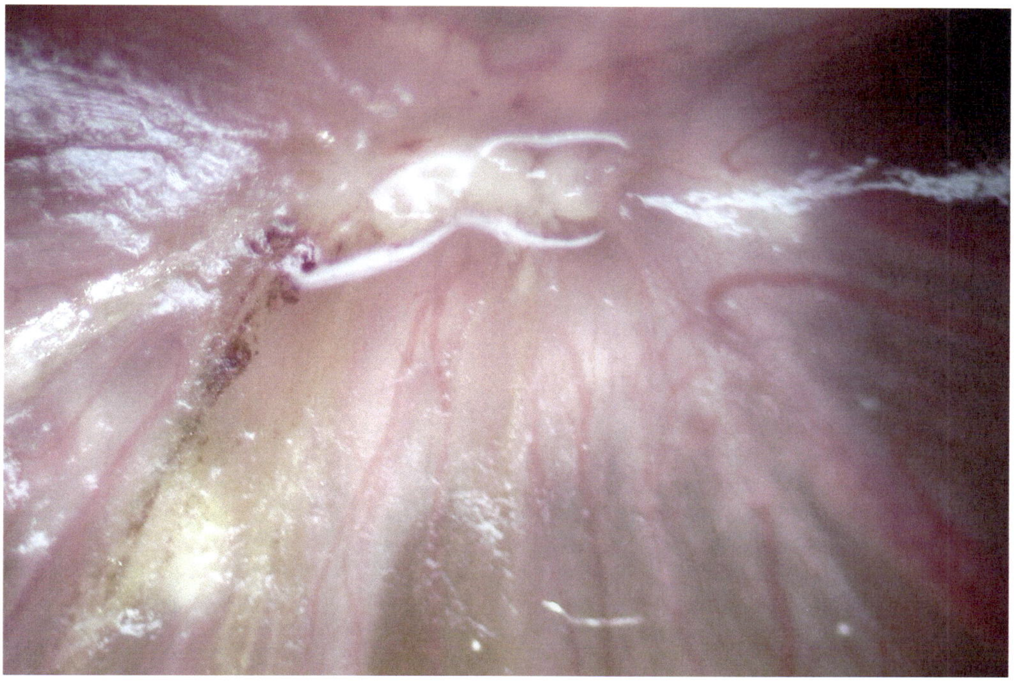

Fig. 2. Tumor nodules were seen on CAM one week after inoculation of U87 cells. Note small satellite tumors apart from the main tumor mass

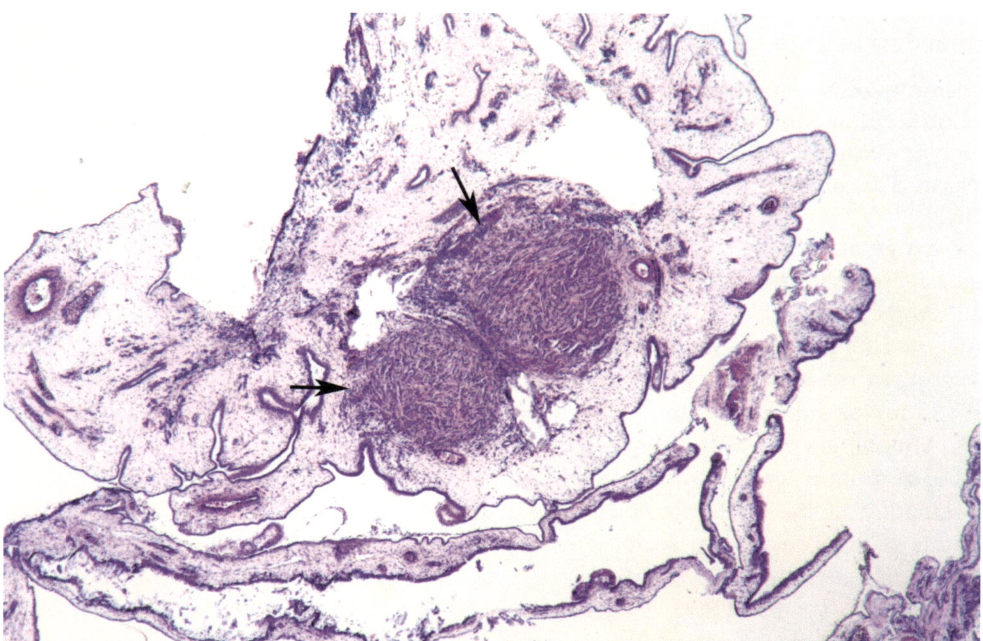

(a)

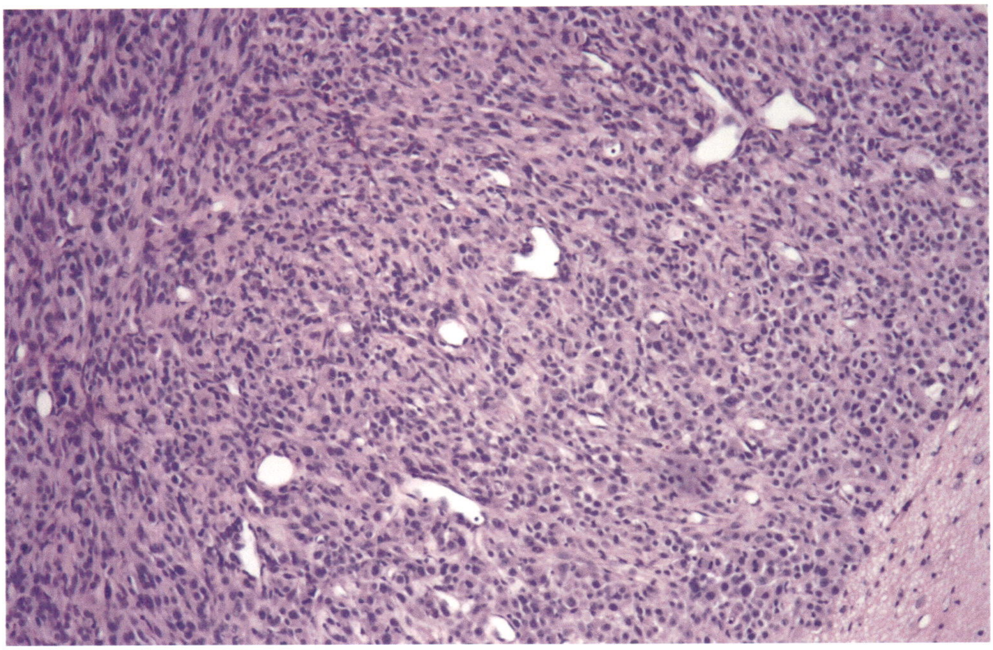

(b)

Fig. 3. Within the CAMs, loosely connective tissue with blood vessels two tumor nodules can be seen (arrows) (H&E, x4) (a); all tumors in rats were sharply demarcated against the surrounding brain tissue (H&E, x40) (b)

The immunohistochemical staining of animal samples was performed for Ki-67, p53, vimentin, glial fibrillary acidic protein (GFAP), S100, CD3, CD20, synaptophysin, cathepsin B, cathepsin L, CD68, vascular endothelial growth factor (VEGF), and leukocyte esterase. The staining of rat brain sections for nestin, musashi and kallikrein 6 was also done.

Ki-67 antigen expression is a measure of the proportion of cellular and, hence, biological aggressiveness in malignancy (Scott et al., 1991; Wilson et al., 1996). The index of proliferation, Ki-67 LI, was high in all samples, but the fraction of Ki-67-positive cells was higher in U87 cell suspension and in rats compared to the spheroids and CAM tumors, indicating increased proliferation in the rat model of tumorigenicity.

The *p53* tumor suppressor gene is frequently mutated in glioblastomas (Newcomb et al., 1993). Mutations within the *p53* gene often results in aberrant expression of the p53 protein, leading to protein accumulation within the nucleus of the cells. The p53 protein is involved in regulation of the cell cycle and it has been speculated that the presence of abnormal amounts of p53 protein is associated with increased rates of proliferation (Cunningham et al., 1997). It was found that the percentage of p53-positive nuclei, which was higher in the tumors grown on the CAM than on rats, did not correlate with the Ki-67 LI. Other researchers have also reported little correlation between this pair of immunohistochemical markers (Cunningham et al., 1997; Balčiūnienė et al., 2009).

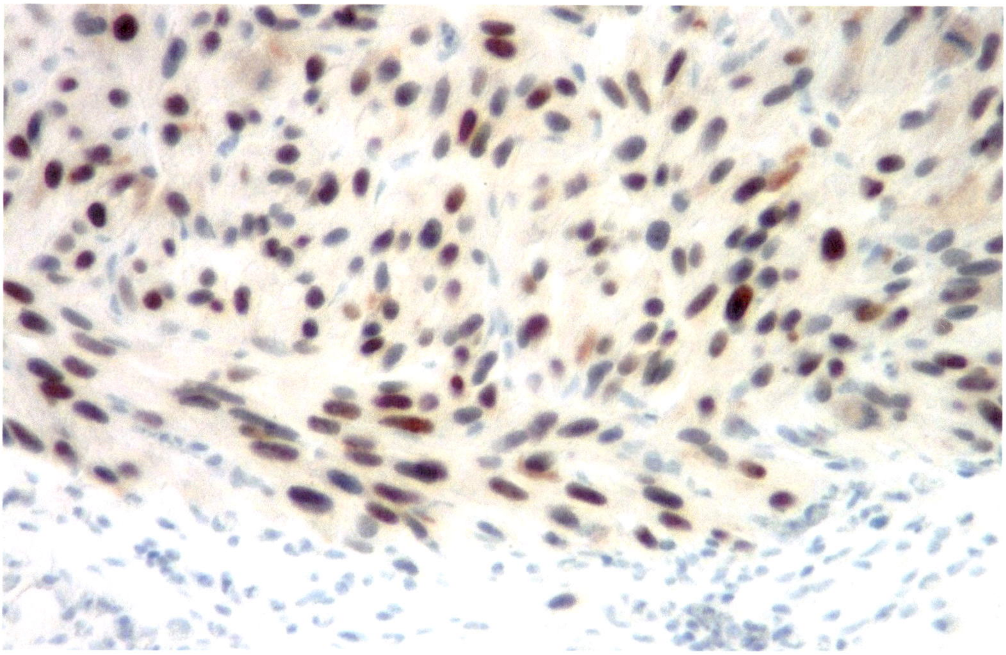

Fig. 4. In tumor grown on CAM many nuclei stained positively for p53 (x40)

Vimentin is an intermediate filament protein, which marks the mesenchymal cell phenotype. In the course of development of the nervous system, vimentin appears first in immature glial cells (Dahl et al., 1981), but rapidly decreases as glial fibrillary acidic protein (GFAP) appears concomitantly with myelination (Dahl, 1981). In mature astroglia, vimentin and GFAP coexist, and normal, reactive and neoplastic astrocytes have been found to contain variable amounts of both (Yung et al., 1985). In our works (Strojnik et al., 2006; Strojnik et al., 2010) it was revealed that high production of vimentin by the tumor cells was preserved in the host in both animal models, thus showing that the U87 clone consists of immature cells. Due to strong and specific staining of the tumor cells, it facilitated visualization of satellite tumors and migrating tumor cells away from the main tumor mass.

GFAP is mostly restricted to mature astrocytes (Lazarides, 1982). In human malignant gliomas, co-expression of GFAP and vimentin has been reported (Herpes, 1996). This was not the case in the animal models used in our study (Strojnik et al., 2010). Although the U87 cell suspension presented a moderate immune reaction for GFAP, this was completely absent from the induced tumors. This does not necessarily mean that a cell is of non-glial origin, but the ability to synthesize GFAP after further dedifferentiation of the U87 cells in the host is gradually lost.

The S100 family of calcium-binding proteins contains approximately 16 members, each of which exhibits a unique pattern of tissue/cell type-specific expression. Although the distribution of these proteins is not restricted to the nervous system, the implication of several members of this family in nervous system development, function, and disease has sparked new interest in these proteins. Different forms of malignant tumors exhibit dramatic changes in the expression of S100 proteins (Sedeghat & Notopoulos, 2008; Sen & Belli, 2007). Only moderate S100 immunoreactivity was detected in the U87 cell suspension and weak expression in the spheroids. Tumors in both animal models were S100 negative, which can be explained by the possible down-regulation of S100 expression following tumor dedifferentiation (Bressler et al., 1985).

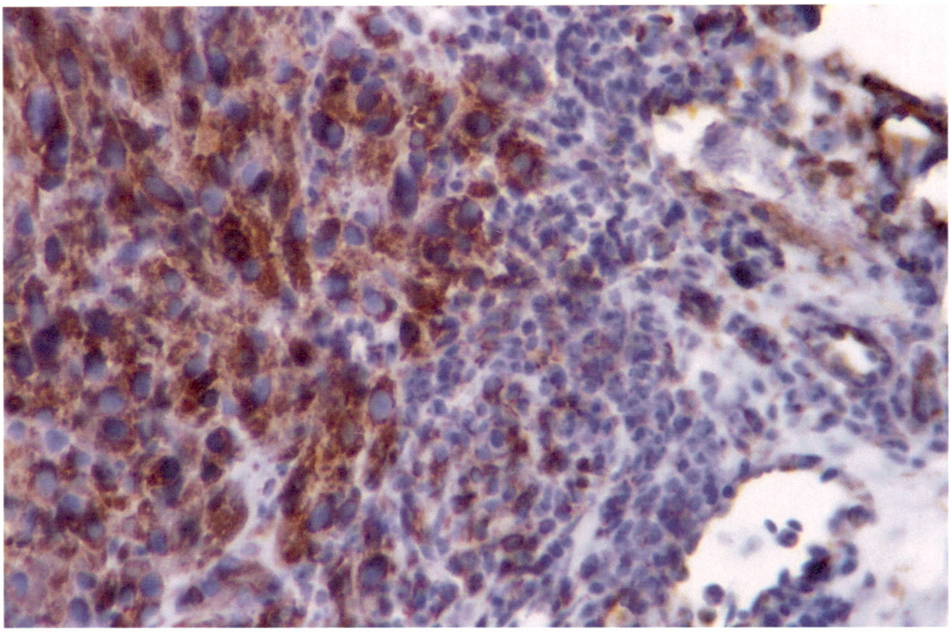

Fig. 5. All of the CAM tumor cells presented a strong and specific immune reaction for vimentin. Vessel walls stained positively for vimentin also (x40)

CD3 is a marker of T lymphocytes. Heterologous transplantation of human tumor cells into animals inevitably leads to immunological response of the host. Cytotoxic T lymphocytes have been implicated as the effectors cell mediating graft rejection (Bierer et al., 1985). Only small numbers of CD3-positive cells were seen in tumor grown on CAM, whereas in rats more CD3-positive cells were seen indicating that some sort of immune response is also present in this immunoincompetent hosts or that these CD3-positive cells might be "T-like" cells, but not actual T-cells, which adopted T lymphocytes phenotype during the dedifferentiation. As expected, no CD3-positive cells were observed in suspension, neither in spheroids nor outside the tumor in the host.

CD20 is expressed on all stages of B cell development, except the first and the last stages. It is also found on skin melanoma cancer stem cells (Fang et al., 2005). No CD20-positive cells were detected in any of the models used in our study. This might be partially explained by the fact that neither B lymphocytes nor antibodies in the circulation nor in the graft itself are required for first-set graft rejection (Hall et al., 1978).

Synaptophysin is a reliable marker for the identification of normal neuroendocrine cells and neuroendocrine neoplasm (McKeever, 1998). Only weak staining was observed in some of the tumor cells in suspension and in spheroids, but no staining was observed in animal tumor models, indicating that tumors induced by U87 clone underwent further dedifferentiation in the host. In humans, pure glial tumors do not usually express synaptophysin.

As expected, our study found strong Cat B staining in culture and in all of the animal models, where not only tumor cells but also endothelial cells stained positively for Cat B. Interestingly, stronger staining for Cat B in tumors was noted in rats than in chicken embryos. This could partially be explained by the relative ease of spreading of the tumor cells in the loose connective tissue of the CAM compared to the brain where more proteolytic activity is needed. We found Cat L staining in tumor cells in culture and in both animal models. Stronger staining for Cat L in tumors was noted in chicken than in rats. Staining with Cat L antibody revealed strong reaction in tumor cells, but there was no staining in the vascular endothelia. Stronger Cat L staining has been noted in the tumor centre, indicating slightly different roles of two cysteine proteases (Cat B and Cat L) in local invasiveness and in the malignant transformation of brain tumor cells.

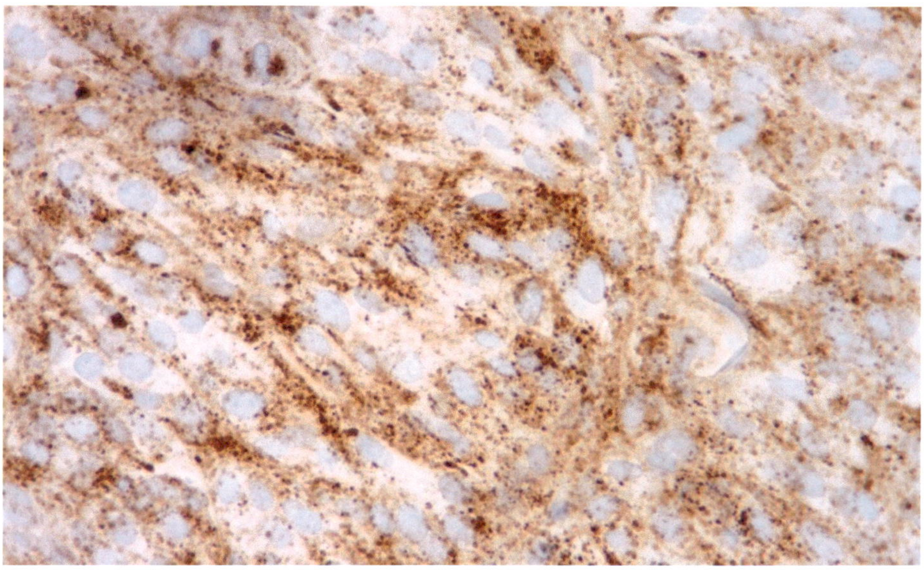

Fig. 6. Strong immunostaining for Cat B was noted in all samples, especially in rats. Vascular endothelia also stained positive for Cat B (40x)

CD68 is a specific marker for macrophage and also resting microglia (Hulette et al., 1992). Considered as immune effector cells of the CNS, the microglia represent a major component of the inflammatory cells found in malignant gliomas (Badie et al., 1999). In accordance to others (Leenstra et al., 1995) our studies also found strong CD68 expression in U87 human glioblastoma cell suspension, in U87 spheroids, as well as in rat and chick embryo U87 tumors (Strojnik et al., 2006; Strojnik et al., 2010). They stained for CD68 in the same way as macrophages do. Again, only minor differences in CD68 expression between animal models were noted. In accordance with the strong immune reaction for CD68 in all our samples we believe, that tumor cells adopted macrophage phenotype due to dedifferentiation.
Vascular endothelial growth factor (VEGF) is a potent mitogen specific for vascular endothelial cells and may directly stimulate the growth of new blood vessels (Leung et al., 1989). Angiogenesis is induced by tumor cell hypoxia and pro-angiogenetic factors (Hendriksen et al., 2009). Both brain tumor models showed only low VEGF expression. The slightly higher levels of vascular endothelial proliferation seen in rat tumors may be

explained by the likelihood of greater hypoxia associated with larger tumor size. It is well known that hypoxia is a potent VEGF trigger.

Leukocyte esterase is an enzyme present in most white blood cells. Neutrophils are present in glioblastoma tissue and not limited to necrotic areas. Researchers reported correlation between tumor grade and the extent of the neutrophil infiltration (Fossati et al., 1999). Their role in glioma progression remains unclear. Extensive leukocyte infiltration was observed in the brain tumor models in our study (Strojnik et al., 2010). This might partially be explained by the fact that xenotransplant acts as a foreign body in both animal models, and perhaps that esterase acts similarly to cathepsins thus contributing to the degradation of extracellular matrix.

Nestin has been detected in primary CNS tumors (Dahlstrand et al., 1992). We showed that nestin could be used as a biological marker for glioma malignancy (Strojnik et al., 2007). Contrary to the weak nestin expression of the U87 clone in cell cultures, immunostaining was absent in the spheroids. A switch to further dedifferentiation in the host might explain the moderate staining in the first generation tumors induced by inoculation of U87 cells or spheroids, as well as in the second and third generations of tumors induced by implantation of tumor tissue. The U87 cell suspension presented a weak immune reaction for musashi and, in contrast to nestin, its expression increased in the tumor cells as the tumor progressed, perhaps related to their malignant growth and dedifferentiation.

Tissue kallikreins have recently been strongly associated with tumor progression (Diamandis et al., 2004). Most of the tumor cells in suspension, spheroids and in tumors of all three generations presented a strong immune reaction for kallikrein 6, whereas the expression in the vascular endothelia of the tumor and in the surrounding brain was weak or absent. Normal and edematous rat brain tissue showed weak expression of kallikrein. Strong kallikrein 6 immunostaining in the U87 cell suspension and in tumors induced by injection of spheroids and implantation of tumor tissue indicated the role of kallikrein in tumor growth.

In conclusion, both animal models, the U-87 human glioblastoma spheroid cell line inoculated in rats or onto the chick embryo CAM, provide a good system for experimental studies of human malignant brain tumors. The panel of marker protein expression was followed in animal tumors. The data from rat study indicated that tumor progression was characterized by increased cell proliferation and tumor cell dedifferentiation, but lower invasiveness of the resulting tumors. Increased angiogenesis indicated high malignancy of the higher tumor generation. Data from the comparison of a panel of immunohistochemical markers between the CAM and rat models indicates that tumor protein expression in the CAM model is sufficiently similar to the rat model. We believe that the chick embryo CAM model is a good alternative to rodent brain tumor models. Anyway, both models may provide the basis for multigenetic and multimolecular glioma tumor cell analyses. They also have a potential use in testing individualized therapies.

2.2 Immunohistochemical staining and prognostic impact of biological markers in glioma

More than hundred patients with primary tumor of central nervous system (CNS), operated at our institution were studied. The histological slides of all cases were reviewed and classified according to the WHO classification of brain tumors (Kleihues & Cavenee, 2000). Patients' clinical and radiological data were collected, including age, sex, date and type of initial operation, clinical neurological examination, computer tomography (CT) features and data of adjuvant therapy. For the survival analyses the follow-up data were registered. Immunohistochemical staining was performed using the standard technique (Strojnik et al, 1999; Strojnik et al., 2005). The staining for markers was scored separately for the tumor cells, the endothelial cells, and/or the macrophages, as described previously (Strojnik et al, 1999; Strojnik et al., 2005; Strojnik et al., 2007; Strojnik et al., 2009). IHC staining was performed for various marker including cathepsins B and L, nestin, musashi, CD68, kallikrein 6 and Ki-67. Statistical analysis was performed using the program Statistica for Windows 6 (StatSoft, Inc., Tulsa, OK, USA). Overall survival probabilities were calculated by the Kaplan-Meier Method (Kaplan & Meier, 1958, as cited in Strojnik et al., 1999); log-rank test was used to evaluate the association between survival and each of the selected markers.

It is unique that the panel of markers was tested on the same group of patients. The fact is that many published biomarker studies in gliomas investigate one, two or maybe three potential markers in their tumor samples. In our successive investigations of numerous markers we were working on the same group of glioma patients, what enables us to compare the prognostic significance of different tumor markers.

2.2.1 Cysteine proteinases cathepsins B and L

Endopeptidases, including cystein proteinase cathepsin (Cat) B, are suggested to be useful prognostic factors in many types of cancer (Lah & Kos, 1998). McCormick first found that Cat B is abundantly secreted in human gliomas in vitro as a latent zymogen requiring activation (McCormick, 1993). Cat B expression at the protein and mRNA levels was later shown to correlate with the malignant progression of gliomas (Rempel et al., 1994; Sivaparvathi et al., 1995). The first immunohistochemical (IHC) study on Cat B in gliomas was performed by Mikkelsen et al. (Mikkelsen et al., 1995), which not only confirmed such an association, but also found high Cat B expression in endothelial cells of new vasculature within the tumors.

In our study we have demonstrated that cathepsin B is expressed in glial tumor cells, macrophages near vessels adjacent to necrotic area, and proliferative endothelial cells of primary tumors of the CNS (Strojnik et al., 1999). Significantly more cases with high Cat B IHC score in tumor and in endothelial cells were observed in malignant compared with benign tumors.

Our results confirm the previous IHC study (Sivaparvathi et al., 1995) which showed more frequent and intense immunostaining for Cat B in more malignant forms of brain tumors. Similarly, another group (Mikkelsen et al., 1995) found the highest Cat B IHC score in GBM, compared with anaplastic astrocytoma and normal brain. Moreover, both groups reported heterogeneity in the staining intensity and its regional distribution, with the proliferative tumor margin staining more intensely than the tumor core. Researchers (Rempel et al., 1994) also observed altered subcellular localization of Cat B. They found Cat B expression to correlate with increased histological and radiological evidence of invasion (Rempel et al., 1994), which is consistent with the strong association of Cat B with the clinical and histological paramaters, indicating advanced tumors in our study. There is, thus, in general agreement that brain tumor progression is associated with increased expression of Cat B in tumor cells (Strojnik et al., 1999). Cat B immunostaining in proliferative endothelial cells was first reported by Mikkelsen et al., 1995, although Cat B immunostaining was lower in endothelial than in tumor cells, as we observed in benign tumors. However, endothelial cell-associated Cat B immunostaining was present in about two-thirds of malignant tumors, compared with less than one-tenth of the benign tumors. Different models of in vivo angiogenesis have been proposed (Paku, 1998) and, according to them, one may speculate that Cat B actively participates in the intracellular lumen formation within the endothelial cell and/or that the secreted forms of Cat B directly degrade the ECM proteins (Buck et al., 1992; Liotta et al., 1991). Irrespective of the mechanism, our data implicate Cat B with brain tumor-induced angiogenesis.

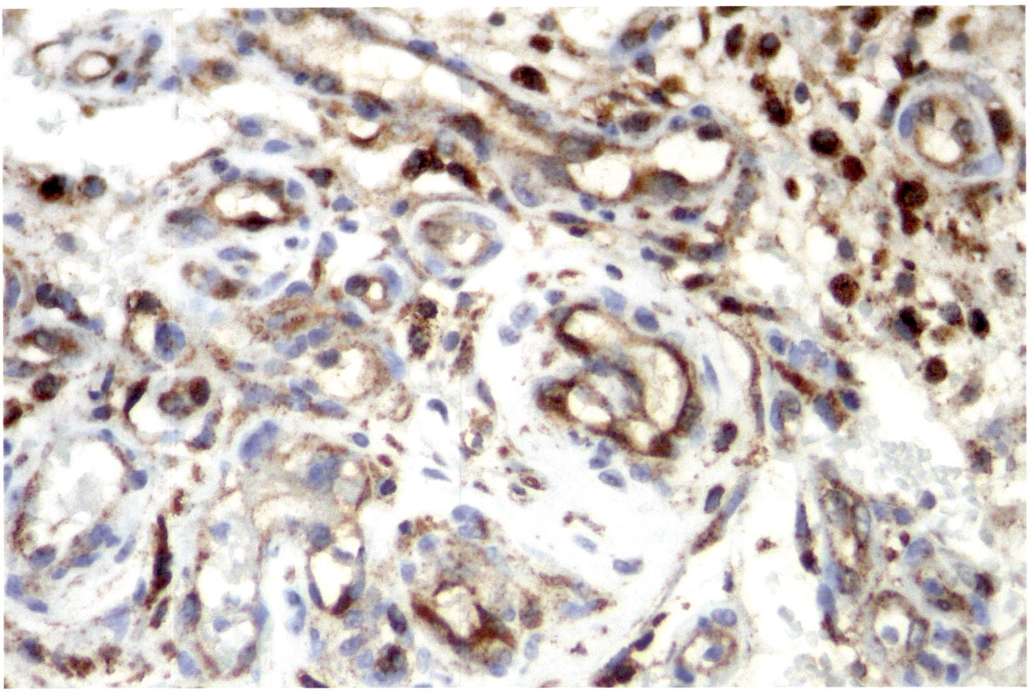

Fig. 7. Glioblastoma multiforme. Cat B antibody shows positively stained tumor cells and strong positive staining in endothelial cells (x40)

Our study (Strojnik et al., 1999) is the first clinical study on prognostic impact of Cat B in tumors of the central nervous system (CNS) and shows that the survival time is significantly longer in patients with low total immunostaining score, as compared with patients with strong staining. Intense Cat B staining of endothelial cells is prognostically important in patients with glioblastoma, indicating significantly shorter survival.

To summarize, we have demonstrated that immunostaining of cathepsin B correlated with high histological score and was significantly associated with poor clinical symptoms. The level of expression of cathepsin B in tumor and endothelial cells is a strong prognostic marker for primary tumors of the CNS. Intense immunostaining of cathepsin B in endothelial cells may be used to predict the survival of glioblastoma patients and, in addition, it indicates the involvement of cathepsin B in tumor-associated angiogenesis. These results suggest that the therapeutic application of cystein proteinase inhibitors should be targeted to both tumor and endothelial cells.

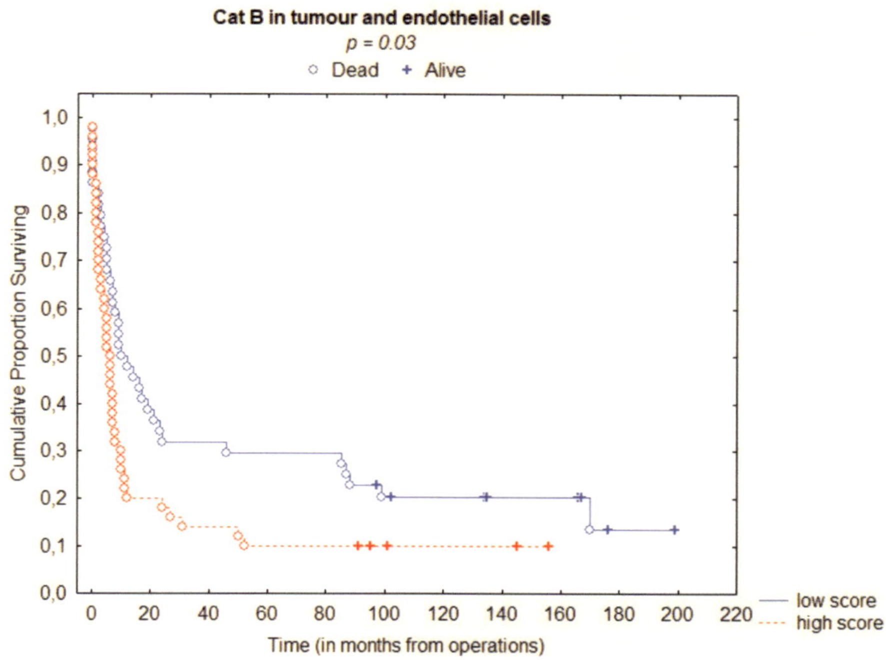

Fig. 8. Cat B in tumor and endothelial cells, and survival in all tumors

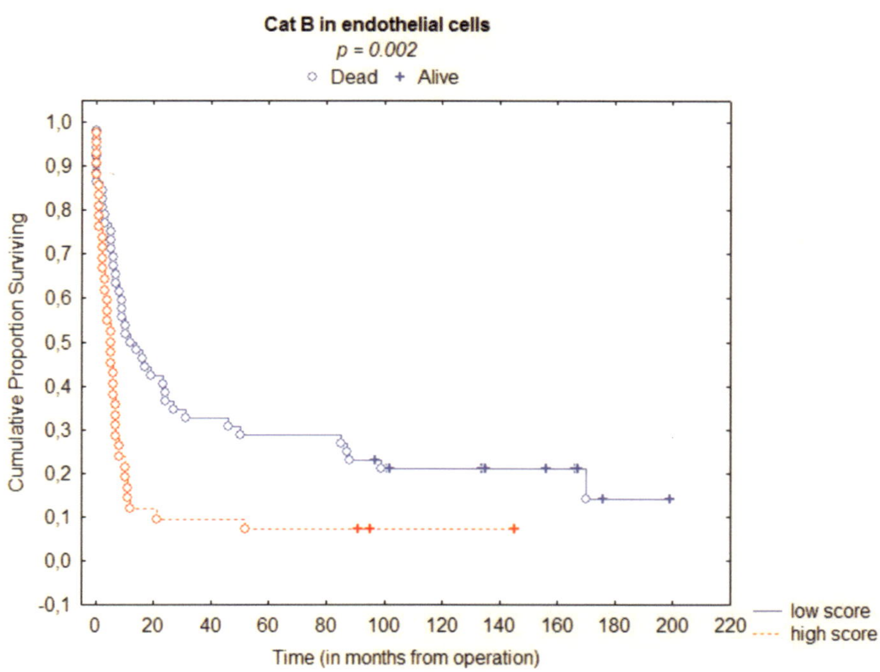

Fig. 9. Cat B in endothelial cells, and survival in glioblastoma multiforme

To complement our work we measured the expression of cathepsin L in the same population of human glioma patients (Strojnik et al., 2005). Cat L expression is also elevated in various types of human tumors (Lah & Kos, 1998) and its levels were prognostic for survival of patients with breast carcinoma (Thomssen et al., 1995). The only previous study of Cat L in brain tumor demonstrated that Cat L expression and activity correlated positively with increased malignancy of human glioma (Sivaparvathi et al., 1996b). We (Strojnik et al., 2005) have confirmed that in gliomas, cathepsin L is found predominantly in the malignant tumor cells. Cat B staining was expressed in both tumor and endothelial cells to the same extent. In contrast, Cat L was expressed significantly more in tumor cells than in the endothelilal cells. Although Cat L concentrations in all tumors appear to be lower than Cat B, we found significantly higher expression of Cat L in malignant than in benign gliomas. This implies a role for Cat L in malignant transformation of brain tumor cells. We also confirmed the correlation between immunostaining of Cat L in tumor cells and the histological score, i.e. the stage of glioma malignancy. Cat L and Cat B IHC staining correlated significantly. However, in contrast to Cat B (Strojnik et al., 1999), another study (Strojnik et al., 2005) did not reveal any prognostic value of Cat L, either in tumor or in endothelial cells.

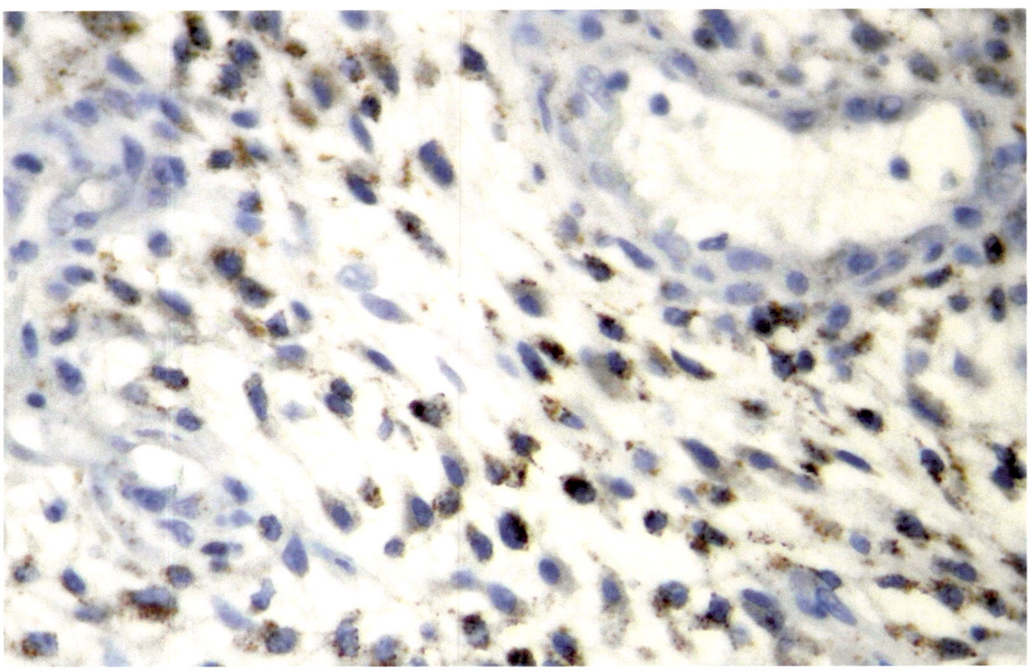

Fig. 10. Immunohistochemical staining of cathepsin L in glioblastoma multiforme (x40); Cat L antibody shows strong positive immunostaining in tumor cells but no staining in endothelial cells

In conclusion, Cat L is preferentially expressed in tumor cells, increasing with glioma progression, but is not significantly associated with new vasculature of glioblastoma. In contrast to Cat B, Cat L has no prognostic impact, suggesting different roles of the two cathepsins in glioma progression.

2.2.2 Neural stem cell markers nestin and musashi proteins

To identify other possible biological markers we studied nestin and musashi proteins, which are expressed by neural progenitor cells during CNS development. Nestin is an intermediate filament (IF) protein involved in the organization of the cytoskeleton, but it has also been implicated in cell signaling, organogenesis, and cell metabolism (Fuchs & Weber, 1994). Class VI IF nestin is expressed abundantly during early embryogenesis in neuroepithelial stem cells but is absent in most cells of the mature CNS (Lendahl et al., 1990). Nestin is down-regulated in mature cells (Steinert & Liem, 1990). It may be expressed in astrocytes of the adult CNS in response to cellular stress, such as neoplastic transformation (Dahlstrand et al., 1992; Tohyama et al., 1992). Nestin has been detected in primary CNS tumor but not in carcinoma metastases (Dahlstrand et al., 1992; Ikota et al., 2006).

The musashi family is an evolutionarily conserved group of neural RNA-binding proteins (Okano et al., 2002, as cited in Strojnik et al., 2007). Musashi 1 is selectively expressed in neural progenitor cells, including neural stem cells (Kaneko et al., 2000, as cited in Strojnik et al., 2007). Its expression is down-regulated with the progression of neurogenesis (Toda et al., 2001). The aim of our study (Strojnik et al., 2007) was to estimate the levels of nestin and musashi in tumor and endothelial cells of low- and high-grade gliomas with a view to correlate the levels to the histopathological score. A comparison was also made to the other prognostic markers, Cat B and L.

Recently, it has been reported that the immunohistochemical detection of nestin expression could be used as indicator of dedifferentiation and progression in astrocytomas (Ehrmann et al., 2005). Nestin is a useful marker for examining the infiltration of malignant cells into surrounding tissue (Kitai et al., 2010). In our study tumor cells from low-grade astrocytomas contain low levels of nestin and most high-grade gliomas express high levels of nestin (Strojnik et al., 2007).

It was proposed that nestin plays a role in tumor invasion of melanomas (Florenes et al., 1994, as cited in Strojnik et al., 2007). Nestin may therefore correlate with other markers of invasiveness, such as cysteine cathepsins B and L, which are both highly up-regulated in high-grade gliomas (Lah et al., 2000; Levičar et al., 2002; Sivaparvathi et al, 1995). In our study, a positive correlation between Cat B and nestin was established in high-grade gliomas, both markers correlating with the malignancy, as defined by histological scores. The exact location of nestin-positive cells was determined by mapping the distribution of nestin in highly invasive human glioma xenograft model. IHC staining of nestin in a xenograft model showed that nestin-positive cells are more abundant at the transition zone of the tumor, as reported for Cat B (Mikkelsen et al., 1995; Rempel et al., 1994). Given that invasion is associated with poor prognostic outcome for glioma patients, it is not surprising that nestin proved a very strong prognostic factor.

It is therefore reasonable to suggest that the switch to malignancy is associated with a significant increase of neural progenitor markers and with high expression of the invasive marker Cat B. Nestin expression correlated with lysosomal Cat L, which has been shown to be associated with glioma cell invasiveness but was not prognostic in our population of patients. This may be due to other biologic functions of Cat L associated, for example, with the cell cycle (Levičar et al., 2003) that may be less favorable for tumor progression. By multivariate Cox regression analysis, only nestin remained a good prognosticator of following variables: patients' age, sex, immunohistochemical scores in tumor and endothelial cells for nestin, cathepsin B and cathepsin L. In previous study (Strojnik et al., 1999), only univariate analysis was performed for Cat B staining in tumor cells, which

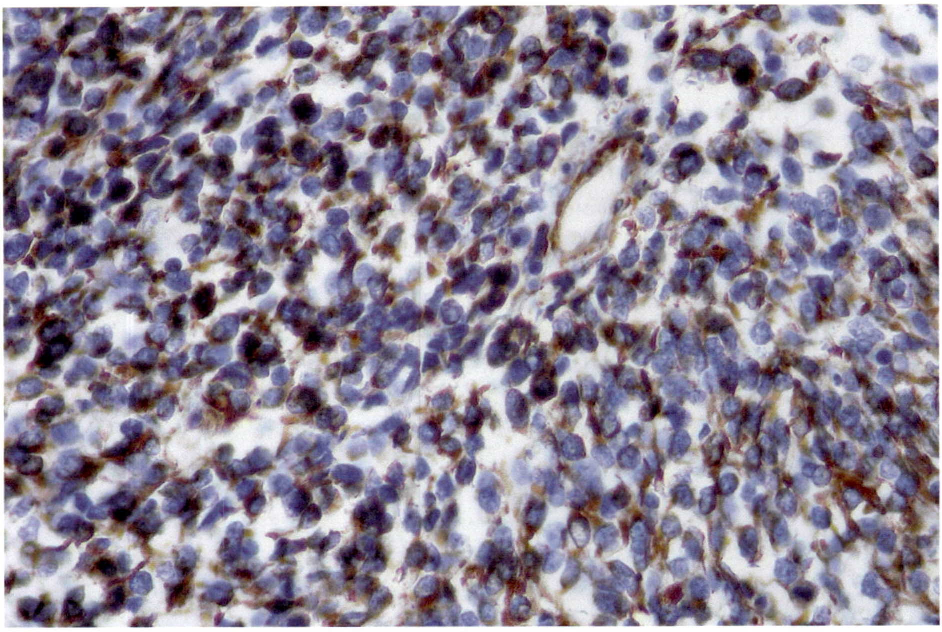

(a)

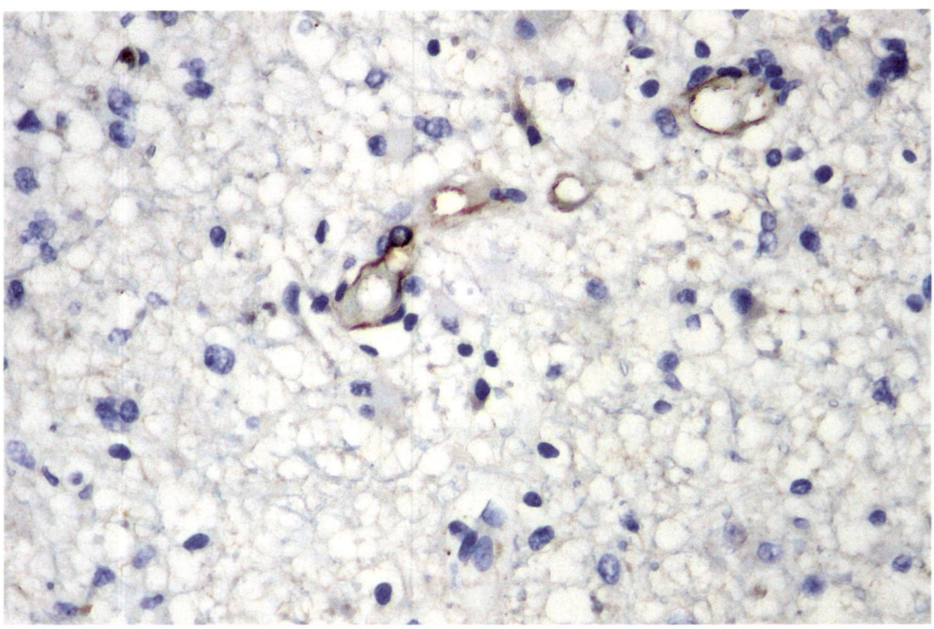

(b)

Fig. 11. Immunohistochemical staining of nestin protein in tumor and endothelial cells in glioblastoma (a) and astrocytoma (b). Intense staining of nestin is seen in the cytoplasm of tumors cells and is more abundant in the high (a) than in the low-grade (b) tumors. The IHC staining of nestin in endothelial cells was the same in the high- and low-grade groups.

showed prognostic significance ($p < 0.03$) but increased to $p < 0.003$ when both tumor and endothelial cells were considered. In multivariate analysis, it is not unusual, that one prognosticator falls out of the significance limits when compared simultaneously with much stronger prognosticator - in our case, the nestin.

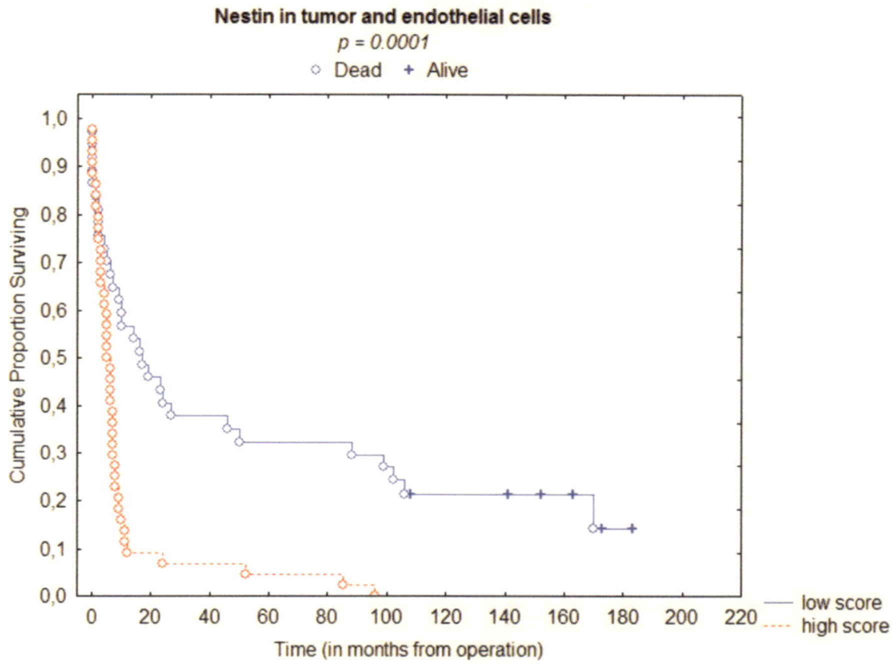

Fig. 12. Survival analyses. Patients stratified according to the median IHC score for nestin (high score or low score) in tumor and endothelial cells combined.

We have shown that the musashi protein is expressed, to a higher extent, in high-grade tumor cells than in those in the low-grade tumors. The expression of musashi was significantly weaker than that of nestin in tumor cells of the high-grade tumors (Strojnik et al., 2007). This differential expression pattern of the two neural progenitor cell markers in gliomas suggests that these two proteins may be stopped early (musashi) and late (nestin) in the BTSC "dedifferentiation" during GBM progression. Musashi is a marker of asymmetric cell division and is probably expressed as an early marker in stem/progenitor cell development. The fact that the musashi expression did not correlate with any prognostic factors may be related to the transformation process where the regulatory function of musashi is lost or changed. The difference in the prognostic impact of both stem cell markers is related to their different functions also. We hypothesize that these functions may be related to the invasiveness of possible stem/progenitor cell subpopulations. This is based on the observations that cathepsins, particularly Cat B - also the marker of glioblastoma cell invasiveness - strongly correlated with the nestin but not with the musashi expression.

It is noteworthy that Cat B and, to a lesser extent, Cat L, as well as nestin, were present in the endothelial cells. The cathepsins have been suggested to play a role in angiogenesis, possibly also assisting endothelial cell invasion during capillary formation (Caserman & Lah, 2004), particularly in GBM (Mikkelsen et al., 1995; Strojnik et al., 1999). Expression of Cat B, but not Cat L, in endothelial cells of high-grade tumors is significantly higher than in low-grade astrocytomas and can be used as a prognostic factor for GBM patients (Strojnik et al., 2005).

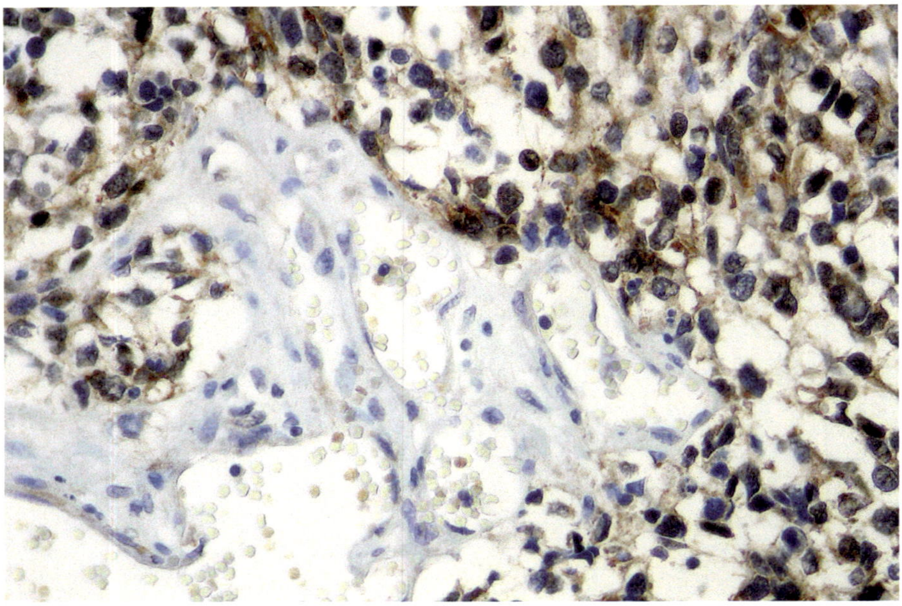

(a)

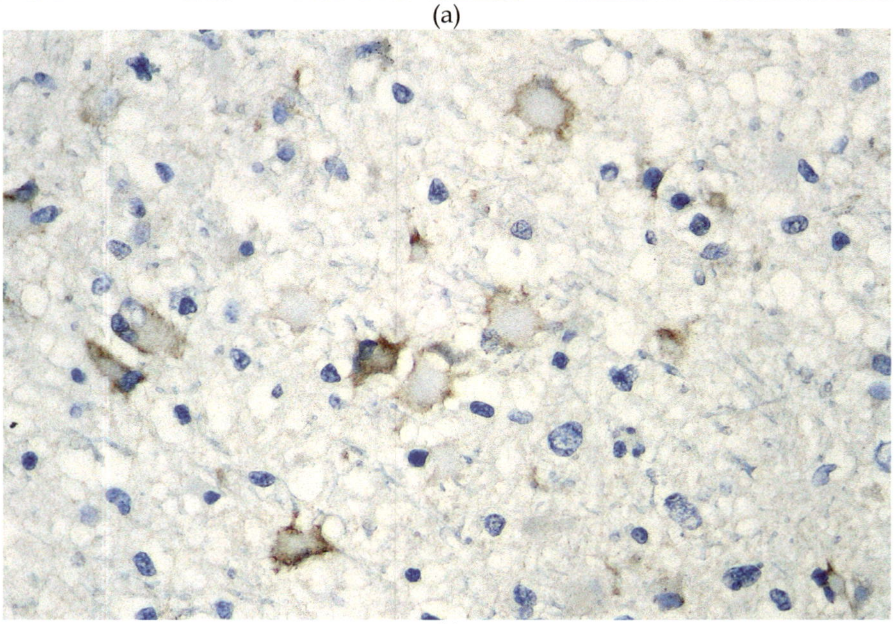

(b)

Fig. 13. Immunohistochemical staining of musashi protein in tumor and endothelial cells in glioblastoma (a) and astrocytoma (b). Musashi immunostaining was weak in endothelial cells of high-grade tumors.

Tumor angiogenesis may be initiated by various mechanisms, for example, "bursting" of new capillaries from the established blood vessels and by attracting angiopoietic stem cells from bone marrow. All the repertoire of protein markers for these stem cells is not known. As the musashi and nestin may be also the markers for the cancer-associated angiopoietic stem cells, we have also paid the attention to the fact that nestin, but, to a much lesser extent, the musashi, was indeed expressed in the endothelial cells. We showed that nestin was expressed in endothelial cells in both low- and high-grade tumors, whereas musashi was expressed only to a limited extent in endothelial cells in the high-grade tumors. We have therefore also estimated their potential impact on the prognosis. The latter was not found significant. However, the further research should confirm the hypothesis derived from our data, that is, that angiogenesis also may result predominantly from the bone marrow stem cells attracted to and differentiating onto blood vessels within the tumor.

On summary, we have confirmed that nestin is expressed in tumor cells and in endothelial cells of primary gliomas to a greater extent than musashi. In our clinical study on the prognostic impact of the neural progenitor cell markers nestin and musashi in tumors of the CNS, the high level of nestin, but not musashi, in tumor cells indicates significantly shorter survival of glioma patients. Intense immunostaining of nestin in tumor cells may be used to predict the risk of death in patients with malignant primary tumors of the CNS. Moreover, by multivariate analysis, nestin presents as the best prognosticator of all the variables. Our data links the invasive glioma cells to CNS precursor cells, indicating that the most malignant cells in the gliomas may well be closely related to the glioma stem cells.

2.2.3 Expression of kallikrein 6 and CD68 in human gliomas

Subsequent study (Strojnik et al., 2009) was designed to evaluate the expression of kallikrein 6 and CD68 in human glioma, and investigate their prognostic significance for survival of brain cancer patients in comparison to previous established prognostic markers.

Kallikreins are expressed by secretory epithelial cells of many organs and have been implicated in a range of normal physiological functions. Some of the kallikreins are known for their clinical application as cancer biomarkers: for example kallikrein 3, which is known as prostate-specific antigen (PSA), is one of the best available biomarkers for monitoring tumor burden in sera of prostate cancer patients and has also been evaluated as a marker for prostate cancer diagnosis and prognosis (Loeb & Catalona, 2007). In vitro data and animal experiments have indicated the role of kallikreins in several steps of tumor progression, such as tumor growth, invasion and metastasis, as well as increased angiogenesis (Borgoño et al., 2004; Borgoño & Diamandis, 2004; Lundwall et al., 2006).

Kallikreins are also widely distributed in various areas of the human brain (Raidoo et al., 1996). It has been suggested that the functional role of kallikreins is to assist in the normal turnover of brain proteins and the processing of peptide hormones, neurotransmitters and nerve growth factors that are essential for normal neuronal function and synaptic transmission (Borgoño et al., 2004; Borgoño & Diamandis, 2004). Kallikrein 6 is among the members of the kallikrein family with high levels of expression in the brain and related fluids (Yousef at al., 2003); however, knowledge of the expression of kallikreins by brain tumors is limited. The objective of our study (Strojnik et al., 2009) was to evaluate the possible prognostic impact of serine protease kallikrein 6 in gliomas. Kallikrein genes/proteins are aberrantly expressed in many cancer types and they may exert diverse and often contrasting effects on the tumor and its microenvironment. Therefore, high kallikrein expression has been associated with either poor or favorable patient prognosis.

Some members of the kallikrein family are listed among the group of tumor-protecting proteases (Lopez-Otin & Matrisian, 2007), but even a single kallikrein may have a dual role in tumor progression. We (Strojnik et al., 2009) demonstrated higher IHC expression of kallikrein 6 in tumor cells of benign human gliomas comparing to malignant tumors.

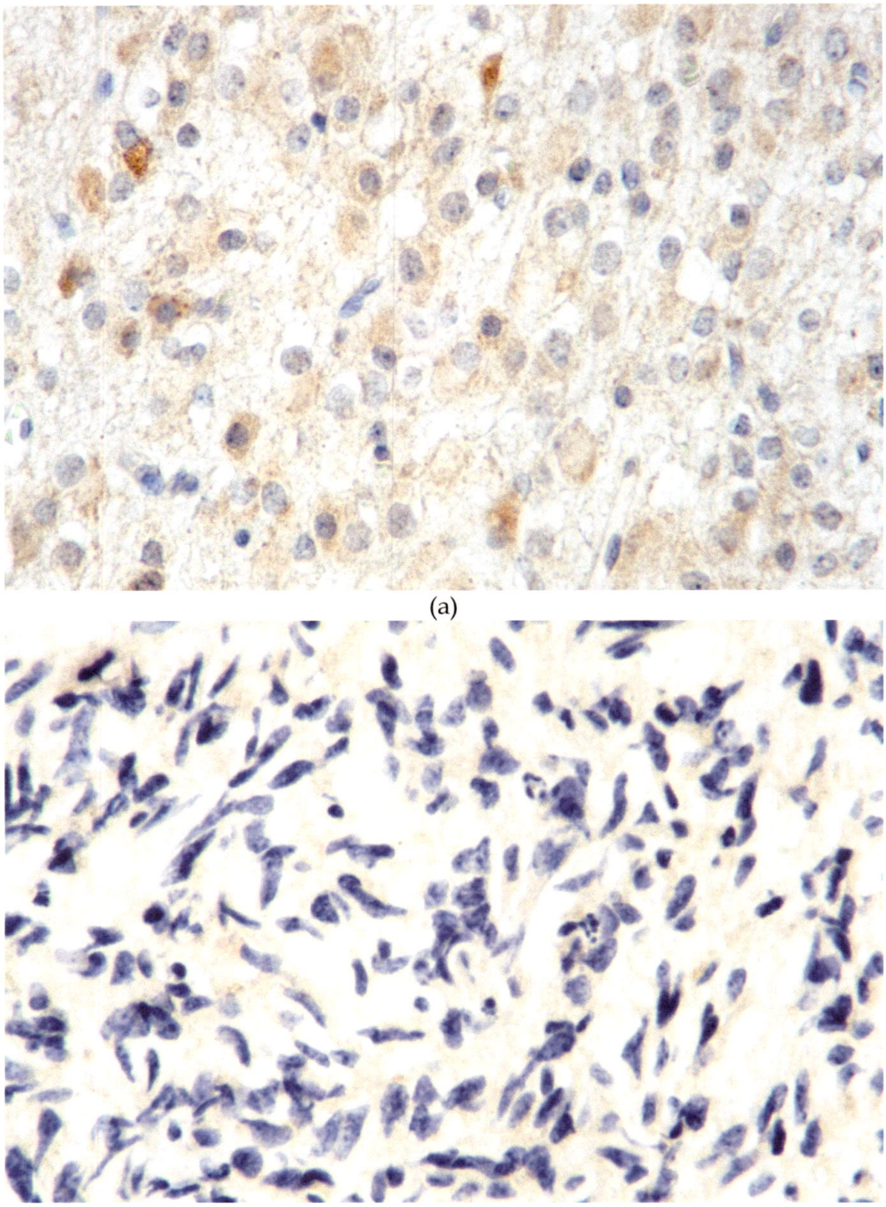

(a)

(b)

Fig. 14. Immunohistochemical staining of astrocytoma with kallikrein 6 antibody revealed strong immunostaining in tumor cells (a) while in glioblastoma staining was weaker (b)

Our data support a potential role of kallikrein 6 in suppression of glioma progression, however, a prognostic value of kallikrein 6 was not revealed by our study. The possibility of a dual role (pro- and antitumor) of kallikrein 6 in tumor growth cannot be overlooked. Clinical studies with larger patient populations are needed to allow further evaluation of kallikrein 6 function in glioma progression.

CD68 is a transmembrane glycoprotein, expressed by monocyte/macrophage lineages and serves as a marker for microglia (Hulette et al., 1992). Microglial cells function as resident immune cells and phagocytes in the CNS. In response to pathology, resident microglia follows a stereotyped pattern of first becoming activated and then phagocytic (Trapp & Herrup, 2004). On one hand, microglia may represent components of the antitumor immune response in the CNS, which is inactivated by local secretion of immunosuppressive factors by glioma cells. On the other hand, taking into account that microglia are capable of secreting a variety of immunomodulatory cytokines, they may be attracted by the gliomas to assist in tumor growth (Badie & Schartner, 2001; Graeber et al., 2002). In human glioma, intratumoral microglia density is higher than in peritumoral and normal brain, and microglia increase in number according to grade of malignancy (Roggendorf et al., 1996; Morris & Esiri, 1991). It has been evidenced that microglia accumulation in diffuse glial tumors does not merely represent a nonspecific reaction to tissue injury but reflects participation of these cells in supporting and promoting the invasive phenotype of astrocytoma cells (Bettinger et al., 2002).

Notably, tumor cells can occasionally be reactive to some macrophage markers (Leenstra et al., 1995). They investigated six specimens of cultured astrocytoma cells and reported that nine macrophage markers, including CD68, were clearly reactive in neoplastic astrocytes, whereas astrocytes in normal brain specimens were not reactive (Leenstra et al., 1995). This study suggested that the demonstration of macrophages within astrocytoma by using macrophage-specific antibodies alone must be cautiously considered. In accordance with quoted studies, we also found strong CD68 expression in tumor cells of U87 human glioblastoma cell suspension, in U87 spheroids (both prepared from the U87 human glioblastoma cell line without microglia), as well as in induced rat tumors (Strojnik et al., 2006). In our CD68 study (Strojnik et al., 2009) we considered the possibility that human malignant astrocytes may adopt a macrophage phenotype and aimed to evaluate the possible prognostic value of CD68 expression for the survival of brain tumor patients. Both microglia and tumor cells expressed CD68. High CD68 staining score was significantly more frequent in the malignant than in the benign tumors.

We evaluated the antigen expression of CD68 in glioma tissue by avoiding any region with necrosis and excluding foamy cells, possibly indicating the presence of macrophage. However, malignant astrocytoma cells were also highly CD68 positive, in accordance with another report (Leenstra et al., 1995). These authors further emphasized that there may be biological properties shared by macrophages and astrocytoma cells, such as phagocytosis and production of the same growth and angiogenic factors. These common properties may be explained: (a) by genetic alterations during malignant transformation of astrocytes; (b) by fusion of astrocytes with macrophages; or (c) by another, as yet unknown, mechanism of gene transfer during glioma progression (Leenstra et al., 1995). These may lead to significantly higher CD68 immunostaining of the malignant glioma.

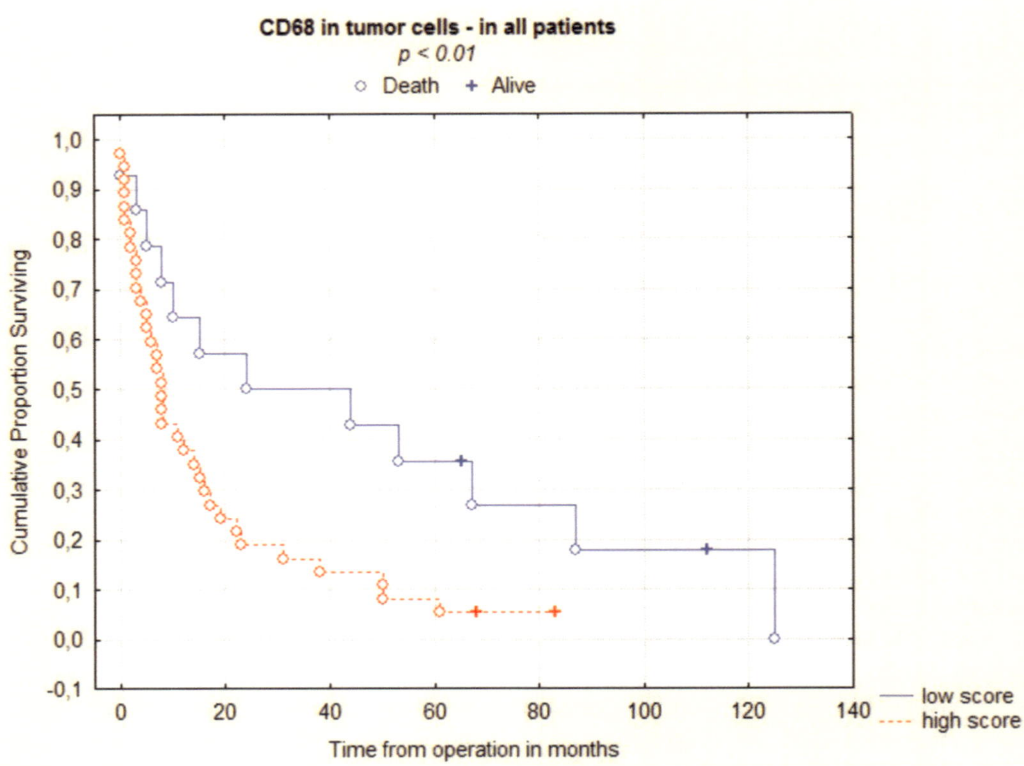

Fig. 15. Prognostic significance of immunolabeling for CD68 (low and high IHC score) for the survival of all patients with primary brain tumors

Survival analysis revealed that CD68 tumor staining has a prognostic value for glioma patients, comparable to that of cathepsin B. Within the malignant group, intense CD68 staining was marginally significant prognosticator for shorter survival. Notably, there was a significant prognostic value of CD68 tumor staining in the group of patients with anaplastic astrocytoma, which may be important for the management of patients with longer survival than these with glioblastoma. Further studies are necessary to investigate the possible mechanisms and consequence of macrophage phenotype expression of malignant astrocytomas, as well as possible role of microglia for tumor progression and patient prognosis.

To resume, kallikrein 6 was down-regulated in malignant glioma, but this differential expression did not have an impact on patient prognosis. In contrast, immunostaining of glioma tissue for CD68, as well as for Cat B and nestin, may be used as prognostic marker for survival of glioma patients. This finding suggests that besides the known role of Cat B in invasion and angiogenesis, nestin and CD68 may be also associated with glioma progression (Strojnik et al., 2007; Strojnik et al., 2009).

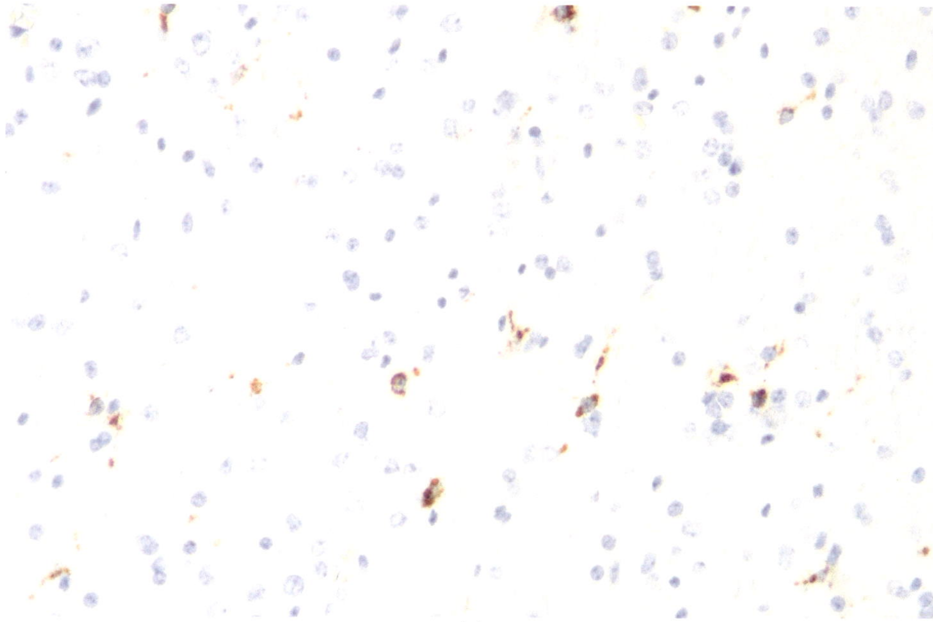

(a)

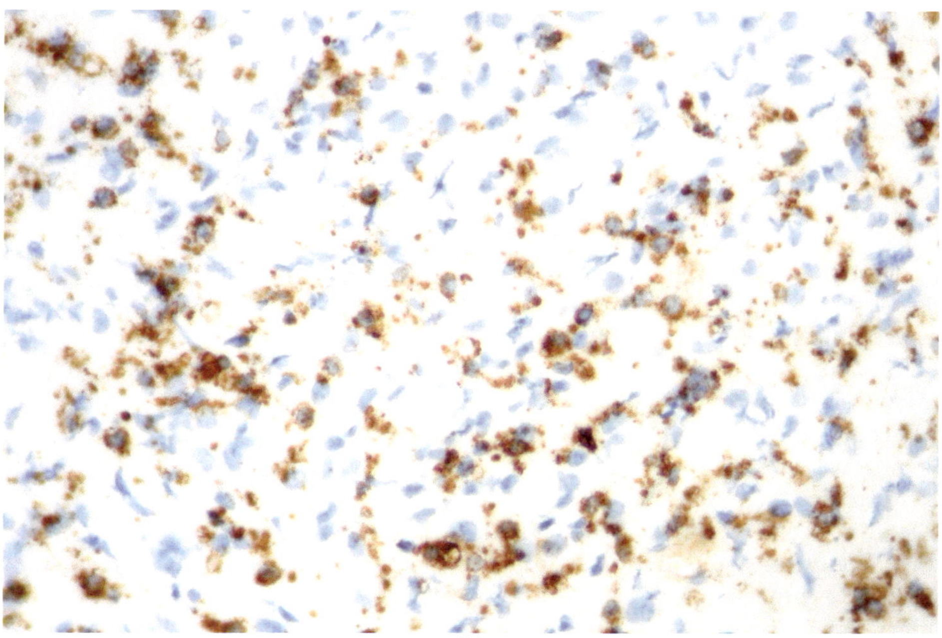

(b)

Fig. 16. Treatment of astrocytoma (x40) with CD68 antibody resulted in a few positively stained tumor cells (a); immunohistchemical staining of CD68 in glioblastoma multiforme (x40) revealed strong reaction in almost all tumor cells (b)

3. Conclusion

In recent years there have been many publications in the area of immunohistochemistry in brain tumor pathology (Takei et al., 2007; Dunbar & Yachnis, 2010; Ikota et al, 2006). Extensive molecular studies have identified diagnostic and prognostic markers in gliomas (Labussiere et al., 2010). They can assist in diagnosis, provide prognostic information and potentially predict response to therapy (Rivera & Pelloski, 2010). As we mentioned above, we combined the clinical work by different experimental glioma models. Animal tumor sections were examined for tumor markers by routine haematoxylin and eosin staining and immunohistochemical analyses. Established animal models provide a basis for further experimental studies of genetic and protein expression fingerprints during human glioma tumorigenesis. Furthermore, in a present paper we reviewed clinical and experimental work in glioma patients operated at our department of neurosurgery. Immunohistochemical studies supplement conventional H&E histology. Immunohistochemically we evaluated the expression of possible biological markers in human gliomas, including proteolytic enzymes (cathepsins B and L), neural stem cell markers (nestin, musashi), marker for microglia (CD68) and others (e.g. kallikrein 6). Differently from other reports, we performed immunohistochemical staining for the panel of markers on the same group of patients. Increased expression of lysosomal cystein proteinases such as cathepsins B and L plays a functional role in tumor cell migration and metastasis (Lah et al., 2000). We found that Cat B expression was highly elevated in GBM compared to lower grade malignant tumors and benign tumors. Cat B was also highly expressed in the endothelial cells of about two third of GBM. The latter finding indicates that Cat B may be associated with the invasion of not only tumor but also endothelial cells in the process of angiogenesis. At the end of the nineties we first published the clinical study on prognostic impact of Cat B in tumors of CNS, revealing that survival time in all patients with weak total immunostaining score is significantly longer compared to survival of patients with strong staining. Intense Cat B staining of endothelial cells is also prognostic important in patients with glioblastoma indicating significantly shorter survival. Cat L is preferentially expressed in tumor cells, increasing with glioma progression, but is not significantly associated with new vasculature of glioblastoma. Nestin is expressed in tumor cells of primary gliomas to a greater extent than musashi. Nestin-positive tumor cells are localized more abundantly in the transition zone of the tumor. Nestin is expressed in the endothelial cells in both low- and high-grade tumors, whereas musashi is expressed only to a limited extent in endothelial cells in the high-grade tumors. The further research should confirm the hypothesis derived from our data, that is, that angiogenesis also may result predominantly from the bone marrow stem cells attracted to and differentiating onto blood vessels within the tumor. Nestin is shown to be a strong prognostic marker for glioma malignancy. Our study revealed that both microglia and tumor cells expressed CD68. Malignant astrocytoma cells were highly CD68 positive in accordance to previous report (Leenstra et al., 1995). We found that some authors recommended to identify macrophages on intraoperative consulatiton to distinguish a neoplastic process from a demyelinating (or other destructive noneoplastic) disorder using IHC staining for CD68 (Dunbar & Yachnis, 2010). We point out that the demonstration of macrophages within the astrocytomas by using macrophage-specific antibodies alone must be cautiously considered. We further conclude that specific immunostaining of CD68 in tumor cells can be used to predict the risk of overall death in patients with glioma.

Noteworthy, we found prognostic value of CD68 immunostaining in tumor cells in anaplastic astrocytoma, which may be important for the management of patients with longer survival than these with GBM.

Taken together our data show that brain tumor progression is associated with increased expression of Cat B, Cat L, nestin and CD68 in tumor cells. We mentioned the role of Cat B and nestin in angiogenesis. IHC studies of biological markers provide important information about gliomagenesis. Biological marker can also assist in diagnosis. Immunohistochemistry has provided us with the ability to differentiate between tumors that are histologically indistinguishable. With this tool, we can now attribute the unpredictable behavior of what was once recognized as one tumor type to the more predictable behaviors of multiple tumors that are distinguishable based on their protein expression. The most challenged is to use findings for target therapy. Screening for the invasiveness of the individual brain tumor might help the neurosurgeon to define his strategy for further postoperative treatment of a given brain tumor.

4. References

Badie, B., Schartner, J.B.S., Klaver, J. & Vorpahl, J. (1999). In vitro modulation of microglia motility by glioma cells is mediated by hepatocyte growth factor/scatter factor. *Neurosurgery,* Vol.44, pp. 1077-1082

Badie, B. & Schartner, J.M. (2001). Role of microglia in glioma biology. *Microscopy Research Technique,* Vol.54, pp. 106-113

Balčiūnienė, N., Tamašauskas, A., Valančiūtė, A., Deltuva, V., Vaitiekaitis, G., Gudinavičienė, I., Weis, J. & von Keyserlingk, D.G. (2009). Histology of human glioblastoma transplanted on chicken chorioallantoic membrane. *Medicina (Kaunas),* Vol.2, pp. 123-131

Bettinger, I., Thanos, S. Paulus, W. (2002). Microglia promote glioma migration. *Acta Neuropathologica,* Vol.103, pp. 351-355

Bierer, B.E., Emerson, S.G., Antin, J., Maziarz, R., Rappeport, J.M., Smith, B.R. & Brakoff, S.J. (1988). Regulation of cytotoxic T lymphocyte-mediated graft rejection following bone marrow transplantation. *Transplantation,* Vol.46, pp. 835-839

Bjerkvig, R., Tønnesen, A., Laerum, O.D. & Backlund, E.O. (1990). Multicellular tumour spheroids from human gliomas maintained in organ culture. *Journal of Neurosurgery,* Vol.72, pp. 463-475

Borgoño, C.A., Michael, I.P. & Diamandis, E.P. (2004). Human tissue kallikreins: physiologic roles and applications in cancer. *Molecular Cancer Research,* Vol.2, pp. 257-280

Borgoño, C.A., & Diamandis, E.P. (2004). The emerging roles of human tissue kallikreins in cancer. *Nature Reviews Cancer,* Vol.4, pp. 876-890

Brem, H. & Sawaya, R. (2004). Brain tumours: general considerations. In: *Youmans Neurological Surgery,* H.R. Winn, (Ed.), pp. 659-660, W.B. Saunders, Philadelphia

Bressler, J., Smith, B.H. & Kornblith, P.L. (1985). Tissue culture techniques in the study of human gliomas, In: *Neurosurgery,* R.H. Wilkins, (Ed.), pp. 542-548, Mc Graw Hill, New York

Buck, M.R., Karustis, D.G., Day, A.N., Honn, K.V. & Sloane, B.F. (1992). Degradation of extracellular matrix proteins by human cathepsin B from normal and tumor tissues. *Biochemical Journal,* Vol.282, pp. 273-278

Calkins, C.C. & Sloane, B.F. (1995). Mammalian cysteine protease inhibitors: biochemical properties and possible roles in tumor progression. *Biological Chemistry Hoppe-Seyler,* Vol.376, pp. 71-80

Caserman, S. & Lah, T.T. (2004). Comparison of expression of cathepsin B and L and MMP2 in endothelial cells and in capillary sprouting in collagen gel. *The International Journal of Biological Markers,* Vol.19, No.2, pp.120-129

Chambers, A.F., Wilson, S.M., Tuck, A.B., Denhardt, G.H. & Cairncross, J.G. (1990). Comparison of metastatic properties of a variety of mouse, rat, and human cells in assay in nude mice and chick embryos. *In Vivo,* Vol.4, pp. 215-219

Cunningham, J.M., Kimmel, D.W., Scheithauer B.W., O'Fallon, J.R., Novotny, P.J. & Jenkins, R.B. (1997). Analysis of proliferation markers and p53 expression in gliomas of astrocytic origin: relationship and prognostic value. *Neurosurgery,* Vol.86, pp. 121-130

Dahl, D. (1981). The vimentin-GFAP protein transition in rat neuroglia cytoskeleton occurs at the time of myelination. *Journal of Neuroscience Research,* Vol.6, pp. 741-748

Dahl, D., Rueger, D.C. & Bignami, A. (1981). Vimentin, the 57,000 molecular weight protein of fibroblast filaments, is the major cytoskeletal component in immature glia. *European Journal of Cell Biology,* Vol.90, pp. 191-196

Dahlstrand, J., Collins, V.P. & Lendahl, U. (1992). Expression of the class VI intermediate filament nestin in human central nervous system tumors. *Cancer Research,* Vol.52, pp. 5334-5341

Diamandis, E.P., Yousef, G.M. & Olsson, A.Y. (2004). An update on human and mouse glandular kallikreins. *Clinical Biochemistry,* Vol.37, pp. 258-260

Dunbar, E. & Yachnis, A.T. (2010). Glioma diagnosis: immunohistochemistry and beyond. *Advances in Anatomic Pathology,* Vol.17, No.3, (May 2010), pp. 187-201

Ehrmann, J., Kolar, Z. & Mokry, J. (2005). Nestin as a diagnostic and prognostic marker: immunohistochemical analysis of its expression in different tumors.*Journal of Clinical Pathology,* Vol.58, pp. 222-223

Engebraaten, O., Hjortland, G.O., Hirschberg, H. & Fodstad, O. (1999). Growth of precultured human glioma specimens in nude rat brain. *Journal of Neurosurgery,* Vol.90, pp. 125-132

Fang, D., Nguyen, T.K., Leishear, K., Finko, R., Kulo, A.N., Hotz, S., Van Belle, P.A., Xu, X., Elder, D.E. & Herlyn, M. (2005). A tumorigenic subpopulation with stem cell properties in melanomas. *Cancer Research,* Vol.65, pp. 9328-9337

Farhadi, H.F. & Rutka J.T. (2008). Molecular markers and pathways in brain tumorigenesis, In: *Neurooncology, The Essentials,* M. Bernstein & M.S. Berger, (Eds.), pp. 32-38, Thieme Medical Publishers, Inc., ISBN 978-3-13-116332-5, New York, Stuttgart

Fossati, G., Ricevuti, G., Edwards, S.W., Walker, C., Dalton, A. & Rossi, M.L. (1999). Neutrophil infiltration into human gliomas. *Acta Neuropathologica,* Vol.98, pp. 349-354

Frosch, B.A. & Sloane, B.F. (1998). The role of proteolytic enzymes in brain tumor invasion, In: *Brain Tumor Invasion,* pp. 275-299, Wiley-Liss Inc., New York

Fuchs, E. & Weber, K. (1994). Intermediate filaments: structure, dynamics, function, and disease. *Annual Review of Biochemistry,* Vol.63, pp. 345-382

Galli, R., Binda, E., Orfanelli, U., Cipelletti, B., Grotto, A., DeVitis, S., Fiocco, R., Foroni, C., Dimeco, F. & Vescovi, A. (2004). Isolation and characterization of tumorigenic, stem-like neural precursors from human glioblastoma. *Cancer Research,* Vol.64, pp. 7011-7021

Gladson, C.L. (1999). The extracellular matrix of gliomas: modulation of cell function. *Journal of Neuropathology and Experimental Neurology,* Vol.58, pp. 1029-1040

Goldbrunner, R.H., Bernstein, J.J. & Tonn, J-C. (1999). Cell-extracellular matrix interaction in glioma invasion. *Acta Neurochirurgica,* Vol.141, pp. 295-305

Graeber, M.B., Scheithauer, B.W. & Kreutzberg, G.W. (2002). Microglia in brain tumors. *Glia,* Vol.40, pp. 252-259

Greenberg, M.S. (2010). *Handbook of Neurosurgery* (7th ed), Greenberg Graphics, Inc., Lakeland, Florida

Hagedorn, M., Javerzat, S., Gilges, D., Meyre, A., de Lafarge, B., Eichmann, A. & Bikfalvi, A. (2000). Accessing key step of human tumour progression in vivo by using an avian embryo model. *PNAS,* Vol.102, pp. 1643-1648

Hall, B.M., Dorsch, S. & Roser, B. (1978). The cellular basis of allograft rejection in vivo. *The Journal of Experimental Medicine,* Vol.148, pp. 878-889

Hendriksen, E.M., Span, P.N., Schuuring, J., Peters, J.P., Sweep, F.C., van der Kogel, A.J. & Bussink, J. (2009). Angiogenesis, hypoxia and VEGF expression during tumour growth in a human xenograft tumour model. *Microvascular Research,* Vol.77, pp. 96-103

Herpers, M.J., Ramaekers, F.C.S., Aldeweireldt, J., Moesker, O. & Slooff, J. (1996). Co-expression of glial acidic protein- and vimentin-type intermediate filaments in human astrocytomas. *Acta Neuropathologica,* Vol.70, pp. 333-339

Hulette, C.M., Downev, B.T. & Burger, P.C. (1992). Macrophage markers in diagnostic neuropathology. *American Journal of Surgical Pathology,* Vol.16, pp. 493-499

Ikota, H., Kinjo, S., Yokoo, H. & Nakazato, Y. (2006). Systematic immunohistochemical profiling of 378 brain tumors with 37 antibodies using tissue microarray technology. *Acta Neuropathologica,* Vol.111, pp. 475-482

Kalkanis, S.N. & Rosenblum, M.L. (2008). Malignant gliomas, In: *Neurooncology, The Essentials,* M. Bernstein & M.S. Berger, (Eds.), pp. 254-265, Thieme Medical Publishers, Inc., ISBN 978-3-13-116332-5, New York, Stuttgart

Kitai, R., Horita, R., Sato, K., Yoshida, K., Arishima, H., Higashino, Y., Hashimoto, N., Takeuchi, H., Kubota, T. & Kikuta, K. (2010). Nestin expression in astrocytic tumors delineates tumor infiltration. *Brain Tumor Pathology,* Vol.27, No.1, (April 2010), pp. 17-21

Kleihues, P. & Cavenee, W.K. (Eds.). (2000). *Pathology & Genetics Tumours of the Nervous System,* International Agency for Research on Cancer (IARC), ISBN 92-832-2409-4, Lyon

Labussiere, M., Wang, X.W., Idbaih, A., Ducray, F. & Sanson, M. (2010). Prognostic markers in gliomas. *Future Oncology,* Vol.6, No.5, (May 2010), pp. 733-739

Lah, T.T. & Kos, J. (1998). Cysteine proteinases in cancer progression and their clinical relevance for prognosis. *Biological Chemistry,* Vol.379, pp. 125-130

Lah, T.T., Strojnik, T., Levičar, N., Bervar, A., Zajc, I., Pilkington, G. & Kos, J. (2000). Clinical and experimental studies of cysteine cathepsins and their inhibitors in human brain tumors. *The International Journal of Biological Markers,* Vol.15, pp. 90-93

Lazarides, E. (1982). Intermediate filaments: a chemically heterogeneous, developmentally regulated class of proteins. *Annual Review of Biochemistry,* Vol.51, pp. 219-250

Leenstra, S., Das, P.K., Troost, D., de Boer, O.J. & Bosch, D.A. (1995). Human malignant astrocytes express macrophage phenotype. *Journal of Neuroimmunology,* Vol.56, pp. 17-25

Lendahl, U., Zimmerman, L.B. & McKay, R.D.G. (1990). CNS stem cells express a new class of intermediate filament protein. *Cell,* Vol.60, pp. 585-595

Leung, D.W., Cachianes, G., Kuang, W.J., Goeddel, D.V. & Ferrara, N. (1989). Vascular endothelial growth factor is a secreted angiogenic mitogen. *Science,* Vol.246, pp. 1306-1309

Levičar, N., Strojnik, T., Kos, J., Dewey, R.A., Pilkington, G.J. & Lah, T.T. (2002). Lysosomal enzymes, Cats in brain tumor invasion. *Journal of Neurooncology,* Vol. 58, pp. 21-32

Levičar, N., Nutall, R.K. & Lah, T. (2003). Proteases in brain tumor progression. *Acta Neurochirurgica,* Vol.145, pp. 825-838

Liotta, L.A., Steeg, P.S. & Stetler-Stevenson, W.G. (1991). Cancer metastasis and angiogenesis: an imbalance of positive and negative regulation. *Cell,* Vol.64, pp. 327-336

Loeb, S. & Catalon, W.J. (2007). Prostate-specific antigen in clinical practice. *Cancer Letters,* Vol.249, pp. 30-39

Lopez-Otin, C. & Matrisian, L.M. (2007). Emerging roles of proteases in tumour suppression. *Nature Reviews Cancer,* Vol.7, pp.800-806

Lundwall, A., Band, V., Blaber, M., Clements, J.A., Courty, Y., Diamandis, E.P., Fritz, H., Lilja, H., Malm, J., Maltais, L.J., Olsson, A.Y., Petraki, C., Scorilas, A., Sotiropoulou, G., Stenman, U.H., Stephan, C., Talieri, M. & Yousef, G.M. (2006). A comprehensive nomenclature for serine proteases with homology to tissue kallikreins. *Biological Chemistry,* Vol.387, pp. 637-641

McCormick, D. (1993). Secretion of cathepsin B by human gliomas in vitro. *Neuropathology and Applied Neurobiology,* Vol.19, pp. 146-151

McKeever, P.E. (1998). Insights about brain tumours gained through immunohistochemistry and in situ hybridization of nuclear and phenotypic markers. *Journal of Histochemistry and Cytochemistry,* Vol.46, pp. 585-594

Merzak, A., Koochekpour, S., Dkhissi, F., Raynal, S., Lawrence, D. & Pilkington, G.J. (1995). Synergism between growth factors in the control of glioma cell proliferation, migration and invasion in vitro. *International Journal of Oncology,* Vol.6. pp. 1079-1085

Mikkelsen, T., Yan, P-S., Ho, K-L., Sameni, M., Sloane, B.F. & Rosenblum, M.L. (1995). Immunolocalization of cathepsin B in human gliomas: implication for tumor invasion and angiogensis. *Journal of Neurosurgery,* Vol.83, pp. 285-290

Minn, Y., Bondy, M. & Wrensch M. (2008). Epidemiology, In: *Neurooncology, The Essentials,* M. Bernstein & M.S. Berger, (Eds.), pp. 3-17, Thieme Medical Publishers, Inc., ISBN 978-3-13-116332-5, New York, Stuttgart

Morris, C.S. & Esiri, M.M. (1991). Immunocytochemical study of macrophages and microglial cells and extracellular matrix components in human CNS disease. 1. Gliomas. *Journal of the Neurological Science,* Vol.101, pp. 47-58

Mueller, M.M. & Fusenig, N.E. (2004). Friends or foes - bipolar effects of the tumour stroma in cancer. *Nature Reviews Cancer,* Vol.4, pp. 839-849

Newcomb, E.W., Madonia, W.J., Pishorody, S., Lang, F.F., Koslow, M. & Miller, D.C. (1993). A correlative study of p53 protein alteration and p53 gene mutation in glioblastoma multiforme. *Brain Pathology,* Vol.3, pp. 229-235

Ossowski, L. & Reich, E. (1980). Experimental model for quantitative study of metastasis. *Cancer Research,* Vol.40, pp. 2300-2309

Paku, S. (1998). Current concepts in tumor-induced angiogenesis. *Pathology Oncology Research,* Vol.4, pp. 62-76

Pilkington, G.J. (1994). Tumor cell migration in the central nervous system. *Brain Pathology,* Vol.4, pp. 157-166

Pilkington, G.J., Bjerkvig, R., De Ridder, L. & Kaaijk, P. (1997). In vitro and in vivo models for the study of brain tumour invasion. *Anticancer Research,* Vol.17, pp. 4107-4110

Raidoo, D.M., Ramsaroop, R., Naidoo, S. & Bhoola, K.D. (1996). Regional distribution of tissue kallikrein in the human brain. *Immunopharmacology,* Vol.32, pp. 39-47

Rempel, S.A., Rosenblum, M.L., Mikkelsen, T., Yan, P-S., Ellis, K.D., Golembieski, W.A., Sameni, M., Rozhin, J., Ziegler, G. & Sloane, B.F. (1994). Cat B expression and localization in glioma progression and invasion. *Cancer Research,* Vol.54, pp. 6027-6031

Rivera, A.L. & Pelloski, C.E. (2010). Diagnostic and prognostic molecular markers in common adult gliomas. *Expert Review of Molecular Diagnostics,* Vol.10, No.5, (July 2010), pp. 637-649

Roggendorf, W., Strupp, S. & Paulus, W. (1996). Distribution and characterization of microglia/macrophages in human brain tumours. *Acta Neuropathologica,* Vol.92, pp. 288-293

Schmitt, M., Janicke, F. & Graeff, F. (1992). Tumor-associated proteinases. *Fibrinolysis,* Vol.6, pp. 3-26

Scott, R., Hall, P. & Haldane, J. (1991). A comparison of immunohistochemical markers of cell proliferation with experimentally determined growth faction. *Journal of Clinical Pathology,* Vol.165, pp. 173-178

Sedeghat, F. & Notopoulos, A. (2007). S100 protein family and its application in clinical practice. *Hippokratia,* Vol.12, pp. 198-204

Sen, J. & Belli, A. (2007). S100B in neuropathologic states: the CRP of the brain? *Journal of Neuroscience Research,* Vol.85, pp. 1373-1380

Singh, S.K., Clarke, I.D., Terasaki, M., Bo, V.E., Hawkins, C., Squire, J. & Dirks, P.B. (2003). Identification of a cancer stem cell in human brain tumors. *Cancer Research,* Vol.63, pp. 5821-5828

Sivaparvathi, M., Sawaya, R., Wang, S.W., Rayford, A., Yamamoto, M., Liotta, L.A., Nicolson, G.L. & Rao, J.S. (1995). Overexpression and localization of cathepsin B during the progression of human glioma. *Clinical & Experimental Metastasis,* Vol.13, pp. 49-56

Sivaparvathi, M., McCutcheon, I.., Sawaya, R., Nicolson, G.L. & Rao, J.S. (1996a). Expression of cysteine protease inhibitors in human gliomas and meningiomas. *Clinical & Experimental Metastasis,* Vol.14, No.4, pp. 344-350

Sivaparvathi, M., Yamamoto, M., Nicolson, G.L., Gokaslan, Z.L., Fuller, G.N., Liotta, L.A., Sawaya, R. & Rao, J.S. (1996b). Expression and immunohistochemical localization of cathepsin L during the progression of human gliomas. *Clinical & Experimental Metastasis,* Vol.14, pp. 27-34

Sloane, B.F., Moin, K. & Lah, T.T. (1994). Regulation of lysosomal endopeptidases in malignant neoplasia, In: *Biochemical and Molecular Aspects of Selected Cancers,* T.G. Pretlow II & T.P. Pretlow (Eds.), pp. 411-466, Academic Press, New York

Steinert, P.M. & Liem, R.K.H. (1990). Intermediate filament dynamics. *Cell,* Vol.60, pp. 521-523

Strojnik, T., Kos, J., Židanik, B., Golouh, R. & Lah, T. (1999). Cathepsin B immunohistochemical staining in tumor and endothelial cells is a new prognostic factor for survival in patients with brain tumors. *Clinical Cancer Research,* Vol.5, (March 1999), pp. 559-567

Strojnik, T., Kavalar, R., Trinkaus, M. & Lah, T.T. (2005). Cathepsin L in glioma progression: comparison with cathepsin B. *Cancer Detection and Prevention,* Vol.29, pp. 448-455

Strojnik, T., Kavalar, R. & Lah, T.T. (2006). Experimental model and immunohistochemical analyses of U87 human glioblastoma cell xenografts in immunosuppressed rat brains. *Anticancer Research,* Vol.26, pp. 2887-2900

Strojnik, T., Røsland, G.V., Sakariassen, P.O., Kavalar, R & Lah, T.T. (2007). Neural stem cell markers, nestin and musashi proteins, in the progression of human glioma: correlation of nestin with prognosis of patient survival. *Surgical Neurology,* Vol.68, pp. 133-144

Strojnik, T., Kavalar, R., Zajc, I., Diamandis, E.P., Oikonomopoulou, K. & Lah, T.T. (2009). Prognostic impact of CD68 and kallikrein 6 in human glioma. *Anticancer Research,* Vol.29, pp. 3269-3280

Strojnik, T., Kavalar, R., Barone, T.A. & Plunkett, R.J. (2010). Experimantal model and immunohistochemical comparison of U87 human glioblastoma cell xenografts on the chicken chorioallantoic membrane and in rat brains. *Anticancer Research,* Vol.30, pp. 4851-4860

Takei, H., Bhattacharjee, M.B., Rivera, A., Dancer, Y. & Powell, S.Z. (2007). New immunohistochemical markers in the evaluation of central nervous system tumors. *Archives of Pathology & Laboratory Medicine,* Vol. 131, pp. 234-241

Thomssen, C., Schmitt, M. & Goretzki, L. (1995). Prognostic value of the cysteine proteases cathepsin B and L in human breast carcinoma. *Clinical Cancer Research,* Vol.1, pp. 741-746

Toda, M., Iizuka, Y., Yu, W., Imai, T., Ikeda, E., Yoshida, K., Kawase, T., Kawakami, Y., Okano, H. & Uyemura, K. (2001). Expression of the neural RNA-binding protein Musashi 1 in human gliomas. *Glia,* Vol.34, pp. 1-7

Tohyama, T., Lee, V.M.-Y., Rorke, L.B., Marvin, M., McKay, R.D.G. & Trajanowski, J.Q. (1992). Nestin expression in embryonic human neuroepithelium and in human neuroepithelial tumor cells. *Laboratory Investigation,* Vol.66, pp. 303-313

Trapp, B.D. & Herrup, K. (2004). Neurons and neuroglia, In: *Youmans Neurological Surgery,* H.R. Winn, (Ed.), pp. 71-96, W.B. Saunders, Philadelphia

Wechsler, W., Szymas, J., Bilzer, T. & Hossmann, K.A. (1989). Experimental transplantation gliomas in the adult cat brain. *Acta Neurochirurgica,* Vol.98, pp. 77-89

Wilson, G., Saunders, M. & Dische, S. (1996). Direct comparison of bromodeoxyuridine and Ki-67 labeling indices in human tumours. *Cell Proliferation,* Vol.29, pp. 141-152

Yousef, G.M., Kishi, T. & Diamandis, E.P. (2003). Role of kallikrein enzymes in the central nervous system. *Clinica Chimica Acta,* Vol.329, pp. 1-8

Yung, W.K.A., Luna, M. & Borit, A. (1985). Vimentin and glial fibrillary acidic protein in human brain tumours. *Journal of Neuroonocolgy,* Vol.3, pp. 35-38

6

Gray or White? – The Contribution of Gray Matter in a Glioma to Language Deficits

Ryuta Kinno[1,2], Yoshihiro Muragaki[3] and Kuniyoshi L. Sakai[2]
[1]*Division of Neurology, Department of Internal Medicine, Showa University Northern Yokohama Hospital*
[2]*Department of Basic Science, Graduate School of Arts and Sciences, The University of Tokyo*
[3]*Department of Neurosurgery, Tokyo Women's Medical University*
Japan

1. Introduction

Symptoms of a glioma include not only headaches and seizures, but cognitive deficits including aphasia. One of the most important regions for aphasia is the anterior speech area, the damage of which causes Broca's aphasia, marked by effortful, distorted articulation, reduced speech output, and agrammatic syntax. These patients show relatively good comprehension of single words and simple sentences, but show trouble understanding sentences with more complex syntactic structures, such as passive sentences and sentences with object relative clauses (Schwartz et al., 1980; Caplan et al., 1985; Grodzinsky, 2000); this aspect of Broca's aphasia is called agrammatic comprehension (Goodglass & Menn, 1985; Menn and Obler, 1990; Pulvermüller, 1995). However, methodological problems have been raised (Badecker & Caramazza, 1985), and general processes of short-term memory or decision-making have been proposed to be disrupted in agrammatic comprehension (Just & Carpenter, 1992; Cupples & Inglis, 1993; Dick et al., 2001). Thus, for appropriately assessing a coginitive deficit, it is crucial to use an experimental task in which general cognitive demands such as the memory load are stricly controlled.
In our recent functional magnetic resonance imaging (fMRI) study with a picture-sentence matching task, we examined the effect of sentence structures strictly controlling general cognitive demands such as the memory load (Kinno et al., 2008), where a sentence was visually presented with a picture representing an action (Fig. 1; the same task and stimuli were used in the present study). The participants indicated whether or not the meaning of each sentence matched the action depicted by the corresponding picture. There were three main conditions with different sentence types: canonical / subject-initial active sentences (AS) (e.g., " Δ-ga ○-o hiiteru", " Δ pulls ○"), noncanonical / subject-initial passive sentences (PS) (e.g., " ○-ga Δ-ni hikareru", " ○ is affected by Δ's pulling it"; see Kinno et al. (2008) for ni direct passive form), and noncanonical / object-initial scrambled sentences (SS) (e.g., " ○-o Δ-ga hiireru", "as for ϒ, ○ pulling it"; this form is allowed not only in Japanese but in German, Finnish, and other languages). Under these conditions, each sentence had a

transitive verb and two arguments (phrases associated with the predicate) with different grammatical relations, i.e., which the subject (S) of a verb (V) is, and which its indirect object (IO) or direct object (DO) is. Sentence comprehension under each condition also explicitly required analysis of two different thematic roles, i.e., who initiates the action, and who is affected by it. In Japanese syntax, the grammatical relations are first marked by case markers (nominative, dative, or accusative in the present stimuli; Fig. 1), which in turn allow the assignment of thematic roles (agent, experiencer, or patient), whereas passiveness is also marked in the verb morphology (-areru). More specifically, the AS, PS, and SS sentences correspond to S-DO-V (agent and patient), S-IO-V (experiencer and agent), and DO-S-V (patient and agent) types, respectively. Therefore, these syntactic analyses for the two-argument relationships were critically required in our paradigm. In the fMRI study, we observed that activations in L. dF3t (extending to L. F3op) and L. LPMC were differentially modulated by these three main conditions. Moreover, we have recently found that a glioma in the opercular and triangular parts of the left inferior frontal gyrus (L. F3op/F3t) or left lateral premotor cortex (L. LPMC) is indeed sufficient to cause agrammatic comprehension that is selective to syntactic decision (Kinno et al., 2009). These findings indicated that our paradigm with three distinct syntactic conditions of AS, PS, and SS would be ideal for appropriately assessing agrammatic comprehension, because the same set of actions depicted by pictures was used under the main conditions, thus controlling semantic comprehension per se. However, it remains to be elucidated whether a cognitive deficit such as agrammatic comprehension is due to the glioma in gray matter (GM) or not, as a glioma extends to both gray and white matter. It is typically supposed that a glioma in a gray matter causes dysfunction of the localized region, whereas a glioma in white matter leads to the disconnection of neural networks. Therefore, a lesion-symptom method, in which brain lesions are precisely divided into gray and white matter, is required to examine the relative contribution of gray matter in a glioma to cognitive deficits.

In this chapter, we firstly propose a modified lesion-symptom method for examining the effect of a GM lesion. Our method is based on the following two methods for processing the structural magnetic resonance imaging (MRI) data and the behavioural data of patients with a glioma: the voxel-based lesion-symptom mapping (VLSM) (Bates et al., 2003) and the "unified segmentation" algorithm (Ashburner & Friston, 2005). The VLSM is a method to analyze the relationship between a lesion location in the structural MRI and behavioural data such as the error rates (ERs) or reaction times (RTs) on a voxel-by-voxel basis. The unified segmentation algorithm is a generative model that combines tissue segmentation, bias correction and spatial normalization in a single unified model. Using our picture-sentence matching task (Fig. 1), we actually applied this new method to real data of patients with a glioma in the left frontal cortex. The tumor locations covered the most of the left frontal regions and thus included L. F3op/F3t and L. LPMC. To precisely localize the glioma, all patients underwent a high-resolution 3D-MRI on the same day as the task examination. All of these results were actually utilized for the preoperative evaluation of detailed language function and for planning a resection of glioma, thereby minimizing the risk of postoperative language deficits (Haglund, Ojemann, & Hochman, 1992). Because neurological data about the real roles of the left frontal regions in syntactic comprehension have been limited, our lesion-symptom method would have both fundamental and clinical implications, which are useful for preserving the quality of life (QOL) for each patient.

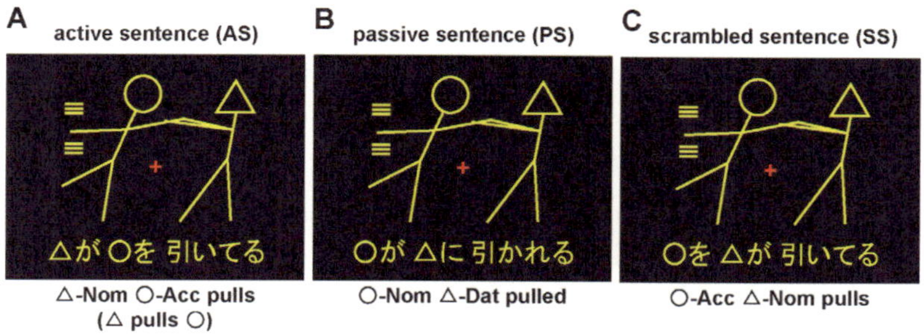

Fig. 1. The three main conditions used in the picture-sentence matching task.

2. Material and methods

2.1 Participants

All patients were native Japanese speakers newly diagnosed as having a glioma in the left frontal region, who were scheduled for surgery at the Department of Neurosurgery of Tokyo Women's Medical University. The following conditions comprised the criteria for inclusion of patients in the present study: (i) right-handedness, (ii) no deficits in verbal / written communication or other cognitive abilities reported by the patients or physicians, (iii) no history of neurological or psychiatric disorders other than glioma and seizures, (iv) freedom from seizures with or without antiepileptic drug, and (v) no medical problems for MRI acquisition. Twenty-one patients (Fig. 2 and Table 1) preoperatively underwent a high-resolution MRI scan and performed the picture-sentence matching task at the University of Tokyo, Komaba. The laterality quotient (LQ) was also determined by the Edinburgh handedness inventory (Oldfield, 1971). The verbal / nonverbal intelligence quotient (IQ) was assessed with the Japanese version of the WAIS-III (1997, 2006; Harcourt Assessment, Inc., San Antonio, TX, USA), including more general and demanding tests than the aphasic tests. All but one patient underwent amytal testing. Following injection of amytal, the patient counted numbers with both hands raised. As soon as the contralateral hemiplegia occurred, a picture naming task was used to determine hemispheric dominance, which was either left or bilateral. The tumour type and grade were postoperatively and pathologically diagnosed by the WHO Classification of Tumours of the Nervous System (2000). Using the same paradigm and parameters, we also tested 21 right-handed participants with no history of neurological or psychiatric disorders. These age-matched normal controls included 12 males and 9 females (age: 20-58; mean: 37 years). Informed consent was obtained from each participant after the nature and possible consequences of the studies were explained. Approval for the experiments was obtained from the institutional review board of the University of Tokyo, Komaba.

Age	LQ	VIQ	non-VIQ	Tumor Volume	GM Ratio
34 ± 10	88 ± 16	98 ± 5.7	99 ± 6.5	44088 ± 21227	55 ± 3.0

Table 1. Characteristics of Patients

Date are shown as mean ± standard deviation MR images were normalized with SPM8 for determination of tumor location and volume (mm^3), as well as the ratio (%) of gray matter (GM) for each tumor. LQ = laterality quotient VIQ = verbal intelligence quotient.

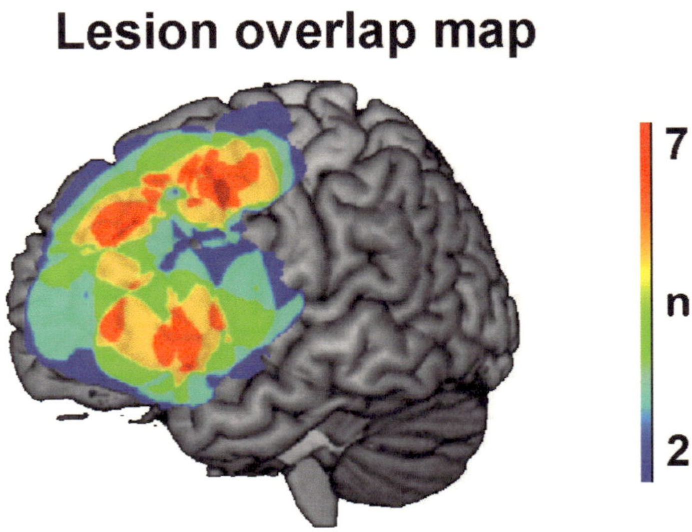

Fig. 2. Lesion overlap map for 21 patients with a glioma in the left frontal cortex

2.2 Stimuli

Each visual stimulus consisted of a picture at the top and a Japanese sentence at the bottom (Fig. 1). The pictures used for AS, PS, and SS were identical (the number of lines used in each picture, mean ± SD: 14 ± 2.4, n = 6). There was one sentence control (SC) condition with intransitive verbs (e.g., "ϒ-to Δ-ga hashitteru", "ϒ and Δ run") and equally complex pictures (14 ± 2.5, n = 6), which were all different from those used under the three main conditions. Half of the pictures depicted action occurring from left to right, and the other half depicted action from right to left. In the pictures, the use of symbols was also counterbalanced for both sides within each condition.

The sentences describing actions were written in a combination of the "hiragana" and "kanji" writing systems, and all sentence stimuli were grammatical in Japanese. Each sentence included two noun phrases and one verb; for example, a noun phrase (ϒ-ga) consisted of a symbol (ϒ) and a hiragana (ga). Two sets of Japanese verbs (six transitive verbs: pull, push, scold, kick, hit, and call; and six intransitive verbs: lie, stand, walk, run, tumble, and cry) were used, each of which, including the passive forms, had either four or five syllables. Note that the verb "call" is used only as a transitive verb in Japanese. There was no significant difference in frequency between the two sets of verbs ($t\ (10) = 0.7$, $p = 0.5$), according to the Japanese lexical database ("Nihongo-no Goitokusei" (Lexical Properties of Japanese), Nippon Telegraph and Telephone Corporation Communication Science Laboratories, Tokyo, Japan, 2003). We prepared eight stimuli for each verb; there were 48 stimuli for each condition.

Each stimulus consisted of one picture (top) and one sentence (bottom). Pictures depicting actions consisted of two stick figures; each stick figure was distinguished by one of three "head" symbols: a circle (○), square (ϒ), or triangle (Δ).The participants indicated whether or not the meaning of each sentence matched the action depicted in the corresponding picture by pressing one of two buttons. (A) Under the active sentence (AS) condition, canonical / subject-initial active sentences were presented ("Δ-ga ○-o hiiteru"). Below each example, a word-by-word translation in English is shown. Nom, nominative case; Acc, accusative case; Dat, dative case. (B) Under the passive sentence (PS) condition, non-canonical / subject-initial passive sentences were presented ("○-ga Δ-ni hikareru"). (C) Under the scrambled sentence (SS) condition, non-canonical / object-initial scrambled sentences were presented ("○-o Δ-ga hiireru"). An identical picture set was used under these three conditions. The sentence stimuli were all grammatical and commonly used in Japanese.All stimuli were presented visually in yellow against a dark background. Each stimulus was presented for 5800 ms followed by a 200 ms blank interval, which was ample time for the patients (see Table 2). For fixation, a red cross was also shown at the center of the screen. Stimulus presentation and behavioural data collection were controlled using the LabVIEW software and interface (National Instruments, Austin, TX, USA).

2.3 Tasks

In the picture-sentence matching task (Fig. 1), the participants read a sentence silently and indicated whether or not the meaning of each sentence matched the action of the corresponding picture by pressing one of two buttons. For AS, PS, and SS, all mismatched sentences were made by exchanging two symbols in the original sentences, e.g., "ϒ pushes ○" instead of "○ pushes ϒ". For SC, symbol-mismatched and action-mismatched sentences were presented equally often, requiring the sentences to be read completely in order for the participants to arrive at a correct judgment.

In addition to the picture-sentence matching task, we used a visual control task (VC), which required neither word nor sentence processing, as a baseline condition (Kinno et al., 2008). For VC, the same sets of pictures used in the picture-sentence matching task were presented, together with a string of jumbled letters taken from a single sentence in which the symbols (○, ϒ, or Δ) and "kanji" appeared at the same positions in the string as in the picture-sentence matching task. The participants were asked to judge whether or not all the symbols in a letter string were the same as those in the picture, irrespective of the order of the symbols. The participants underwent practice sessions before testing to become fully familiarized with the tasks.

A single run of the testing sessions contained 24 "trial events" of the picture-sentence matching task (six times each for AS, PS, SS, and SC), with variable inter-trial intervals of 6 and 12 s (one and two VC, respectively), pseudorandomized within a run. Since meaningless letter strings were presented throughout VC while sentences were presented only in the trial events, the participants could switch from VC to the trial events according to the stimulus type. The order of AS, PS, SS, and SC was pseudorandomized in each run to prevent any condition-specific strategy. Eight runs were tested in a day per one participant. Half of the stimuli consisted of matched picture-sentence pairs (24 trials for each condition), and the other half consisted of mismatched pairs (24 trials for each condition). All patients underwent the testing sessions inside the scanner while they received three to six fMRI runs, and then they completed the rest of the eight runs outside the scanner. Because the number of fMRI runs was limited by the patients' medical conditions, here we focused on the behavioural data and the anatomical MRI scans alone. All of the behavioural data from normal controls were acquired outside the scanner.

2.4 MRI data acquisition and analyses

The MRI scans were conducted on a 1.5 T scanner (Stratis II, Premium; Hitachi Medical Corporation, Tokyo, Japan), and a high-resolution T1-weighted 3D image (repetition time:

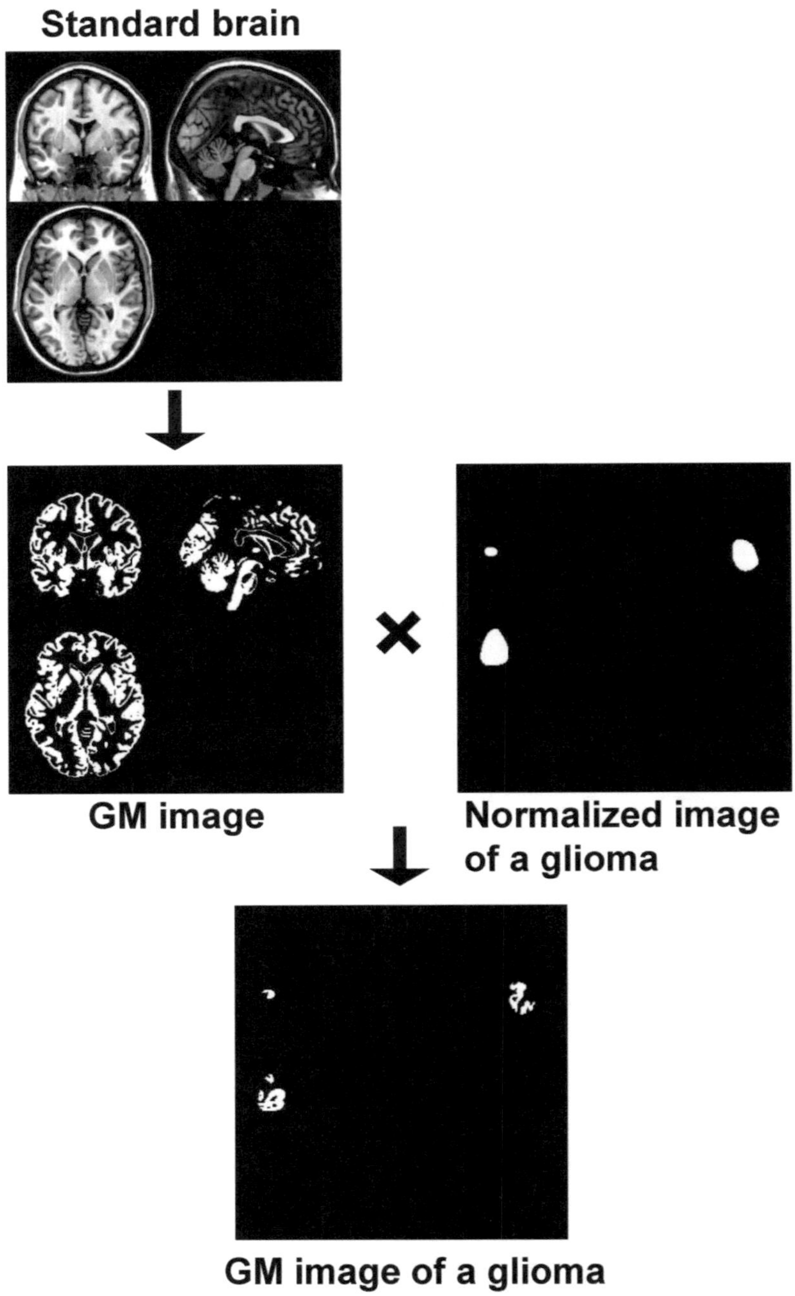

Fig. 3. Schematic representation of methods for making GM images.

30 ms, acquisition time: 8 ms, flip angle: 60°, field of view: 192 × 192 mm^2, resolution: 0.75 × 0.75 × 1 mm^3) was acquired for each patient. The location of the glioma was first identified on this MR image, and the glioma boundary was semi-automatically determined using MRIcroN software (http://www.mricro.com/) (Rorden & Brett, 2000). T2-weighted MR images (Department of Neurosurgery of Tokyo Women's Medical University) and positron-emission tomography (PET) data (Chubu Medical Center for Prolonged Traumatic Brain Dysfunction, Mino-Kamo-shi, Japan) were also used to assist the precise determination of the boundary. Each individual's structural image was spatially normalized to the standard brain space as defined by the Montreal Neurological Institute (MNI) using the "unified segmentation" algorithm, which is a generative model that combines tissue segmentation, bias correction and spatial normalization in a single unified model (Ashburner & Friston, 2005), which was resampled to 1 × 1 × 1 mm^3 voxel size using statistical parametric mapping SPM8 software (Wellcome Department of Cognitive Neurology, London, UK) (Friston et al., 1995) on MATLAB (Math Works, Natick, MA, USA).

These resultant individually normalized images were divided into gray and white matters as follows (Fig. 3). Firstly, a GM image was made by dividing the standard brain into gray and white matters using MRIcroN software. This GM image was used as a mask, which applied to the individually normalized image of each glioma.

Using the resultant GM image of each glioma, we next employed voxel-based lesion-symptom mapping (VLSM) to analyze the relationship between glioma location and the error rates on a voxel-by-voxel basis (Bates et al., 2003). The patients were divided into two groups according to whether they did or did not have a glioma including that voxel. The error rates for each condition or the difference in error rates between two conditions (e.g., PS - AS) were then compared for these two groups by a t-test, in which the statistical threshold was set to $p = 0.05$ after correction for multiple comparisons using the false discovery rate (FDR). To minimize the effects of outlier observations, the voxels used in the VLSM analysis were within the gliomas of at least two patients. Finally, the result of VLSM was projected onto a standard brain using MRIcroN software.

3. Results

In our paradigm with three main conditions of AS, PS, and SS, under which two-argument relationships were critically required (see the Introduction), the same set of actions depicted by pictures was used, thus controlling semantic comprehension per se. In contrast, a different set of pictures were used under the SC condition (e.g., "ϒ and Δ run"), which basically required matching between words (symbols and verbs) and pictures alone, without syntactic analyses for the two-argument relationships. Thus, the SC condition was syntactically less complex and easier to comprehend than other conditions. It was therefore mandatory to analyze the three main conditions and SC separately. Moreover, the analyses also match with our fMRI study (Kinno et al., 2008), in which SC was used as a separate control. In the sections 3.1-3.3, we focus on the main conditions of AS, PS, and SS, and the results of SC are presented in the section 3.4.

3.1 Behavioral analyses

The ERs for the patients and the normal controls are shown in Table 2. A repeated-measures analysis of variance (rANOVA) with two factors (group [patients, normal controls] ×

condition [AS, PS, SS]) revealed significant main effects of group (F (1, 40) = 16, p = 0.0003) and condition (F (2, 80) = 8.9, p = 0.0003), as well as a significant interaction of group by condition (F (2, 80) = 9.2, p = 0.0003). The patients showed significantly higher error rates than the normal controls for each of AS, PS, and SS (t-test; AS: t (40) = 2.5, p = 0.016; PS: t (40) = 2.9, p = 0.0055; SS: t (40) = 4.1 p = 0.0002). According to paired t-tests on the three main conditions, the patients' error rates were significantly higher for SS than for AS and PS (AS: t (20) = 3.8, p = 0.0010; PS: t (20) = 2.5, p = 0.021), whereas the difference was marginal between AS and PS (t (20) = 1.9, p = 0.07). However, there was no significant difference among the normal controls' error rates under the main conditions (p > 0.7). The resuls from the normal controls is consistent with our previous results (Kinno et al 2008).

These significant errors were observed in spite of the patient's normal verbal and nonverbal IQs (Table 1; range: 86-113 within 1 SD of ± 15; one sample t-test for the difference from 100: verbal, t (20) =1.2, p = 0.25 and nonverbal, t (20) = 0.51, p = 0.62). According to correlation analyses, the error rates for each condition could not be attributed to their ages, verbal / nonverbal IQs, or tumor volumes and GM ratio (all, p > 0.1). These results corresponded with our previous findings (Kinno et al., 2009), demonstrating that the tumor locations affected the actual performance of the three main conditions.

The RTs for the patients and the normal controls are also shown in Table 2. An rANOVA with two factors (group [patients, normal controls] × condition [AS, PS, SS]) showed that neither a main effect of group (F (1, 40) = 2.1, p = 0.2) nor that of condition was significant (F (2, 80) = 2.8, p = 0.1), with no significant interaction of group by condition (F (2, 80) = 0.30, p = 0.7). Because there was a significant main effect of condition regarding the error rates, the error rates were better indicators than RTs for estimating condition-selective effects. Therefore, we used error rates as indicators in the following VLSM analyses.

Participant	Error Rate (%)				RT (ms)			
	AS	PS	SS	SC	AS	PS	SS	SC
Normal controls	1.8 ± 2.6	2.1 ± 2.4	2.4 ± 2.6	1.8 ± 1.4	3334 ± 470	3524 ± 466	3599 ± 405	2712± 535
Patients	8.1 ± 7.4	12 ± 12	22 ± 21	2.4 ± 2.3	3372 ± 423	3476 ± 453	3499 ± 455	2760± 298

Table 2. Behavioral Data under Each Condition. ERs and RTs (for correct trials only) are shown as mean ± standard deviation.

3.1.1 VLSM analyses for gray and white matters

To identify any critical regions for the main conditions of AS, PS, and SS, we first conducted VLSM analyses, in which error rates for each condition were evaluated among the left frontal-damaged patients (n = 21). We found that significantly higher error rates for AS were associated with lesions in L. IFG, including L. dorsal F3op/F3t, as well as isolated lesions in L. LPMC (Fig. 4A). Moreover, significantly higher error rates for PS were associated with lesions in L. dorsal F3op/F3t, further extending to ventral F3op/F3t (Fig. 3B). In contrast, significantly higher error rates for SS were associated with lesions in L. LPMC and ventral IFG (Fig. 3C). These results indicate that both of L. F3op/F3t and L. LPMC are the critical regions for AS, PS, and SS.

Next we examined which regions were critically involved in the comprehension of syntactically complex sentences. For this purpose, we conducted VLSM analyses, in which the difference in error rates between the conditions of noncanonical vs. canonical sentences, i.e., PS - AS or SS - AS, was evaluated among the left frontal-damaged patients. We found that the significantly larger difference in PS - AS was associated with lesions in L. F3op/F3t (Fig. 4D). In contrast, we found that the significantly larger difference in SS - AS was associated mostly with lesions in L. LPMC (Fig. 4E). These results are consistent with our previous results (Kinno et al., 2009) with better sensitivity, indicating that both of L. F3op/F3t and L. LPMC are sufficient to cause agrammatic comprehension.

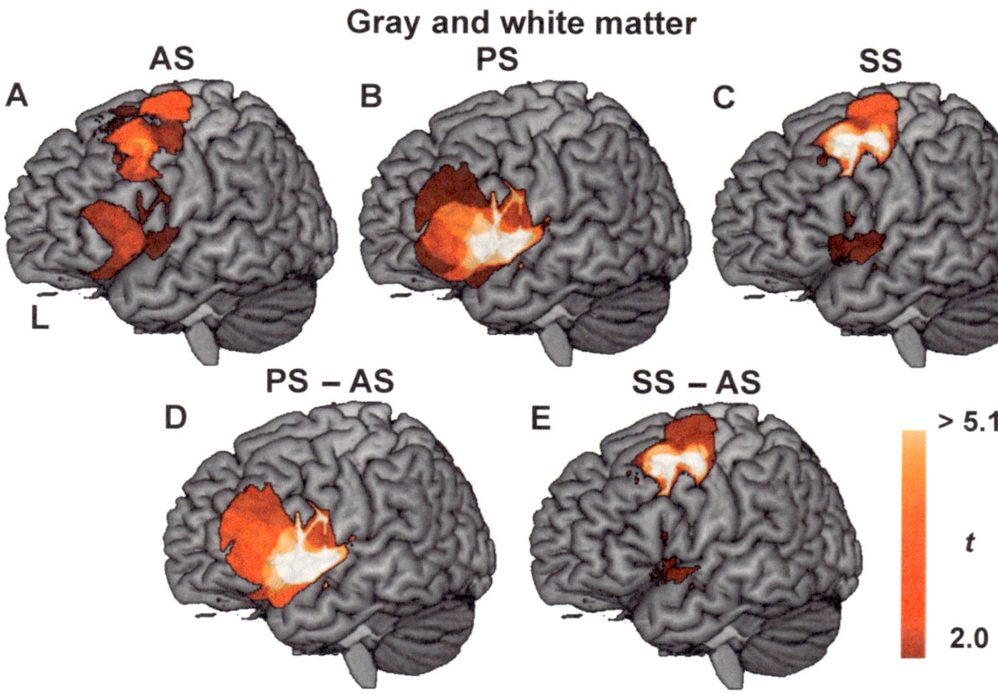

Fig. 4. Brain regions identified by the VLSM analysis for gray and white matters

Brain regions identified by the VLSM analysis for gray and white matters among the left frontal-damaged patients (n = 21) for AS, PS, SS, PS - AS, and SS - AS, respectively. The resultant t-map is projected on the left (L) lateral surface; the threshold was established at $t > 2.0$ (FDR corrected $p < .05$).

3.1.2 VLSM analyses for gray matter

We performed the modified VLSM analyses to identify the relateve contribution of gray matter to syntactic processing required for the main conditions of AS, PS, and SS, in which a GM image of each glioma was used. We found that significantly higher error rates for AS were associated with ventral lesions in L. IFG, as well as isolated lesions in L. LPMC (Fig. 5A).

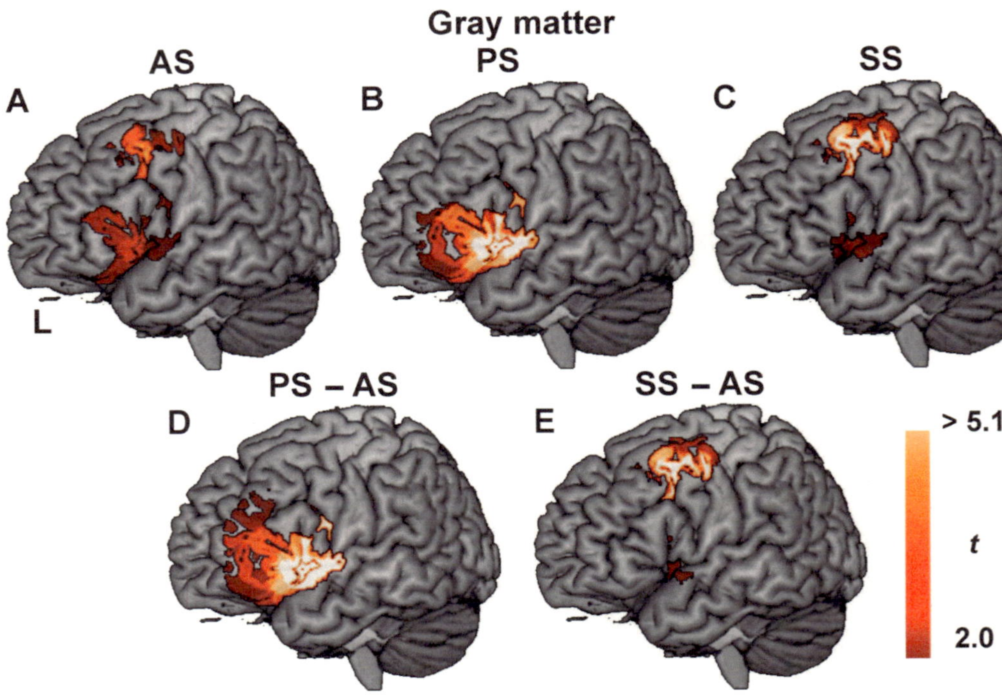

Fig. 5. Brain regions identified by the VLSM analysis for gray matter.

Moreover, significantly higher error rates for PS were associated with lesions in L. ventral F3op/F3t, further extending to dorsal F3op/F3t (Fig. 5B). In contrast, significantly higher error rates for SS were associated with lesions in L. LPMC (Fig. 5E) and ventral IFG (Fig. 5C). These results are compatible to our previous findings.

Next we examined the effect of gray matter on the comprehension of syntactically complex sentences. We found that the significantly larger difference in PS - AS was associated with lesions in L. F3op/F3t (Fig. 5D). In contrast, we found that the significantly larger difference in SS - AS was associated mostly with lesions in L. LPMC. These results indicate that the gray matter of L. F3op/F3t as well as L. LPMC are critically involved in the comprehension of syntactically complex sentences.

3.2 The analyses of the SC condition

We compared the performance data for SC between all patients and the normal controls to examine whether or not such basic comprehension of sentences was affected for the patients. The patients showed no significant difference in error rates for SC when compared with the normal controls ($t(40) = 0.87$, $p = 0.4$) (Table 2). Regarding RTs for SC, there was no significant difference between the patients and normal controls ($t(40) = 0.36$, $p = 0.7$). Moreover, paired t-tests showed that the patients' error rates were significantly lower for SC than for AS, PS, and SS (AS: $t(20) = 3.6$, $p = 0.020$; PS: $t(20) = 3.4$, $p = 0.0029$; SS: $t(20) = 4.5$, $p = 0.0002$), whereas the normal controls' error rates for SC were not significantly different from those for the three main conditions ($p > 0.7$). For both the patients and normal controls, RTs were significantly shorter for SC than for the three main conditions (all, $p < 0.0001$). These results indicate that basic comprehension of sentences under the SC condition was preserved among the patients.

4. Discussion

In this chapter, we have presented the modified VLSM method that can directly examine the effect of a GM lesion on a cognitive process. The present study successfully demonstrates that GM of L. F3op/F3t and L. LPMC are actually essential for AS, PS, and SS (Fig. 5), and that both regions are indeed critically involved in the comprehension of syntactically complex sentences. The patients with a lesion in GM of L. F3op/F3t or L. LPMC had significant deficits in syntactic analyses for the two-argument relationships required for the three main conditions, but without deficits in any factors required for SC. These results provide crucial evidence that GM of L. F3op/F3t and L. LPMC subserves syntactic comprehension.

The condition-selectivity in error rates for the patients with a GM lesion in either L. F3op/F3t or L. LPMC cannot be explained by general disorders of the patients, including visual / memory / motor impairment, attention disturbance due to drowsiness or dizziness, and perseveration for a particular sentence type. It is natural to assume that the patients with normal verbal IQ would not otherwise experience or exhibit difficulty in language comprehension with such simple sentences; however the patients indeed exhibited clear deficits even for canonical sentences for AS in the present study. In daily conversation, pragmatic information about word use resolves syntactic difficulty (e.g., "The officer chased the thief" is more acceptable than "The thief chased the officer."). The use of appropriate syntactic judgment tests is thus necessary for a proper assessment of syntactic comprehension. The importance of GM of L. F3op/F3t and L. LPMC has been underpinned by accumulating results from fMRI studies, which demonstrated the selectivity for syntactic processing in L. F3op/F3t and /or L. LPMC (Dapretto & Bookheimer, 1999; Embick et al., 2000; Hashimoto & Sakai, 2002; Bornkessel et al., 2005; Grewe et al., 2006), indicating the critical role of the two left frontal regions on the language network for syntactic processing (Sakai, 2005). Moreover, the present results are consistent with another recent fMRI study, in which both L. dF3t and L. LPMC were selectively activated for the syntactic comprehension of honorification, in which two-argument relationships of either subject honorifics or object honorifics were critically involved (Momo, Sakai, & Sakai, 2008). Further research is required for understanding both anatomical and functional bases for the differential roles of these two critical regions.

It has been well known that the left temporal cortex is also engaged during sentence comprehension. In our fMRI study with the same paradigm, we have reported that a localized activation in the left posterior superior / middle temporal gyrus (L. pSTG/MTG) was also enhanced for SS when compared with AS and PS (Kinno et al., 2008). Other fMRI studies have also reported that this region was activated by contrasting object-initial vs. subject-initial sentences (Bornkessel et al., 2005), as well as by contrasting sentences with syntactic / semantic anomaly and normal sentences (Suzuki & Sakai, 2003). A lesion in L. pSTG/MTG may thus result in the SS-selective deficit. A recent intraoperative electrocorticography study in humans showed bidirectional connectivity between L. IFG and L. pSTG/MTG (Matsumoto et al., 2004), and additional evidence for this connectivity has been reported in studies using MRI to investigate structural connectivity (Catani, Jones, & Ffytche, 2005; Friederici et al., 2006). Therefore, it is possible that this network subserves syntactic integration, thereby combining multiple linguistic information. Further lesion studies are required to examine whether or not a lesion in gray or white matter of the left temporal region is sufficient to cause deficits in such a linguistic process. Our lesion-symptom method would be useful for this purpose.

Compared with a cerebrovascular disease such as an infarct or a hemorrhage, a glioma has both advantages and disadvantages in neuropsychological and neurolinguistic research. First, it is advantageous that the location of a glioma is basically random in the cerebrum and not restricted by the cerebrovascular distribution. Indeed, damage to the middle cerebral artery affects the perisylvian cortex including F3op/F3t, but it spares more dorsal regions including LPMC. Using the lesion data with a glioma, we successfully showed the functional roles of L. F3op/F3t and L. LPMC. Second, the precise determination of the location and extent of a glioma is often difficult, because a glioma may induce edemas, abnormalities by compressing its peripheral region, and infiltration. In the present study, we used both T2-weighted MR images and PET data, which enabled us to determine precise boundary of lesions including brain edemas and abnormalities of perfusion. Third, some neural functions may be still preserved within a glioma, as indicated by cortical stimulation and fMRI studies (Ojemann, Miller, & Silbergeld, 1996; Krainik et al., 2003). It has been also reported that patients with tumors in the left hemisphere showed less language impairment than their counterparts with stroke (Anderson, Damasio, & Tranel, 1990). In the present study, however, we regarded an entire glioma as a lesion, and clear language deficits were observed despite such residual functions. Fourth, the onset and time course of a glioma is difficult to determine; a glioma develops gradually without apparent symptoms such as hemiplegia or dysarthria. In the present study, the patients were at least 21 years old at their start of medication, and had no prior history of benign or malignant brain tumors, indicating an adult-onset glioma. For evaluating the real function of a cortical region, it is thus important to compare the lesion symptom data from our lesion-symptom method with the functional neuroimaging data from normal controls.

It has been recently demonstrated that slow-growing lesions like WHO grade II gliomas, but not high-grade gliomas, may induce cortical reorganization even before operation (Desmurget, Bonnetblanc, & Duffau, 2007). Moreover, the grade II gliomas undergo anaplastic transformation over the years, i.e., the progression into grade III gliomas (Behin et al., 2003), which may be enough time for cortical reorganization. Such a functional

reshaping might affect the observation of the present study, because the tumor types of the patients were heterogeneous including WHO grade II (n = 10), and III (n = 11), with different biological processes for each tumor. However, it should be noted that the patients with a glioma in either L. F3op/F3t or L. LPMC showed marked deficits in syntactic comprehension, which had not been rescued by any functional reshaping. It is possible that the reorganization of other cortical regions due to a lesion in L. F3op/F3t or L. LPMC is entirely different each other, thus leading to the differential patterns of condition-selective deficits. Further functional neuroimaging studies for brain-damaged patients are required to clarify real mechanisms of cortical reorganization.
Understanding cortical networks for a cognitive process requires knowledge of functional as well as anatomical connections between brain regions. Not only lesion symptom mapping but also functional imaging studies of patients with a well-defined lesion are useful for understanding cortical networks by revealing abnormal activations: overactivity (i.e., regions where patients activate more than normal controls) or underactivity (i.e., regions where patients activate less than normal controls) (Price & Friston, 1999; Price, Crinion , & Friston, 2006). These differential activations can imply a change in cognitive or neuronal implementation. Changes in cognitive implementation occur when a patient uses a different set of cognitive processes either because a new cognitive strategy has been learned, or because of increased demands on normal processing due to a brain damage. Changes in neuronal implementation are mediated by changes in the strength of pre-existing connections. Abnormal activations distant to the lesion location suggest the dysfunctional region has been disconnected from its normal inputs. This disconnection may result in overactivity, due to disinhibition of an inhibitory network, or underactivity, due to a failure to activate a cortical region. These abnormal activations can reveal a duplicate system for a cognitive process, in which the dominant system inhibits the others. Within the duplicate system, the less dominant systems are able to respond when the dominant system is damaged. This duplication of functionality renders a function immune from the effects of focal damage. Functional imaging studies of patients, therefore, have an important role to play in the identification of a duplicate system—the multiplicity of sufficient brain systems for a cognitive function. Further study is required to investigate the language-specific system for the human brain.

5. Conclusion

In this chapter, we have presented a lesion-symptom mapping method that can directly examine the effect of a GM lesion on a cognitive process. As a glioma extends to both gray and white matter, it remains to be elucidated whether the cognitive deficits are due to the glioma in gray or white matter. It is typically supposed that a glioma in GM causes dysfunction of the localized region, whereas a glioma in white matter leads to the disconnection of neural networks. Therefore, the effect of GM lesion should be assessed precisely; for this purpose, our method would be useful. While a glioma in the cerebral cortex causes a deficit in cognitive function, the severity and course of such a dysfunction need to be thoroughly assessed (Wefel, Kayl, & Meyers, 2004). An extensive study of tumors with multiple neuropsychological tests have confirmed that patients with left hemispheric tumors exhibited poorer verbal fluency and verbal learning than those with right hemispheric tumors (Hahn et al., 2003). The present study demonstrated the severity of dysfunction, such that a GM lesion in L. F3op/F3t and/or L. LPMC can cause clear deficits in syntactic comprehension. Our language task would be thus sensitive enough and useful for a general assessment of linguistic knowledge. Our findings further indicate that brain surgery for a glioma in the left frontal cortex requires careful assessment for maintaining syntactic abilities, which are indeed the source of the creative faculty for producing infinite expressions (Hauser, Chomsky, & Fitch, 2002), and thus for ensuring the best possible QOL for individual patients.

6. Acknowledgment

We thank M. Kawamura for his suggestion regarding neurological issues, N. Komoro for her technical assistance, H. Matsuda for her administrative assistance. This research was supported by a research grant from the Narishige Neuroscience Research Foundation (R. K.) and a Core Research for Evolutional Science and Technology (CREST) grant from the Japan Science and Technology Agency (JST) (K. L. S.).

7. References

Anderson, S. W., Damasio, H., & Tranel, D. (1990). Neuropsychological impairments associated with lesions caused by tumor or stroke. Archives of Neurology 47, 397-405.

Ashburner, J & Friston, K. J. (2005). Unified segmentation., NeuroImage 26: 839– 851.

Badecker, W. & Caramazza, A. (1985). On considerations of method and theory governing the use of clinical categories in neurolinguistics and cognitive neuropsychology: The case against agrammatism., Cognition 20: 97-125.

Bates, E., Wilson, S. M., Saygin, A. P., Dick, F., Sereno, M. I., Knight, R. T., & Dronkers, N. F. (2003). Voxel-based lesion-symptom mapping., Nature Neuroscience 6: 448-450.

Behin, A., Hoang-Xuan, K., Carpentier, A. F., & Delattre, J.-Y. (2003). Primary brain tumours in adults. Lancet 361, 323-331.

Bornkessel, I., Zysset, S., Friederici, A. D., von Cramon, D. Y., & Schlesewsky, M. (2005). Who did what to whom? The neural basis of argument hierarchies during language comprehension. Neuroimage 26, 221-233.

Caplan, D., Baker, C., & Dehaut, F. (1985). Syntactic determinants of sentence comprehension in aphasia. Cognition 21, 117-175.

Catani, M., Jones, D. K., & Ffytche, D. H. (2005). Perisylvian language networks of the human brain. Annals of Neurology 57, 8-16.

Cupples, L. & Inglis, A. L. (1993). When task demands induce "asyntactic" comprehension: A study of sentence interpretation in aphasia. Cognitive Neuropsychology 10, 201-234.

Dapretto, M. & Bookheimer, S. Y. (1999). Form and content: Dissociating syntax and semantics in sentence comprehension. Neuron 24, 427-432.

Desmurget, M., Bonnetblanc, F., & Duffau, H. (2007). Contrasting acute and slow-growing lesions: A new door to brain plasticity. Brain 130, 898-914.

Dick, F., Bates, E., Wulfeck, B., Utman, J. A., Dronkers, N., & Gernsbacher, M. A. (2001). Language deficits, localization, and grammar: Evidence for a distributive model of

language breakdown in aphasic patients and neurologically intact individuals. Psychological Review 108, 759-788.
Embick, D., Marantz, A., Miyashita, Y., O'Neil, W., & Sakai, K. L. (2000). A syntactic specialization for Broca's area. Proceedings of the National Academy of Sciences of the United States of America 97, 6150-6154.
Friederici, A. D., Bahlmann, J., Heim, S., Schubotz, R. I., & Anwander, A. (2006). The brain differentiates human and non-human grammars: Functional localization and structural connectivity. Proceedings of the National Academy of Sciences of the United States of America 103, 2458-2463.
Friston, K. J., Holmes, A. P., Worsley, K. J., Poline, J.-P., Frith, C. D., & Frackowiak, R. S. J. (1995). Statistical parametric maps in functional imaging: A general linear approach. Human Brain Mapping 2, 189-210.
Goodglass, H. & Menn, L. (1985) Is agrammatism a unitary phenomenon? In M.-L. Kean (Ed), Agrammatism (pp. 1-26). Orlando, FL: Academic Press.
Grewe, T., Bornkessel, I., Zysset, S., Wiese, R., von Cramon, D. Y., & Schlesewsky, M. (2006). Linguistic prominence and Broca's area: The influence of animacy as a linearization principle. Neuroimage 32, 1395-1402.
Grodzinsky, Y. (2000). The neurology of syntax: Language use without Broca's area. Behavioral and Brain Sciences 23, 1-71.
Haglund, M. M., Ojemann, G. A., & Hochman, D. W. (1992). Optical imaging of epileptiform and functional activity in human cerebral cortex. Nature 358, 668-671.
Hahn, C. A., Dunn, R. H., Logue, P. E., King, J. H., Edwards, C. L., & Halperin, E. C. (2003). Prospective study of neuropsychologic testing and quality-of-life assessment of adults with primary malignant brain tumors. International Journal of Radiation Oncology*Biology*Physics 55, 992-999.
Hashimoto, R. & Sakai, K. L. (2002). Specialization in the left prefrontal cortex for sentence comprehension. Neuron 35, 589-597.
Hauser, M. D., Chomsky, N., & Fitch, W. T. (2002). The faculty of language: What is it, who has it, and how did it evolve? Science 298, 1569-1579.
Just, M. A. & Carpenter, P. A. (1992). A capacity theory of comprehension: Individual differences in working memory. Psychological Review 99, 122-149.
Kinno, R., Kawamura, M., Shioda, S., & Sakai, K. L. (2008). Neural correlates of noncanonical syntactic processing revealed by a picture-sentence matching task. Human Brain Mapping 29, 1015-1027.
Kinno, R., Muragaki, Y., Hori, T., Maruyama, T, Kawamura, M, Sakai. K. L. (2009). Agrammatic comprehension caused by a glioma in the left frontal cortex. Brain and Language 110, 71-80.
Krainik, A., Lehéricy, S., Duffau, H., Capelle, L., Chainay, H., Cornu, P., Cohen, L., Boch, A.-L., Mangin, J.-F., Le Bihan, D., & Marsault, C. (2003). Postoperative speech disorder after medial frontal surgery: Role of the supplementary motor area. Neurology 60, 587-594.
Matsumoto, R., Nair, D. R., LaPresto, E., Najm, I., Bingaman, W., Shibasaki, H., & Lüders, H. O. (2004). Functional connectivity in the human language system: A cortico-cortical evoked potential study. Brain 127, 2316-2330.

Menn, L. & Obler, L. K. (1990) Theoretical motivations for the cross-language study of agrammatism. In L. Menn & L. K. Obler (Eds.), Agrammatic Aphasia: A Cross-Language Narrative Sourcebook (pp. 3-12). Amsterdam: John Benjamins Publishing Company.

Momo, K., Sakai, H., & Sakai, K. L. (2008). Syntax in a native language still continues to develop in adults: Honorification judgment in Japanese. Brain and Language 107, 81-89.

Ojemann, J. G., Miller, J. W., & Silbergeld, D. L. (1996). Preserved function in brain invaded by tumor. Neurosurgery 39, 253-259.

Oldfield, R. C. (1971). The assessment and analysis of handedness: The Edinburgh inventory. Neuropsychologia 9, 97-113.

Price, C. J., & Friston, K. J. (1999). Scanning patients with tasks they can perform. Human Brain Mapping 8,102–108.

Price, C. J., Crinion J., & Friston, K. J. (2006). Design and Analysis of fMRI Studies With Neurologically Impaired Patients. Journal of magnetic resonance imaging 23, 816–826 (2006)

Pulvermüller, F. (1995). Agrammatism: Behavioral description and neurobiological explanation. Journal of Cognitive Neuroscience 7, 165-181.

Rorden, C. & Karnath, H. O. (2004). Using human brain lesions to infer function: A relic from a past era in the fMRI age? Nature Reviews Neuroscience 5, 813-819.

Sakai, K. L. (2005). Language acquisition and brain development. Science 310, 815-819.

Schwartz, M. F., Saffran, E. M., & Marin, O. S. M. (1980). The word order problem in agrammatism. I. Comprehension. Brain and Language 10, 249-262.

Suzuki, K. & Sakai, K. L. (2003). An event-related fMRI study of explicit syntactic processing of normal/anomalous sentences in contrast to implicit syntactic processing. Cerebral Cortex 13, 517-526.

Van Valin, R. D., Jr. & LaPolla, R. J. (1997). Syntax: Structure, Meaning, and Function. Cambridge, UK: Cambridge University Press.

Wefel, J. S., Kayl, A. E., & Meyers, C. A. (2004). Neuropsychological dysfunction associated with cancer and cancer therapies: A conceptual review of an emerging target. British Journal of Cancer 90, 1691-1696.

Part 2

Novel Imaging and Diagnostic Modalities

7

3D TrueFISP MRI Provides Accurate Longitudinal Measurements of Glioma Volumes in Mice

Emeline Julie Ribot[1,2], Line Pourtau[1,3], Philippe Massot[1,3], Pierre Voisin[1,3], Eric Thiaudiere[1,3], Jean- Michel Franconi[1,3] and Sylvain Miraux[1,3]
[1]*Centre de Résonance Magnétique des Systèmes Biologiques, Université Bordeaux Segalen, CNRS*
[2]*Imaging Research Laboratories, Robarts Research Institute, The University of Western Ontario*
[3]*Laboratory of Excellence TRAIL, Translational Research and Advanced Imaging Laboratory, University of Bordeaux*
[1,3]*France*
[2]*Canada*

1. Introduction

One of the most common models used in pre-clinical studies is nude mice implanted with brain tumors. In fact, owing to a deficiency in their immune systems, nude mice allow many tumor models to be studied and a wide range of therapeutic treatments to be investigated.

The best way to evaluate the efficiency of a treatment is to compare the kinetics of the tumor volume between a control group and a treatment group [1-3]. Since brain tumors generally evolve very quickly (7 to 15 days) in mice, the tumor must be detected early and characterized daily.

The advantages of non-invasive imaging methods are evident compared with conventional methods such as histochemistry, where animal sacrifice, end-point analysis only, and 2D tumor-diameter measurement are mandatory.

However, obtaining images of high spatial resolution and high contrast for the same animal in a longitudinal study is not trivial.

As in clinical MR imaging, the tumor can be detected in two possible ways. The first consists of using a gadolinium-based contrast agent injected intravenously to visualize the breakdown of the blood–brain barrier. Using a T1-weighted 3D gradient-echo sequence, high-resolution images can be obtained in a reasonable acquisition time. Nevertheless, because of the injuries caused by repeated injection of contrast agent into the tail vein, experiments cannot be performed frequently [1]. The other way consists of using T2-weighted sequences. RARE imaging, with or without magnetization transfer preparation [3–5], allows small tumors to be detected noninvasively. The sequence is usually acquired in multi-slice 2D imaging in order to limit the total acquisition time. However, high-resolution,

accurate 3D information is very important in longitudinal studies such as, for instance, the evaluation of a therapeutic treatment.
An alternative to RARE T2 [6] or 3D contrast-enhanced T1 imaging is fully balanced SSFP imaging (also called bSSFP, TrueFISP or FIESTA) [7]. In fact, it has recently been shown that this sequence can be used at high field, in 3D, to detect tumors of very small size [8]. The advantage of this sequence is the ability to combine the speed of 3D gradient echo and T1/T2 contrast.
The purpose of this study is to demonstrate that a 3D TrueFISP MRI sequence is applicable, at high magnetic field, to glioma-bearing mouse models in longitudinal studies. Theoretical considerations of tumor contrast and signal-to-noise ratio as a function of sequence parameters (TE/TR/flip angle) were carried out and compared with experimental data.
The 3D TrueFISP MRI sequence was also compared with the sequence most widely used in clinical applications: 2D RARE. Finally, the sequence was used to perform accurate longitudinal measurements of glioma volumes in mice.

2. Materials and methods

2.1 MRI system

Magnet

NMR machines to image small animals are becoming more and more widespread. The various manufacturers have developed systems for use in studies using small animals by adapting their components (magnet, gradients, antennae, monitoring system and animal handling solutions).
The main component of an MRI system is the magnet, which generates an intense static magnetic field. While for clinical imaging 1.5-T and 3-T magnets are used, for rats and mice a magnetic field between 4.7 T and 11.6 T is generally used. The magnets can be positioned either horizontally or vertically. This type of magnetic fields provides an increased signal-to-noise ratio (S/N), required for the acquisition of highly spatially resolved images. However, a theoretical increase in signal causes problems which must be considered when high-quality images are to be obtained. In this way, an increase in magnetic field leads to a reduced natural contrast between the tissues in T2 or T1-weighted scans. In addition, susceptibility effects are enhanced and may lead to artifacts with gradient-echo sequences.
Most of the images presented here were acquired at 4.7 T. This level of magnetic field provides a compromise between signal-to-noise ratio, contrast and sensitivity to susceptibility artifacts. The use of a more intense magnetic field will also be addressed.

2.2 Gradient system

The second essential component of an MRI system is the magnetic field gradient. Gradients allow the image to be spatially encoded. When imaging small animals, the spatial resolution required is much greater than for human imaging. For example, in anatomic imaging of rats, a voxel size of at least 400 µm is required in all three dimensions (3D); in mice, a size of at least 200 µm is needed.
In MRI, the digital resolution, i.e. pixel size, is inversely proportional to the gradient intensity, G, and application time, tG (Eq. [1]).

$$\Delta y = \frac{\pi}{t_G \gamma G} \quad (1)$$

The actual resolution is inversely proportional to the relaxation time, T2*, and to the gradient intensity and application time (Eq. [2]).

$$\text{Resolution} = \frac{2}{\gamma G T_2^*} \quad (2)$$

The advantages of using intense magnetic field gradients are thus obvious, particularly at strong magnetic fields, with very short T2*.

Commercial gradient systems have been developed with intensities of greater than 400 mT/m over 10 cm, up to 1 T/m over 3 cm. Because the target diameter of these gradient systems is spatially limited, they can only be used to study animals such as rats or mice.

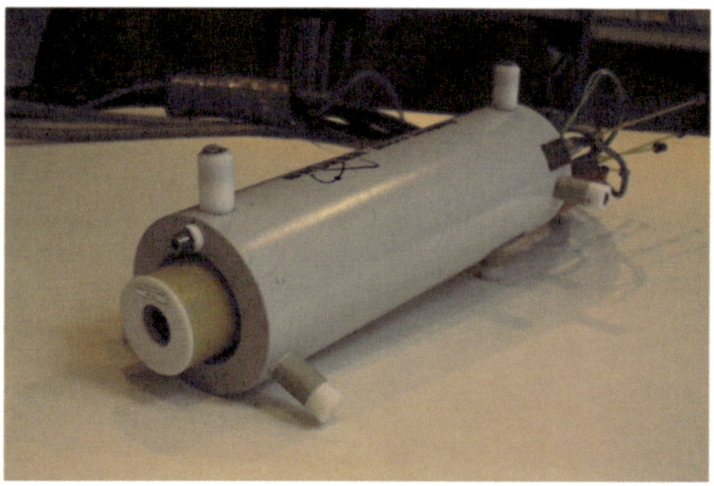

Fig. 1. Photograph of a 1-T/m gradient system. The system can be inserted into a magnet equipped with a 12-cm-diameter tunnel and can contain an antenna up to 6 cm in diameter. The gradient is linear over a distance of approximately 3 cm.

2.3 Coil

Image quality is also significantly affected by the choice of antenna. The S/N depends entirely on this component as it is proportional to the square root of the antenna's quality factor, Q. Thus, a well-designed antenna is recommended. In addition, the S/N is directly proportional to the filling factor for the antenna, represented by η in Eq. [3].

$$S/N \propto (Q)^{1/2} \eta \quad (3)$$

Optimal image quality will therefore be obtained using an antenna with a size and shape perfectly adapted to the zone to be imaged. Several types of antennae have been developed and can be used to meet these criteria. Volumetric emission/reception antennae are the most common. They provide a very homogeneous radio-frequency field, often required when using spin-echo sequences. However, their filling factor is relatively low, which can penalize the S/N. This sensitivity problem can be partially mitigated by using cross-polarized antennae. This type of volumetric antenna is the easiest to use, and was used for the images presented in this chapter.

Surface antennae can also be used, offering an excellent quality factor combined with a very high filling factor. This type of antenna therefore provides a higher S/N than the antennae described previously.

However, due to their configuration, the flip angle applied varies depending on the depth of the zone to be imaged within the sample, making the use of spin-echo sequences impossible. In addition, with this type of antenna, contrast can vary depending on the depth of the zone observed within the sample.

Finally, in clinical imaging, and increasingly for small-animal imaging, volumetric emission antennae coupled to an array of surface reception antennae are the most commonly used. This setup offers the advantages of the two types of antennae described above: excellent B1 emission homogeneity associated with an excellent signal-to-noise ratio.

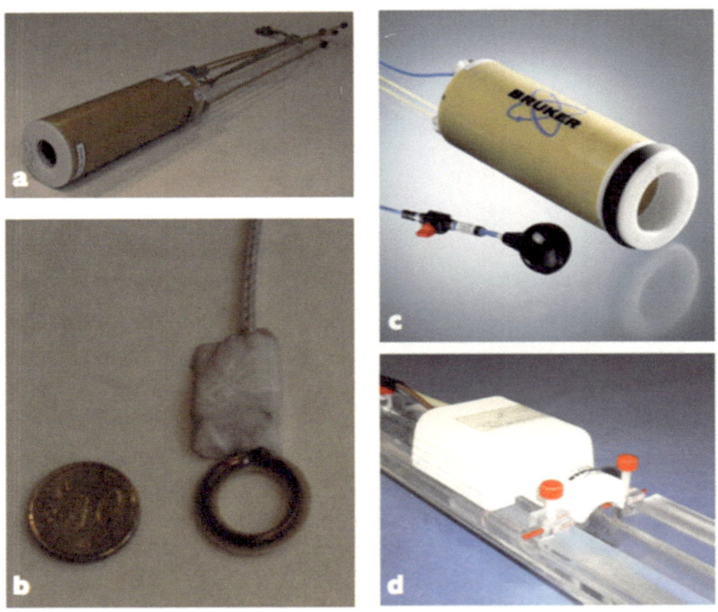

Fig. 2. a) Cross-polarized 25-mm-diameter volumetric antenna; b) 16-mm-diameter surface emission/reception antenna; c) & d) antenna system combining volumetric emission (80 mm in diameter) and phased-array reception.

These three types of antennae are exclusively used for mouse brain imaging and were tuned to 200 MHz in the experiments described here.

2.4 Animal handling/monitoring

Finally, quality imaging in small animals requires a specific component to position and monitor the animal. This component must allow the animal to be maintained in a stable and

fairly reproducible position. In particular, it must allow imaging to be applied repeatedly (approximately once a day) to particularly fragile animals.
A tooth bar assembly is generally used to position the animal's head based on the position of its teeth. Ear bars may be added but are not always necessary. This type of stereotactic positioning is often used for brain imaging in animals.
The animal is monitored by measuring its respiratory rate using an air balloon placed on the abdomen or back of the animal and connected to a pressure sensor linked to a computer via an optical fiber during imaging sessions. The respiratory rate can thus be followed on a computer screen in real time.
Isoflurane inhalation-based anesthesia is used, with adaptation of the percentage of isoflurane mixed with air to maintain the animal's respiration rate at greater than 70 and less than 110 breaths/min. Isoflurane can be recycled through a capture system.
The animal's body temperature is maintained constant either with an electric blanket, or by using circulating hot water to maintain the gradient system at 32 °C.

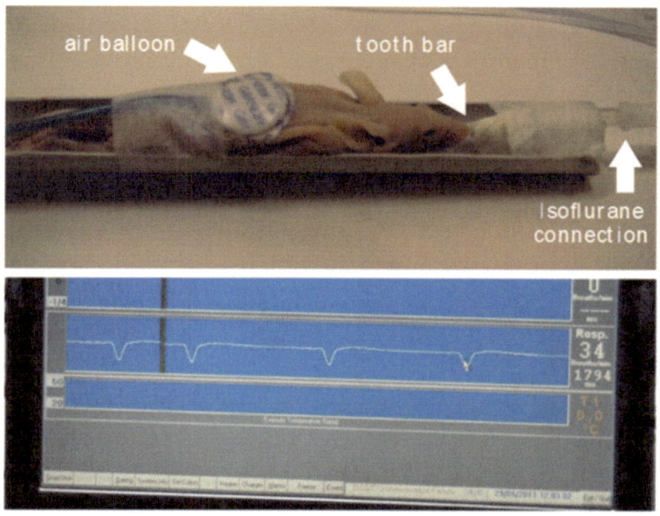

Fig. 3. Nude mouse in a home-made bed. A tooth-bar assembly holds the animal in position and a 1-2% air/isoflurane mixture is delivered in the region of the nose. A balloon is placed on the animal's back to measure its respiration rate. The SA Instruments system is linked to a computer, where the animal's respiration can be visualized on-screen.

2.5 Animal model

U87 human brain tumor cells were implanted in nude mice (18-20 g, n = 20, Charles Rivers, L'Arbresle, France) by stereotactic injection into the striatum. Mice were anesthetized with isoflurane (1.5% in air) and secured in the stereotactic apparatus (Stoelting Europe, Dublin, Ireland). The scalp was cleaned with Betadine (MEDA Pharma, Paris, France) and the skull was exposed by midline scalp excision. A small hole (0.5 mm in diameter) was then drilled 0.1 mm posterior and 2.3 mm left to the bregma. Five hundred thousand U87 cells dissolved in 2 mL of Minimum Essential Medium were injected using a 10-mL Hamilton syringe into the left hemisphere at a depth of 3 mm below the brain's surface. On withdrawal of the injection needle, the hole in the skull was sealed with bone wax and the scalp was sutured.

3. Sequence

3.1 RARE 2D

T2-weighted sequences are the most widely used for imaging-based tumor detection. These are accelerated spin-echo sequences (RARE, or Rapid Acquisition with Refocused Echoes) which are generally acquired in two dimensions (2D), in multi-slice mode. When these sequences are used for clinical imaging, pulses are often added to suppress fluid signals (FLAIR, or Fluid-Attenuated Inversion Recovery).

To image small animals, the following parameters are used:

in 2D

TE/TR = 70/5,000 ms; FOV: 22.5 x 22.5 mm; matrix: 192 x 128; spatial resolution: 117 x 175 µm; slice thickness: 750 µm; excitation pulse: Hermite 1 ms, 90°; refocusing pulse: Hermite 1 ms, 180°; reception bandwidth: 260 Hertz/pixel; RARE factor: 32; number of averages: 32, total acquisition time: 10 min 40 sec; transverse orientation.

3.2 TrueFISP

The specificity of bSSFP (balanced Steady-State Free Precession) type sequences, also known as TrueFISP or FIESTA, is their perfect symmetry, with an echo time (TE) equal to half the repetition time (TR). This maintains the magnetization in the transverse plane. Due to spin dephasing, the signal generated is more intense than with gradient-echo sequences. This allows 3D images to be constructed with good spatial resolution within a reasonable acquisition time. Besides, the tissue contrast generated is proportional to the T1/T2 ratio. The alternating phase RF pulse method must be used with 4 or 8 $\Delta\varphi$ phase values (180°, 0°, 90°, 270°; 45°, 135°, 225°, 315°). Image reconstruction is based on the Sum-Of-Square (SOS) method, i.e. calculation of the square root of the sum of squares of the magnitude signal.

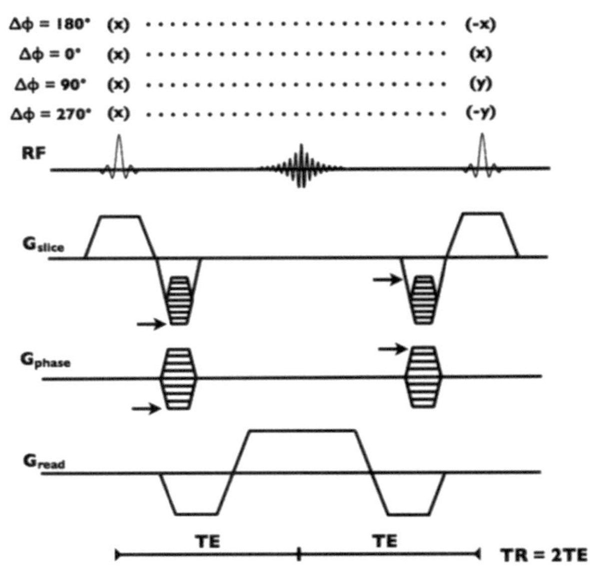

Fig. 4. 3D TrueFISP sequence chronogram. The RF pulse phase indicated generates images corresponding to the following $\Delta\varphi$ values: 180°, 0°, 90°, 270°. The sequence is perfectly symmetrical about the center of the echo. Thus, the echo time (TE) is equal to half the repetition time (TR).

The following sequence parameters are used:

- TE/TR = 2.5/5 ms; FOV: 32 x 18 x 18 mm; matrix: 192 x 96 x 80; spatial resolution: 166 x 187 x 225 μm; excitation pulse: Hermite 0.4 ms; reception bandwidth: 260 Hertz/pixel; number of averages (NA): 16 (including 4 $\Delta\varphi$ values), total acquisition time: 2 min 34 sec x4 = 10 min 16 sec; transverse orientation.
- TE/TR = 1.5/3 ms;
- TE/TR = 5/10 ms;
- TE/TR = 10/20 ms;

3.3 Theory

Simulations of the state of magnetization with TrueFISP, gradient-echo and spin-echo sequences were performed in Igor Pro using well-known equations (Eq. [4], [5] and [6)]. They were performed as a function of flip angle α, TR, TE or the T1 and T2 values of tissues. At 4.7 T, the T1 and T2 values of brain was equal to 1,295 ms and 53 ms, respectively, and for tumors, 1,525 and 72 ms, respectively [8].

- TrueFISP

$$S_{TrueFISP} = \frac{(1 - \exp^{-TR/T1}) \sin\alpha}{1 - (\exp^{-TR/T1} - \exp^{-TR/T2}) \cos\alpha - (\exp^{-TR/T1} \exp^{-TR/T2})} \exp^{-0.5TR/T2} \quad (4)$$

- Gradient echo

$$S_{GE} = \frac{(1 - \exp^{-TR/T1}) \sin\alpha}{1 - \cos\alpha (\exp^{-TR/T1})} \exp^{-TE/T2^*} \quad (5)$$

with TE = 2.5 ms and T2* = 25 ms

- Spin echo

A 1/6.32 correction factor was applied to 2D RARE (Eq. [6]), corresponding to the voxel size, the number of averages and the number of k-space samples by comparison with 3D TrueFISP acquisition.

$$S_{SE} = (1 - 2\exp^{(TE/2-TR)/T1}) + \exp^{-TR/T1}) \exp^{-TE/T2} \quad (6)$$

S/N was simulated for the brain and tumor, and contrast was evaluated according to Eq. [7].

$$\text{Contrast} = S_{Tumor} - S_{Brain} \quad (7)$$

The signal-to-noise ratio was evaluated for both tumor and brain tissues. For the TrueFISP sequence, the maximal signal was obtained with the shortest possible TE and a flip angle between approximately 15° and 35°, as shown in Figs. 5ab. The slight S/N difference between the healthy brain and the tumor is also observable. The gradient-echo sequence generates a much lower S/N compared with the TrueFISP sequence for all flip angles.

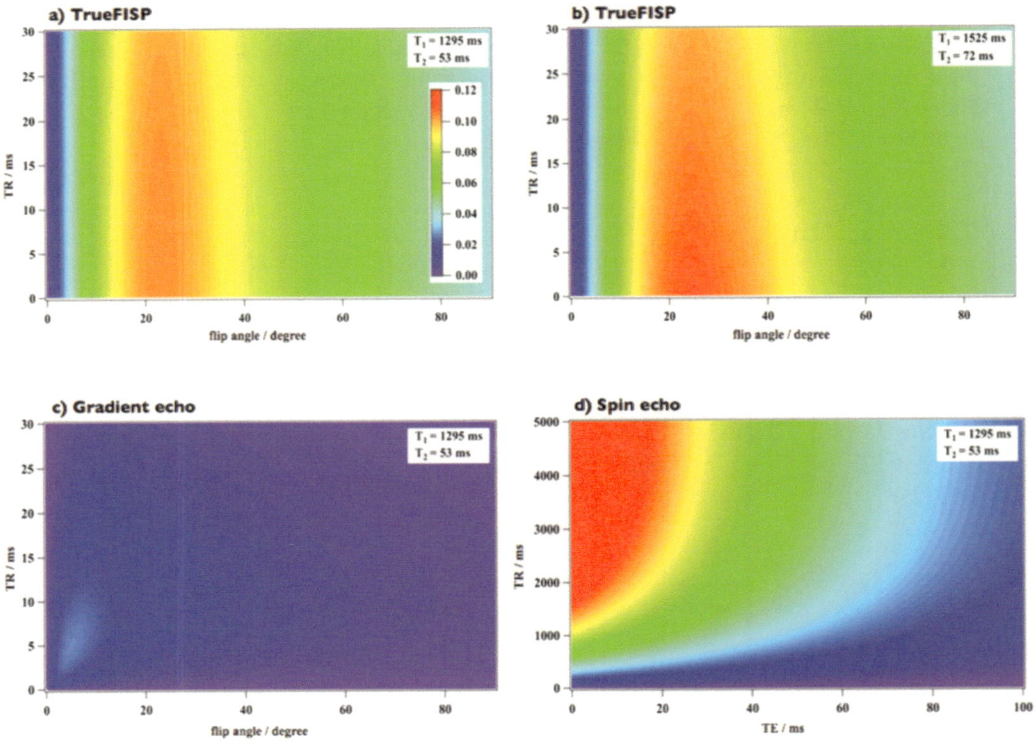

Fig. 5. Modeling of the signal-to-noise ratio using the above equations for: ab) the TrueFISP sequence, c) the gradient-echo sequence, and d) the spin-echo sequence. The signal was estimated as a function of the flip angle and TR for a), b), and c). For the spin-echo sequence, the signal was estimated as a function of the TEs and TRs of the sequence. The T1 and T2 values for the brain (1,295 ms and 53 ms, respectively) were used in a), c), and d). The T1 and T2 values for the tumor (1,525 ms and 72 ms, respectively) were used in b). The same color scale was used in the 4 simulations. To allow for the 2-dimensional nature of the spin-echo sequence, a correction factor was applied.

The spin-echo sequence should provide a high S/N, provided the TR is long and TE very short. However, these acquisition conditions do not provide sufficient contrast, as shown in the following figure.

We can thus clearly see the advantage of the TrueFISP sequence, as far as the S/N is concerned, for an equivalent total acquisition time, compared with both a standard 3D gradient-echo sequence and a 2D RARE spin-echo sequence.

3.4 Contrast

The contrast was then assessed theoretically, based on the signal difference between the tumor and the healthy brain. For the TrueFISP sequence (Fig. 6a), optimal contrast was achieved with a short TE and a flip angle between 25° and 50°.

The gradient-echo sequence provided almost no contrast compared with the TrueFISP sequence, while the spin-echo sequence provided improved contrast for TRs over 3,500 ms and TEs greater than 50 ms.

To conclude on these simulations (S/N and contrast), a very high S/N can be expected with the TrueFISP sequence. This method provides adequate contrast between the brain and tumor with flip angles around 30° and short TEs. Yet, contrast should be improved with the T2-weighted accelerated spin-echo sequence (RARE), but this method is generally used to acquire 2D images only, thus limiting its capacity to measure tumor volumes. Using it for 3D imaging can produce artifacts due to movements, and the acquisition time is much longer than with the TrueFISP sequence.

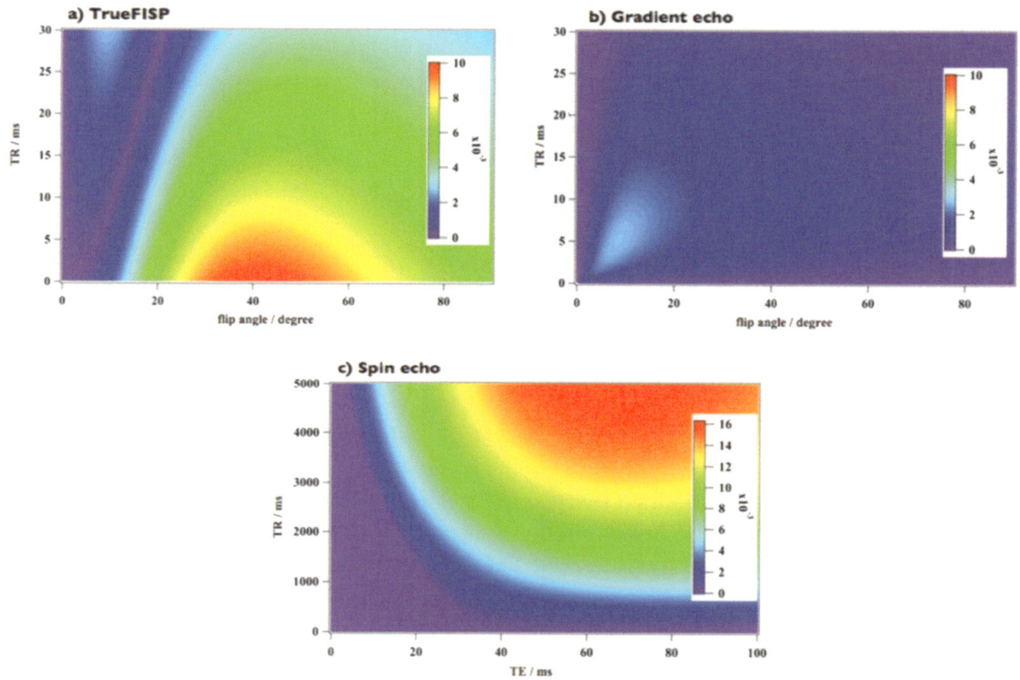

Fig. 6. Simulation of the contrast between tumor and brain using a) the 3D TrueFISP sequence, b) the 3D gradient-echo sequence, and c) the 2D spin-echo sequence. The contrast is estimated as a function of the flip angle and TR for the TrueFISP and gradient-echo sequences, and as a function of TE and TR for the spin-echo sequence.

4. Results

4.1 Correction of TrueFISP banding artifacts

TrueFISP images were acquired at 4.7 T using a cross-polarized antenna. A U87 glioma was implanted in a mouse, and imaging was performed 4 days later.

Fig. 7.a shows the image acquired using the TrueFISP sequence with a TE of 2.5 ms, a flip angle of 35°, and a $\Delta\varphi$ value of 180°. As expected, black-signal bands are clearly visible in the image. These hinder visualization of parts of the animal's brain. Modifying the $\Delta\varphi$ value (to 0°, 90°, and 270°) shifts the positions of the null-signal bands. For some of these values ($\Delta\varphi$ = 270°), the tumor is clearly visible, while for others ($\Delta\varphi$ = 90°), the null-signal zone covers the area containing the tumor, making all subsequent analyses of the tumor impossible.

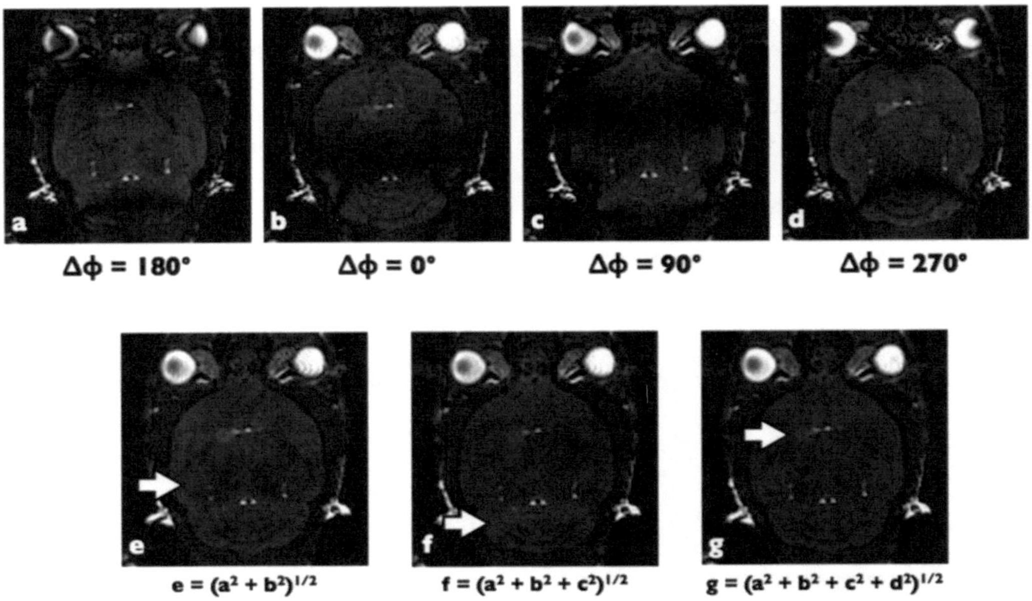

Fig. 7. Brain images from a mouse with an implanted tumor on day 4 after implantation. Images were obtained using the 3D TrueFISP sequence at 4.7 T and $\Delta\varphi$ = 180° (a), 0° (b), 90° (c), 270° (d). Null-signal bands are clearly visible and shift in position. Image e was obtained by SOS reconstruction from a) and b). The arrow indicates a non-compensated low-signal-intensity band. Image f was obtained by reconstruction from a), b), and c). The arrow indicates a high-signal-intensity band. Finally, Image g was obtained from the 4 images a), b), c), and d). The arrow shows the tumor, with a volume of less than 2 μL.

To eliminate these null-signal bands, the images acquired in a), b), c), and d) can be combined. To do so, various methods have been described in the literature, such as the sum of k-spaces, the sum of magnitude images, or the square root of the sum of squares of magnitude images. The latter method will be used here as it has been shown to be the most effective [14].

As shown in Images a-b, the black-signal bands do not appear to overlap. These two images were therefore combined to produce Image e. This eliminated the very pronounced null-signal bands, and the tumor became clearly visible. Nevertheless, the signal was not homogeneous throughout the brain, and a band (indicated by the white arrow in Image e) shows a reduced signal intensity compared with other areas of the brain. This type of artifact appears in various positions for all types of combinations of 2 images (ac, ad, bc, etc.).

This low-signal-intensity band could be eliminated by adding a third image to the combination (a, b, and c). However, a band of slightly higher signal intensity (white arrow in Image f) appeared. The position of this band corresponds to the black-signal band in Image d.

Finally, by adding Image d to the final combination, Image g was obtained (g = (a2 + b2 + c2 + d2)1/2. In this case, the brain appears perfectly homogeneous and the tumor is clearly visible.

4.2 Influence of flip angle on S/N and contrast on TrueFISP imaging

As shown in the simulations, for a TR of 5 ms, the S/N should be optimal with a flip angle between 15° and 35°. On the other hand, contrast between tumor and brain should be optimal with a flip angle between 25° and 55°. For a fixed TE, TrueFISP images were acquired with a flip angle between 8° and 35°. Above this range, the S/N is reduced and, more importantly, signals from sub-cutaneous fat and fluids (such as cerebrospinal fluid) become very intense. This leads to a strong reduction in signal dynamics for the brain and tumor, and generates images which are more difficult to interpret.

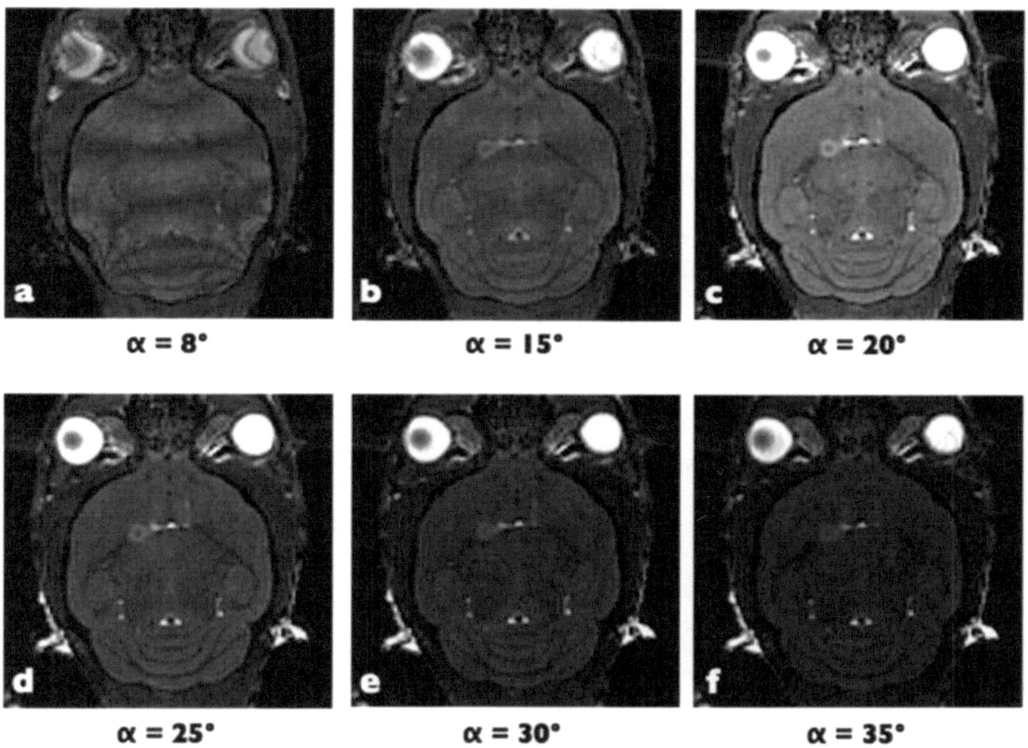

Fig. 8. Images obtained using the 3D TrueFISP sequence after correction of banding artifacts according to the α flip angle. TE was set to 2.5 ms.

The best contrast between brain and tumor was achieved at 35°. For α = 25 and 30°, good contrast was maintained, providing easy tumor detection, and the S/N was increased. Below this, the signal for healthy brain was increased and the tumor became difficult to distinguish. An 8° angle gave rise to more TrueFISP artifacts in different positions. At this value, reconstruction could not generate an image without null-signal bands, and the tumor became indistinguishable from the surrounding brain.

The table below gives the S/N and contrast between the brain and tumor for the various flip angles. To summarize, flip angles between 25 and 35° allow tumors to be segmented semi-automatically based on tissue contrast.

TE = 2.5 ms flip angle (°)	S/N Brain	S/N Tumor	Contrast
35	26.0	37.7	11.7
30	29.8	40.3	10.5
25	33.3	43.5	10.2
20	46.3	56.6	10.3
15	51	60.5	9.5
8	57.6	57.8	0.2

Table 1. S/N and contrast for brain and tumor, as a function of the flip angle, α. TE was set to 2.5 ms.

4.3 Influence of TE on S/N and contrast in TrueFISP imaging

Using a low bandwidth generates images with a high S/N. However, a decrease in bandwidth causes an increase in the sequence's TE. The influence of this was measured over the range between 1.5 and 10 ms (with the flip angle set at 35°). With a low TE (1.5 ms), the contrast appeared better than in the reference image acquired at 2.5 ms, but the S/N was significantly reduced, and the signal from fatty tissue was increased due to its relatively low T1. This resulted in a lower-quality image. Interestingly, at higher TEs (5 and 10 ms), the TrueFISP sequence generated few susceptibility artifacts compared with a FLASH sequence with the same TE (data not shown). However, at TE = 10 ms, the tumor was no longer visible due to a strongly reduced contrast between brain and tumor.
As described in the table below, only a TE value of 2.5 ms provides a contrast greater than 10, allowing the tumor to be segmented semi-automatically.

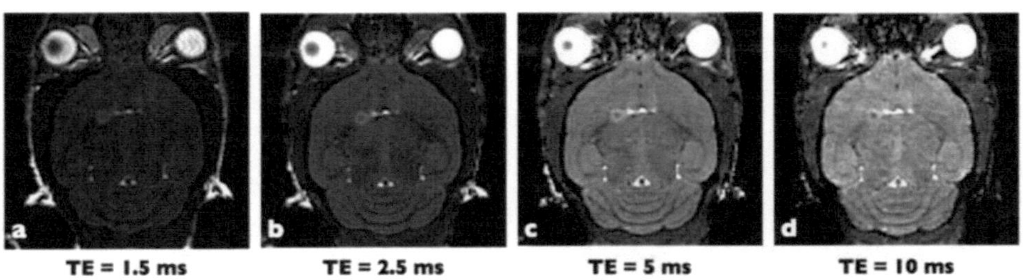

Fig. 9. Images acquired using the 3D TrueFISP sequence after correction of banding artifacts based on TE. The flip angle was set to 35°.

flip angle = 35° TE	S/N Brain	S/N Tumor	Contrast
1.5	22.46	28.53	6
2.5	26.0	37.7	11.7
5	46.7	54.4	7.7
10	38.6	41.9	3.3

Table 2. S/N and contrast for brain and tumor, as a function of the echo time. The flip angle α was set at 35°.

4.4 Comparison between RARE and TrueFISP imaging

The reference method for tumor detection by anatomic imaging is T2-weighted spin-echo imaging. Images were therefore acquired with a T2-weighted 2D RARE sequence. This sequence detects the tumor despite its small size (see Fig. 10d). In addition, as expected from simulations, contrast between the tumor and healthy brain is higher than with the TrueFISP sequence (Fig. 10a). The total acquisition time for the 2D RARE sequence was comparable with that for the 3D TrueFISP sequence. However, as the images were acquired in 2D by multi-slice imaging, reconstruction in other dimensions generates images with poor resolution and low quality (Figs. 10ef) compared with the 3D TrueFISP sequence (Figs. 10bc).
The two imaging methods were next used to measure tumor volume. With the TrueFISP sequence, the volume was estimated at 2.4 µL, while with the RARE sequence it was estimated at 4.3 µL. This overestimation of the volume with the RARE sequence is due to the low spatial resolution of this sequence in the third dimension. Actually, significant partial-volume effects are generated by this sequence and lead to volume-measurement errors.
A 3D RARE sequence validated the 2.4 µL volume determined using the TrueFISP sequence. The 3D RARE image was acquired over 45 minutes.

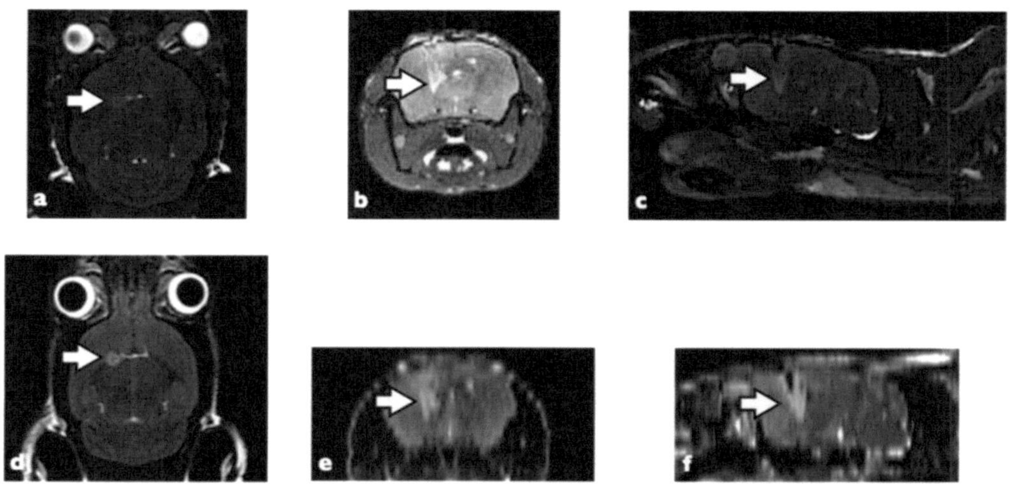

Fig. 10. 3D TrueFISP (a, b, and c) and multi-slice 2D RARE imaging (d, e, and f) of a mouse with implanted glioma: a) & d) sagittal sections; b) & e) reconstruction of transverse sections; c) & f) reconstruction of coronal sections. The white arrows indicate the tumor.

Volume overestimation based on 2D imaging was confirmed by using the two sequences to image a phantom consisting of a known volume of water. With the 2D RARE sequence, the error in volume measurement was around 20%, while with the TrueFISP sequence the error was only 4%.

4.5 Imaging at 9.4T

Images were acquired with the same 2 sequences at 9.4 T on a mouse model of glioma. To suppress banding artifacts with the TrueFISP sequence, 8 images had to be acquired with 8 different Δφ values (180°, 0°, 90°, 270°, 45°, 135°, 225°, 315°).

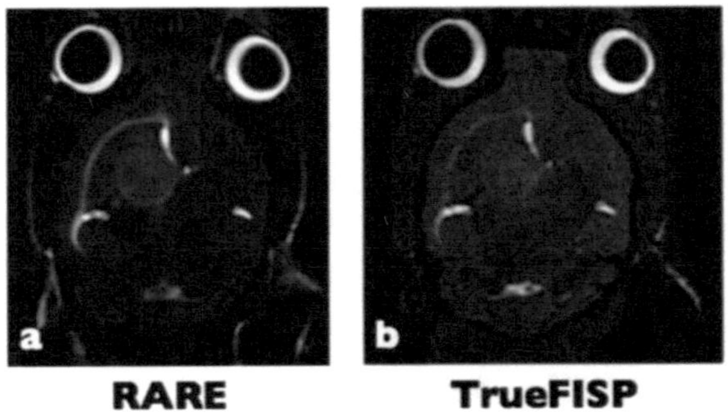

Fig. 11. 2D RARE (a) and 3D TrueFISP (b) imaging at 9.4 T. With RARE imaging, the tumor is clearly visible, while TrueFISP provides a lower tumor/brain contrast.

With the RARE sequence, the tumor is clearly detectable and contrast is comparable with that of an image acquired at 4.7 T (Fig. 10a). For the TrueFISP sequence, the contrast is reduced, making it very difficult to distinguish the tumor from the remainder of the brain, except from the presence of structural heterogeneity. In this case, it is not possible to semi-automatically segment the tumor, and it is therefore impossible to measure its volume with good reproducibility. In addition, as demonstrated previously, small tumors may turn out to be undetectable.

TE	S/N Brain	S/N Tumor	Contrast
TrueFISP 4.7 T	26.0	37.7	11.7
RARE 4.7 T	25.4	38.5	13.1
TrueFISP 9.4 T	24.6	28.3	3.7
RARE 9.4 T	18.9	32.2	13.3

Table 3. S/N and contrast for brain and tumor, at 4.7 T and 9.4 T, with RARE and TrueFISP sequences.

4.6 Longitudinal follow up of glioma volume at 4.7T

The simulations and experiments performed above show that an implanted tumor can be unambiguously distinguished by 3D TrueFISP imaging when a TE of 2.5 ms is combined with a flip angle of 35° for imaging at 4.7 T. These parameters were therefore used for the longitudinal follow-up of tumor volume in an animal implanted with a U87-type glioma. Images were also acquired with the 2D RARE sequence to compare volume measurements.

The tumor was easily detectable 7 days after implantation despite its small volume (2 μL). The images obtained with the TrueFISP sequence are shown from day 9 after implantation. The animal was then followed up for approximately 30 days, with a 2 or 3-day interval between MRI scans. The increase in tumor diameter is visible in the images (Fig. 12). From d25, zones of black signal appear in the tumor's center, these are probably due to necrotic areas.

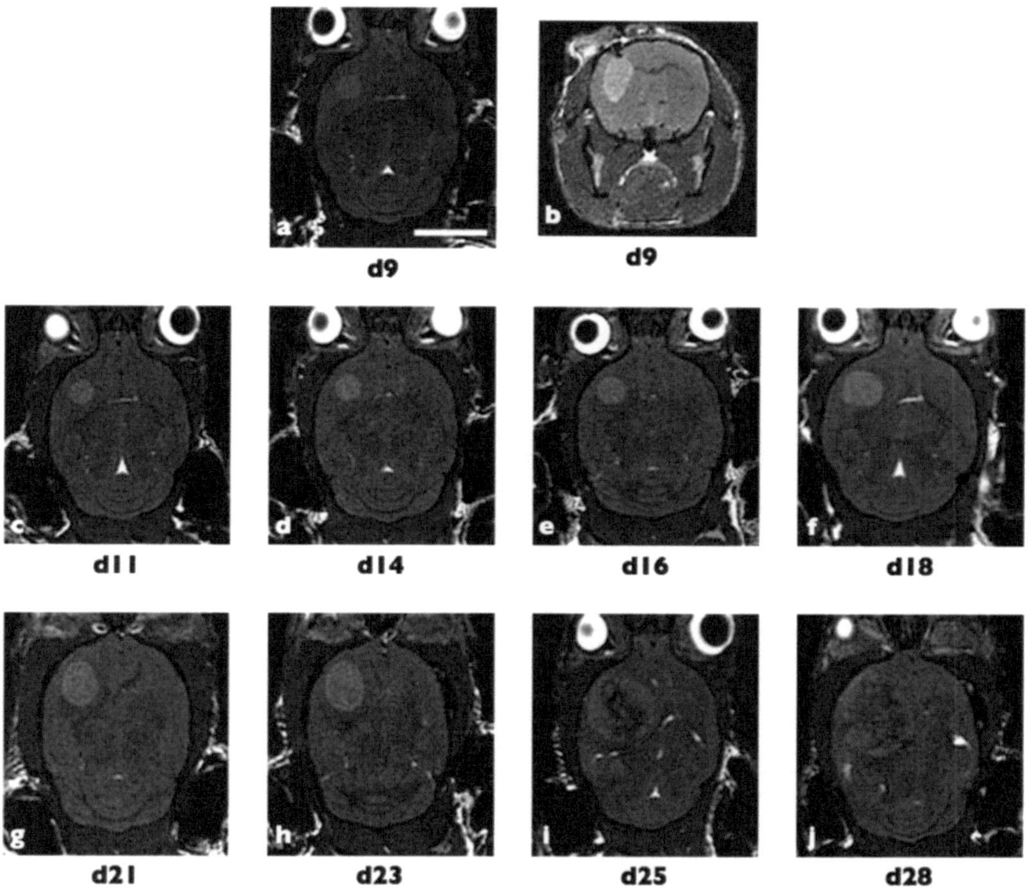

Fig. 12. Longitudinal follow-up of tumor progression by 3D TrueFISP imaging at 4.7 T. Images ab show the sagittal and transverse sections of the mouse brain at d9 after implantation. Images cj show tumor progression between d11 and d28.

Based on these 3D images (a-h), the tumor can readily be semi-automatically segmented, and the 3D volume could be reconstructed (Fig. 13). In Images i-j, the tumor/brain contrast is lower, but the tumor can still be manually delimited and its volume measured.
Based on these 3D reconstructions, tumor volume progression was reported as a function of time (Fig. 14). Tumor growth could thus be assessed, from its initial approximately 4μL volume up to its final 100μL volume, i.e. approximately one quarter of the animal's total brain volume.

On the other hand, with the 2D RARE sequence, the tumor is also visible from day 7 after implantation. However, the volume measured based on images acquired with the RARE sequence is always greater than that measured by TrueFISP, and, importantly, very little difference is observed over the first 4 analysis times (d9, d11, d14, d16). This is probably due to a less precise measurement of the tumor volume, which, as indicated above, is due to very low spatial resolution in the third dimension.

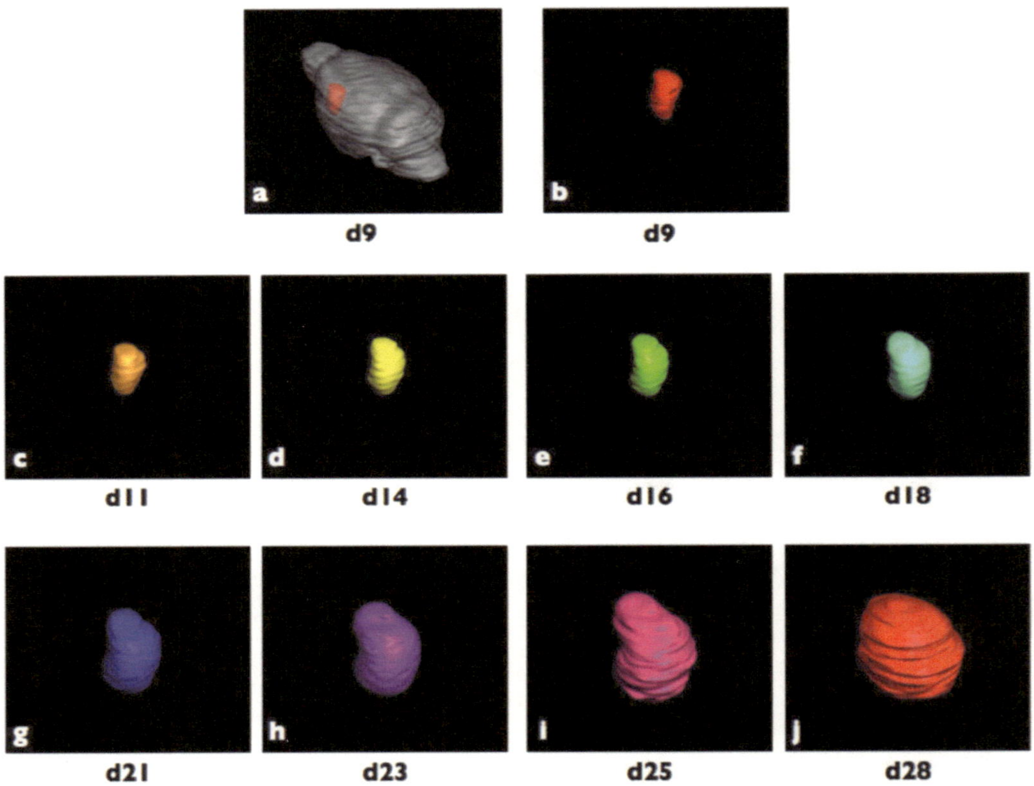

Fig. 13. 3D reconstruction of the tumor by semi-automatic segmentation from the images shown in Figure 11. Image a: reconstruction of the whole brain (gray) and the tumor (red) at d9. Images bj: 3D representation of the tumor over time. The same arbitrary scale is used in all images.

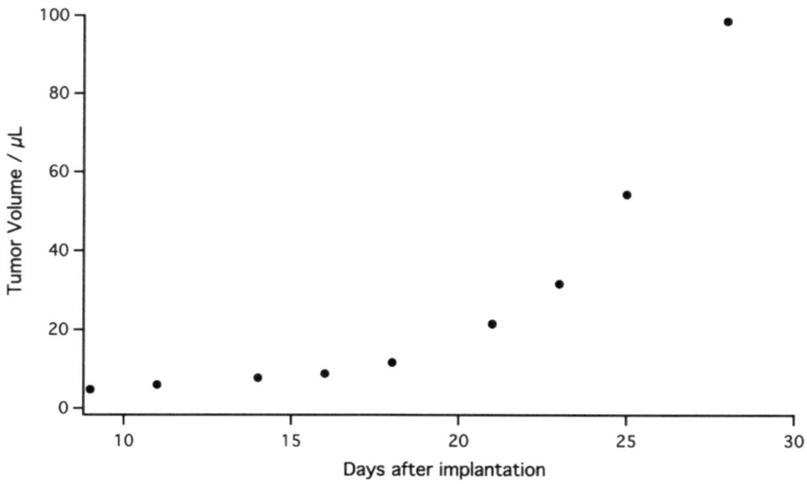

Fig. 14. Progression of tumor volume over time based on the volumes shown in Figure 13.

5. Discussion and conclusion

The aim of this chapter was to show how the 3D TrueFISP sequence can improve longitudinal follow-up of glioma volume in a given animal model.

This sequence is rarely used at high magnetic fields as it generates numerous artifacts known as banding artifacts [10-12]. However, the S/N and contrast provided by this sequence can be useful in imaging small animals at high fields.

It has been shown that these artifacts can be easily corrected at 4.7 T and 9.4 T when studying mouse brains, and also for areas which are much more sensitive to movements and susceptibility artifacts, such as the heart [8,13]. To do so, the so-called 'alternating-phase RF pulse' method is used, in combination with reconstruction through calculation of the square root of the sum of squares of the magnitude signal [14]. As shown here, 4 phase steps are necessary to suppress artifacts at 4.7 T, while at least 8 steps are required at 9.4 T [8]. The resulting image appears perfectly homogeneous in terms of signal, and no longer displays artifacts. The requirement for 4 images increases the total acquisition time, but this nevertheless remains much shorter than with a T2-weighted 3D RARE sequence (12 min vs. 45 min) [8,15].

The 3D TrueFISP imaging sequence was compared, in terms of S/N and contrast, with the more commonly used gradient-echo and spin-echo sequences. Simulations, which were confirmed by experimental results, indicate a clear superiority of this sequence in terms of S/N. As the sequence can be used with short TRs (like a gradient-echo sequence), it is perfectly adapted to 3D imaging, unlike spin-echo sequences which require long TRs. A high S/N is obtained with the magnetization maintained in the transverse plane, thanks to a zero gradient sum at the end of each TR. This is much better than 'spoiling', which is used with the more common gradient-echo or FLASH sequences.

The TrueFISP sequence provides a much higher signal-to-noise ratio than a 2D accelerated spin-echo sequence. This is associated with better spatial resolution in the third dimension. Yet, the RARE sequence can also be used in 3D and also provides very high S/Ns. However, additional spatial encoding for the T2-weighted RARE spin echo has a drastic effect on the total acquisition time: good T2 weighting is required for tumor detection, and can only be obtained with TRs greater than 3,500 ms. This leads to a total acquisition time on the order of 1 hour, whereas around 10 minutes is adequate with the 2D sequence or the 3D TrueFISP sequence.

The TrueFISP sequence provides adequate contrast, allowing even very small tumors to be detected clearly, and semi-automatically segmented using generic image-analysis tools. However, as shown in both simulations and images, the contrast between the healthy brain and the tumor remains lower than that provided by the spin-echo sequence. This is due to TrueFISP-sequence weighting, which relies on the T1/T2 ratio, while the RARE sequence only uses T2 weighting. This has several consequences. In some cases, e.g. when the tumor becomes very large and heterogeneous, semi-automatic segmentation becomes difficult due to inadequate contrast with the healthy brain. Manual segmentation therefore becomes necessary, which may be both tedious and subjective. Nevertheless, the error rate when estimating even large volumes remains low.

Another consequence is that it is almost impossible to detect a glioma in the brain at fields higher than 4.7 T based on natural contrast. This is because the T1 and T2 values for the brain and tumor become almost identical, which limits the contrast at very high magnetic fields. The T2-weighted RARE sequence still works perfectly at these higher fields.

Thus, for this type of application, the TrueFISP sequence at 9.4 T or greater provides little advantage over other, more commonly used sequences. However, at low fields, the S/N and contrast provided by the TrueFISP sequence make it particularly interesting. It has already been shown with specific instruments that it allows tumors to be easily detected in mice based on natural contrast, and that it provides an excellent signal-to-noise ratio at clinical magnetic fields (1.5 T and 3 T) [16,17].

In terms of spatial resolution, the advantages of 3D compared with 2D imaging are obvious. Three-dimensional imaging results in much smaller voxel sizes with comparable acquisition times, while maintaining a high S/N. This requires the addition of a phase-encoding table in the slice direction, i.e. a much greater number of lines read in the Fourier volume. The advantages of sequences with short TRs thus become obvious. As shown, the TrueFISP sequence also provides a much greater precision when measuring tumor volume, in particular for small tumors. With the 2D RARE sequence, it is impossible to precisely measure volume changes in the first days following tumor implantation. With the 3D TrueFISP sequence, this information is readily available.

In addition, as the sequence is relatively rapid in terms of total acquisition time, it can be repeated at very short intervals to follow tumor progression, even in relatively fragile mice. The total examination, between preparation of the animal and imaging, lasts less than 20 minutes. This makes it possible to study animals on a daily basis. This is much more difficult when contrast agents must be injected, or with acquisition times of around 1 hour, as with 3D RARE sequences [15].

To conclude, the 3D TrueFISP sequence can be easily used to follow tumor progression in a small animal model imaged at 4.7 T. Thanks to a particularly high S/N, artifact-free images can be acquired, with excellent spatial resolution and good tumor/healthy brain contrast. The total acquisition time remains under 15 minutes, thus offering precise longitudinal follow-up of tumor volume. Thus, this sequence could be used to noninvasively validate the efficacy of new genetic or pharmacological treatments for glioma.

At lower magnetic fields, the sequence has also demonstrated its efficacy. In contrast, it is currently not applicable at 9.4 T or higher to precisely measure tumor volumes.

6. References

[1] Bock NA, Zadeh G, Davidson LM, et al. High-resolutionlongitudinal screening with magnetic resonance imaging in a murine brain cancer model. Neoplasia 2003;5:546–554.

[2] Moats RA, Velan-Mullan S, Jacobs R, et al. Micro-MRI at 11.7T of a murine brain tumor model using delayed contrast enhancement. Mol Imaging 2003;2:150–158 [erratum: Mol Imaging 2003;2(4)].

[3] Miraux S, Lemiere S, Pineau R, et al. Inhibition of FGF receptor activity in glioma implanted into the mouse brain using the tetra- cyclin-regulated expression system. Angiogenesis 2004;7:105–113.

[4] Sun Y, Mulkern RV, Schmidt K, et al. Quantification of water dif- fusion and relaxation times of human U87 tumors in a mouse model. NMR Biomed 2004;17:399–404.

[5] Quesson B, Bouzier AK, Thiaudiere E, Delalande C, Merle M, Ca- nioni P. Magnetization transfer fast imaging of implanted glioma in the rat brain at 4.7T: interpretation using a binary spin-bath model. J Magn Reson Imaging 1997;7:1076–1083.

[6] Hennig J, Nauerth A, Friedburg H. RARE imaging: a fast imaging method for clinical MR. Magn Reson Med 1986;3:823–833.

[7] Oppelt A, Graumann R, Barfu H, Fischer H, Hartl W, Schajor W. FISP—a new fast MRI sequence. Electromedica 1986;54:15–18.

[8] Miraux S, Massot P, Ribot EJ, Franconi JM, Thiaudiere E. 3D TrueFISP imaging of mouse brain at 4.7T and 9.4T. J Magn Reson Imaging 2008;28:497–503.

[9] De Coene B, Hajnal JV, Gatehouse P, Longmore DB, White SJ, Oatridge A, Pennock JM, Young IR, Bydder GM. MR of the brain using fluid-attenuated inversion recovery (FLAIR) pulse sequences. AJNR Am J Neuroradiol. 1992 Nov-Dec;13(6):1555-64.

[10] Haacke EM, Wielopolski PA, Tkach JA, Modic MT. Steady-state free precession imaging in the presence of motion: application for im- proved visualization of the cerebrospinal fluid. Radiology 1990;175: 545–552.

[11] Zur Y, Wood ML, Neuringer LJ. Motion-insensitive, steady-state free precession imaging. Magn Reson Med 1990;16:444 - 459.

[12] Vasanawala SS, Pauly JM, Nishimura DG. Linear combination steady-state free precession MRI. Magn Reson Med 2000;43:82–90. 11. Casselman JW, Kuhweide R, Deimling M, Ampe W, Dehaene I, Meeus L. Constructive interference in steady state-3DFT MR imaging of the inner-ear and cerebellopontine angle. AJNR Am J Neuroradiol 1993;14:47–57.

[13] Miraux S, Calmettes G, Massot P, Lefrancois W, Parzy E, Muller B, Arsac LM, Deschodt-Arsac V, Franconi JM, Diolez P, Thiaudie`re E. 4D retrospective black blood trueFISP imaging of mouse heart. Magn Reson Med 2009; 62: 1099–1105.

[14] Vasanawala SS, Pauly JM, Nishimura DG. Linear combination steady-state free precession MRI. Magn Reson Med 2000; 43: 82–90.

[15] Natt O, Watanabe T, Boretius S, Radulovic J, Frahm J, Michaelis T. High-resolution 3D MRI of mouse brain reveals small cerebral structures in vivo. J Neurosci Methods 2002;120:203–209.

[16] Bernas LM, Foster PJ, Rutt BK. Imaging iron-loaded mouse glioma tumors with bSSFP at 3 T. Bernas LM, Foster PJ, Rutt BK. Magn Reson Med. 2010 Jul;64(1):23-31.

[17] Ribot EJ, Martinez-Santiesteban FM, Simedrea C, Steeg PS, Chambers AF, Rutt BK, Foster PJ, In Vivo Single Scan Detection of Both Iron-Labeled Cells and Breast Cancer Metastases in the Mouse Brain Using Balanced Steady-State Free Precession Imaging at 1.5 T. J Magn Reson Imaging 2011 Jul;34(1):231-8.

8

Clinical Microdialysis in Glioma

Hani Marcus and Dipankar Nandi
Imperial College London
United Kingdom

1. Introduction

Microdialysis is a technique that may be used to directly investigate brain chemistry in-vivo. Although initially developed over 35 years ago (Ungerstedt and Pycock 1974), it is only relatively recently that studies have begun to utilise microdialysis in patients with glioma and other brain tumours. In this chapter we will review the general principles of microdialysis, the use of the technique to investigate glioma pathogenesis and evaluate chemo- and radiotherapy, and the potential utilisation of retrograde microdialysis to administer chemotherapeutic agents directly to the tumour bed.

2. Microdialysis

Present-day microdialysis is the result of several decades of technological advancement. An understanding of the principles underlying the technique is an essential prerequisite to appreciating its potential uses and limitations.

2.1 Principles, uses and limitations

2.1.1 Principles

Microdialysis enables sampling of the extracellular fluid (ECF). A microdialysis catheter or probe with a semi-permeable membrane at its tip is placed into the tissue of interest. Perfusate with a similar composition to the ECF is then slowly and continuously infused through the catheter. Substances of interest diffuse across the semi-permeable membrane into the catheter, and the resulting dialysate is collected in microvials, which are changed at regular intervals and subsequently analysed (see Figure 1).

Diffusion of substances from the ECF, across the membrane, and into the flowing perfusate, is often incomplete. Thus, the concentration of a substance within the dialysate represents a fraction of that in the ECF. The *extraction fraction* or *relative recovery* is defined as the ratio of a substance's concentration in the dialysate ($C_{dialysate}$) compared to the actual concentration in the ECF (C_{ECF}).

$$\text{Relative Recovery} = C_{dialysate} / C_{ECF} \times 100\%$$

A number of variables may influence the relative recovery including the flow rate, the semi-permeable membranes length and pore size, and the properties of the substance of interest itself (see Table 1) (de Lange et al. 1997, de Lange, de Boer and Breimer 1999, Hutchinson et al. 2000, Benjamin et al. 2004, Helmy et al. 2009, Chefer et al. 2009, Blakeley et al. 2009).

Reducing the perfusate flow rate increases the time available for diffusion of substances across the semi-permeable membrane, and in turn increases the relative recovery of a substance (Tossman and Ungerstedt 1986, Hutchinson et al. 2000). This must be balanced against the reduced dialysate volumes obtained over time, which usually necessitate longer sampling intervals. Increasing the length of the semi-permeable membrane along which diffusion can occur also increases the relative recovery of a substance (Tossman and Ungerstedt 1986, Hutchinson et al. 2000) but the dimensions of the tissue being probed may limit this. Increasing the pore size of the semi-permeable membrane increases the size of molecules that are able to diffuse across it. Most microdialysis catheters used clinically are low molecular weight cut-off (LWCO) with a membrane pore size permitting molecules of approximately 20kDa (such as glucose and its metabolites) to diffuse across them. Recently high molecular weight cut-off (HWCO) catheters have been utilised with a larger membrane pore size permitting molecules of approximately 100kDa (such as cytokines) to diffuse across them. There are a number of methodological difficulties with using such catheters to measure the concentration of macromolecules (Helmy et al. 2009). One concern is that the increased membrane pore size used may lead to net efflux of fluid from the perfusate into the ECF thus influencing the composition of the ECF itself and compromising the validity of data obtained. There have been efforts to counter this net fluid efflux with the addition of a colloid to the perfusate. Various properties of the molecule being measured may also influence its relative recovery such as its shape, charge, hydrophobicity or hydrophilicity, hydrodynamic radius, and interaction with other molecules, such as dimerisation. The effect of these factors is that even molecules of a similar molecular weight may have considerably different relative recoveries in-vivo. Other factors may also alter the relative recovery. The diffusion coefficient has been estimated to increase by 1-2% for every degree Celsius increase in temperature. The diffusion coefficient within an aqueous solution is almost always greater than in tissue due to the increased diffusional path (or "tortousity") of the latter (Blakeley and Portnow).

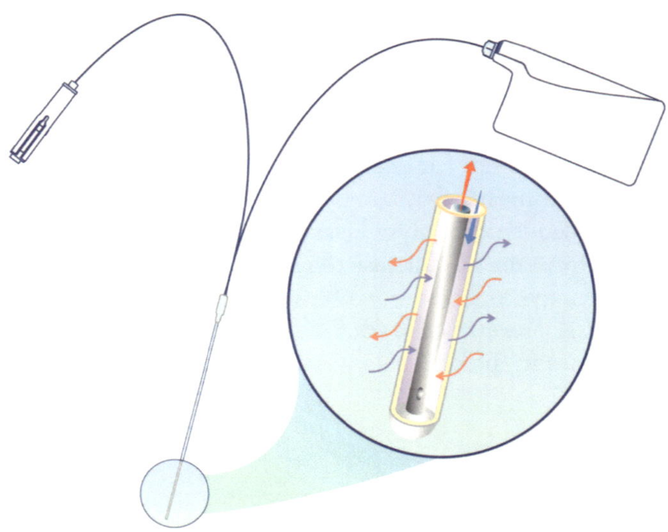

Fig. 1. Microdialysis components. micropump is seen on the right, microdialysis catheter in the centre, and microvials on the left.

Factor	Effect
Microdialysis dependent	
Perfusate flow rate	Decreasing recovery with faster flow rate
Membrane length	Increasing recovery with larger membrane
Membrane pore size	Larger molecules recovered with increasing pore size
Context dependent	
Analyte properties	Recovery of molecules of similar size may be very different
Solution properties	Recovery in-vitro and in-vivo may be very different
Temperature	Increasing recovery with temperature

Table 1. Factors affecting relative recovery

In-vitro studies have calculated the relative recovery for specific molecules under different experimental conditions in which the concentration of a substance in the external medium is known or directly measurable. Using such methods the in-vitro recovery for glucose and its metabolites using a LWCO catheter with a 10mm membrane at a flow rate of 0.3microl/min has been estimated at between 70-100% (Hutchinson et al. 2000, Blakeley and Portnow). The in-vitro recoveries of macromolecules such as cytokines using similar methods with a HWCO catheter are variable but usually far lower (Helmy et al. 2009). Although some investigators have used these calculated relative recoveries to correct dialysate concentrations measured, this has proved unreliable because, as mentioned previously, diffusion within aqueous test solutions differs significantly from diffusion within tissue in-vivo.

Several methods of determining relative recovery in-vivo have been described in attempt to overcome the shortcomings of in-vitro estimates (see Table 2) (Benjamin et al. 2004, Chefer et al. 2009, Blakeley and Portnow). These methods include the no-net-flux method, the flow-rate method, and the use of standards whose concentration is known (both exogenous and endogenous). In the no-net-flux method, perfusate containing several different concentrations of the analyte of interest (both above and below the anticipated concentration in the ECF) is perfused through the microdialysis probe and the amount of this analyte gained or lost from the probe is determined. Using this method the relative recovery may be calculated as the gradient of the linear regression that describes the dialysate concentration of the analyte being studied as a function of experimenter controlled variations in the perfusate concentration. In the flow-rate method, it is assumed that at a flow rate of zero (i.e. stasis) equilibrium between perfusate and the ECF is eventually achieved and that increasing the flow rate leads to a reduced relative recovery in a predictable but non-linear fashion. By infusing at different flow-rates and measuring the concentration of the analyte of interest, it is therefore possible to calculate the relative recovery (Hutchinson et al. 2000). Other methods rely on the use of an internal standard to estimate in-vivo relative recovery. Often, the perfusate contains a known concentration of a radiolabelled molecule similar to the analyte of interest. By determining the loss of this molecule during microdialysis it is possible to calculate its relative recovery. Alternatively, some investigators have made use of urea – which is assumed to have the same concentration throughout all water compartments in the body – as an endogenous standard. By determining the difference between the concentration of urea in plasma, and the concentration in dialysate collected, an estimate of the relative recovery of similar small molecules may be obtained (Brunner et al. 2000, Sorg et al. 2005).

Method	Principle
No-net-flux	When analyte concentrations within perfusate and ECF are equal, there is no-net-flux
Variable flow rate	When flow rate is zero (i.e. stasis) equilibrium occurs between perfusate and ECF
Internal standard (Exogenous e.g. radiolabelled)	Fraction of exogenous standard lost from perfusate is equal to fraction of analyte extracted from ECF
Internal standard (Endogenous e.g. urea)	Fraction of endogenous standard and analyte extracted from ECF is equal

Table 2. In-vivo methods of determining relative recovery

There are a number of methodological difficulties in estimating relative recovery using these described in-vivo techniques, particularly in the context of glioma research. The no-net-flux method requires an accurate estimation of the concentration of analytes in-vivo but the concentration of the cytokines and growth factors involved in gliomagenesis can vary by several orders of magnitude. The flow-rate method requires very slow flow rates to increase the accuracy of the regression analysis, which in turn necessitates long collection periods to obtain sufficient sample volume. The use of an internal standard relies on the assumption that it has a similar relative recovery to the analyte of interest, which, for the reasons mentioned above, may not be valid. These methodological difficulties in estimating relative recovery using in-vivo techniques have led some commentators to the conclusion that the ratio of the concentration of related physiological substances (such as the ratio of lactate/pyruvate, or pro-/anti-inflammatory cytokines) may be a more robust and valuable measurement than attempts to determine the absolute concentration of these molecules in the ECF (Helmy et al. 2009).

2.1.2 Uses

Until relatively recently few studies had applied microdialysis to patients undergoing surgical biopsy or resection of their brain tumours. To this end, clinical studies using microdialysis in patients with brain tumours offer a number of potential advantages over other methodological approaches. First, in contrast to traditional in-vitro studies, clinical microdialysis studies permit the assessment of brain tumours in-vivo, recognising the complex interactions between tumour- and host-related factors, and the role these interactions play in tumourogenesis. Second, by applying microdialysis to patients with brain tumours, rather than animal models of such tumours, clinical microdialysis eliminates the possibility of erroneous interpretation of interspecies differences or of limitations of the brain tumour model itself. Third, clinical microdialysis provides a direct measure of analytes within the ECF when compared with imaging techniques. Fourth, microdialysis easily allows repeated evaluation over an extended time course. Microdialysis therefore provides a unique method of continuously measuring brain and tumour chemistry allowing investigation of metabolites and macromolecules involved in tumourogenesis, the dynamic changes in the concentration these molecules over time, and their response to chemo- and radiotherapy. Finally, retrograde microdialysis offers the potential for the direct administration of chemotherapeutic agents to brain tumours.

2.1.3 Limitations

Several confounding factors must be considered when performing or interpreting studies that utilise microdialysis to investigate brain tumours. First, although microdialysis is a direct measure of analytes within the ECF, the concentration of a substance within the dialysate still represents only a fraction of that in the ECF. As discussed above, this relative recovery depends upon a large number of variables and estimation by in-vitro and in-vivo techniques has proved unreliable. Second, the invasive nature of microdialysis probe insertion may result in trauma artefact. A recent consensus meeting on microdialysis in neuro-intensive care recognised that data was unreliable for at least one hour after insertion (Bellander et al. 2004). In patients with brain tumour undergoing resection or debulking, the trauma artefact may be considerably longer, particularly if the macromolecules such as growth factors and cytokines are being monitored. Third, the precise location of the catheter tip may greatly influence the data obtained by microdialysis. Studies that have applied microdialysis to patients with brain tumour have demonstrated significantly different metabolic profiles at the tumour centre, tumour periphery or border, and grossly normal peri-tumoural tissue (Roslin et al. 2003, Marcus et al.).

These confounding factors are at least partially mitigated by the use of physiologically meaningful ratios (rather than absolute concentrations), the omission of the first few hours of data obtained post-insertion, and the careful note of catheter locations intra-operatively and using post-operative imaging (see Table 3). The combination of microdialysis with other research methods such as animal studies, in-vitro techniques and imaging provides a powerful research paradigm.

Limitation	Strategy
Relative recovery variable	Use physiological ratios rather than absolute concentrations
Trauma artefact	Minimise trauma and wait for data to normalise
Location of probe	Note location intra-operatively and image post-operatively to confirm

Table 3. Limitations of microdialysis and strategies to avoid

2.2 Equipment and technique

2.2.1 Equipment

The equipment required for microdialysis includes perfusion fluid, microdialysis syringes, microinfusion pumps, microdialysis catheters, and microvials (See Figure 1). Not all commercially available microdialysis equipment is suitable or certified for human use and this must be carefully considered before selecting study apparatus. Perfusion fluid should be as close to the cerebral ECF as possible and CMA CNS perfusion fluid composed of NaCl

(147 mM), KCl (2.7 mM), CaCl2 (1.2 mM), and MgCl2 (0.85 mM) in water, is often used. Perfusion fluid is contained in microdialysis syringes with a capacity of approximately 2.5ml. Microinfusion pumps are portable battery driven pumps that compress syringes at a slow predefined rate, which is usually fixed (0.3microl/min) but may be adjustable (0.1microl/min to 5microl/min). Microdialysis catheters vary in their membrane length (10-30mm) and pore size (LWCO/20kDa or HWCO/100kDa), and by their physical properties (such as shaft size). Conventional clinical microdialysis uses LWCO catheters. Clinical microdialysis studies investigating macromolecules such as cytokines or growth factors require HWCO catheters to maximise recovery of these substances. Fluid is collected in microvials designed to collect micro volume samples and minimise evaporation.

2.2.2 Technique

All patients must be thoroughly counselled beforehand about the potential (but very low) additional risk of haemorrhage and infection, and written informed consent obtained. Pre-operatively all the microdialysis equipment should be checked. Particular attention must be paid to the microdialysis catheter, syringe and perfusion fluid to ensure that their packaging remains intact and sterility maintained. Many clinicians advocate priming the catheter so that the system is already functional prior to insertion. This ensures constant fluid flow at the catheter tip and theoretically reduces sedimentation and non-specific binding of proteins to the catheter membrane. The microdialysis syringe is filled with CNS perfusion fluid, and connected to the microdialysis catheter using strict aseptic technique. The microdialysis syringe is placed in the microinfusion pump and a microvial placed at the distal end of the microdialysis catheter to collect the dialysate. Upon closing the lid of the microinfusion pump a 5-minute flush cycle is initiated followed by an automatic decrease to the preset flow rate.

Operative insertion of the microdialysis catheter into cerebral parenchyma may be via a closed or an open technique following tumour biopsy or resection respectively. In the closed technique stereotactic biopsy of brain tumour tissue is performed and then the microdialysis catheter inserted so that the catheter tip lies in the region of interest. Multiple catheters can be placed through a single burr hole using multiple different trajectories. The advantage of this technique is that traumatic artefact is minimised. In the open technique the brain tumour is resected and then the microdialysis catheter placed into the region of interest. Intra-operative real-time three-dimensional ultrasound probes have been used to assist catheter placement (Homapour et al.). Although there is greater traumatic resection artefact associated with open placement the risk of inadvertent complications, such as intracerebral haematoma, is theoretically lower because the catheter is inserted under direct visualisation and blood vessels can be avoided. The precise position of catheters within the brain is critical to interpreting clinical microdialysis studies but a number of terms have been used in the literature with conflicting and overlapping definitions. To avoid confusion during subsequent discussion we will define catheter locations in the following way: Tumour (T) catheters are either within grossly affected tumour tissue, or within 5mm of the resection margin of such tissue; Peritumour (PT) catheters are within 5mm-20mm of the tumour or resection margin; Brain Around Tumour (BAT) catheters are within grossly unaffected brain at least 20mm away from the tumour or resection margin. Once in place the catheter may be secured using a commercial "bolt" or by tunnelling the catheter and stitching it into place, depending on whether a closed or open approach insertion technique is used respectively.

Term	Definition
Tumour (T)	Within grossly affected tumour tissue, or within 5mm of the resection margin of such tissue
Peritumour (PT)	Within 5mm-20mm of the tumour or resection margin
Brain Around Tumour (BAT)	Within grossly unaffected brain at least 20mm away from the tumour or resection margin

Table 4. Definitions on the location of microdialysis catheters

Imaging should be performed to confirm the catheter position post-operatively. Most commercially available microdialysis catheters are fashioned with a "gold-tip" that is visible on CT to facilitate their identification. The initial microvial (containing flush) is not analysed. Subsequent microvials are numbered and exchanged sequentially at predefined intervals. Microvials are either analysed immediately or stored in -80c for subsequent analysis. Studies have shown that the concentration of glucose and its metabolites within microdialysate is equivalent with measured immediately or after storage in this manner (Hutchinson et al. 2000).

Glucose and its metabolites are frequently measured using commercial point-of-care analysers such as the ISCUS or CMA 600 (CMA Microdialysis AB, Solna, Sweden), which employ an enzyme-kinetic technique. Several techniques can also be used to analyse the macromolecules present within dialysate. Because the volumes of liquid are small and the concentrations of substances very low, techniques such as Enzyme-Linked Immunosorbent Assay (ELISA), High Performance Liquid Chromatography (HPLC), or Mass Spectroscopy (MS) are often employed.

2.2.3 Troubleshooting

Although microdialysis is generally a robust technique if difficulties do arise and dialysate is not obtained, a systematic approach is advocated. The micropump should be examined and new batteries placed (if not already done). The catheter insertion site should be examined to check that the catheter remains secure and is not obviously displaced. The microvials can be removed and replaced to ensure that they click into place appropriately. Once confident these components are satisfactory the system may be flushed by re-opening and then closing the lid of the micropump.

3. In vivo assessment of pathogenesis

To date, almost a dozen clinical studies have utilised microdialysis in patients with cerebral tumours; with approximately half of these devoted to investigating gliomagenesis, and the remaining to evaluating treatment with chemo- and radiotherapy. Studies investigating gliomagenesis may be further subdivided into those utilising LWCO or HWCO microdialysis catheters.

3.1 Low molecular weight cut off

In a landmark Swedish study in 2003 Roslin et al studied the baseline concentration of glucose and its metabolites, glycerol and glutamate in patients with high grade glioma

(HGG) (Roslin et al. 2003). The group performed an in-vitro recovery experiment, which confirmed relative recoveries of greater than 90% of the substrates of interest. Fifteen patients with HGG undergoing brain biopsy were recruited and two LWCO catheters were placed stereotactically: one within the tumour (T), and one 10mm outside the contrast enhancing region in the peritumour region (PT). Surprisingly, the only significant difference between dialysates obtained from T and PT was lactate, which was more concentrated in T than PT ($p<0.05$). This is in contrast to in-vitro studies (Klegeris, Walker and McGeer 1997), animal studies (Behrens et al. 2000), and subsequent clinical microdialysis studies (Marcus et al.), all of which demonstrate an increased concentration of glutamate and other metabolites within tumour cell lines and tissue respectively. The possible reasons for this incongruity are discussed below (see Section 3.2)

Investigators in Italy also used LWCO microdialysis catheters to establish the baseline concentration of other small molecules including amino acids, adenosine, and choline in 21 patients with HGG (Melani et al. 2003, Bianchi et al. 2004). An in-vitro recovery experiment was carried out and demonstrated the relative recovery of adenosine estimate to be $43.4 \pm 5.1\%$ (relative recovery was not calculated for amino acids and choline). Unlike the Swedish study patients underwent tumour resection and three microdialysis catheters were placed using an open technique: one into the tumour resection margin (T), one into peritumoural tissue 10mm away from the resection margin (PT), and one into grossly normal brain around the tumour at least 20mm away from the resection margin (BAT). Samples were analysed using various methods including HLPC. The group found that concentration of adenosine and glutamate were significantly reduced in T compared with BAT ($p<0.05$), the concentration of aspartate was unchanged, and the concentration of the remaining amino acids and choline were all significantly increased in T compared with BAT ($p<0.01$). Interestingly epilepsy, which occurs in approximately a third of patients with brain tumours (Villemure and de Tribolet 1996), was found to be an important confounding variable when the concentrations of aspartate, glutmate and GABA were considered.

3.2 High molecular weight cut off

Flannery et al were the first group to take advantage of HWCO catheters to assess the cysteine protease Cathepsin S (CatS) in gliomagenesis (Flannery et al. 2007). In total 11 patients with suspected HGG were recruited. Of these 11 patients, one was subsequently found to be a low-grade glioma (LGG), 2 were cerebral metastases, and the remaining 8 cases confirmed HGGs. A further patient with suspected hydrocephalus that was undergoing intracranial pressure monitoring was also included as a control. All patients underwent tumour resection with insertion of a single microdialysis catheter at the tumour resection margin (T). Analysis of CatS was by activity and ELISA concentration assays. Unfortunately, the absence of paired catheter data makes interpretation of the study's findings difficult but there was no significant relationship between CatS concentration and function, and the grade of brain tumours investigated.

A more recent study utilising HWCO catheters in patients undergoing surgery for intrinsic brain tumours set out to first to repeat earlier measurements of glucose and its metabolites, glycerol and glutamate, and second to assess the concentration of macromolecules such as growth factors, cytokines and other proteins involved in the pathogenesis of HGGs (Marcus et al.). Eight patients with suspected HGG were recruited. Of these 8 patients, one was found to have a lymphoma, and the remaining 7 cases confirmed HGGs. A further patient with traumatic brain injury was included as a non-tumour control. All but one of the patients with cerebral tumours underwent surgical resection with the first microdialysis catheter placed at the tumour resection margin (T) and the second inserted at least 20mm away in macroscopically unaffected brain around tumour (BAT). The remaining one patient had an image-guided biopsy of their tumour with stereotactic insertion of a catheter into the tumour margin (T). Microdialysates were first assessed for small molecules using the CMA 600 or ISCUS analyser. Tumour microdialysates were found to have a significantly lower glucose, higher lactate/pyruvate (L/P) ratio, higher glycerol and higher glutamate compared to the brain around tumour. These findings suggest that the tumour margin of HGGs is particularly metabolically active and are consistent with previously published in-vitro and animal studies, but differ from the previous clinical microdialysis study by Roslin et al. There are a several reasons that may account for the discrepancy between these studies. First, the small number of cases in both studies necessitates cautious interpretation of their findings as variation in patients, their pathology and tumour heterogeneity may all have influenced the concentration of glucose and its metabolites, glycerol and glutamate. Second, Roslin et al introduced catheters following biopsy using a closed stereotactic technique while Marcus et al introduced catheters after tumour resection using an open technique. Trauma artefact may therefore have influenced findings (though in the Marcus et al study measurements were taken at least 4 hours post-operatively to try and reduce this effect). Third, while Roslin et al placed the tumour catheters in the tumour centre, Marcus et al placed tumour catheters at the tumour resection margin or tumour periphery. It is possible that the core of the tumour, which is often necrotic, may be less metabolically active than the brain-tumour interface.

In the same study Marcus et al analysed all the remaining microdialysate samples for macromolecules using a sandwich ELISA like procedure. There was great variability in the dialysate concentrations of the various growth factors (TGF-alpha, VEGF, EGF), cytokines (IL-1a, IL -1b, IL-1ra, IL-6, IL-8) and matrix metalloproteases and their tissue inhibitors (MMP2, MMP9, TIMP1, TIMP9). Nevertheless, microdialysates were found to have significantly raised MMP2/TIMP1 and IL-8 in T compared to BAT samples suggesting an environment favouring invasion and angiogenesis respectively.

4. In vivo assessment of therapies

In addition to using microdialysis to evaluate the baseline concentration of molecules involved glioma pathogenesis, several studies have also made use of the technique to investigate the response to treatment with chemo- and radiotherapy.

4.1 Chemotherapy

Microdialysis may be used to evaluate both chemotherapeutic pharmacokinetics and pharmacodynamics. Interestingly, the earliest example of clinical microdialysis in patients with brain tumours to investigate a drug's pharmacology focused not on chemotherapy but on the antimicrobial rifampicin. Mindermann et al recruited 5 patients with HGG and 3 patients with LGG (Mindermann 1999). All patients received a single pre-operative dose of 600mg rifampicin 3 hours before skin incision. Patients then underwent craniotomy and tumour resection with a single microdialysis catheter placed distantly from the resection margin in grossly unaffected brain around tumour (BAT). A LWCO catheter was infused with two solutions of different concentrations of rifampin at a rate of 3μl/m. The loss or gain of rifampin from the two solutions was determined and rifampin concentration then calculated using the no-net-flux method. Intra-operatively solid tissue samples were also taken from tumour tissue, peri-tumour tissue and unaffected brain around tumour tissue. The concentration of rifampin was greatest within solid tissue samples from tumour and peritumour, followed by BAT microdialysates, and then solid tissue samples from unaffected brain around tumour. The rifampin concentration in all compartments exceeded the minimum inhibitory concentration (MIC) for staphylococci and streptococci.

Blakeley et al used clinical microdialysis to investigate the pharmacokinetics of high dose methotrexate (12g/m^2) (Blakeley et al. 2009). The group performed an in-vitro recovery experiment, which demonstrated a relative recovery of 43.6 ± 2.6%. Four patients with recurrent HGG were recruited and underwent biopsy or resection as clinically indicated. A LWCO microdialysis catheter was then placed into either the contrast-enhancing or non-enhancing residual tumour (T). Samples were analysed using liquid chromatography/mass spectroscopy. Methotrexate penetration in T was found to be variable with the highest concentrations measured within the contrast-enhancing regions. Nevertheless, the concentration of methotrexate in all regions exceeded the minimum concentration required for 50% cell kill against glioma cell lines in vitro.

Portnow et al used clinical microdialysis to investigate the pharamcokinetics of another chemotherapeutic drug temozolamide (TMZ) (Portnow et al. 2009). Contemporary post-operative management of patients with a HGG is with daily TMZ tablets and concurrent radiotherapy. Phase I studies of TMZ suggested that peak levels in blood occurred approximately an hour after ingestion and patients are therefore typically instructed to take their tablets an hour prior to radiotherapy to potentiate their oncotoxic effects (Dhodapkar et al. 1997). The group first performed an in-vitro recovery experiment, which demonstrated a relative recovery of 87 ± 5.5%. Portnow et al then recruited 9 patients of which 6 patients had HGG, and 3 had non-small cell lung cancer. All patients underwent resection and a single LWCO microdialysis catheter was placed within 5mm of the tumour resection margin (T). Post-operatively one patient refused TMZ, and in another the microdialysis catheter was occluded. In the remaining 7 patients microdialysates were analysed using HPLC to determine the concentration of TMZ. Concentrations of temozolamide in the brain measured in their study were consistent with previous studies but it was noted that the mean time to reach peak level in the brain was 2.0 ± 0.8 hour. The clinical corollary of their findings is that current chemoradiation regimens may be improved by advising patients to take their tablets 2 hours before radiotherapy sessions.

4.2 Radiotherapy

A series of studies by a group in Sweden have used microdialysis to monitor patients undergoing radiotherapy. The focus of their first study was Boron Neutron Capture Therapy (BNCT), an experimental technique in which patients are injected with boron, which preferentially binds to tumour cells, and then treated with neutron beam radiotherapy generating oncotoxic alpha particles and Lithium ions. The technique is theoretically attractive because of the short path length of alpha particles (approximately one cell diameter) compared to conventional gamma radiation. Bergenheim et al used clinical microdialysis to determine the pharmacokinetics of boronophenylalanine (BPA) with a view to optimising the timing of radiation (Bergenheim et al. 2005). An in-vitro experiment determined a mean BPA recovery of 66.8 ± 8.8%. The group also monitored glucose and its metabolites, glutamate and glycerol throughout the procedure. Four patients with WHO grade IV glioblastoma multiforme (GBM) were recruited. One patient underwent gross total resection, one a subtotal resection, and two stereotactic biopsies. In the patients that underwent resection a microdialysis catheter was placed within 5mm of the resection margin (T), and in the patients undergoing biopsy catheters were placed within viable tumour tissue (T). In all patients a second catheter was placed at least 20mm outside of the radiological bulk of the tumour in macroscopically normal brain around tumour (BAT). Microdialysates were analysed using the CMA 600 analyser, except for boron that was measured using an inductively coupled atomic emission spectrometer. The concentrations of boron varied considerably depending on the tissue sampled: in T samples the pharmacokinetic profile of BPA followed that of blood, while in BAT uptake was generally very low with a delay of up to 8 hours in relation to blood levels. No significant changes in glucose and its metabolites were noted during BNCT treatment. An increase in the concentration of glycerol was noted in T and PT 1-3 days after BNCT treatment while BAT levels were low and unchanged. Glutamate also showed high levels in PT compared to BAT, although no obvious changes were observed over time.

In their second study the Swedish group evaluated the levels of glucose and its metabolites, glycerol and glutamate in patients with HGG undergoing conventional post-operative radiotherapy (Tabatabaei et al. 2008). Thirteen patients with HGG were recruited with one catheter placed within the tumour (T), and a second 10mm outside the contrast-enhancing area in the peritumour region (PT). Samples were obtained at least 20 hours before radiotherapy commenced, and then continued for at least 20 hours after the fifth radiotherapy session. Baseline levels of glucose were significantly lower, and the L/P ratio significantly higher, in dialysates from T compared with PT. Radiotherapy did not influence glucose and its metabolites, or glycerol or glutamate.

Bergenheim's group subsequently extended their approach to utilise HWCO catheters enabling evaluation of macromolecules during conventional radiotherapy (Wibom et al.). Eleven patients with HGG were underwent stereotactic biopsy with insertion of two microdialysis catheters: one placed into the contrast enhancing tumour (T), and a second outside it in the peritumour region (PT). Reference samples were also collected subcutaneously from patients' abdomen. Microdialysates were analysed using gas chromatography - time-of-flight mass spectroscopy. Marked differences in metabolomic patterns were noted between T and PT, and between brain and abdominal microdialysates. In addition, dynamic changes occurred with radiotherapy in T and PT microdialysates.

5. Retrograde microdialysis

A novel use of clinical microdialysis is to deliver chemotherapeutic agents through a process termed retrograde microdialysis. The technique offers a number of potential advantages. First, the precise placement of catheters allows chemotherapy to bypass the blood-brain barrier and be administered directly to the tumour bed. Second, equilibration occurs across a semi-permeable membrane ensuring the therapeutic concentration is maintained. Third, simultaneous measurement of metabolism allows direct assessment of a drug's effects. The therapeutic principle was first explored by Ungerstedt's group in Sweden who treated three patients with GBM by adding the oncotoxic non-physiological amino acid L-2, 4 daminobutyric acid (DAB) to perfusate (Ronquist et al. 1992). This was extended by Bergenheim et al who recruited 10 patients with GBM that underwent stereotactic biopsy with the insertion of two microdialysis catheters: one in the contrast enhancing tumour (T), and the second 10mm outside the contrast enhancing region in the peritumour region (PT) (Bergenheim et al. 2006). Catheters inserted into T were LWCO with 30mm membranes, and were perfused with 80 or 120mmol/l DAB at a rate of 2µl/m. Samples were analysed for metabolites using a CMA 600 analyser, and for amino acids using HPLC. During treatment with DAB a significant increase in a number of amino acids including glutamate was observed suggesting cellular toxicity. PT samples were unaffected suggesting treatment effects was localised to the tumour compartment. Although the sample size was too small to determine whether there was an effect on clinical outcome, the study nevertheless provides evidence to support the feasibility of the technique.

6. Conclusion

In the last decade there has been a surge of interest in the application of clinical microdialysis to neuro-oncology. In this chapter we have reviewed the principles of microdialysis, and systematically appraised studies on the use of the technique to investigate gliomagenesis, the effect of treatment with chemotherapy and radiotherapy, and the potential for administration of drugs with retrograde microdialysis. The utility of the technique lies in its use alongside other methods such as in-vitro, animal and imaging studies.

7. Acknowledgments

We thank Keri Carpenter, Stephen Price, and Peter Hutchinson for their continued advice on clinical microdialysis.

8. References

Behrens, P. F., H. Langemann, R. Strohschein, J. Draeger & J. Hennig (2000) Extracellular glutamate and other metabolites in and around RG2 rat glioma: an intracerebral microdialysis study. *J Neurooncol,* 47, 11-22.

Bellander, B. M., E. Cantais, P. Enblad, P. Hutchinson, C. H. Nordstrom, C. Robertson, J. Sahuquillo, M. Smith, N. Stocchetti, U. Ungerstedt, A. Unterberg & N. V. Olsen (2004) Consensus meeting on microdialysis in neurointensive care. *Intensive Care Med,* 30, 2166-9.

Benjamin, R. K., F. H. Hochberg, E. Fox, P. M. Bungay, W. F. Elmquist, C. F. Stewart, J. M. Gallo, J. M. Collins, R. P. Pelletier, J. F. de Groot, R. C. Hickner, I. Cavus, S. A. Grossman & O. M. Colvin (2004) Review of microdialysis in brain tumors, from concept to application: first annual Carolyn Frye-Halloran symposium. *Neuro Oncol,* 6, 65-74.

Bergenheim, A. T., J. Capala, M. Roslin & R. Henriksson (2005) Distribution of BPA and metabolic assessment in glioblastoma patients during BNCT treatment: a microdialysis study. *J Neurooncol,* 71, 287-93.

Bergenheim, A. T., M. Roslin, U. Ungerstedt, A. Waldenstrom, R. Henriksson & G. Ronquist (2006) Metabolic manipulation of glioblastoma in vivo by retrograde microdialysis of L-2, 4 diaminobutyric acid (DAB). *J Neurooncol,* 80, 285-93.

Bianchi, L., E. De Micheli, A. Bricolo, C. Ballini, M. Fattori, C. Venturi, F. Pedata, K. F. Tipton & L. Della Corte (2004) Extracellular levels of amino acids and choline in human high grade gliomas: an intraoperative microdialysis study. *Neurochem Res,* 29, 325-34.

Blakeley, J. & J. Portnow Microdialysis for assessing intratumoral drug disposition in brain cancers: a tool for rational drug development. *Expert Opin Drug Metab Toxicol,* 6, 1477-91.

Blakeley, J. O., J. Olson, S. A. Grossman, X. He, J. Weingart & J. G. Supko (2009) Effect of blood brain barrier permeability in recurrent high grade gliomas on the intratumoral pharmacokinetics of methotrexate: a microdialysis study. *J Neurooncol,* 91, 51-8.

Brunner, M., C. Joukhadar, R. Schmid, B. Erovic, H. G. Eichler & M. Muller (2000) Validation of urea as an endogenous reference compound for the in vivo calibration of microdialysis probes. *Life Sci,* 67, 977-84.

Chefer, V. I., A. C. Thompson, A. Zapata & T. S. Shippenberg (2009) Overview of brain microdialysis. *Curr Protoc Neurosci,* Chapter 7, Unit7 1.

de Lange, E. C., M. Danhof, A. G. de Boer & D. D. Breimer (1997) Methodological considerations of intracerebral microdialysis in pharmacokinetic studies on drug transport across the blood-brain barrier. *Brain Res Brain Res Rev,* 25, 27-49.

de Lange, E. C., B. A. de Boer & D. D. Breimer (1999) Microdialysis for pharmacokinetic analysis of drug transport to the brain. *Adv Drug Deliv Rev,* 36, 211-227.

Dhodapkar, M., J. Rubin, J. M. Reid, P. A. Burch, H. C. Pitot, J. C. Buckner, M. M. Ames & V. J. Suman (1997) Phase I trial of temozolomide (NSC 362856) in patients with advanced cancer. *Clin Cancer Res,* 3, 1093-100.

Flannery, T., R. S. McConnell, S. McQuaid, G. McGregor, M. Mirakhur, L. Martin, C. Scott, R. Burden, B. Walker, C. McGoohan & P. G. Johnston (2007) Detection of cathepsin S cysteine protease in human brain tumour microdialysates in vivo. *Br J Neurosurg,* 21, 204-9.

Helmy, A., K. L. Carpenter, J. N. Skepper, P. J. Kirkpatrick, J. D. Pickard & P. J. Hutchinson (2009) Microdialysis of cytokines: methodological considerations, scanning electron microscopy, and determination of relative recovery. *J Neurotrauma,* 26, 549-61.

Homapour, B., J. E. Bowen, E. J. Want, K. O'Neill, V. Apostolopoulos, D. Nandi, J. R. Van Dellen & F. Roncaroli Intra-operative, real-time, three-dimensional ultrasound assisted positioning of catheters in the microdialysis of glial tumours. *J Clin Neurosci,* 17, 506-10.

Hutchinson, P. J., M. T. O'Connell, P. G. Al-Rawi, L. B. Maskell, R. Kett-White, A. K. Gupta, H. K. Richards, D. B. Hutchinson, P. J. Kirkpatrick & J. D. Pickard (2000) Clinical cerebral microdialysis: a methodological study. *J Neurosurg,* 93, 37-43.

Klegeris, A., D. G. Walker & P. L. McGeer (1997) Regulation of glutamate in cultures of human monocytic THP-1 and astrocytoma U-373 MG cells. *J Neuroimmunol,* 78, 152-61.

Marcus, H. J., K. L. Carpenter, S. J. Price & P. J. Hutchinson In vivo assessment of high-grade glioma biochemistry using microdialysis: a study of energy-related molecules, growth factors and cytokines. *J Neurooncol*, 97, 11-23.

Melani, A., E. De Micheli, G. Pinna, A. Alfieri, L. D. Corte & F. Pedata (2003) Adenosine extracellular levels in human brain gliomas: an intraoperative microdialysis study. *Neurosci Lett*, 346, 93-6.

Mindermann, T. (1999) Pressure gradients within the central nervous system. *J Clin Neurosci*, 6, 464-6.

Portnow, J., B. Badie, M. Chen, A. Liu, S. Blanchard & T. W. Synold (2009) The neuropharmacokinetics of temozolomide in patients with resectable brain tumors: potential implications for the current approach to chemoradiation. *Clin Cancer Res*, 15, 7092-8.

Ronquist, G., R. Hugosson, U. Sjolander & U. Ungerstedt (1992) Treatment of malignant glioma by a new therapeutic principle. *Acta Neurochir (Wien)*, 114, 8-11.

Roslin, M., R. Henriksson, P. Bergstrom, U. Ungerstedt & A. T. Bergenheim (2003) Baseline levels of glucose metabolites, glutamate and glycerol in malignant glioma assessed by stereotactic microdialysis. *J Neurooncol*, 61, 151-60.

Sorg, B. S., C. D. Peltz, B. Klitzman & M. W. Dewhirst (2005) Method for improved accuracy in endogenous urea recovery marker calibrations for microdialysis in tumors. *J Pharmacol Toxicol Methods*, 52, 341-9.

Tabatabaei, P., P. Bergstrom, R. Henriksson & A. T. Bergenheim (2008) Glucose metabolites, glutamate and glycerol in malignant glioma tumours during radiotherapy. *J Neurooncol*, 90, 35-9.

Tossman, U. & U. Ungerstedt (1986) Microdialysis in the study of extracellular levels of amino acids in the rat brain. *Acta Physiol Scand*, 128, 9-14.

Ungerstedt, U. & C. Pycock (1974) Functional correlates of dopamine neurotransmission. *Bull Schweiz Akad Med Wiss*, 30, 44-55.

Villemure, J. G. & N. de Tribolet (1996) Epilepsy in patients with central nervous system tumors. *Curr Opin Neurol*, 9, 424-8.

Wibom, C., I. Surowiec, L. Moren, P. Bergstrom, M. Johansson, H. Antti & A. T. Bergenheim Metabolomic patterns in glioblastoma and changes during radiotherapy: a clinical microdialysis study. *J Proteome Res*, 9, 2909-19.

PET Imaging of Gliomas

Aditya Bansal[1], Terence Z. Wong[2] and Timothy R. DeGrado[1]
[1]*Division of Nuclear Medicine and Molecular Imaging, Brigham and Women's Hospital, Harvard Medical School, Boston, MA*
[2]*Department of Radiology, Nuclear Medicine Division, Duke University Medical Center, Durham, NC,*
USA

1. Introduction

Noninvasive imaging methods, including positron emission tomography (PET), have become essential for diagnosis and staging of gliomas, and monitoring of treatment response. The utility of these techniques have been found to be highly dependent on tumor grade. According to the World Health Organization (WHO) classification of tumors (Kleihues and Sobin 2000), gliomas are classified into 3 main histological types: astrocytoma, oligodendroglioma and glioblastoma. These histological types are further classified on the basis of anaplasia and degree of malignancy as: grade I, noninvasive glioma (pilocytic astrocytoma); grade II, less-invasive glioma (astrocytomas and oligodendrogliomas); grade III, invasive glioma (analplastic astrocytoma/oligodendrogliomas); and grade IV, highly invasive glioma (glioblastoma, or GBM).

Low-grade gliomas (grade I and II) typically affect younger patients. Grade I glioma is the most common form of glioma in children and is less frequent in adults (Burkhard et al. 2003) while grade II gliomas are common in adults (mean age of onset is 40 years) (Hagerstrand et al. 2008). Median survival for low-grade glioma is varied but prognosis and treatment require regular follow ups. Low-grade gliomas grow slowly or stabilize spontaneously and with surgical resection, median survival can be 20 years or more (Burkhard et al. 2003). For high-grade gliomas, the mean age of onset is 40 years for grade III glioma and 61 years for GBM (Ohgaki and Kleihues 2005). GBM is the most malignant and most common glioma, accounting for 45% - 50% of all adult gliomas. Median survival for grade III glioma is 2-3 years and for GBM is 1 year (Chen 2007). For optimal disease prognosis, treatment and follow up, one should be able to delineate the tumor lesion and most importantly, differentiate benign lesions from neoplastic lesions, low-grade from high grade tumors, and tumor progression from therapy induced necrosis. As will be discussed later, efforts are also being directed toward defining early imaging predictors of response to therapy.

Conventional imaging with magnetic resonance imaging (MRI) provides excellent anatomical definition of brain tumors. MRI is highly sensitive in identifying lesions, mass effect, edema, hemorrhage, necrosis and signs of increased intracranial pressure (Chen 2007). Pathologic changes are characterized on MRI by increased water content (edema) and blood-brain barrier (BBB) disruption, visualized as contrast enhancement (Grosu et al. 2002). Most tumors (low-grade or high-grade) have prolonged T1 and T2 relaxation times and thus appear hypointense on T1-weighted images but hyperintense on T2-weighted images relative to normal brain (Grosu et al. 2002; Sartor 1999). In low-grade gliomas, peritumoral edema is minimal or absent and no contrast enhancement is seen due to intact BBB. Whereas, in high-grade gliomas, peritumoral edema is frequently seen and the tumor lesions usually show contrast enhancement, correlated with the extent of neovascularization and loss of integrity of the BBB owing to tumor infiltration and production of vascular endothelial growth factor. The anatomical features obtained by MRI are not sufficient to differentiate low-grade from high-grade gliomas with intact BBB, tumor lesions from inflammatory or vascular processes, and post-operative residual/relapse from necrosis (Chen 2007).

In contrast to MRI, positron emission tomography (PET) provides unique functional information of tumors on a range of biological processes such as glucose metabolism, protein/DNA synthesis, cell proliferation, membrane synthesis, angiogenesis and oxygen tension that can reflect the changes in neoplasm (Basu and Alavi 2009). Assessment of the status of these processes in areas of interest in brain has been shown to be helpful in detection and grading of gliomas, delineation of tumor margins, disease prognosis and treatment. PET has also been useful in differentiating post-operative residual tumor from therapy induced necrosis and edema. This review discusses radiopharmaceuticals and progress in the development of PET techniques for imaging of gliomas in the following areas: glucose uptake, amino acid transport, cellular proliferation rate, choline uptake, somatostatin receptor density, angiogenesis and hypoxia.

2. Glucose-based probes

Increased glucose uptake and glycolysis are hallmark characteristics of a variety of neoplasms (Pedersen 2007; Warburg 1956). This makes radiolabeled glucose analogs logical tracers of choice for imaging of tumors. The radiofluorinated analog of glucose, [^{18}F]fluorodeoxyglucose, or [^{18}F]FDG, is the most common PET tracer for clinical PET oncology studies. A practical synthesis, suitable half-life ($T_{1/2}$=109.7 min), negligible circulating metabolites, and well-established kinetics of uptake and retention of [^{18}F]FDG makes it a preferred imaging probe in cancer imaging (Spence et al. 1998). [^{18}F]FDG is transported into cancer cells by glucose transporters (GLUT1 and GLUT3) and, like glucose, it is phosphorylated via hexokinase to form [^{18}F]fluorodeoxyglucose-6-phosphate. However, in contrast to glucose-6-phosphate, [^{18}F]fluorodeoxyglucose-6-phosphate is very slowly metabolized further and hence is effectively trapped in the cancer cell (Spence et al. 1998). The trapped [^{18}F]FDG-6-phosphate can be detected by [^{18}F]FDG-PET thereby allowing non-invasive evaluation of glucose uptake and glycolysis. In general, [^{18}F]FDG-PET performs well in identifying highly malignant, high-grade gliomas because they typically exhibit higher glycolysis rates than the normal cerebral cortex (Di Chiro et al. 1982, 1987a). Di Chiro et al. (1985, 1987a, 1987b) were first to correlate [^{18}F]FDG uptake with WHO grading of gliomas on the basis of a semiquantitative index of the ratio of [^{18}F]FDG uptake in tumor to the average [^{18}F]FDG uptake in normal cerebral cortex. [^{18}F]FDG uptake ratio in high-grade glioblastoma was almost twice that of low-grade gliomas. In a different study, Delbeke et al. (1995) reported that high-grade gliomas can be detected with high sensitivity of 94% and specificity of 77% when tumor-to-white matter ratios exceed 1.5, and tumor-to-grey matter ratios exceed 0.6. In addition,[^{18}F]FDG-PET was able to indicate anaplastic transformation of grade II gliomas into grade III gliomas by an increase in ^{18}F-FDG uptake (Chen 2007).

[18F]FDG-PET has also been useful to differentiate hypoglycolytic non-malignant toxoplasmosis common in AIDS patients from hyperglycolytic CNS lymphoma (Hoffman et al. 1993).

Assessment of [18F]FDG uptake in gliomas has high prognostic value (Di Chiro 1987). De Witte et al. (1996) studied 28 patients with histologically proven low-grade gliomas with [18F]FDG–PET and followed progression of disease for a mean of 27 months. All 19 patients with tumors that were hypoglycolytic on PET were alive at the end of the follow-up period, whereas 6 of 9 patients with hyperglycolytic patterns on PET died. The prognostic utility of [18F]FDG–PET has been confirmed in several other studies (Alavi et al. 1988; Barker et al. 1997; Padma et al. 2003; Patronas et al. 1985).

Although [18F]FDG-PET is accurate to detect high-grade gliomas, it has limited usefulness in detection of low-grade gliomas and some high-grade gliomas such as post-operative residual and recurrent glioma (Olivero et al. 1995; Ricci et al. 1998). Since glucose is the preferred fuel in normal brain, high [18F]FDG uptake in surrounding normal tissues in brain is unavoidable (Di Chiro et al. 1982). Low grade gliomas tend to have the same or lower [18F]FDG uptake as compared to average [18F]FDG uptake in white matter, thus resulting in false negative readings (Kawai et al. 2005). This is also true for certain high-grade gliomas, especially hypoglycolytic residual (Padma et al. 2003) and recurrent tumors (Chao et al. 2001) that may exhibit less or similar [18F]FDG uptake to average [18F]FDG uptake in grey matter. In addition, in the case of patients with Alzheimer disease and epilepsy, affected regions in brain can show decreased [18F]FDG uptake compared to background (Fazekas et al. 1989; McGeer et al. 1986). On the other hand, brain regions with abscess or acute necrosis occurring hours of weeks after radiotherapy, chemotherapy can show increased [18F]FDG uptake compared to background leading to false positive readings (Floeth et al. 2006). Thus, low tumor-to-normal background radioactivity concentration (T/N) ratios and difficult to interpret contrasts between normal and pathological regions limit the specificity of [18F]FDG-PET to detect low-grade and residual or relapsed high-grade brain tumors.

Given these concerns, attempts have been made to improve the accuracy of [18F]FDG for imaging of gliomas. In cases where T/N (white or grey matter) ratios for [18F]FDG uptake are not useful for delineating low-grade, residual or relapsed high-grade glioma, two strategies have been reported to help: (1) co-registration of [18F]FDG–PET images with MR images (Chao et al. 2001; Wang et al. 2006) and (2) delayed [18F]FDG–PET imaging (Spence et al. 2004). Co-registration and interpretation of [18F]FDG–PET images with MR images can improve the performance of [18F]FDG–PET **(Figure 1)** for detecting low-grade (Borgwardt et al. 2005; Wong et al. 2004), residual or relapsed high-grade gliomas (Chao et al. 2001; Wang et al. 2006). Low grade gliomas can be identified by similar [18F]FDG uptake to white matter in regions with increased signal on T2-weighted MRI (Borgwardt et al. 2005; Wong et al. 2004), while recurrent high grade gliomas are often indicated as [18F]FDG uptake in regions with contrast enhancement on T1-weighted MRI (Chao et al. 2001; Wang et al. 2006). Delayed PET imaging, as proposed by Spence et al. (2004), is another strategy to improve the contrast between tumor lesion and background. In this study, nineteen patients with gliomas were imaged from 0 to 90 min and once or twice at 3–8 h after injection. In 12 of 19 patients, visual analysis of delayed images up to 8 h after injection showed these images to better distinguish relapsed tumors in grey matter (**Figure 2**). Standardized uptake values (SUVs) were also greater in tumors than in normal grey or white matter on delayed imaging. Using kinetic modeling, they demonstrated that the rate constant of

[18F]fluorodeoxyglucose-6-phosphate degradation (k4) was not significantly different between tumor and normal brain tissue for shorter datasets but was lower in tumor than in normal brain tissue for the longer dataset (8 h), suggesting that higher [18F]Fluorodeoxyglucose-6-phosphate degradation rates are present in normal brain tissue than tumor. Since this report, other studies have shown the utility of delayed PET imaging for delineating brain tumors (Farid et al. 2009; Kim et al. 2010).

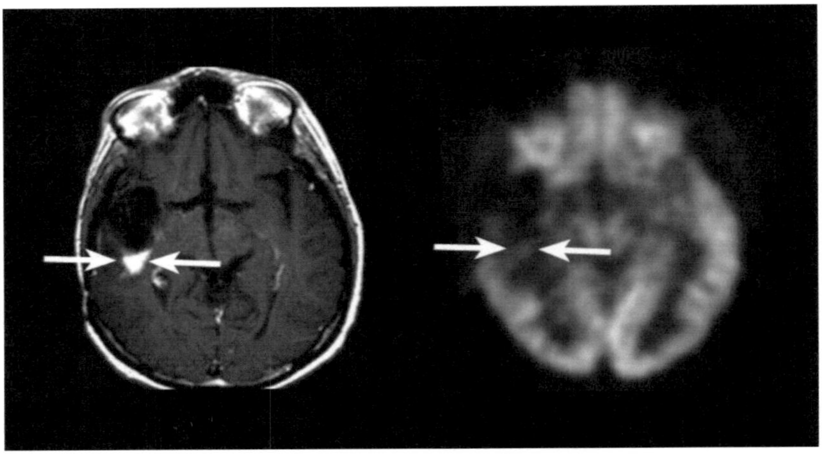

Fig. 1. A patient who had received surgery, radiation, and chemotherapy for anaplastic astrocytoma. Axial gadolinium-enhanced T1-weighted image (left) demonstrates nodular enhancement posterior to the surgical resection cavity. Co-registered [18F]FDG-PET image demonstrates increased [18F]FDG activity corresponding to this region, similar to gray matter, compatible with recurrent tumor. Correlation of the MRI and PET imaging findings is necessary to make this determination, and accurate image co-registration is essential.

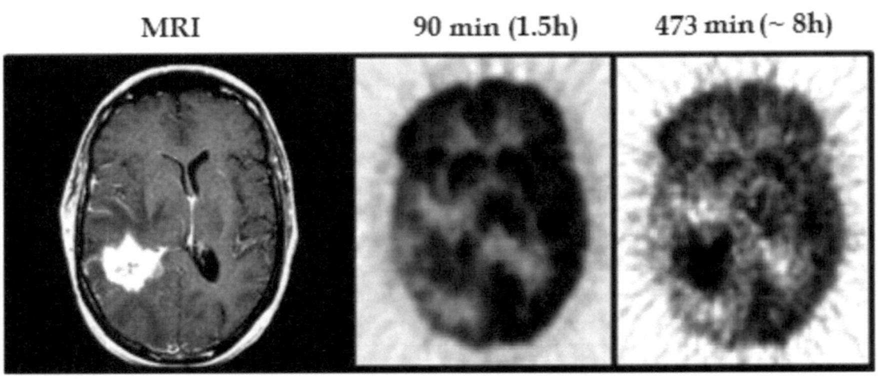

Fig. 2. A 45-year-old woman with recurrent right temporal GBM. T1-weighted gadolinium-enhanced (T1Gd) MRI showing contrast enhancement in right temporal region of the brain. [18F]FDG-PET scan with much more prominent T/N delineation in this right temporal region at the later time point, 473 min (~8 h), compared to 90 min (1.5 h). *Image reproduced from work by Spence et al. (2004) and used with permission.*

3. Amino acid-based probes

Amino acids play a central role in protein synthesis and intermediary metabolism (Cellarier et al. 2003; Morowitz et al. 2000). The enhanced uptake of essential amino acids into neoplasms through specific amino acid transporters has motivated the design and evaluation of a large number of positron-labeled essential amino acid analogs. In addition, the low uptake of essential amino acids in normal brain tissue relative to tumor tissue renders amino acid tracers advantageous for imaging gliomas (Lilja et al. 1985). The most studied essential amino acid tracers are [^{11}C]methionine ([^{11}C]MET), [^{18}F]fluoroethyl-L-tyrosine ([^{18}F]FET) and 3,4-dihydroxy-6-^{18}F-fluoro-L-phenylalanine ([^{18}F]FDOPA).

3.1 [^{11}C]MET

Increased uptake of methionine by cancer cells results from increased transport flux, primarily by L-amino acid transporters, enhanced protein synthesis, increased need for polyamines, and a high rate of trans-methylation and trans-sulfuration reactions (Leskinen-Kallio et al. 1991). [^{11}C]MET uptake in tumor lesions is not dependent on disruption of the BBB (Roelcke et al. 1995; Sasajima et al. 2004). This is a major advantage compared to MRI where contrast enhancement for detection of tumor lesions is dependent on BBB disruption. Studies with [^{11}C]MET-PET have shown that amino acid tracer, [^{11}C]MET, accumulates in all gliomas, including low-grade glioma that are difficult to detect on contrast-enhanced MRI and [^{18}F]FDG-PET (Ogawa et al. 1993).

[^{11}C]MET-PET can be used to predict histological grades of gliomas. Lilja et al. (1985) evaluated 14 patients with gliomas and found that [^{11}C]MET-PET could differentiate high-grade glioma from low-grade glioma on the basis of T/N ratio. The ratio of the uptake of [^{11}C]MET in high-grade tumors was 1.9-4.8 and low-grade tumor was 0.8-1.0. Derlon et al. (1989) too confirmed positive correlation of T/N ratio with the histological grade of gliomas. Later study with large set of 196 patients, Herholz et al. (1998) showed that [^{11}C]MET could differentiate among high-grade gliomas, low-grade gliomas, and chronic or subacute nontumoral lesions. In this study, [^{11}C]MET-PET was also useful in detecting recurrent or residual tumors as they showed higher [^{11}C]MET uptake than primary gliomas.

[^{11}C]MET-PET has been shown to have high prognostic potential. Kaschten et al. (1998) performed [^{18}F]FDG-PET and [^{11}C]MET-PET in 54 patients with gliomas. [^{11}C]MET was superior to [^{18}F]FDG in predicting the histologic grade and prognosis of gliomas. With a larger set of 85 patients, De Witte et al. (2001) applied qualitative and quantitative scoring systems for [^{11}C]MET uptake. Both scoring systems confirmed the prognostic importance of [^{11}C]MET-PET. In this study, gliomas were histologically graded following [^{11}C]MET-PET guided resection (42 cases) or stereotactic biopsy (43 cases). Uptake of [^{11}C]MET was present in 98% of the gliomas studied. The T/N ratio was significantly correlated with the histological grade of glioma. A statistically poor patient outcome was demonstrated during follow-up when this ratio was higher than a threshold of 2.2 for grade II gliomas and 2.8 for grade III gliomas. A high [^{11}C]MET uptake was statistically associated with short survival times. Better prognostic utility of [^{11}C]MET-PET relative to [^{18}F]FDG-PET was also shown in other studies (Kim et al. 2005; Van Laere et al. 2005).

[^{11}C]MET-PET is also useful to differentiate recurrent tumor from post-operative radiation injury (Gehrke et al. 1991; Ogawa et al. 1991; Sonoda et al. 1998). Tsuyuguchi et al. (2003) examined 21 adult patients with [^{11}C]MET-PET to differentiate radiation necrosis from recurrent metastatic brain tumor following stereotactic radiosurgery. They observed mean

T/N ratio and mean SUV for [^{11}C]MET to be 1.15 and 1.78, respectively, in the radiation necrosis group (12 cases); and 1.62 and 2.5, respectively, in the tumor recurrence group (9 cases). The sensitivity and specificity of [^{11}C]MET-PET for detection of tumor recurrence were determined to be 77.8% and 100%, respectively. In a separate study, [^{11}C]MET-PET was shown to be superior to [^{18}F]FDG-PET in detecting recurrent brain lesions (Chung et al. 2002). A recent study by Okamoto et al. (2010) further confirmed the utility of [^{11}C]MET-PET to detect recurring lesions. Mean T/N ratio of all recurrent tumors and necrosis were 1.98 ± 0.62 and 1.27 ± 0.28, respectively ($p < 0.01$) (Okamoto et al. 2010). In smaller lesions (20 - 30 mm), T/N ratio for recurrent tumor (1.72 ± 0.44) was also significantly higher than that for necrosis (1.20 ± 0.11) ($p < 0.01$) (Okamoto et al. 2010). Thus, [^{11}C]MET-PET provides high diagnostic value for recurring tumor lesions, with particular value in early diagnosis of recurrence.

3.2 [^{18}F]FET

Wester et al. (1999) were the first to introduce the fluorinated tyrosine analog [^{18}F]FET for imaging gliomas. The longer half-life of ^{18}F (109.7 min) relative to ^{11}C (20 min) is more practical for production and distribution to multiple PET scanning facilities. The high *in vivo* stability of [^{18}F]FET, fast brain and tumor uptake kinetics, low accumulation in non-tumor tissue, and ease of synthesis strongly supported evaluation of [^{18}F]FET as an amino acid tracer for imaging gliomas.

Weber et al. (2000) compared uptakes of [^{18}F]FET and [^{11}C]MET by gliomas in 13 patients. On the basis of the [^{11}C]MET-PET, viable tumor tissue were delineated in all 13 patients. The same tumors showed rapid uptake of [^{18}F]FET with high image contrast. The mean uptake (SUV) of [^{11}C]MET was slightly higher than [^{18}F]FET in normal grey matter (1.4 ± 0.2 for [^{11}C]MET and 1.1 ± 0.2 for [^{18}F]FET); normal white matter (0.9 ± 0.1 for [^{11}C]MET and 0.8 ± 0.2 for [^{18}F]FET); and tumor lesions (3.3 ± 1.0 for [^{11}C]MET, 2.7 ± 0.8 for [^{18}F]FET). However, contrast between tumor and normal tissue background was not significantly different between [^{11}C]MET and [^{18}F]FET (**Figure 3**). In comparison to [^{18}F]FDG-PET, a recent study found [^{18}F]FET-PET was more accurate to detect malignant brain lesions, especially low-grade gliomas (Lau et al. 2010).

Although there is doubt on the potential of [^{18}F]FET-PET for grading gliomas (Popperl et al. 2004), a clinical study by Pauleit et al. (2005) showed that co-registration of [^{18}F]FET-PET and MRI could significantly improve the sensitivity and specificity of tumor detection and correlation to histological grade of tumor. In addition, a separate study showed have shown that the kinetic profile of [^{18}F]FET uptake for high- and low-grade lesions may be useful in grading tumors (Spence et al. 2004). In their study, tumors were classified into low (grade I and II) and high grade (grade III and IV) prior to [^{18}F]FET-PET scans. A significant difference ($p<0.05$) in T/N ratio was observed between high-grade (ratio = 3.2) and low-grade tumors (ratio = 2.0) in early time points (0-10 min post-injection). No significant differences were found at later time points (30-40 min post-injection). The importance of the kinetics of [^{18}F]FET is not limited to grading primary tumor lesions. Low-grade recurrent tumors associated with good prognosis were differentiated from high-grade recurrent tumor associated with poor prognosis on the basis of kinetics of [^{18}F]FET uptake (Popperl et al. 2006).

A major strength of [^{18}F]FET-PET is that it reliably distinguishes post-operative benign lesions from recurrent tumors (Popperl et al. 2004; Popperl et al. 2006). Popperal et al. (2004)

studied 53 patients with low grade (1 grade I, 9 grade II) or high grade gliomas (16 grade III, 27 grade IV) and clinically suspected recurrent tumors. The patients underwent [^{18}F]FET-PET scans 4-180 months after various treatments. In the 42 patients with confirmed recurrence, there was additional distinct focal [^{18}F]FET uptake with significantly higher values compared with those in the 11 patients without clinical signs of recurrence.

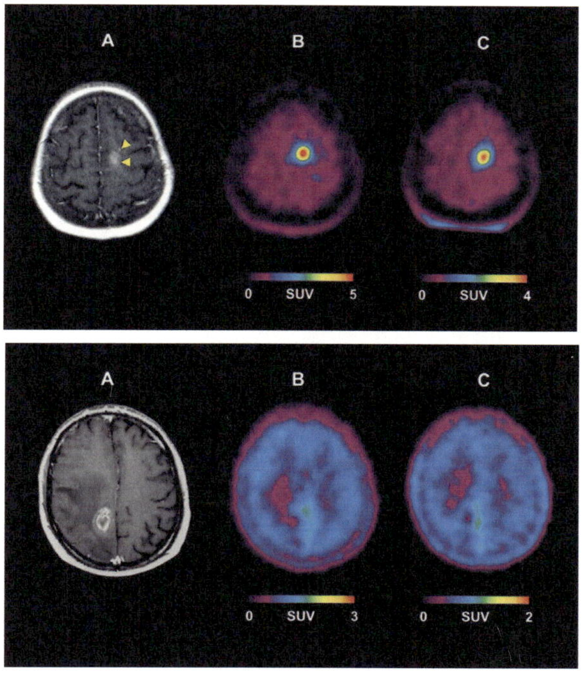

Fig. 3. Patient with residual tumor after subtotal resection of GBM (top) and a patient with radiation induced changes after radiotherapy for metastatic melanoma (bottom). T1-weighted contrast-enhanced MRI showing contrast enhancement in both residual tumor (A, top) and radiation induced injury (A, bottom). In the patient with residual GBM, [^{11}C]MET-PET (B, top) and [^{18}F]FET-PET (C, top) shows markedly increased tracer uptake. However, there is no increased uptake of [^{11}C]MET (B, bottom) and [^{18}F]FET (C, bottom) in radiation induced injury. *Image reproduced from work by Wolfgang A. Weber et al. (2000) and used with permission.*

3.3 [^{18}F]FDOPA

In mammalian cells, L-DOPA is synthesized from the amino acid, L-tyrosine, by the enzyme tyrosine hydroxylase (Kaufman 1995). L-DOPA is a precursor of the neurotransmitters: dopamine, norepinephrine, and epinephrine (Nagatsu 1995). L-DOPA is taken up by the brain through the blood-brain barrier (BBB) mediated by large neutral amino acid transporters (Lemmens et al. 2005). The [^{18}F]fluorinated L-DOPA analog, [^{18}F]FDOPA was initially developed as a radiotracer for use in patients with movement disorders (Heiss et al. 1996). In an early study, [^{18}F]FDOPA-PET of a 57 y old patient revealed pathologically increased [^{18}F]FDOPA accumulation in the right frontal lobe (Heiss et al. 1996). Unexpectedly, further PET examinations demonstrated increased [^{11}C]MET uptake and low [^{18}F]FDG uptake in this

right frontal region, suggesting a low-grade glioma lesion. MRI, ^{1}H-MRSI and histological examination later confirmed presence of a grade II oligo-astrocytoma in the lesion.
Following this incidental discovery, various studies were performed to evaluate the potential of [^{18}F]FDOPA-PET for imaging of gliomas. Chen et al. (2006) compared [^{18}F]FDOPA-PET with [^{18}F]FDG-PET to evaluate the potential of [^{18}F]FDOPA-PET to detect tumor lesions in patients with newly diagnosed or previously treated brain tumors. The [^{18}F]FDOPA-PET images were acquired for 10–30 min post-injection. In this study, [^{18}F]FDOPA-PET demonstrated excellent visualization of both low-grade and high-grade tumors, although the absolute uptake was not significantly different between the different tumor grades. [^{18}F]FDOPA-PET was more sensitive and specific than [^{18}F]FDG-PET for evaluating and distinguishing recurrent tumors from radiation necrosis. Specific transport of [^{18}F]FDOPA (Lemmens et al. 2005) independent of disruption of BBB and low background activity rendered it superior to MRI and [^{18}F]FDG for detecting recurrent gliomas.
A number of subsequent studies have suggested that tumor grade does not significantly affect [^{18}F]FDOPA uptake (**Figure 4**) (Chen et al. 2006; Duan et al. 2004; Jager et al. 2001; Li and Zhang 2004; Ono et al. 2004). However, Schiepers et al. (2007) used kinetic modeling of [^{18}F]FDOPA time courses out to 75 min to show that high-grade tumors had significantly higher transport rate constant, k1, equilibrium distribution volumes, and influx rate constant K than did low-grade tumors ($P< 0.01$). A 3-compartment model with corrections for tissue blood volume, metabolites, and partial volume, suggested that [^{18}F]FDOPA was transported but not trapped in tumors. The shape of the uptake curve appeared to be related to tumor grade. After an early maximum, high-grade tumors had a steep descending branch, whereas low-grade tumors had a slowly declining curve, like that for the cerebellum but on a higher scale. A high correlation was found between SUV in tumors and influx rate constant K, indicated that simple uptake measurements at 60-70 min should be sufficient in clinical practice for grading tumors.

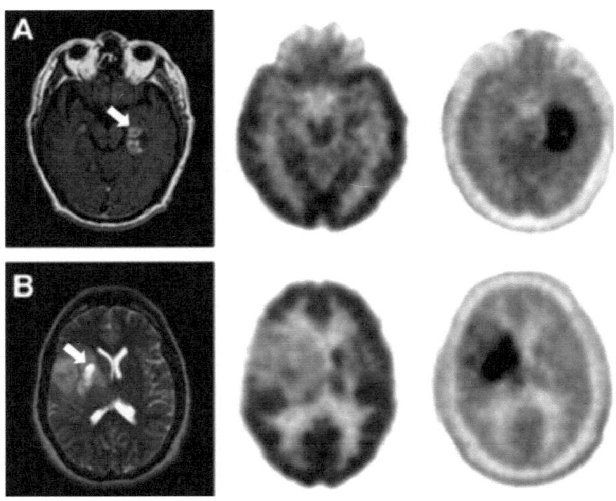

Fig. 4. Patient with newly diagnosed (A) GBM (B) Grade II oligodendroglioma. Tumor lesion shown as region with contrast enhancement in T1-weighted MRI (left). This region is not visible in [^{18}F]FDG-PET scan (middle) but a prominent [^{18}F]FDOPA uptake is seen in this region in [^{18}F]FDOPA-PET scan (right). *Image adapted from work by Wei Chen et al. (2006) and used with permission.*

Potential use of [^{18}F]FDOPA in tumor grading was also supported by a recent study by Chen et al. (2006) that showed significantly higher uptake in high-grade than in low-grade tumors in newly diagnosed tumors. This correlation was not seen in recurrent tumors that had been treated previously. In summary, [^{18}F]FDOPA-PET has been found useful in detecting and differentiating recurrent tumors from radiation necrosis and may also have potential in grading newly diagnosed tumors, although more studies are needed to fully define the potential of [^{18}F]FDOPA-PET.

A number of other positron-labeled amino acid analogs have been developed for imaging of brain tumors, although having fewer clinical trials to determine their characteristics for imaging of gliomas. These include [^{124}I]iodophenylalanine (Farmakis et al. 2008), [^{18}F]fluoromethylphenylalanine (FMP), [^{18}F]fluoroboronophenylalanine (FBP) (Hsieh et al. 2005; Imahori et al. 1998), [^{18}F]fluoroethylphenylalanine (FEP) (Wang et al. 2011) and [^{18}F]fluoropropylphenylalanine (FPP) (Wang et al. 2011), and 1-Aminocyclobutane-1-[^{11}C]carboxylic acid (1-[^{11}C]-ACBC) (Hubner et al. 1998).

4. Choline-based probes

In recent years, choline metabolism has received a growing interest in cancer research. Choline is incorporated into membrane phospholipid in the form of phosphatidylcholine through the multistep Kennedy pathway. Phosphatidylcholine is one of the major lipid components of plasma membranes in mammalian cells and is essential for membrane structural stability and cell proliferation. Following its transport into the cell, choline undergoes ATP-dependent phosphorylation to form phosphocholine, a reaction catalyzed by choline kinase. High levels of choline uptake and increased choline kinase activity relative to normal tissues have been reported in various cancers including brain tumors (Fulham et al. 1992). This has motivated the development of choline based PET imaging for noninvasive evaluation of gliomas.

Shinoura et al. (1997) were the first to use choline as a PET tracer of brain tumor imaging. They evaluated 20 patients with brain tumors using [^{11}C]choline PET. Progressive uptake of [^{11}C]choline was observed in brain tumors, while uptake by surrounding normal cerebral cortex was 10-fold lower. Later, Ohtani et al. (2001) compared [^{11}C]choline-PET with [^{18}F]FDG-PET in 22 patients with histopathologically confirmed benign lesions and brain tumors from grade I-IV. Higher uptake of [^{11}C]choline relative to [^{18}F]FDG was observed in high-grade grade III and grade IV gliomas. Furthermore, [^{11}C]choline was able to detect the extent of tumor better than MRI and could differentiate high-grade from low-grade lesions, but could not differentiate low-grade lesions from benign lesions.

The short half-life of [^{11}C]choline limits the use of this tracer to facilities having an on-site cyclotron. In view of this, a choline radiotracer with a longer half-life is highly desirable. [^{18}F]Fluorinated analogs of choline [^{18}F]FCH are promising options for choline based PET tumor imaging.

DeGrado et al. (2001) first reported brain tumor imaging with [^{18}F]FCH in a patient with previously resected anaplastic astrocytoma. The maximal T/N ratio of ~10:1 was attained within 5 min after injection. [^{18}F]FDG -PET revealed a corresponding area of increased [^{18}F]FDG uptake; however, the tumor boundaries were difficult to assess with FDG because of high uptake by normal cortex. Hara et al. (2003) performed studies with [^{18}F]fluoroethylcholine (FECH) in 12 glioma patients. The T/N ratio of [^{18}F]FECH was 10.5-12 in anaplastic astrocytoma and 13.2-21 in glioblastoma. These ratios were slightly higher

than those obtained with [^{11}C]choline in the same patients. A preliminary study by Kwee et al. (2004) in 2 patients suggested that [^{18}F]FCH uptake was significantly higher in glioblastoma multiforme (GBM) than benign demyelinating disease. Subsequently, Kwee et al. (2007) performed a more extensive [^{18}F]FCH PET study on 30 consecutive patients (14 women, 16 men; age range, 26-79 years) with solitary brain lesions defined by MRI. In this study, the order of SUV and T/N ratios were benign lesions < high-grade gliomas < metastases from distant tumors with appreciable separation of these classes. [^{18}F]FCH is also useful in detecting recurrent GBMs (**Figure 5**).
Pre-clinical studies on the *in vivo* kinetics and metabolism of [^{18}F]FCH and choline in a 9L glioma allograft tumor model showed marked washout from the tumor possibly resulting from the hypoxic nature of these tumors. However, a strong association of [^{18}F]FCH uptake and angiogenesis was found in the C6 glioma xenograft model (Wyss et al. 2007) and increased [^{18}F]FCH uptake was observed in a multidrug resistant U87MG glioma tumor model (Vanpouille et al. 2009).

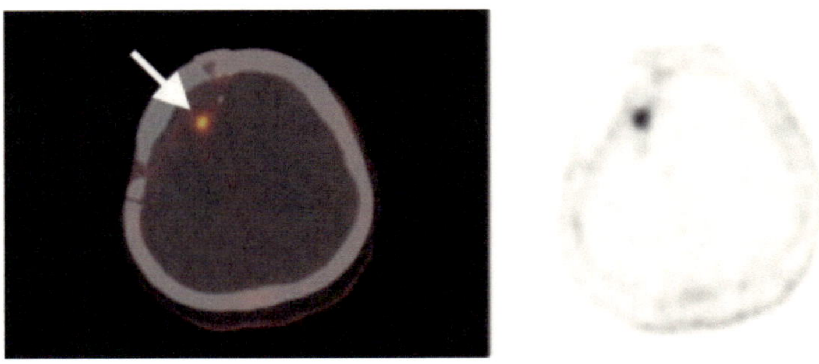

Fig. 5. [^{18}F]FCH uptake in recurrent GBM. PET/CT (left) and [^{18}F] FCH-PET (right) image shows a 6 mm focus of increased [^{18}F]FCH uptake along a right frontal lobe resection cavity. This lesion was noted to increase in size on serial brain MRI consistent with the diagnosis of recurrent tumor. A post-craniotomy defect is evident on the PET/CT image. [^{18}F] FCH-PET is potentially advantageous for imaging brain tumors such as GBM given the low amounts of physiologic cerebral [^{18}F]FCH uptake. *Image Courtesy of Dr. Sandi A. Kwee, MD, Nuclear Medicine Department, Queen's Medical Center, Honolulu, HI, USA.*

5. Integrin-based probes

Angiogenesis is a crucial process for tumor growth and metastasis (Kountouras et al. 2005). This process requires intracellular and extracellular interactions in which integrins play an important role (Brooks et al. 1994). Antagonists against alpha$_v\beta_3$ integrin have been shown to block angiogenesis and reduce tumor growth in preclinical animal models (MacDonald et al. 2001) and clinical trials (Carter 2010). This integrin is a membrane bound receptor that mediates intracellular signal transduction by recognizing and binding to Arg-Gly-Asp (RGD) containing proteins in the extracellular matrix (Main et al. 1992). On binding to different types of RGD containing protein, it senses the external microenvironment and accordingly regulate cellular shape, mobility and cell cycle progression along with angiogenesis and metastatsis (Brooks et al. 1994). Alpha$_v\beta_3$ integrin is expressed at low levels on epithelial cells and mature endothelial cells but highly expressed on activated endothelial cells of the neovasculature of gliomas (Liu 2009). Its expression correlates well with tumor progression and invasiveness of gliomas (Bello et al. 2001). Therefore, this integrin has received attention as a target for imaging probe development.

The most common integrin-targeting radiopharmaceuticals are radiolabeled RGD containing peptides. Cyclic RGD peptides (cRGD peptides) are preferred over linear RGD peptides due to their higher metabolic stability (Bogdanowich-Knipp et al. 1999). However, radiolabeled cRGD peptides (^{18}F-FB-cRGDs (Chen et al. 2004) and ^{64}Cu-DOTA-cRGDs (Chen et al. 2004)) commonly suffer the drawback of poor tumor retention and high renal and/or hepatic uptake. To improve the tumor imaging properties of these tracers, dimeric (Chen et al. 2004) and tetrameric (Wu et al. 2005) cyclic RGD congeners have been developed. The multimeric cyclic RGD probes showed higher tumor uptake but nevertheless exhibited rapid uptake by liver and kidneys. To decrease uptake in liver and kidneys, modifications such as glycosylation (Schnell et al. 2009) or PEGylation (Chen et al. 2004) have helped to achieve higher uptake in tumors along with decreased uptake in liver and kidney in U87MG glioblastoma models (Chen et al. 2004; Chen et al. 2004; Wu et al. 2005) and in patients with *de novo* or recurrent GBM (Schnell et al. 2009).

New developments to integrin imaging are in progress. Recently, a new generation of RGD containing probes have been designed that show better potential for imaging gliomas. The new approach is based on cystine knot proteins or knottins that are relatively stable in physical, chemical and biological environments due to presence of scaffold of disulfide-bonded framework and a triple-stranded ß-sheet fold (Kimura et al. 2009). The Knottin family members also possess one or more surface-exposed loops that can tolerate sequence diversity. RGD peptides have been grafted into these surface-exposed loops, while radiolabeling accomplished with conjugation of PET radionuclide, ^{18}F-FB or ^{64}Cu-DOTA. In a U87MG glioblastoma model, a knottin based probe demonstrated rapid and high tumor accumulation, fast clearance from blood and normal organs, and low uptake in the kidney and liver (Miao et al. 2009).

6. Cellular proliferation probes

Increased cellular proliferation is an integral part of the cancer phenotype (Bading and Shields 2008). The primary requirement for cell proliferation is replication of nuclear DNA. Of the 4 nucleotides (adenine, guanine, cytosine and thymidine) required for DNA synthesis, thymidine is the only one that is specific for DNA. In cells, thymidine is derived either *de novo* or through the salvage pathway (Bading and Shields 2008). The *de novo* pathway is not a viable alternative for monitoring DNA synthesis in proliferating cells because the relevant precursors (deoxyuridine, uridine, and uracil) are routed into both DNA and RNA (Bading and Shields 2008). Thus, thymidine salvage pathway is a better choice for indication of proliferation. PET radiotracers of thymidine have been developed, including [^{11}C]thymidine ([^{11}C]TdR) (De Reuck et al. 1999) and 3'-deoxy-3'-fluorothymidine ([^{18}F]FLT). These probes are currently being evaluated for their potential for imaging cellular proliferation in gliomas. The thymidine-based tracers are transported into cells and subsequently phosphorylated by thymidine kinase-1 (TK-1), thereby rendering them trapped within the cell. Since TK-1 activity correlates to a significant extent with the cellular proliferation rate, the PET-measurement of tissue retention of radioactivity is a non-invasive indicator of proliferation. The advantage of using the fluorinated thymidine tracer [^{18}F]FLT over [^{11}C]TdR is twofold. First, replacement of the hydroxy group of

deoxyribose with radiofluorine makes it resistant to degradation (Shields et al. 1998) and second, the longer half-life of ^{18}F is more practical for clinical imaging.
Increased glucose metabolism in inflammatory tissues and other non-specific lesions is the main source of false-positive [^{18}F]FDG-PET findings in oncology. Van Waarde et al. (2004) used a rodent model with C6 glioma tumor and inflammatory lesion to show that [^{18}F]FLT was more specific than [^{18}F]FDG for uptake by glioma lesions relative to inflammation. However, the ability of [^{18}F]FLT to detect tumors was dependent on disruption of the BBB (Muzi et al. 2006), rendering it more suitable for detecting high-grade gliomas than low-grade ones. In a separate clinical study (Chen et al. 2005), [^{18}F]FLT–PET was more sensitive than [^{18}F]FDG-PET for imaging recurrent high-grade tumors, correlated better with the Ki-67 proliferation index and was a more powerful predictor of tumor progression and survival. The reason for superiority of [^{18}F]FLT–PET over [^{18}F]FDG–PET was low [^{18}F]FLT uptake in the normal brain tissue leading to higher T/N contrast (**Figure 6**). When compared with [^{11}C]MET, Jacobs et al. (2005) showed that [^{18}F]FLT was less sensitive in detecting tumors than [^{11}C]MET, especially for low-grade astrocytomas. Nevertheless, Kawai et al. (2009) found a high correlation between histological tumor grade and [^{18}F]FLT uptake in gliomas. A significant difference in SUV_{max} of [^{18}F]FLT was observed between grade II (0.27 ± 0.06, n=6) and grade IV (2.18 ± 0.93, n=10) gliomas ($P < 0.0001$), and grade III (0.70 ± 0.45, n=7) and grade IV gliomas ($P < 0.001$). Importantly, [^{18}F]FLT uptake correlated significantly better with the Ki-67 index ($r = 0.86$, $P < 0.0001$) than did methionine uptake in gliomas. Studies have also reported the use of [^{18}F]FLT-PET in investigating the effectiveness of therapy and prognosis of gliomas (Chen et al. 2007; Kawai et al. 2009). Increased [^{18}F]FLT accumulation is also observed in other brain tumors including malignant lymphoma (Kawai et al. 2009).

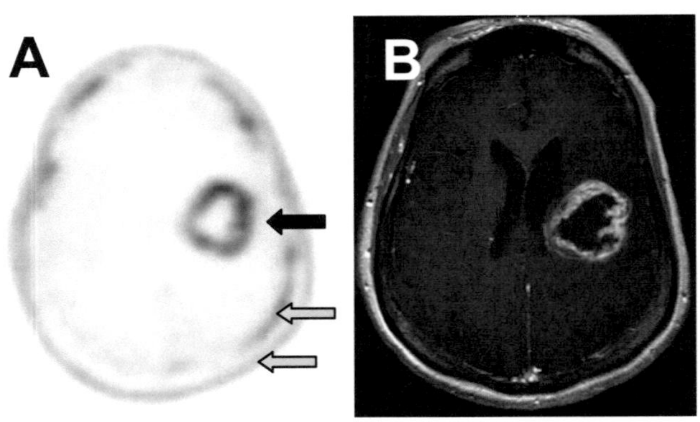

Fig. 6. Patient with glioblastoma. FLT-PET scan (A) and contrast-enhanced MRI (B) of biopsy-proven glioblastoma multiforme (GBM) in a 58 year-old female, just prior to the initiation of chemoradiation. Thick black arrow points to the highly proliferative rim of tumor surrounding a photopenic region of central necrosis. FLT uptake in the normal brain parenchyma is minimal, allowing a favorable lesion-to-background ratio. Physiologic uptake is also seen within the bone marrow (short thin arrow) and scalp (long thin arrow) *Image Courtesy of Dr. Laura Horky, Brigham and Women's Hospital, Boston.*

Another strategy for imaging of cell proliferation in tumor lesions involves non-invasive assessment of the concentration of sigma receptors in cells using sigma-receptor ligands

(Wheeler et al. 2000). Sigma-receptors are expressed more in proliferating tumor cells than in quiescent tumor cells (Wheeler et al. 2000). Using a preclinical tumor model, Van Waarde et al. (2004) were the first to report feasibility of using sigma-receptor binding ligands, [^{11}C]SA4503 and [^{18}F]FE-SA5845 for detecting gliomas. It is known that tumors are heterogenous in nature, including areas of low and high proliferation rates. The proportion of cells with low proliferation rate increases with increase in tumor size, especially in the necrotic center. In the C6 glioma rat model, tumor uptake of [^{18}F]FE-SA5845 showed a negative correlation with tumor size ($P < 0.0001$), in contrast to that of [^{11}C]SA4503, suggesting that tissue binding of [^{18}F]FE-SA5845 is solely related to cellular proliferation. Later Van Waarde et al. (2006) compared the bio-distribution of 4 PET tracers ([^{11}C]SA4503, [^{18}F]FE-SA5845, [^{11}C]choline and [^{11}C]MET) with previously published bio-distribution data of [^{18}F]FLT and [^{18}F]FDG in C6 glioma rat tumor model. In their study, sigma-receptor ligands and [^{18}F]FLT were more tumor selective than [^{18}F]FDG, [^{11}C]choline, or [^{11}C]MET in the C6 glioma model. However, [^{11}C]SA4503 and [^{18}F]FE-SA5845 were less sensitive than were [^{11}C]choline, [^{11}C]MET, and [^{18}F]FDG. Clinical PET studies for evaluation of sigma receptor expression in gliomas are ongoing.

7. Somatostatin-based probes

Meningiomas are the most common non-glial primary tumors of the central nervous system accounting for approximately 15% of all intracranial tumors (Buetow et al. 1991). More than 90% of intracranial meningiomas are slow growing and histopathologically benign but malignant meningiomas are not rare (Buetow et al. 1991; Goldsmith et al. 1994). [^{18}F]FDG uptake in tumor lesions is dependent on glycolytic rate and disruption of blood brain barrier (Roelcke et al. 1995). High expression of the somatostatin receptor (SSTR) subtype 2 (Dutour et al. 1998) in meningiomas offer the possibility of receptor-targeted imaging (Henze et al. 2005; Henze et al. 2001) of meningiomas. In the case of meningiomas with low glycolytic rate and intact BBB (Roelcke et al. 1995), somatostatin receptor based tracers might be more useful for tumor detection and disease management than [^{18}F]FDG. In a clinical study, a somatostatin receptor analog, ^{68}Ga-DOTA-D-Phe^{1}-Tyr^{3}-octreotide (DOTA-TOC) labeled with the positron emitter ^{68}Ga (half-life, 68 min) was evaluated for imaging meningioma (Henze et al. 2001). In contrast to [^{18}F]FDG, this ligand showed higher T/N uptake ratios. The initial results are encouraging but more clinical studies are needed to fully assess the potential of somatostatin receptor based tracers for imaging meningiomas.

8. Hypoxia-based probes

Hypoxia, a hallmark of aggressive tumor behavior often noted in high grade glioblastomas, is associated with resistance to therapy, poorer survival, invasion and aggressiveness (Szeto et al. 2009). Estimation of hypoxia could be an important determinant of overall survival in several tumors including gliomas. PET imaging with the hypoxia radiotracer [^{18}F]fluoromisonidazole ([^{18}F]FMISO) presents a possible means of noninvasively detecting tumor hypoxia in gliomas (Rasey et al. 2000; Valk et al. 1992). In a preclinical C6 glioma tumor model study (Tochon-Danguy et al. 2002), [^{18}F]FMISO uptake was significantly higher in tumor tissue compared to normal brain and the uptake was independent of tumor size. [^{18}F]FMISO uptake was observed homogeneously throughout viable glioma tissue in tumor sizes ranging from 2 mm to almost 1 cm. Quantitation of uptake of [^{18}F]FMISO showed a tumor-to-brain ratio of 1.9 and a tumor-to-blood ratio of 2.6 at 2 hours post-injection. In a recent clinical study by Shibahara et al. (2010), 8 patients with gliomas of different grades underwent PET studies with a new imidazole based hypoxia imaging agent, 1-(2-[^{18}F]fluoro-1-[hydroxymethyl]ethoxy)methyl-2-nitroimidazole ([^{18}F]FRP-170). The new agent showed higher image contrast and faster clearance than [^{18}F]FMISO. [^{18}F]FRP-170 images showed positive correlation with HIF-1α expression, a weak correlation with [^{18}F]FDG-PET and MR, but no correlation with [^{11}C]MET-PET. The [^{18}F]FRP-170-PET images showed marked uptake in the 3 GBM, and moderate uptake in recurrent anaplastic astrocytoma and oligodendroglioma, but no uptake in the other tumors (oligodendroglioma and diffuse astrocytoma). It is suggested that the use of hypoxia markers in patients with primary or recurrent gliomas could potentially assist in defining hypoxic tumor regions and predicting response to radiotherapy, but is not effective for grading tumors.

9. Acetate-based probes

Acetate is transported into the cell via the monocarboxylic acid transporter where it is converted in mitochondria to acetyl-coenzyme A (acetyl-CoA) (Lopresti and Mason 2009). Acetyl-CoA is a substrate for several biochemical pathways, most notably the tricarboxylic acid (TCA) cycle, and for glutamine and lipid synthesis. Additional studies have demonstrated that the preferential use of acetate by astrocytes is mediated by transport, although the exact mechanism is not fully understood (Lopresti and Mason 2009). In a clinical study, Yamamoto et al. (2008) evaluated [^{11}C]acetate for detecting brain gliomas and differentiating high-grade gliomas. Sensitivities of [^{11}C]acetate, [^{11}C]MET, and [^{18}F]FDG were 90%, 100%, and 40%, respectively. The T/N ratios of [^{11}C]acetate and [^{11}C]MET were significantly higher than that of [^{18}F]FDG. With respect to tumor grades, uptakes (SUVs) of [^{11}C]acetate and [^{18}F]FDG in high-grade gliomas were significantly higher than those in low-grade gliomas while no significant differences were observed with [^{11}C]MET. In another clinical study (Tsuchida et al. 2008), [^{11}C]acetate was superior to [^{18}F]FDG in differentiating high-grade tumors from low-grade tumors. In a recent preclinical animal study (Marik et al. 2009), the fluorinated form of acetate, [^{18}F]fluoroacetate, was evaluated for the assessment of several neuropathologies including glioblastoma represented by the orthotopic U87 xenografts, ischemia associated with stroke or hypoxia. In this study, [^{18}F]fluoroacetate showed the highest T/N ratio in glioblastoma followed by stroke-ischemia and hypoxia-ischemia.

10. Conclusions

PET imaging offers a growing "toolbox" of molecular imaging probes for noninvasive evaluation of gliomas. In general, [^{18}F]FDG-PET has high prognostic value, performs well in identifying anaplastic transformations and detecting malignant high grade gliomas. But due to high normal cerebral uptake, it has limited use in detection of low-grade gliomas and residual/recurrent gliomas. Amino acid based probes (e.g, [^{11}C]MET, [^{18}F]FET and [^{18}F]FDOPA) have low normal cerebral uptake, resulting in improved detection of low-grade lesions. They have shown utility for grading of gliomas and they can differentiate residual/recurrent tumor from post-operative radiation injury. Preclinical studies with sigma receptor ligands suggest them to be more selective but less sensitive for tumor lesions than [^{18}F]FDG, [^{11}C]MET and [^{11}C]choline. Use of somatostatin receptor ligands may be limited to detecting meningiomas, while hypoxia markers are best suited for disease prognosis and predicting response to radiotherapy. Recent studies with choline-, acetate- and integrin-based PET probes seem encouraging but more work is needed to fully appreciate their potential. In conclusion, positron-labeled amino acids are showing highest general utility for staging and therapy management of gliomas, while other metabolic probes are undergoing validation to answer selected clinical questions such as assessment of hypoxia and angiogenesis.

11. Acknowledgement

The authors thank Drs. Sandi A. Kwee and Laura Horky for their contributions. The work was supported by the US Department of Energy (DE-FG02-10ER41691, (TRD)) and NIH (R21 EB0110085 (TRD)).

12. References

Alavi, J. B.; Alavi, A.; Chawluk, J.; Kushner, M.; Powe, J.; Hickey & W., Reivich, M. (1988). Positron emission tomography in patients with glioma. A predictor of prognosis, *Cancer*, Vol. 62, No. 6, pp. 1074-1078, ISSN 0008-543X

Bading, J. R. & Shields, A. F. (2008). Imaging of cell proliferation: status and prospects, *J Nucl Med*, Vol. 49 Suppl. 2, pp. 64S-80S, ISSN 0161-5505

Barker, F. G. ; Chang, S. M.; Valk, P. E.; Pounds, T. R. & Prados, M. D. (1997). 18-Fluorodeoxyglucose uptake and survival of patients with suspected recurrent malignant glioma, *Cancer*, Vol. 79, No. 1, pp. 115-126, ISSN 0008-543X

Basu, S. & Alavi, A. (2009). Molecular imaging (PET) of brain tumors, *Neuroimaging Clin N Am*, Vol. 19, No. 4, pp. 625-646, ISSN 1557-9867

Bello, L.; Francolini, M.; Marthyn, P.; Zhang, J.; Carroll, R. S.; Nikas, D. C. & Black, P. M. (2001). Alpha(v)beta3 and alpha(v)beta5 integrin expression in glioma periphery, *Neurosurgery*, Vol. 49, No. 2, pp. 380-389; discussion 390, ISSN 0148-396X

Bogdanowich-Knipp, S. J.; Jois, D. S. & Siahaan, T. J. (1999). The effect of conformation on the solution stability of linear vs. cyclic RGD peptides, *J Pept Res*, Vol. 53, No. 5, pp. 523-529, ISSN 1397-002X

Borgwardt, L.; Hojgaard, L.; Carstensen, H.; Laursen, H.; Nowak, M.; Thomsen, C. & Schmiegelow, K. (2005). Increased fluorine-18 2-fluoro-2-deoxy-D-glucose (FDG) uptake in childhood CNS tumors is correlated with malignancy grade: a study with FDG positron emission tomography/magnetic resonance imaging coregistration and image fusion, *J Clin Oncol*, Vol. 23, No. 13, pp. 3030-3037, ISSN 0732-183X

Brooks, P. C.; Montgomery, A. M.; Rosenfeld, M.; Reisfeld, R. A.; Hu, T.; Klier, G. & Cheresh, D. A. (1994). Integrin alpha v beta 3 antagonists promote tumor regression by inducing apoptosis of angiogenic blood vessels, *Cell*, Vol. 79, No. 7, pp. 1157-1164, ISSN 0092-8674

Buetow, M. P.; Buetow, P. C. & Smirniotopoulos, J. G. (1991). Typical, atypical, and misleading features in meningioma, *Radiographics*, Vol. 11, No. 6, pp. 1087-1106, ISSN 0271-5333

Burkhard, C.; Di Patre, P. L.; Schuler, D.; Schuler, G.; Yasargil, M. G.; Yonekawa, Y.; Lütolf, U. M.; Kleihues, P. & Ohgaki, H. (2003). A population-based study of the incidence and survival rates in patients with pilocytic astrocytoma, *J Neurosurg*, Vol. 98, No. 6, pp. 1170-1174, ISSN 0022-3085

Carter, A. (2010). Integrins as target: first phase III trial launches, but questions remain, *J Natl Cancer Inst*, Vol. 102, No. 10, pp. 675-677, ISSN 1460-2105

Cellarier, E.; Durando, X.; Vasson, M. P.; Farges, M. C.; Demiden, A.; Maurizis, J. C.; Madelmont, J. C. & Chollet, P. (2003). Methionine dependency and cancer treatment, *Cancer Treat Rev*, Vol.29, No.6, pp. 489-499, ISSN 0305-7372

Chao, S. T.; Suh, J. H.; Raja, S.; Lee, S. Y. & Barnett, G. (2001). The sensitivity and specificity of FDG PET in distinguishing recurrent brain tumor from radionecrosis in patients treated with stereotactic radiosurgery, *Int J Cancer*, Vol. 96, No. 3, pp. 191-197, ISSN 0020-7136

Chen, W. (2007). Clinical applications of PET in brain tumors, *J Nucl Med*, Vol. 48, No. 9, pp. 1468-1481, ISSN 0161-5505

Chen, W.; Cloughesy, T.; Kamdar, N.; Satyamurthy, N.; Bergsneider, M.; Liau, L.; Mischel, P.; Czernin, J.; Phelps, M. E. & Silverman, D. H. (2005). Imaging proliferation in brain tumors with 18F-FLT PET: comparison with 18F-FDG, *J Nucl Med*, Vol.46, No.6, pp. 945-952, ISSN 0161-5505

Chen, W.; Delaloye, S.; Silverman, D. H.; Geist, C.; Czernin, J.; Sayre, J.; Satyamurthy, N.; Pope, W.; Lai, A.; Phelps. M. E. & Cloughesy T. (2007). Predicting treatment response of malignant gliomas to bevacizumab and irinotecan by imaging proliferation with [^{18}F] fluorothymidine positron emission tomography: a pilot study, *J Clin Oncol*, Vol. 25, No. 30, pp. 4714-4721, ISSN 1527-7755

Chen, W.; Silverman, D. H.; Delaloye, S.; Czernin, J.; Kamdar, N.; Pope, W.; Satyamurthy, N.; Schiepers, C. & Cloughesy, T. (2006). 18F-FDOPA PET imaging of brain tumors: comparison study with 18F-FDG PET and evaluation of diagnostic accuracy, *J Nucl Med*, Vol.47, No.6, pp. 904-911, ISSN 0161-5505

Chen, X.; Hou, Y.; Tohme, M.; Park, R.; Khankaldyyan, V.; Gonzales-Gomez, I.; Bading, J. R.; Laug, W. E. & Conti, P. S. (2004). Pegylated Arg-Gly-Asp peptide: 64Cu labeling and PET imaging of brain tumor alphavbeta3-integrin expression, *J Nucl Med*, Vol.45, No.10, pp. 1776-1783, ISSN 0161-5505

Chen, X.; Park, R.; Shahinian, A. H.; Tohme, M.; Khankaldyyan, V.; Bozorgzadeh, M. H.; Bading, J. R.; Moats, R.; Laug, W. E. & Conti, P. S. (2004). 18F-labeled RGD peptide: initial evaluation for imaging brain tumor angiogenesis, *Nucl Med Biol*, Vol.31, No.2, pp. 179-189, ISSN 0969-8051

Chen, X.; Park, R.; Tohme, M.; Shahinian, A. H.; Bading, J. R. & Conti, P. S. (2004). MicroPET and autoradiographic imaging of breast cancer alpha v-integrin expression using 18F- and 64Cu-labeled RGD peptide, *Bioconjug Chem*, Vol.15, No.1, pp. 41-49, ISSN 1043-1802

Chen, X.; Tohme, M.; Park, R.; Hou, Y.; Bading, J. R. & Conti, P. S. (2004). Micro-PET imaging of alphavbeta3-integrin expression with 18F-labeled dimeric RGD peptide, *Mol Imaging*, Vol.3, No.2, pp. 96-104, ISSN 1535-3508

Chung, J. K.; Kim, Y. K.; Kim, S. K.; Lee, Y. J.; Paek, S.; Yeo, J. S.; Jeong, J. M.; Lee, D. S.; Jung, H. W. & Lee, M. C. (2002). Usefulness of 11C-methionine PET in the evaluation of brain lesions that are hypo- or isometabolic on 18F-FDG PET, *Eur J Nucl Med Mol Imaging*, Vol.29, No.2, pp. 176-182, ISSN 1619-7070

De Reuck, J.; Santens, P.; Goethals, P.; Strijckmans, K.; Lemahieu, I.; Boon, P.; Achten, E.; Lemmerling, M.; Vandekerckhove, T. & Caemaert, J. (1999). [Methyl-11C]thymidine positron emission tomography in tumoral and non-tumoral cerebral lesions, *Acta Neurol Belg*, Vol.99, No.2, pp. 118-125, ISSN 0300-9009

De Witte, O.; Goldberg, I.; Wikler, D.; Rorive, S.; Damhaut, P.; Monclus, M.; Salmon, I.; Brotchi, J. & Goldman, S. (2001). Positron emission tomography with injection of methionine as a prognostic factor in glioma, *J Neurosurg*, Vol. 95, No. 5, pp. 746-750, ISSN 0022-3085

De Witte, O.; Levivier, M.; Violon, P.; Salmon, I.; Damhaut, P.; Wikler, D.; Hildebrand, J.; Brotchi, J. & Goldman, S. (1996). Prognostic value positron emission tomography with [^{18}F]fluoro-2-deoxy-D-glucose in the low-grade glioma, *Neurosurgery*, Vol. 39, No. 3, pp. 470-476; discussion 476-477, ISSN 0148-396X

DeGrado, T. R.; Baldwin, S. W.; Wang, S.; Orr, M. D.; Liao, R. P.; Friedman, H. S.; Reiman, R.; Price, D. T. & Coleman, R. E. (2001). Synthesis and evaluation of (18)F-labeled choline analogs as oncologic PET tracers, *J Nucl Med*, Vol. 42, No. 12, pp. 1805-1814, ISSN 0161-5505

Delbeke, D.; Meyerowitz, C.; Lapidus, R. L.; Maciunas, R. J.; Jennings, M. T.; Moots, P. L. & Kessler, R. M. (1995). Optimal cutoff levels of F-18 fluorodeoxyglucose uptake in the differentiation of low-grade from high-grade brain tumors with PET, *Radiology*, Vol.195, No.1, pp. 47-52, ISSN 0033-8419

Derlon, J. M.; Bourdet, C.; Bustany, P.; Chatel, M.; Theron, J.; Darcel, F. & Syrota, A. (1989). [^{11}C]L-methionine uptake in gliomas, *Neurosurgery*, Vol. 25, No. 5, pp. 720-728, ISSN 0148-396X

Di Chiro, G.; DeLaPaz, R. L.; Brooks, R. A.; Sokoloff, L.; Kornblith, P. L.; Smith, B. H.; Patronas, N. J.; Kufta, C. V.; Kessler, R. M.; Johnston, G. S.; Manning, R. G. & Wolf, A. P. (1982). Glucose utilization of cerebral gliomas measured by [18F] fluorodeoxyglucose and positron emission tomography, *Neurology*, Vol.32, No.12, pp. 1323-1329, ISSN 0028-3878

Di Chiro, G. (1985). Brain imaging of glucose utilization in cerebral tumors, *Res Publ Assoc Res Nerv Ment Dis*, Vol. 63, pp. 185-197, ISSN 0091-7443

Di Chiro, G. (1987a). Positron emission tomography using [^{18}F]fluorodeoxyglucose in brain tumors. A powerful diagnostic and prognostic tool, *Invest Radiol*, Vol. 22, No. 5, pp. 360-371, ISSN 0020-9996

Di Chiro, G.; Hatazawa, J.; Katz, D. A.; Rizzoli, H. V. & De Michele, D. J., (1987b). Glucose utilization by intracranial meningiomas as an index of tumor aggressivity and probability of recurrence: a PET study, *Radiology*, Vol. 164, No. 2, pp. 521-526, ISSN 0033-8419

Duan, L.; Aoyagi, M.; Tamaki, M.; Yoshino, Y.; Morimoto, T.; Wakimoto, H.; Nagasaka, Y.; Hirakawa, K.; Ohno, K. & Yamamoto, K. (2004). Impairment of both apoptotic and cytoprotective signalings in glioma cells resistant to the combined use of cisplatin and tumor necrosis factor alpha, *Clin Cancer Res*, Vol.10, No.1 Pt 1, pp. 234-243, ISSN 1078-0432

Dutour, A.; Kumar, U.; Panetta, R.; Ouafik, L.; Fina, F.; Sasi, R. & Patel, Y. C. (1998). Expression of somatostatin receptor subtypes in human brain tumors, *Int J Cancer*, Vol. 76, No. 5, pp. 620-627, ISSN 0020-7136

Farid, K.; Sibon, I.; Fernandez, P.; Guyot, M.; Jeandot, R. & Allard, M. (2009). Delayed acquisition and hyperglycemia improve brain metastasis detection on F-18 FDG PET, *Clin Nucl Med*, Vol.34, No.8, pp. 533-534, ISSN 1536-0229

Farmakis, G.; Brandau, W.; Hellwig, D.; Wollenweber, F.; Schaefer, A.; Kirsch, C. M. & Samnick, S. (2008). PET imaging with p-[I-124]iodo-l-phenylalanine as a new tool for diagnosis and postoperative control in patients with glioma, *Clin Nucl Med*, Vol.33, No.6, pp. 441-442, ISSN 1536-0229

Fazekas, F.; Alavi, A.; Chawluk, J. B.; Zimmerman, R. A.; Hackney, D.; Bilaniuk, L.; Rosen, M.; Alves, W. M.; Hurtig, H. I.; Jamieson, D. G. & et al. (1989). Comparison of CT, MR, and PET in Alzheimer's dementia and normal aging, *J Nucl Med*, Vol.30, No.10, pp. 1607-1615, ISSN 0161-5505

Floeth, F. W.; Pauleit, D.; Sabel, M.; Reifenberger, G.; Stoffels, G.; Stummer, W.; Rommel, F.; Hamacher, K. & Langen, K. J. (2006). 18F-FET PET differentiation of ring-enhancing brain lesions, *J Nucl Med*, Vol.47, No.5, pp. 776-782, ISSN 0161-5505

Fulham, M. J.; Bizzi, A.; Dietz, M. J.; Shih, H. H.; Raman, R.; Sobering, G. S.; Frank, J. A.; Dwyer, A. J.; Alger, J. R. & Di Chiro, G. (1992). Mapping of brain tumor metabolites with proton MR spectroscopic imaging: clinical relevance, *Radiology*, Vol.185, No.3, pp. 675-686, ISSN 0033-8419

Gehrke, J.; Haring, C.; Konig, H.; Marin, H.; Schmidt, H. & Stolze, G. (1991). [Use of a computer in a clinical-toxicological laboratory with a fuzzy search], *Z Med Lab Diagn*, Vol.32, No.3-4, pp. 197-203, ISSN 0323-5637

Goldsmith, B. J.; Wara, W. M.; Wilson, C. B. & Larson, D. A., (1994). Postoperative irradiation for subtotally resected meningiomas. A retrospective analysis of 140 patients treated from 1967 to 1990, *J Neurosurg*, Vol. 80, No. 2, pp. 195-201, ISSN 0022-3085

Grosu, A. L.; Feldmann, H.; Dick, S.; Dzewas, B.; Nieder, C.; Gumprecht, H.; Frank, A.; Schwaiger, M.; Molls, M. & Weber, W. A. (2002). Implications of IMT-SPECT for postoperative radiotherapy planning in patients with gliomas, *Int J Radiat Oncol Biol Phys*, Vol.54, No.3, pp. 842-854, ISSN 0360-3016

Hagerstrand, D.; Smits, A.; Eriksson, A.; Sigurdardottir, S.; Olofsson, T.; Hartman, M.; Nister, M.; Kalimo, H. & Ostman, A. (2008). Gene expression analyses of grade II gliomas and identification of rPTPbeta/zeta as a candidate oligodendroglioma marker, *Neuro Oncol*, Vol.10, No.1, pp. 2-9, ISSN 1522-8517

Hara, T.; Kondo, T. & Kosaka, N., (2003). Use of ^{18}F-choline and ^{11}C-choline as contrast agents in positron emission tomography imaging-guided stereotactic biopsy sampling of gliomas, *J Neurosurg*, Vol. 99, No. 3, pp. 474-479, ISSN 0022-3085

Heiss, W. D.; Wienhard, K.; Wagner, R.; Lanfermann, H.; Thiel, A.; Herholz, K. & Pietrzyk, U. (1996). F-Dopa as an amino acid tracer to detect brain tumors, *J Nucl Med*, Vol.37, No.7, pp. 1180-1182, ISSN 0161-5505

Henze, M.; Dimitrakopoulou-Strauss, A.; Milker-Zabel, S.; Schuhmacher, J.; Strauss, L. G.; Doll, J.; Mäcke, H. R.; Eisenhut, M.; Debus, J. & Haberkorn, U. (2005). Characterization of 68Ga-DOTA-D-Phe1-Tyr3-octreotide kinetics in patients with meningiomas, *J Nucl Med*, Vol. 46, No. 5, pp. 763-769, ISSN 0161-5505

Henze, M.; Schuhmacher, J.; Hipp, P.; Kowalski, J.; Becker, D. W.; Doll, J.; Mäcke, H. R., Hofmann, M., Debus, J., Haberkorn, U. (2001). PET imaging of somatostatin receptors using [^{68}GA]DOTA-D-Phe1-Tyr3-octreotide: first results in patients with meningiomas, *J Nucl Med*, Vol. 42, No. 7, pp. 1053-1056, ISSN 0161-5505

Herholz, K.; Holzer, T.; Bauer, B.; Schroder, R.; Voges, J.; Ernestus, R. I.; Mendoza, G.; Weber-Luxenburger, G.; Löttgen, J.; Thiel, A.; Wienhard, K. & Heiss WD. (1998). ^{11}C-methionine PET for differential diagnosis of low-grade gliomas, *Neurology*, Vol. 50, No. 5, pp. 1316-1322, ISSN 0028-3878

Hoffman, J. M.; Waskin, H. A.; Schifter, T.; Hanson, M. W.; Gray, L.; Rosenfeld, S. & Coleman, R. E. (1993). FDG-PET in differentiating lymphoma from nonmalignant central nervous system lesions in patients with AIDS, *J Nucl Med*, Vol.34, No.4, pp. 567-575, ISSN 0161-5505

Hsieh, C. H.; Chen, Y. F.; Chen, F. D.; Hwang, J. J.; Chen, J. C.; Liu, R. S.; Kai, J. J.; Chang, C. W. & Wang, H. E. (2005). Evaluation of pharmacokinetics of 4-borono-2-(18)F-fluoro-L-phenylalanine for boron neutron capture therapy in a glioma-bearing rat model with hyperosmolar blood-brain barrier disruption, *J Nucl Med*, Vol.46, No.11, pp. 1858-1865, ISSN 0161-5505

Hubner, K. F., Thie, J. A., Smith, G. T., Kabalka, G. W., Keller, I. B., Kliefoth, A. B., Campbell, S. K., Buonocore, E. (1998). Positron Emission Tomography (PET) with 1-Aminocyclobutane-1-[(11)C]carboxylic Acid (1-[(11)C]-ACBC) for Detecting Recurrent Brain Tumors, *Clin Positron Imaging*, Vol. 1, No. 3, pp. 165-173, ISSN 1095-0397

Imahori, Y.; Ueda, S.; Ohmori, Y.; Kusuki, T.; Ono, K.; Fujii, R. & Ido, T. (1998). Fluorine-18-labeled fluoroboronophenylalanine PET in patients with glioma, *J Nucl Med*, Vol.39, No.2, pp. 325-333, ISSN 0161-5505

Jacobs, A. H.; Thomas, A.; Kracht, L. W.; Li, H.; Dittmar, C.; Garlip, G.; Galldiks, N.; Klein, J. C.; Sobesky, J.; Hilker, R.; Vollmar, S.; Herholz, K.; Wienhard, K. & Heiss, W. D. (2005). 18F-fluoro-L-thymidine and 11C-methylmethionine as markers of increased transport and proliferation in brain tumors, *J Nucl Med*, Vol.46, No.12, pp. 1948-1958, ISSN 0161-5505

Jager, P. L.; Vaalburg, W.; Pruim, J.; de Vries, E. G.; Langen, K. J. & Piers, D. A. (2001). Radiolabeled amino acids: basic aspects and clinical applications in oncology, *J Nucl Med*, Vol.42, No.3, pp. 432-445, ISSN 0161-5505

Kaschten, B.; Stevenaert, A.; Sadzot, B.; Deprez, M.; Degueldre, C.; Del Fiore, G.; Luxen, A. & Reznik, M. (1998). Preoperative evaluation of 54 gliomas by PET with fluorine-18-fluorodeoxyglucose and/or carbon-11-methionine, *J Nucl Med*, Vol. 39, No. 5, pp. 778-785, ISSN 0161-5505

Kaufman, S. (1995). Tyrosine hydroxylase, *Adv Enzymol Relat Areas Mol Biol*, Vol.70, pp. 103-220, ISSN 0065-258X

Kawai, N.; Kagawa, M.; Miyake, K.; Nishiyama, Y.; Yamamoto, Y. & Shiraishi, H. (2009). Use of ^{18}F-fluorothymidine positron emission tomography in brain tumor, *No Shinkei Geka*, Vol. 37, No. 7, pp. 657-664, ISSN 0301-2603

Kawai, N.; Kawanishi, M.; Tamiya, T. & Nagao, S. (2005). Crossed cerebellar glucose hypermetabolism demonstrated using PET in symptomatic epilepsy--case report, *Ann Nucl Med*, Vol.19, No.3, pp. 231-234, ISSN 0914-7187

Kim, D. W.; Jung, S. A.; Kim, C. G. & Park, S. A. (2010). The efficacy of dual time point F-18 FDG PET imaging for grading of brain tumors, *Clin Nucl Med*, Vol.35, No.6, pp. 400-403, ISSN 1536-0229

Kim, S.; Chung, J. K.; Im, S. H.; Jeong, J. M.; Lee, D. S.; Kim, D. G.; Jung, H. W. & Lee, M. C. (2005). 11C-methionine PET as a prognostic marker in patients with glioma: comparison with 18F-FDG PET, *Eur J Nucl Med Mol Imaging*, Vol.32, No.1, pp. 52-59, ISSN 1619-7070

Kimura, R. H.; Cheng, Z.; Gambhir, S. S. & Cochran, J. R. (2009). Engineered knottin peptides: a new class of agents for imaging integrin expression in living subjects, *Cancer Res*, Vol.69, No.6, pp. 2435-2442, ISSN 1538-7445

Kleihues, P. & Sobin, L. H. (2000). World Health Organization classification of tumors, *Cancer*, Vol.88, No.12, pp. 2887, ISSN 0008-543X

Kountouras, J.; Zavos, C. & Chatzopoulos, D. (2005). Apoptotic and anti-angiogenic strategies in liver and gastrointestinal malignancies, *J Surg Oncol*, Vol.90, No.4, pp. 249-259, ISSN 0022-4790

Kwee, S. A.; Coel, M. N.; Lim, J. & Ko, J. P., (2004). Combined use of F-18 fluorocholine positron emission tomography and magnetic resonance spectroscopy for brain tumor evaluation, *J Neuroimaging*, Vol. 14, No. 3, pp. 285-289, ISSN 1051-2284

Kwee, S. A.; Ko, J. P.; Jiang, C. S.; Watters, M. R. & Coel, M. N., (2007). Solitary brain lesions enhancing at MR imaging: evaluation with fluorine 18 fluorocholine PET, *Radiology*, Vol. 244, No. 2, pp. 557-565, ISSN 0033-8419

Lau, E. W.; Drummond, K. J.; Ware, R. E.; Drummond, E.; Hogg, A.; Ryan, G.; Grigg, A.; Callahan, J. & Hicks, R. J. (2010). Comparative PET study using F-18 FET and F-18 FDG for the evaluation of patients with suspected brain tumour, *J Clin Neurosci*, Vol.17, No.1, pp. 43-49, ISSN 1532-2653

Lemmens, K. P.; Abraham, C.; Hoekstra, T.; Ruiter, R. A.; De Kort, W. L.; Brug, J. & Schaalma, H. P. (2005). Why don't young people volunteer to give blood? An investigation of the correlates of donation intentions among young nondonors, *Transfusion*, Vol.45, No.6, pp. 945-955, ISSN 0041-1132

Leskinen-Kallio, S.; Nagren, K.; Lehikoinen, P.; Ruotsalainen, U. & Joensuu, H. (1991). Uptake of 11C-methionine in breast cancer studied by PET. An association with the size of S-phase fraction, *Br J Cancer*, Vol.64, No.6, pp. 1121-1124, ISSN 0007-0920

Li, G. Q. & Zhang, H. F. (2004). Mad2 and p27 expression profiles in colorectal cancer and its clinical significance, *World J Gastroenterol*, Vol.10, No.21, pp. 3218-3220, ISSN 1007-9327

Lilja, A.; Bergstrom, K.; Hartvig, P.; Spannare, B.; Halldin, C.; Lundqvist, H. & Langstrom, B. (1985). Dynamic study of supratentorial gliomas with L-methyl-11C-methionine and positron emission tomography, *AJNR Am J Neuroradiol*, Vol.6, No.4, pp. 505-514, ISSN 0195-6108

Liu, S. (2009). Radiolabeled cyclic RGD peptides as integrin alpha(v)beta(3)-targeted radiotracers: maximizing binding affinity via bivalency, *Bioconjug Chem*, Vol.20, No.12, pp. 2199-2213, ISSN 1520-4812

Lopresti, B. J. & Mason, N. S., (2009). 2-^{18}F-fluoroacetate: a useful tool for assessing gliosis in the central nervous system?, *J Nucl Med*, Vol. 50, No. 6, pp. 841-843, ISSN 0161-5505

MacDonald, T. J.; Taga, T.; Shimada, H.; Tabrizi, P.; Zlokovic, B. V.; Cheresh, D. A. & Laug, W. E. (2001). Preferential susceptibility of brain tumors to the antiangiogenic effects of an alpha(v) integrin antagonist, *Neurosurgery*, Vol.48, No.1, pp. 151-157, ISSN 0148-396X

Main, A. L.; Harvey, T. S.; Baron, M.; Boyd, J. & Campbell, I. D. (1992). The three-dimensional structure of the tenth type III module of fibronectin: an insight into RGD-mediated interactions, *Cell*, Vol.71, No.4, pp. 671-678, ISSN 0092-8674

Marik, J.; Ogasawara, A.; Martin-McNulty, B.; Ross, J.; Flores, J. E.; Gill, H. S.; Tinianow, J. N.; Vanderbilt, A. N.; Nishimura, M.; Peale, F.; Pastuskovas, C.; Greve, J. M.; van Bruggen, N. & Williams, S.P. (2009). PET of glial metabolism using 2-^{18}F-fluoroacetate, *J Nucl Med*, Vol. 50, No. 6, pp. 982-990, ISSN 0161-5505

McGeer, P. L.; Kamo, H.; Harrop, R.; McGeer, E. G.; Martin, W. R.; Pate, B. D. & Li, D. K. (1986). Comparison of PET, MRI, and CT with pathology in a proven case of Alzheimer's disease, *Neurology*, Vol.36, No.12, pp. 1569-1574, ISSN 0028-3878

Miao, Z.; Ren, G.; Liu, H.; Kimura, R. H.; Jiang, L.; Cochran, J. R.; Gambhir, S. S. & Cheng, Z. (2009). An engineered knottin peptide labeled with 18F for PET imaging of integrin expression, *Bioconjug Chem*, Vol.20, No.12, pp. 2342-2347, ISSN 1520-4812

Morowitz, H. J.; Kostelnik, J. D.; Yang, J. & Cody, G. D. (2000). The origin of intermediary metabolism, *Proc Natl Acad Sci U S A*, Vol.97, No.14, pp. 7704-7708, ISSN 0027-8424

Muzi, M.; Spence, A. M.; O'Sullivan, F.; Mankoff, D. A.; Wells, J. M.; Grierson, J. R.; Link, J. M. & Krohn, K.A. (2006). Kinetic analysis of 3'-deoxy-3'-^{18}F-fluorothymidine in patients with gliomas, *J Nucl Med*, Vol. 47, No. 10, pp. 1612-1621, ISSN 0161-5505

Nagatsu, T. (1995). Tyrosine hydroxylase: human isoforms, structure and regulation in physiology and pathology, *Essays Biochem*, Vol.30, pp. 15-35, ISSN 0071-1365

Ogawa, T.; Kanno, I.; Shishido, F.; Inugami, A.; Higano, S.; Fujita, H.; Murakami, M.; Uemura, K.; Yasui, N. & Mineura, K. (1991). Clinical value of PET with 18F-fluorodeoxyglucose and L-methyl-11C-methionine for diagnosis of recurrent brain tumor and radiation injury, *Acta Radiol*, Vol.32, No.3, pp. 197-202, ISSN 0284-1851

Ogawa, T.; Shishido, F.; Kanno, I.; Inugami, A.; Fujita, H.; Murakami, M.; Shimosegawa, E.; Ito, H.; Hatazawa, J. & Okudera, T. (1993). Cerebral glioma: evaluation with methionine PET, *Radiology*, Vol.186, No.1, pp. 45-53, ISSN 0033-8419

Ohgaki, H. & Kleihues, P. (2005). Population-based studies on incidence, survival rates, and genetic alterations in astrocytic and oligodendroglial gliomas, *J Neuropathol Exp Neurol*, Vol.64, No.6, pp. 479-489, ISSN 0022-3069

Ohtani, T.; Kurihara, H.; Ishiuchi, S.; Saito, N.; Oriuchi, N.; Inoue, T. & Sasaki T. (2001). Brain tumour imaging with carbon-11 choline: comparison with FDG PET and gadolinium-enhanced MR imaging, *Eur J Nucl Med*, Vol. 28, No. 11, pp. 1664-1670, ISSN 0340-6997

Okamoto, S.; Shiga, T.; Hattori, N.; Kubo, N.; Takei, T.; Katoh, N.; Sawamura, Y.; Nishijima, K.; Kuge, Y. & Tamaki, N. (2010). Semiquantitative analysis of C-11 methionine PET may distinguish brain tumor recurrence from radiation necrosis even in small lesions, *Ann Nucl Med*, ISSN 1864-6433

Olivero, W. C.; Dulebohn, S. C. & Lister, J. R. (1995). The use of PET in evaluating patients with primary brain tumours: is it useful?, *J Neurol Neurosurg Psychiatry*, Vol.58, No.2, pp. 250-252, ISSN 0022-3050

Ono, Y.; Ito, T.; Watanabe, T.; Koshio, O.; Tansho, S.; Ikeda, T.; Kawakami, S. & Miyazawa, Y. (2004). Opsonic activity assessment of human intravenous immunoglobulin preparations against drug-resistant bacteria, *J Infect Chemother*, Vol.10, No.4, pp. 234-238, ISSN 1341-321X

Padma, M. V.; Said, S.; Jacobs, M.; Hwang, D. R.; Dunigan, K.; Satter, M.; Christian, B.; Ruppert, J.; Bernstein, T.; Kraus, G. & Mantil, J. C. (2003). Prediction of pathology and survival by FDG PET in gliomas, *J Neurooncol*, Vol.64, No.3, pp. 227-237, ISSN 0167-594X

Patronas, N. J.; Di Chiro, G.; Kufta, C.; Bairamian, D.; Kornblith, P. L.; Simon, R. & Larson, S. M. (1985). Prediction of survival in glioma patients by means of positron emission tomography, *J Neurosurg*, Vol.62, No.6, pp. 816-822, ISSN 0022-3085

Pauleit, D.; Floeth, F.; Hamacher, K.; Riemenschneider, M. J.; Reifenberger, G.; Muller, H. W.; Zilles, K.; Coenen, H. H. & Langen, K. J. (2005). O-(2-[^{18}F]fluoroethyl)-L-tyrosine PET combined with MRI improves the diagnostic assessment of cerebral gliomas, *Brain*, Vol. 128, No. Pt 3, pp. 678-687, ISSN 1460-2156

Pedersen, P. L. (2007). Warburg, me and Hexokinase 2: Multiple discoveries of key molecular events underlying one of cancers' most common phenotypes, the "Warburg Effect", i.e., elevated glycolysis in the presence of oxygen, *J Bioenerg Biomembr*, Vol.39, No.3, pp. 211-222, ISSN 0145-479X

Popperl, G.; Gotz, C.; Rachinger, W.; Gildehaus, F. J.; Tonn, J. C. & Tatsch, K. (2004). Value of O-(2-[18F]fluoroethyl)- L-tyrosine PET for the diagnosis of recurrent glioma, *Eur J Nucl Med Mol Imaging*, Vol.31, No.11, pp. 1464-1470, ISSN 1619-7070

Popperl, G.; Kreth, F. W.; Herms, J.; Koch, W.; Mehrkens, J. H.; Gildehaus, F. J.; Kretzschmar, H. A.; Tonn, J. C. & Tatsch, K. (2006). Analysis of 18F-FET PET for grading of recurrent gliomas: is evaluation of uptake kinetics superior to standard methods?, *J Nucl Med*, Vol.47, No.3, pp. 393-403, ISSN 0161-5505

Rasey, J. S.; Casciari, J. J.; Hofstrand, P. D.; Muzi, M.; Graham, M. M. & Chin, L. K. (2000). Determining hypoxic fraction in a rat glioma by uptake of radiolabeled fluoromisonidazole, *Radiat Res*, Vol.153, No.1, pp. 84-92, ISSN 0033-7587

Ricci, P. E.; Karis, J. P.; Heiserman, J. E.; Fram, E. K.; Bice, A. N. & Drayer, B. P. (1998). Differentiating recurrent tumor from radiation necrosis: time for re-evaluation of positron emission tomography?, *AJNR Am J Neuroradiol*, Vol.19, No.3, pp. 407-413, ISSN 0195-6108

Roelcke, U.; Radu, E. W.; von Ammon, K.; Hausmann, O.; Maguire, R. P. & Leenders, K. L. (1995). Alteration of blood-brain barrier in human brain tumors: comparison of [18F]fluorodeoxyglucose, [11C]methionine and rubidium-82 using PET, *J Neurol Sci*, Vol.132, No.1, pp. 20-27, ISSN 0022-510X

Sartor, K. (1999). MR imaging of the brain: tumors, *Eur Radiol*, Vol.9, No.6, pp. 1047-1054, ISSN 0938-7994

Sasajima, T.; Miyagawa, T.; Oku, T.; Gelovani, J. G.; Finn, R. & Blasberg, R. (2004). Proliferation-dependent changes in amino acid transport and glucose metabolism in glioma cell lines, *Eur J Nucl Med Mol Imaging*, Vol.31, No.9, pp. 1244-1256, ISSN 1619-7070

Schnell, O.; Krebs, B.; Carlsen, J.; Miederer, I.; Goetz, C.; Goldbrunner, R. H.; Wester, H. J.; Haubner, R.; Popperl, G.; Holtmannspotter, M.; Kretzschmar, H. A.; Kessler, H.; Tonn, J. C.; Schwaiger, M. & Beer, A. J. (2009). Imaging of integrin alpha(v)beta(3) expression in patients with malignant glioma by [18F] Galacto-RGD positron emission tomography, *Neuro Oncol*, Vol.11, No.6, pp. 861-870, ISSN 1523-5866

Shibahara, I.; Kumabe, T.; Kanamori, M.; Saito, R.; Sonoda, Y.; Watanabe, M.; Iwata, R.; Higano, S.; Takanami, K.; Takai, Y. & Tominaga, T. (2010). Imaging of hypoxic lesions in patients with gliomas by using positron emission tomography with 1-(2-[^{18}F]fluoro-1-[hydroxymethyl]ethoxy)methyl-2-nitroimidazole, a new ^{18}F-labeled 2-nitroimidazole analog, *J Neurosurg*, Vol. 113, No. 2, pp. 358-368, ISSN 1933-0693

Shields, A. F.; Grierson, J. R.; Dohmen, B. M.; Machulla, H. J.; Stayanoff, J. C.; Lawhorn-Crews, J. M.; Obradovich, J. E.; Muzik, O. & Mangner, T. J. (1998). Imaging proliferation in vivo with [F-18]FLT and positron emission tomography, *Nat Med*, Vol. 4, No. 11, pp. 1334-1336, ISSN 1078-8956

Schiepers, C.; Chen, W.; Cloughesy, T.; Dahlbom, M. & Huang, S. (2007). 18F-FDOPA Kinetics in Brain Tumors, *J Nucl Med*, Vol. 48, pp. 1651–1661, ISSN 0161-5505

Shinoura, N.; Nishijima, M.; Hara, T.; Haisa, T.; Yamamoto, H.; Fujii, K.; Mitsui, I.; Kosaka, N. & Kondo, T. (1997). Brain tumors: detection with C-11 choline PET, *Radiology*, Vol.202, No.2, pp. 497-503, ISSN 0033-8419

Sonoda, Y.; Kumabe, T.; Takahashi, T.; Shirane, R. & Yoshimoto, T. (1998). Clinical usefulness of ^{11}C-MET PET and 201T1 SPECT for differentiation of recurrent glioma from radiation necrosis, *Neurol Med Chir (Tokyo)*, Vol. 38, No. 6, pp. 342-347; discussion 347-348, ISSN 0470-8105

Spence, A. M.; Muzi, M.; Graham, M. M.; O'Sullivan, F.; Krohn, K. A.; Link, J. M.; Lewellen, T. K.; Lewellen, B.; Freeman, S. D.; Berger, M. S. & Ojemann, G. A. (1998). Glucose metabolism in human malignant gliomas measured quantitatively with PET, 1-[C-11]glucose and FDG: analysis of the FDG lumped constant, *J Nucl Med*, Vol.39, No.3, pp. 440-448, ISSN 0161-5505

Spence, A. M.; Muzi, M.; Mankoff, D. A.; O'Sullivan, S. F.; Link, J. M.; Lewellen, T. K.; Lewellen, B.; Pham, P.; Minoshima, S.; Swanson, K. & Krohn, K. A. (2004). 18F-FDG PET of gliomas at delayed intervals: improved distinction between tumor and normal gray matter, *J Nucl Med*, Vol.45, No.10, pp. 1653-1659, ISSN 0161-5505

Szeto, M. D.; Chakraborty, G.; Hadley, J.; Rockne, R.; Muzi, M.; Alvord, E. C., Jr.; Krohn, K. A.; Spence, A. M. & Swanson, K. R. (2009). Quantitative metrics of net proliferation and invasion link biological aggressiveness assessed by MRI with hypoxia assessed by FMISO-PET in newly diagnosed glioblastomas, *Cancer Res*, Vol.69, No.10, pp. 4502-4509, ISSN 1538-7445

Tochon-Danguy, H. J.; Sachinidis, J. I.; Chan, F.; Chan, J. G.; Hall, C.; Cher, L.; Stylli, S.; Hill, J.; Kaye, A. & Scott, A. M. (2002). Imaging and quantitation of the hypoxic cell fraction of viable tumor in an animal model of intracerebral high grade glioma using [18F]fluoromisonidazole (FMISO), *Nucl Med Biol*, Vol.29, No.2, pp. 191-197, ISSN 0969-8051

Tsuchida, T.; Takeuchi, H.; Okazawa, H.; Tsujikawa, T. & Fujibayashi, Y. (2008). Grading of brain glioma with 1-^{11}C-acetate PET: comparison with ^{18}F-FDG PET, *Nucl Med Biol*, Vol. 35, No. 2, pp. 171-176, ISSN 0969-8051

Tsuyuguchi, N.; Sunada, I.; Iwai, Y.; Yamanaka, K.; Tanaka, K.; Takami, T.; Otsuka, Y.; Sakamoto, S.; Ohata, K.; Goto, T. & Hara M. (2003). Methionine positron emission tomography of recurrent metastatic brain tumor and radiation necrosis after stereotactic radiosurgery: is a differential diagnosis possible?, *J Neurosurg*, Vol. 98, No. 5, pp. 1056-1064, ISSN 0022-3085

Valk, P. E.; Mathis, C. A.; Prados, M. D.; Gilbert, J. C. & Budinger, T. F. (1992). Hypoxia in human gliomas: demonstration by PET with fluorine-18-fluoromisonidazole, *J Nucl Med*, Vol. 33, No. 12, pp. 2133-2137, ISSN 0161-5505

Van Laere, K.; Ceyssens, S.; Van Calenbergh, F.; de Groot, T.; Menten, J.; Flamen, P.; Bormans, G. & Mortelmans, L. (2005). Direct comparison of 18F-FDG and 11C-methionine PET in suspected recurrence of glioma: sensitivity, inter-observer variability and prognostic value, *Eur J Nucl Med Mol Imaging*, Vol.32, No.1, pp. 39-51, ISSN 1619-7070

van Waarde, A.; Cobben, D. C.; Suurmeijer, A. J.; Maas, B.; Vaalburg, W.; de Vries, E. F.; Jager, P. L.; Hoekstra, H. J. & Elsinga, P. H. (2004). Selectivity of 18F-FLT and 18F-

FDG for differentiating tumor from inflammation in a rodent model, *J Nucl Med*, Vol.45, No.4, pp. 695-700, ISSN 0161-5505

van Waarde, A.; Cobben, D. C.; Suurmeijer, A. J.; Maas, B.; Vaalburg, W.; de Vries, E. F.; Jager, P. L.; Hoekstra, H. J. & Elsinga, P. H. (2004). Selectivity of ^{18}F-FLT and ^{18}F-FDG for differentiating tumor from inflammation in a rodent model, *J Nucl Med*, Vol. 45, No. 4, pp. 695-700, ISSN 0161-5505

van Waarde, A.; Jager, P. L.; Ishiwata, K.; Dierckx, R. A. & Elsinga, P. H., (2006). Comparison of sigma-ligands and metabolic PET tracers for differentiating tumor from inflammation, *J Nucl Med*, Vol. 47, No. 1, pp. 150-154, ISSN 0161-5505

Vanpouille, C.; Le Jeune, N.; Kryza, D.; Clotagatide, A.; Janier, M.; Dubois, F. and Perek, N. (2009). Influence of multidrug resistance on (18)F-FCH cellular uptake in a glioblastoma model, *Eur J Nucl Med Mol Imaging*, Vol. 36, No. 8, pp. 1256-1264, ISSN 1619-7089

Wang, L.; Qu, W.; Lieberman, B. P.; Plossl, K. & Kung, H. F., (2011). Synthesis, uptake mechanism characterization and biological evaluation of (18)F labeled fluoroalkyl phenylalanine analogs as potential PET imaging agents, *Nucl Med Biol*, Vol. 38, No. 1, pp. 53-62, ISSN 1872-9614

Wang, S. X.; Boethius, J. & Ericson, K. (2006). FDG-PET on irradiated brain tumor: ten years' summary, *Acta Radiol*, Vol. 47, No. 1, pp. 85-90, ISSN 0284-1851

Warburg, O. (1956). On the origin of cancer cells, *Science*, Vol. 123, No. 3191, pp. 309-314, ISSN 0036-8075

Weber, W. A.; Wester, H. J.; Grosu, A. L.; Herz, M., Dzewas, B.; Feldmann, H. J.; Molls, M.; Stöcklin, G. & Schwaiger, M. (2000). O-(2-[^{18}F]fluoroethyl)-L-tyrosine and L-[methyl-^{11}C]methionine uptake in brain tumours: initial results of a comparative study, *Eur J Nucl Med*, Vol. 27, No. 5, pp. 542-549, ISSN 0340-6997

Wester, H. J.; Herz, M.; Weber, W.; Heiss, P.; Senekowitsch-Schmidtke, R.; Schwaiger, M., et al. & Stöcklin G. (1999). Synthesis and radiopharmacology of O-(2-[^{18}F]fluoroethyl)-L-tyrosine for tumor imaging, *J Nucl Med*, Vol. 40, No. 1, pp. 205-212, ISSN 0161-5505

Wheeler, K. T.; Wang, L. M.; Wallen, C. A.; Childers, S. R.; Cline, J. M.; Keng, P. C. & Mach, R. H. (2000). Sigma-2 receptors as a biomarker of proliferation in solid tumours, *Br J Cancer*, Vol. 82, No. 6, pp. 1223-1232, ISSN 0007-0920

Wong, T. Z.; Turkington, T. G.; Hawk, T. C. & Coleman, R. E. (2004). PET and brain tumor image fusion, *Cancer J*, Vol. 10, No. 4, pp. 234-242, ISSN 1528-9117

Wu, Y., Zhang, X.; Xiong, Z.; Cheng, Z.; Fisher, D. R.; Liu, S.; Gambhir, S. S. & Chen, X. (2005). microPET imaging of glioma integrin {alpha}v{beta}3 expression using (64)Cu-labeled tetrameric RGD peptide, *J Nucl Med*, Vol. 46, No. 10, pp. 1707-1718, ISSN 0161-5505

Wyss, M. T.; Spaeth, N., Biollaz, G.; Pahnke, J.; Alessi, P.; Trachsel, E.; Treyer, V.; Weber, B.; Neri, D. & Buck A. (2007). Uptake of ^{18}F-Fluorocholine, ^{18}F-FET, and ^{18}F-FDG in C6 gliomas and correlation with ^{131}I-SIP(L19), a marker of angiogenesis, *J Nucl Med*, Vol. 48, No. 4, pp. 608-614, ISSN 0161-5505

Yamamoto, Y.; Nishiyama, Y.; Kimura, N.; Kameyama, R.; Kawai, N.; Hatakeyama, T.; Kaji, M. & Ohkawa, M. (2008). ^{11}C-acetate PET in the evaluation of brain glioma: comparison with ^{11}C-methionine and ^{18}F-FDG-PET, *Mol Imaging Biol*, Vol. 10, No. 5, pp. 281-287, ISSN 1536-1632

10

Visualization and Photodynamic Therapy in Malignant Glioma - An Overview and Perspectives

Rainer Ritz
Department of Neurosurgery, Eberhard Karls University Tübingen, Tübingen Germany

1. Introduction

Photodynamic therapy (PDT) is a relatively new modality of cancer treatment. Actual ongoing clinical era started with the studies of Dougherty in the 1970s. PDT is based on the application of a so called photosensitizer (PS), which preferably enriches in the tumor tissue. The application of light at an appropriate wavelength excites the PS molecules from their ground state S_0 to an electronically excited singlet state S_x. The energy of the excited state can be dissipated via several relaxation pathways. By this, so called cytotoxic reactive oxygen species (ROS) are generated. ROS react with various biomolecules inducing cell death by different mechanims.(Dougherty et al. 1998b)

2. History of PDT

The newer history of PDT starts with the observations of Von Tappeiner and Raab at the Maximilian Ludwig University in Munich. In 1900, Raab first reported on the chemical sensitisation of tissue by light.(Raab 1900) Von Tappeiner described in 1904 the so called "photodynamic reaction".(Tappeiner & Jodlbauer 1904) He believed that this effect was based on fluorescence. In contrast Neiser (Breslau) and Dreyer (Finsen Institue in Kopenhagen) described a sensitisation by light for photodynamic reaction.(Dreyer 1903;Neisser & Halberstaedtter 1904) At this time Ledoux-Lebards already proved the concept of the presence of oxygen as a condition for PDT at the Institute Pasteur in Paris (1902).(Ledoux-Lebards 1902) In this era skin diseases were treated with chinidin, acridin and eosin with unsatisfying results.
Already from the beginning of PDT, haematoporphyrin (Hp) was of special interest. Hausmann used Hp for photodynamic investigations in mice in 1911.(Hausmann 1911) In 1913, Meyer-Betz studied Hp to determine its biological effects on himself. After exposition to sunlight he suffered from extensive phototoxic reactions.(Meyer-Betz 1913) Policard detected 1924 in rat sarcoma a red fluorescence after Hp administration.(Policard 1924) In 1942 Auler and Banzer reported on the affinity of neoplastic tissues for Hp in tumor, metastases and lymphatic vessels in patients suffering cancer.(Auler & Banzer 1942) Further investigations were performed by Figge et al. in 1948; they demonstrated the properties of Hp to localize tumors.(Figge, Weiland, & Manganiello 1948) Due to high toxic reactions of

Hp, in 1955 a hematoporphyrin derivat (HpD) was developed by Schwartz et al..(Schwartz, Absolon, & Vermund 1955) This derivat also contained many components of hematoporphyrins. Lipson et al. used the HpD *in vivo* and in patients for tumor detection and localisation in the early sixties.(Lipson, Baldes, & Olsen 1964)
A milestone in PDT was done by Dougherty in 1973.(Dougherty 1973) Dougherty postulated the criteria for PSs and for PDT. Essential for a successful PS is less or no toxicity without light, selective enrichment in the tumor or affected tissue and activation by light with a wavelength of 600 nm or more.(Dougherty et al. 1978;Dougherty et al. 1998a) HpD was further purified by Dougherty's group to Photofrin®. Photofrin is up to now for PDT drug approved.

2.1 First and second generation photosensitizers

HpD and Photofrin® are first generation PSs. The maximum of absorption of HpD is 628 to 632 nm. Penetration depth is about 5 mm. *In vivo* the concentration of HpD is twelve times higher compared to normal brain tissue. In clinical investigations the concentration was 1:2.5 to 1:4 fold. (Kostron, Obwegeser, & Jakober 1996) This first generation PSs have some disadvantages, e.g. high impurity, prolonged skin photosensitivity about several weeks and low absorbance at 630 nm, where tissue penetration of light is low. To improve this, second generation photosensitizers (phthalocyanines, naphthalocyanins, benzoporphyrins, chlorines, purpurins, texaphyrins, porphycenes, pheophobides, bacteriochlorins, etc.) were introduced (Juzeniene, Peng, & Moan 2007). Second generation PSs have a high absorbance in the region of 650-850 nm and produce adequate singlet oxygen. Meta-tetra hydroxyphenylchlorin (m-THPC; Foscan®, Biolitec AG) and benzoporphyrin derivative monoacid A (BPD-MA; Visudyne®, QLT Inc. and Novartis Opthalmics) are approved drugs for clinical use. The second generation PS mTHPC has its maximum absorption at 652 nm. Phototoxic reaction had been observed up to a depth of 15 mm. For meta-tetrahydroxyphenylchlorin (mTHPC) a ratio tumor to normal tissue of more than 80:1 has been described *in vivo* after implantation of C6 glioma in Spraque-Dawley rats. In clinical applications the ratio tumor to normal brain tissue was 20:1.(Dougherty, Gomer, Henderson, Jori, Kessel, Korbelik, Moan, & Peng 1998a;Obwegeser, Jakober, & Kostron 1998) Several more PSs are available, but have been less usage in neurosurgery. Third generation PSs are second generation photosensitizers bound to carriers for selective accumulation in the tumor.

2.2 Prodrug: 5-aminolevulinic acid derived protoporphyrin IX

5-aminolevulinic acid (5-ALA) a prodrug transformed to 5-aminolevulinic acid-derived protoporphyrin IX (5-ALA PpIX) is especially used for photodiagnosis (PD) although properties for as a PS are known. In 1955 Scott described the transitory hypersensitivity to sunlight following exogenous administration of 5-ALA.(Scott 1955) First description about the use of 5-ALA as a porphyrin precursor in PDT was done by Malik and Lugaci, who demonstrated, that exogenous 5-ALA PpIX in combination with light led to inactivation of leukemic cells.(Malik & Lugaci 1987) Kennedy et al. reported about successful treatment of malignant and precancerous skin diseases in 1990.(Kennedy, Pottier, & Pross 1990) The use of 5-ALA PpIX in neurosurgery for fluorescence guided resection of glioblastoma was a milestone. Stummer et al. demonstrated convincingly that the radicality of tumor resection and thus the outcome of patients improves significantly by intraoperative tumor visualisation.(Stummer et al. 2000;Stummer et al. 2006;Stummer et al. 2008) 5-ALA is a precursor, converted in malignant cells to PpIX, the fluorescent substance. 5-ALA is the first substrate in the heme biosynthesis. Heme biosynthesis consists of eight discrete enzymes catalysed steps which involve the mitochondrial (the first and the last three steps) and cytosolic (the other four intermediate steps) compartments of the cell. In the first step 5-ALA is produced by ALA synthetase in the mitochondria. This is the rate-limiting step in heme biosynthesis. 5-ALA is actively transported to the cytoplasm. After reentry into the mitochondrion, PpIX is produced. PpIX is the last step in the heme pathway before forming heme by insertion of ferrous iron by the enzyme ferrochelatase. Mitochondrial ferrochelatase is dependent on mitochondrial energy generation. In malignant tissue ferrochelatase is reduced, therefore PpIX, a strongly fluorescent and effective tissue PS accumulates in higher concentrations after application of 5-ALA in gliomas.(Kemmner et al. 2008) Some more reasons for higher accumulation of PSs should be mentioned. On the surface of tumour cells more low-density lipoprotein (LDL) receptors are found than on the surface of normal cells.(Maziere, Morliere, & Santus 1991) Increased porphobilinogendeaminase activity in malignant glioma cells also leads to higher PpIX concentration. (Berkovitch-Luria et al. 2011;Greenbaum et al. 2002) At least slightly elevated temperature increases also the rate of biosynthesis of PpIX.

3. Photodiagnosis and photodynamic therapy in neurosurgery

Currently, standard treatment of glioblastoma is based on microsurgical tumour resection, radiation and chemotherapy. Overall prognosis of glioblastoma patients remains poor; therefore, new therapeutical options are necessary. Glioblastomas are diffuse infiltrating tumors, with growth patterns according to Scherer as follows: (i)perineuronal growth (perineuronal satellitosis); (ii) surface (subpial) growth; (iii) perivascular growth and (iv) intrafascicular growth.(Peiffer & Kleihues 1999) Due to the fact that tumor recurrence occurs most frequently at the resection margins, PDT of malignant glioma might be a promising treatment option as a local therapy. Additionally PDT might be able to reach the so called Guerilla cells(Claes, Idema, & Wesseling 2007), tumor cells localized in the brain adjacent to tumor region (BAT region) by local therapy at the end of the resection and perhaps by PDT stimulated anti-tumor immunity. Stimulation of anti-tumor immunity by PDT is off increasing relevance, an opportunity for PDT to become quite more than another local glioma treatment method. This topic will be discussed later in the chapter.

In the 1970s, when lasers and optical light delivery systems became available, the therapeutic use of Hp maintained interest also in neurosurgery. In 1972, Diamond et al. studied the photodynamic effects of Hp in glioma cell cultures where addition of 10^{-5} M Hp and exposure to light caused cell death.(Diamond et al. 1972) In 1975 the same group investigated the photodynamic effect of Hp *in vivo* in Fisher rats and subcutaneous implanted glioma cells; the authors demonstrated a time dependent cell death of glioma cells increasing by time of light exposure. For clinical use of PDT in Neurosurgery mainly HpD and mTHPC are currently in use.

3.1 Photodiagnosis (PD) and PDT with 5-ALA PpIX

Introduction of 5-ALA fluorescence guided resection was a milestone in neurosurgery in the last fifteen years. Great contribution was done by Stummer and coworkers. 5-ALA is orally applied about 4 hours before surgery. Surgery is performed under operating microscope, during resection the surgeon is able to switch between the white light mode and the fluorescent mode (blue light), where the tumour appears red fluorescent, see also figure 1.

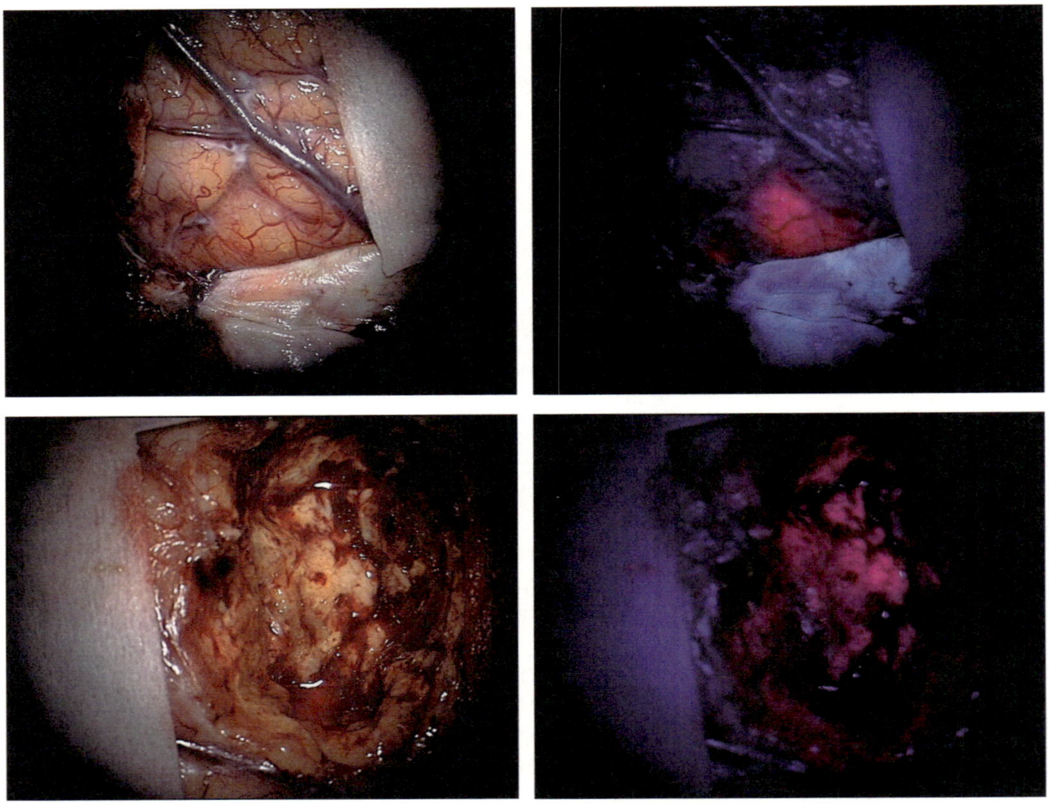

Fig. 1. Glioblastoma WHO IV at the beginning of resection in white light mode (upper row left) and under fluorescence mode (upper row right) after opening of the dura. Note the red shining PpIX fluorescence. During resection under white light conditions residual tumor (bottom row left) can be clearly detected under fluorescence mode (bottom row right).

The first results of improvement of the radicality of resection by 5-ALA fluorescence guided surgery were published in the nineties. The results of a randomised controlled multicentre phase III trial performed are summerized. The German study group investigated 322 patients enrolled by 32 investigators at 17 study centres. 161 patients were treated by fluorescence-guided surgery with 5-ALA, (20 mg/kg bodyweight; medac, Wedel, Germany), 161 were resected under conventional white light mode. In the fluorescence guided resection group tumor was resected completely in 65%, in the white light group complete tumor resection was achieved only in 36% of patients, as investigated by early postsurgical MRI. The difference between the groups was 29% [95% Confidence interval (CI) 17-40], p<0.0001. Table 1 gives a short overview about the results depending to surgery (5-ALA fluorescence guided vs. resection under white light mode).(Stummer, Pichlmeier, Meinel, Wiestler, Zanella, & Reulen 2006)

	5-ALA	White light
PFS (median)	5.1 mon.	3.6 mon.
PFS-6 months	41.0 %	21.1 %
SR age > 55 years	14.1 mon.	11.5 mon.
SR age < 55 years	18 mon.	17.5 mon.
SR 5-ALA vs. whitelight	17,9 mon.	12,9 mon
PFS: progression free survival; SR: survival rate		

Table 1. Summary of the randomised controlled multicentre phase III trial, fluorescence-guided surgery with 5-ALA versus white light surgery. Stummer et al. 2006

Stratification by postoperative MRI findings showed that patients without residual contrast-enhancing tumor had higher overall median survival than did those with residual-enhancing tumour (**17.9** months [CI 14.3-19.4] vs **12.9** months [CI 10.6-14.0]). Although *in vivo* experience demonstrated the feasibility to perform 5-ALA PDT, 5-ALA PDT is not established up to now in clinical practice without exceptions of some groups. Beck et al. 2007 treated 10 patients with small and circumscribed recurrent malignant gliomas by implantation of up to six light diffusers with a distance of 9mm.(Beck et al. 2007) By this method a mean tumor volume of 5.9 cm^3 could be treated. The median survival was 15 months, without side effects in the treated patients.

3.2 PDT in neurosurosurgery clinical studies – an overview

Currently Kostron (2010) reviewed clinical investigations of PDT in a meta analysis, median survival of primary GBM with PDT was 22 months vs 15, in recurrent GBM 9 months vs. 3 months.(Kostron 2010) A brief overview about the relevant clinical investigations in the last decade is given by table 2. For PDT the PSs Hpd (Photofrin®) and mTHPC (Foscan) were

Author, Publication year	Photosensitizer	Light dose	Number of patients	Results
Stylli 2005 (Stylli et al. 2005)	HpD 5 mg/kg bw	70-260 J/cm^2	145	Mean survival 14.3 mon. 2-year survival 28% for newly diagnosed GBM
Kostron 2006(Kostron, Fiegele, & Akatuna 2006)	mTHPC 0.15 mg/kg bw	20 J/cm^2	26	Median survival 9 mon. Control 3.5 mon.
Muller 2006(Muller & Wilson 2006)	HpD 2 mg/kg bw		96	Survival time 7.5 mon., 1-year survival 44%, 2-year survival 22%
Eljamel 2008 (Eljamel 2008)	ALA and Photofrin (HpD)	500 J/cm^2	27, 13 study group 14 control group	Tumor progression 8.6 mon. vs. 4.8 mon.

Table 2. Short overview - clinical investigations with PDT

used, the survival time was enlarged in newly and also in patients with tumor recurrence. Side effects of PDT were modest, including skin sensitivity against sunlight and sometimes increased intracranial pressure.

Due to the small penetration depth of 5-ALA derived PpXI of 2-3mm, Eljamel et al. combined fluorescence guided resection and PDT.(Eljamel 2008) They used 5-ALA PpXI for resection and HpD for PDT. In respect to the limitation of these PSs we were encouraged to investigate a new PS combining both positive properties.

4. Hypericin – high potential for PD and PDT

Hypericin, a Naphtodianthron is a naturally occurring compound of the plant *Hypericum perforatum*, better known as St. John's wort. St. John's wort is a plant that has been used since the Middle Ages to treat wounds and depression. It grows bushy and has its peak season between May and August, see figure 2. St. John's wort contains the following active ingredients: essential oils, flavonoids (Biapigenin, hyperoside, Isoquercitin, rutin), tannins, glycosides, resins, Naphtodianthrone (hypericin, Pseudohyericin) and phloroglucinol (hyperforin). In 1942 by Pace a pronounced sensitization of the skin by light for grazing animals taken St. John's wort containing feed was described. The changes in the skin were reversible after the animals were protected from sun exposure. The phenomenon was described as hypericism.(Pace 1942) Hypericin is a lipophilic molecule that is incorporated into the phospholipid bilayer of cell membranes and has already in the dark versatile pharmacological activities. These include antiviral, anticancer and antiangiogenic properties. Takahashi et al. could show an inhibitory effect on proteinkinase C, which is involved in cell proliferation.(Takahashi et al., 1989) Malignant gliomas have, compared to glial cells, a high proteinkinase C activity.(Couldwell et al. 1991) Hypericin has excellent properties as a PS. It has a high triplet quantum yield and a high efficiency in the formation of ROS.(Diwu & Lown 1993;Ehrenberg, Anderson, & Foote 1998;Hadjur et al. 1996)

The excessive production of the so called ROS leads to oxidative stress to many biomolecules, e.g. proteins, causing cell death by induction of apoptosis, necrosis or autophagy associated cell death.(Buytaert, Dewaele, & Agostinis 2007)

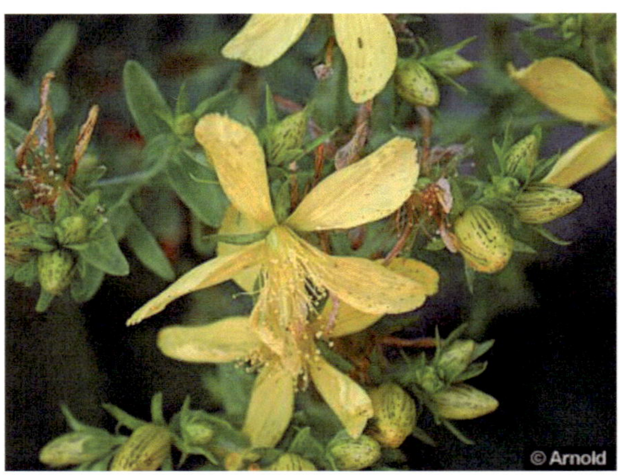

Fig. 2. *St. John's wort, also known as Hypericum perforatum;* [www.awl.ch/heilpflanzen/hypericum-perforatum/index.htm].

4.1 Hypericin differentiating neurons and glioma cell lines in vitro

For selective PDT it would be advantageous when the PS enriches in the malignant cells more compared to neurons or glial cells. In 2005 we investigated eight human glioma cell lines (L; LN-18,LN-229, U87MG, U373MG, D247MG, U251MG, U251MG,T98G) and twelve primary human glioma cell cultures (P) and compared the hypericin uptake with human astrocytes (AC; SV-FHAS) and cerebellar granule neurons (N) prepared from 8-day-old Sprague-Dawley rat pups (Charles River, Sulzfeld, Germany). Long term glioma cell lines and primary human glioma cell cultures showed significant higher hypericin uptake compared to neurons. Hypericin uptake in astrocytes was higher compared to glioma cells and to neurons.(Ritz et al. 2005) Another investigation done by fluorescence microscopy showed that hypericin was predominately localized in the glial envelope surrounding the neuron in a model with crayfish neuron and surrounding glia. Uzdensky et al. found a minor fraction of hypericin in the neuron compared to the glia in this model.(Uzdensky et al. 2003)

4.2 Subcellular distribution of hypericin

Predominantly perinuclear localization of hypericinis is in common concordance.(Uzdensky et al. 2001) The more detailed description of subcellular distribution of hypericin is not uniform. Due to the very short life span of the singlet-oxygen for cytotoxic reactions, the subcellular distribution of hypericin is off interest to understand PDT mechanisms in more detail. Many investigators studied in different cultured cell lines with different methods the subcellular hypericin localisation. According to our studies hypericin enriches particularly in the endoplasmatic reticulum (ER) and the Golgi apparatus (GA) in U37MG glioblastoma cells after incubation with noncytotoxic hypericin (1µM, 2h incubation time). ER is predominantly found in the perinuclear region while the GA is more distant to the nucleus, see figure 3.(Ritz et al. 2007b;Ritz et al. 2008)

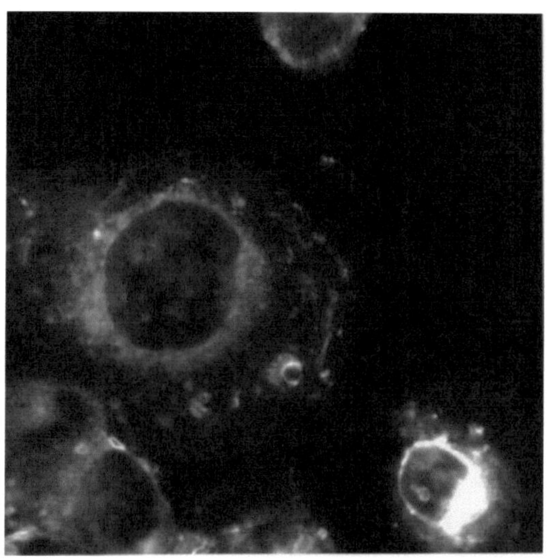

Fig. 3a. Long-term glioblastoma, incubated with 20µM Hypericin. Note the perinuclear granular enrichment.

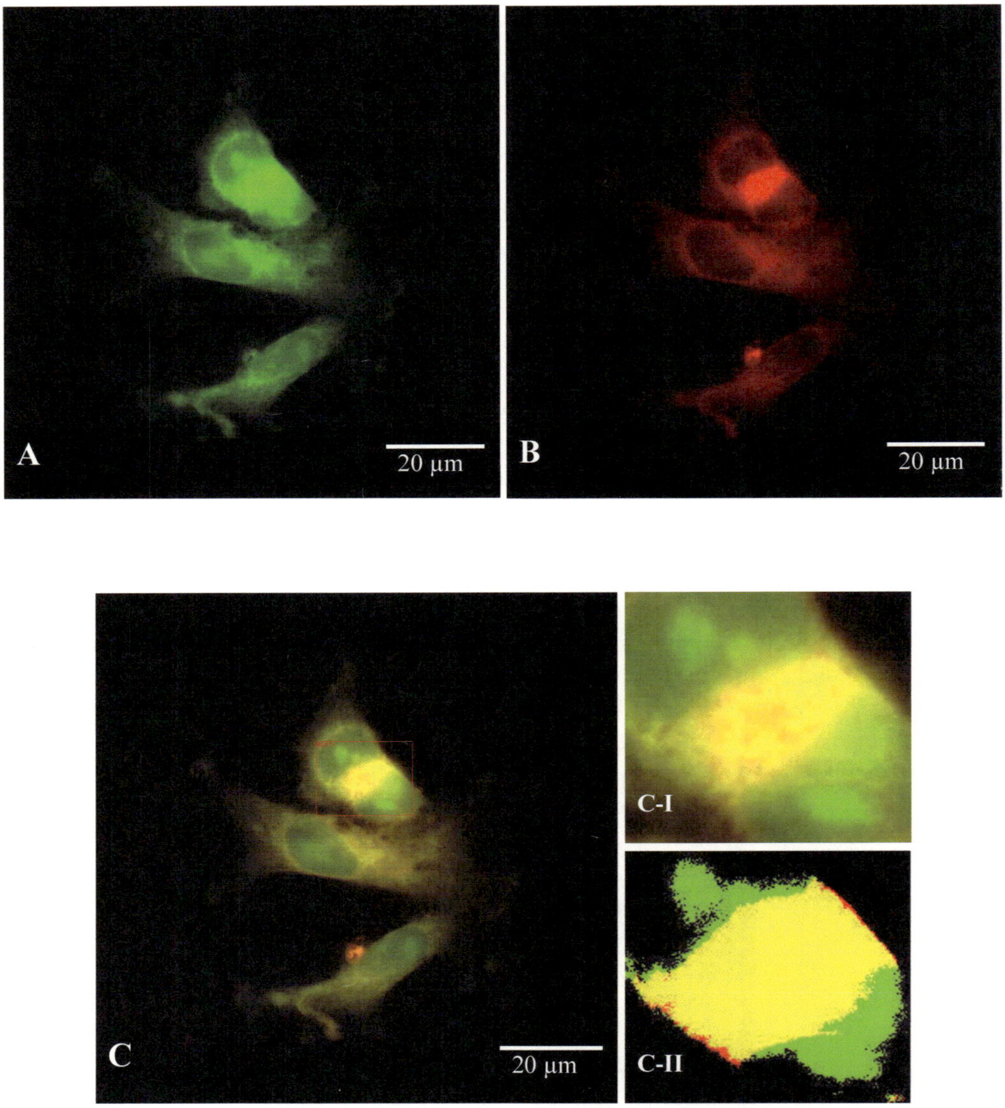

Fig. 3b. Fluorescence microscopic images of U373 MG glioblastoma cells, co stained with ER-Tracker (2 M/20 min) and Hypericin (1µM/2h). (A) staining for ER, (B) hypericin fluorescence. (C) demonstrates the costaining image. C-I original image, C-II after image processing.

4.3 Kinetic of intracellular accumulation of hypericin

The cellular accumulation of hypericin in glioma cell culture is time and concentration dependent. Short incubation times of 2 h lead to saturation up to 5µM hypericin, higher concentrations do not increase hypericin accumulation. Cellular hypericin uptake is subjected by active temperature dependent transport mechanism, although details are not clear at all (Fig. 4).(Ritz, Wein, Dietz, Schenk, Roser, Tatagiba, & Strauss 2007b)

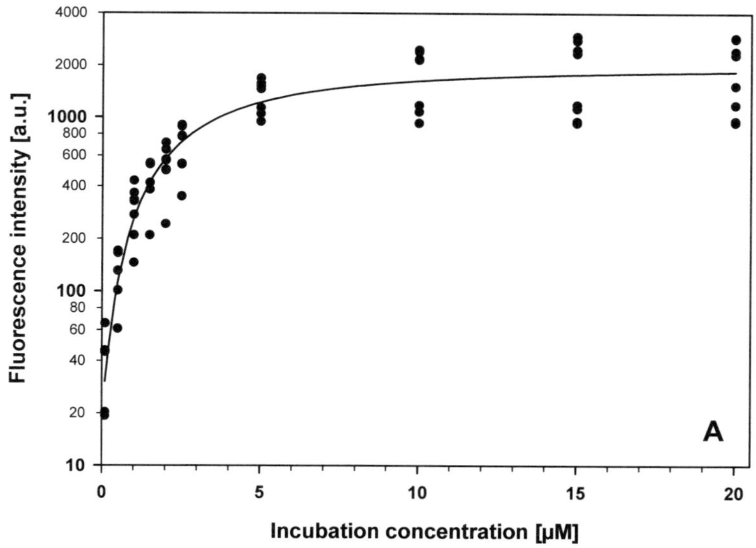

Fig. 4a. Incubation concentration dependent hypericin uptake in U373 MG cells. Cells were incubated for 2 hours; up to 5 µM cellular fluorescence increased. No further increase was found at higher incubation concentrations.

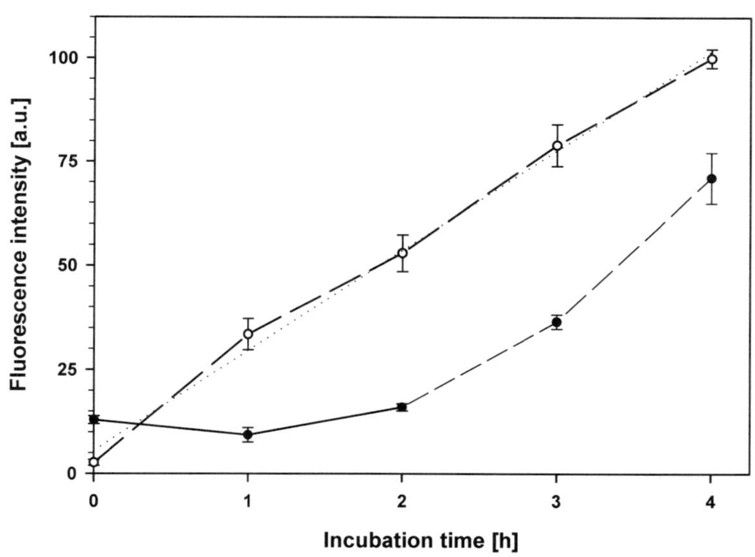

Fig. 4b. Cellular accumulation of hypericin in U373MG glioblastoma cells (incubation concentration 2.5µM) dependent on incubation temperature [(4°C for 2h and subsequently 37°C for further 2 h (•) vs. 37°C for 4h (o)] measured by flow cytometry.

4.4 Photodynamic therapy with hypericin in glioma

Hypericin exhibits high phototoxicity combined with weak to negligible dark cytotoxicity, as reported previously.(Ritz et al. 2007a) Optimal illumination wavelength for PDT is at 595nm. In our *in vitro* studies on glioma cells, a dosis of 0.15-0.2 J/cm² resulted in cell survival to 50% (ID_{50}-value); after exposure to 0.4 J/cm² cell survival was reduced to about 10% as compared to non-illuminated controls. In comparison other investigators applied light doses between 2 J/cm² (ID_{50} in U373 MG) up to 15J/cm² for 5-ALA PDT.(Blake & Curnow 2010)

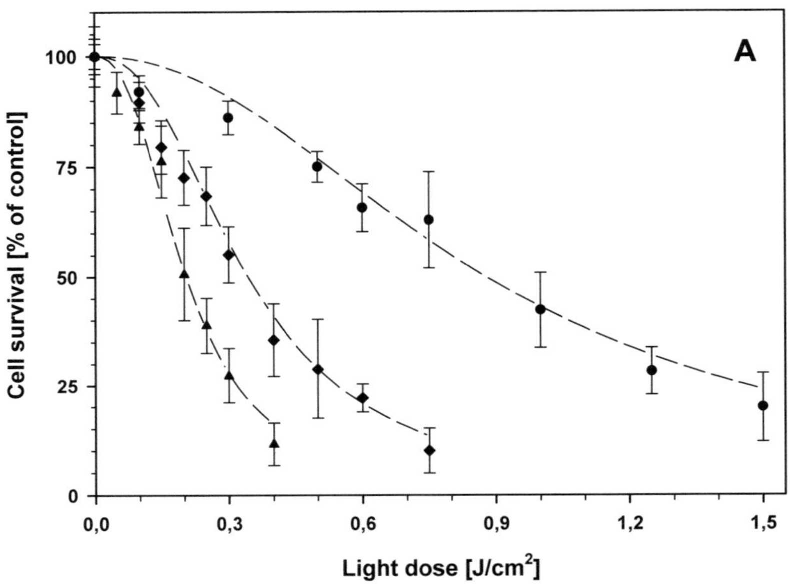

Fig. 5. Phototoxicity of hypericin in T98G cell line. Phototoxicity depends on incubation concentration (incubation time of 2h) and light dose. Cells were incubated with 0.5 µM (●) 1.5 µM (♦) and 2.5 µM (▲). Illumination was performed at 595 nm, light was delivered at 5-10 mW/cm². Cell viability is given on the ordinate.

4.5 Tumor selectivity of hypericin *in vivo*

Basical for a successful clinical application of hypericin for fluorescence guided resection and PDT is a selective enrichment in tumor tissue without enrichment in normal brain tissue. For this we evaluated in a C6 rat glioma model selective hypericin accumulation in tumor tissue compared to BAT zone and normal brain tissue. By these experiments it could be demonstrated that ratios of hypericin in rat glioma compared to BAT and normal brain tissue were 19.8:2.5:1 (Fig. 6).(Noell et al. 2011) Hypericin was found in a high concentration in tumor tissue, BAT zone was also enriched by hypericin in contrast to normal brain tissue were no hypericin was found.

Our first clinical results demonstrated also a high potential of hypericin for fluorescence guided surgery in malignant glioma, data are submitted for publication.

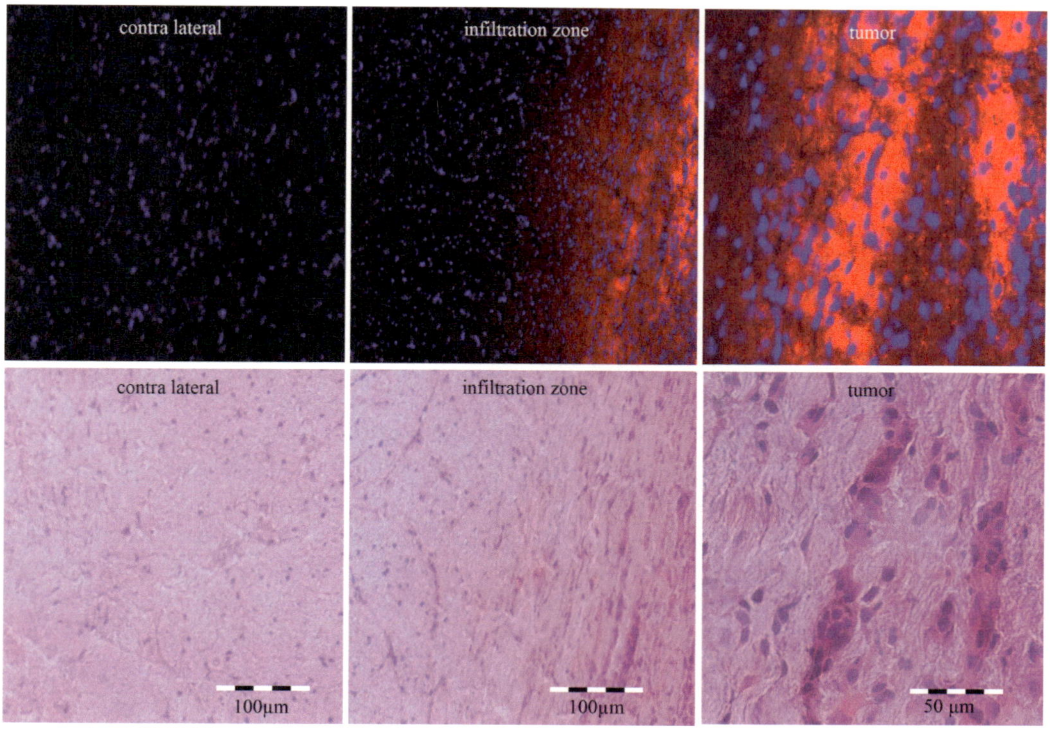

Fig. 6. Cryosections of the C6 glioma in rat brain. Contralateral hemisphere without tumor (left), BAT zone (middle) and tumor (right). Selective hypericin accumulation (red fluorescence) in the tumor and tumor infiltration zone co-stained with DAPI (blue) is demonstrated in the upper row. Corresponding sections stained by hematotoxylin and eosin (lower row).

5. Photodynamic therapy and anti-tumor immunity – A chance for PDT to be more than a local cancer therapy?

In malignant brain tumors standard therapy is based on surgery, radiation and chemotherapy. The prognosis of patients is still dismal. There is no doubt about the necessitiy of other treatment options. As mentioned in this chapter PDT represents an interesting therapy option in addition to the modern therapeutical strategies described in this book. At the first moment PDT seems only as one additional tool of local tumor treatment, with all advantages, e.g. low costs compared to modern biotechnical products, selective and repetitive application. Therapy resistancy has been seldom observed. PDT is able to occluse tumor associated vessels, mainly PDT induces apoptosis and necrosis, also autophagy plays a role. Great hope lies in the modulation of immune system by PDT. Fluorescence guided tumor resection is able to eradicate tumor locally. In combination with

induced systemic anti-tumor immune reactions distant tumor cells, e.g. Guerilla cells could be treated. Several mechanisms contribute therefore. Cells killed by PDT produce signals, increasing antigen presentation by dendric cells (DCs) and recruit antigen-specific cytotoxic T lymphocytes (CTLs).(Mroz et al. 2011)
Great importance is also given to so called damage-associated molecular patterns (DAMPs). DAMPs are intracellular molecules in living cells, exposed by sudden cell damage as initialized for example by PDT. Up to date it is generally accepted that PDT activates the immune system. Complete understanding of the processes and how to influence them for improvement the immune responses is mandatory and could be advanced by closer cooperation of researchers in PDT and immunology.

6. Conclusion and future directions

PDT for malignant gliomas is an interesting additional therapeutic tool with low side effects. By fundamentally distinct mechanisms compared to radiochemotherapy PDT also offers new opportunities for patients with tumor relapse. Hypericin seems to be a quite effective fluorescence marker for the detection of glioma. Since hypericin exhibits excellent photosensitizing properties, as demenostrated in detail *in vitro,* it might also be a promising PS in glioma therapy. Further *in vivo* investigations will proof this hypothesis in future. Due to high induction of apoptosis by hypericin mediated PDT, further investigations should focus on anti-tumor immunity by hypericin PDT, a chance to be more than only a local therapeutic tool.

7. References

Auler, H. & Banzer, G. Untersuchungen über die Rolle der Porphyrine bei geschwulstkranken Menschen und Tieren. Z Krebsforsch 53[65], 68. 1942.
Ref Type: Journal (Full)

Beck, T. J., Kreth, F. W., Beyer, W., Mehrkens, J. H., Obermeier, A., Stepp, H., Stummer, W., & Baumgartner, R. 2007, "Interstitial photodynamic therapy of nonresectable malignant glioma recurrences using 5-aminolevulinic acid induced protoporphyrin IX", *Lasers Surg.Med.*, vol. 39, no. 5, pp. 386-393.

Berkovitch-Luria, G., Weitman, M., Nudelman, A., Rephaeli, A., & Malik, Z. 2011, "Multifunctional 5-aminolevulinic acid prodrugs activating diverse cell-death pathways 1", *Invest New Drugs*.

Blake, E. & Curnow, A. 2010, "The hydroxypyridinone iron chelator CP94 can enhance PpIX-induced PDT of cultured human glioma cells 1", *Photochem.Photobiol.*, vol. 86, no. 5, pp. 1154-1160.

Buytaert, E., Dewaele, M., & Agostinis, P. 2007, "Molecular effectors of multiple cell death pathways initiated by photodynamic therapy 2", *Biochim.Biophys.Acta*, vol. 1776, no. 1, pp. 86-107.

Claes, A., Idema, A. J., & Wesseling, P. 2007, "Diffuse glioma growth: a guerilla war", *Acta Neuropathol.*, vol. 114, no. 5, pp. 443-458.

Couldwell, W. T., Uhm, J. H., Antel, J. P., & Yong, V. W. 1991, "Enhanced protein kinase C activity correlates with the growth rate of malignant gliomas in vitro

41", *Neurosurgery*, vol. 29, no. 6, pp. 880-886.

Diamond, I., Granelli, S. G., McDonagh, A. F., Nielsen, S., Wilson, C. B., & Jaenicke, R. 1972, "Photodynamic therapy of malignant tumours 2", *Lancet*, vol. 2, no. 7788, pp. 1175-1177.

Diwu, Z. & Lown, J. W. 1993, "Photosensitization with anticancer agents. 17. EPR studies of photodynamic action of hypericin: formation of semiquinone radical and activated oxygen species on illumination", *Free Radic.Biol.Med.*, vol. 14, no. 2, pp. 209-215.

Dougherty, T. J. Photoradiation therapy. Abstracts of the American Chemical Society Meeting 1973, Chicago, Il. 1973. Ref Type: Abstract

Dougherty, T. J., Gomer, C. J., Henderson, B. W., Jori, G., Kessel, D., Korbelik, M., Moan, J., & Peng, Q. 1998a, "Photodynamic therapy", *J.Natl.Cancer Inst.*, vol. 90, no. 12, pp. 889-905.

Dougherty, T. J., Gomer, C. J., Henderson, B. W., Jori, G., Kessel, D., Korbelik, M., Moan, J., & Peng, Q. 1998b, "Photodynamic therapy 4", *J Natl.Cancer Inst.*, vol. 90, no. 12, pp. 889-905.

Dougherty, T. J., Kaufman, J. E., Goldfarb, A., Weishaupt, K. R., Boyle, D., & Mittleman, A. 1978, "Photoradiation therapy for the treatment of malignant tumors 14", *Cancer Res.*, vol. 38, no. 8, pp. 2628-2635.

Dreyer, G. Lichtbehandlung nach Sensibilisierung. Dermatol Z 10, 6. 1903.

Ehrenberg, B., Anderson, J. L., & Foote, C. S. 1998, "Kinetics and yield of singlet oxygen photosensitized by hypericin in organic and biological media", *Photochem.Photobiol.*, vol. 68, no. 2, pp. 135-140.

Eljamel, M. S. 2008, "Brain photodiagnosis (PD), fluorescence guided resection (FGR) and photodynamic therapy (PDT): past, present and future", *Photodiagnosis. Photodyn.Ther.*, vol. 5, no. 1, pp. 29-35.

Figge, H. J., Weiland, G. S., & Manganiello, L. J. Cancer detection and therapy, affinity of neoplastic, embryonic, and traumatized tissues for porphyrins and metalloporphyrins. Proc Soc Exp Biol Med 68, 640-641. 1948.

Greenbaum, L., Gozlan, Y., Schwartz, D., Katcoff, D. J., & Malik, Z. 2002, "Nuclear distribution of porphobilinogen deaminase (PBGD) in glioma cells: a regulatory role in cancer transformation? 4", *Br.J Cancer*, vol. 86, no. 6, pp. 1006-1011.

Hadjur, C., Richard, M. J., Parat, M. O., Jardon, P., & Favier, A. 1996, "Photodynamic effects of hypericin on lipid peroxidation and antioxidant status in melanoma cells", *Photochem.Photobiol.*, vol. 64, no. 2, pp. 375-381.

Hausmann, W. Die sensibilisierende Wirkung des Hämatoporphyrins. Biochem Z 30, 276-316. 1911.

Juzeniene, A., Peng, Q., & Moan, J. 2007, "Milestones in the development of photodynamic therapy and fluorescence diagnosis 12", *Photochem.Photobiol.Sci.*, vol. 6, no. 12, pp. 1234-1245.

Kemmner, W., Wan, K., Ruttinger, S., Ebert, B., Macdonald, R., Klamm, U., & Moesta, K. T. 2008, "Silencing of human ferrochelatase causes abundant protoporphyrin-IX accumulation in colon cancer 1", *FASEB J*, vol. 22, no. 2, pp. 500-509.

Kennedy, J. C., Pottier, R. H., & Pross, D. C. 1990, "Photodynamic therapy with endogenous protoporphyrin IX: basic principles and present clinical experience 16", *J Photochem.Photobiol.B*, vol. 6, no. 1-2, pp. 143-148.

Kostron, H. 2010, "Photodynamic diagnosis and therapy and the brain 4", *Methods Mol.Biol*, vol. 635, pp. 261-280.

Kostron, H., Fiegele, T., & Akatuna, E. Combination of FOSCAN mediated fluorescence guided resection and photodynamic treatment as new therpeutic concept for malignant brain tumors. Med Las Appl 21, 285-290. 2006.

Kostron, H., Obwegeser, A., & Jakober, R. 1996, "Photodynamic therapy in neurosurgery: a review 19", *J Photochem.Photobiol.B*, vol. 36, no. 2, pp. 157-168.

Ledoux-Lebards, C. Annales de l'Institut Pasteur 16, 593. 1902.

Lipson, L., Baldes, E. J., & Olsen, A. M. A further evaluation of the use of hematoporphyrin derivative as a new aid for the endoscopic detection of malignan disease. Dis Chest 46, 676-679. 1964.

Malik, Z. & Lugaci, H. 1987, "Destruction of erythroleukaemic cells by photoactivation of endogenous porphyrins 2", *Br.J Cancer*, vol. 56, no. 5, pp. 589-595.

Maziere, J. C., Morliere, P., & Santus, R. 1991, "The role of the low density lipoprotein receptor pathway in the delivery of lipophilic photosensitizers in the photodynamic therapy of tumours 11", *J Photochem.Photobiol.B*, vol. 8, no. 4, pp. 351-360.

Meyer-Betz, F. Untersuchungen über die biologische (photodynamische) Wirkung des Hämatoporphyrins und anderer Derivate des Blut- und Gallenfarbstoffes. Dtsch Arch Klin Med 112, 476-503. 1913.

Mroz, P., Hashmi, J. T., Huang, Y. Y., Lange, N., & Hamblin, M. R. 2011, "Stimulation of anti-tumor immunity by photodynamic therapy 4", *Expert.Rev.Clin.Immunol.*, vol. 7, no. 1, pp. 75-91.

Muller, P. J. & Wilson, B. C. Photodynamic therapy of brain tumors-A work in progress. Lasers Surg.Med. 38, 384-389. 2006.

Neisser, A. & Halberstaedtter, L. Mitteilung über Lichtbehandlung nach Dreyer. Dtsch Med Wochenschr 8, 265-269. 1904.

Noell, S., Mayer, D., Strauss, W. S., Tatagiba, M. S., & Ritz, R. 2011, "Selective enrichment of hypericin in malignant glioma: Pioneering in vivo results 2", *Int.J Oncol.*, vol. 38, no. 5, pp. 1343-1348.

Obwegeser, A., Jakober, R., & Kostron, H. 1998, "Uptake and kinetics of 14C-labelled meta-tetrahydroxyphenylchlorin and 5-aminolaevulinic acid in the C6 rat glioma model 14", *Br.J Cancer*, vol. 78, no. 6, pp. 733-738.

Pace, N. 1942, "The etiology of hypericism, a photosensitivity produced by St. Johnswort", *Am J Physiol*, vol. 136, pp. 650-565.

Peiffer, J. & Kleihues, P. 1999, "Hans-Joachim Scherer (1906-1945), pioneer in glioma research 11", *Brain Pathol.*, vol. 9, no. 2, pp. 241-245.

Policard, A. Etude sur les aspects offerts pa des tumeurs expérimentales examinées à la lumière de Wood. C R Soc Biol 91, 1423-1424. 1924.

Raab, O. Über die Wirkung fluoreszierender Stoffe auf Infusoria. Z Biol 39, 524-566. 1900.

Ritz, R., Muller, M., Weller, M., Dietz, K., Kuci, S., Roser, F., & Tatagiba, M. 2005, "Hypericin: a promising fluorescence marker for differentiating between glioblastoma and neurons in vitro", *Int.J.Oncol.*, vol. 27, no. 6, pp. 1543-1549.

Ritz, R., Roser, F., Radomski, N., Strauss, W. S., Tatagiba, M., & Gharabaghi, A. 2008, "Subcellular colocalization of hypericin with respect to endoplasmic reticulum and Golgi apparatus in glioblastoma cells", *Anticancer Res.*, vol. 28, no. 4B, pp. 2033-2038.

Ritz, R., Wein, H. T., Dietz, K., Schenk, M., Roser, F., Tatagiba, M., & Strauss, W. S. 2007a, "Photodynamic therapy of malignant glioma with hypericin: comprehensive in vitro study in human glioblastoma cell lines", *Int.J Oncol.*, vol. 30, no. 3, pp. 659-667.

Ritz, R., Wein, H. T., Dietz, K., Schenk, M., Roser, F., Tatagiba, M., & Strauss, W. S. 2007b, "Photodynamic therapy of malignant glioma with hypericin: comprehensive in vitro study in human glioblastoma cell lines", *Int.J.Oncol.*, vol. 30, no. 3, pp. 659-667.

Schwartz, S., Absolon, K., & Vermund, H. Some relationships of porphyrins, x-rays and tumors. Med Bull 27, 7-13. 1955.

Scott, J. The Biosynthesis of Porphyrins and Porphyrin metabolism. Ciba foundation Symposium, London, Churchill , 43. 1955.

Stummer, W., Novotny, A., Stepp, H., Goetz, C., Bise, K., & Reulen, H. J. 2000, "Fluorescence-guided resection of glioblastoma multiforme by using 5-aminolevulinic acid-induced porphyrins: a prospective study in 52 consecutive patients", *J.Neurosurg.*, vol. 93, no. 6, pp. 1003-1013.

Stummer, W., Pichlmeier, U., Meinel, T., Wiestler, O. D., Zanella, F., & Reulen, H. J. 2006, "Fluorescence-guided surgery with 5-aminolevulinic acid for resection of malignant glioma: a randomised controlled multicentre phase III trial", *Lancet Oncol.*, vol. 7, no. 5, pp. 392-401.

Stummer, W., Reulen, H. J., Meinel, T., Pichlmeier, U., Schumacher, W., Tonn, J. C., Rohde, V., Oppel, F., Turowski, B., Woiciechowsky, C., Franz, K., & Pietsch, T. 2008, "Extent of resection and survival in glioblastoma multiforme: identification of and adjustment for bias", *Neurosurgery*, vol. 62, no. 3, pp. 564-576.

Stylli, S.S., Kaye, A.H., MacGregor, L., Howes, M., Rajendra, P.J. 2005, "Photodynamic therapy of high grade glioma - long term survival." Clin Neurosci., vol. 12no. 4, pp. 389-98.

Takahashi, I., Nakanishi, S., Kobayashi, E., Nakano, H., Suzuki, K., & Tamaoki, T. 1989, "Hypericin and pseudohypericin specifically inhibit protein kinase C: possible relation to their antiretroviral activity", *Biochem.Biophys.Res.Commun.*, vol. 165, no. 3, pp. 1207-1212.

Tappeiner, H. v. & Jodlbauer, A. Über die Wirkung der photodynamischen (fluoreszierenden) Stoffe auf Infusorien. Dtsch Arch Klin Med 80, 427-487. 1904.

Uzdensky, A. B., Bragin, D. E., Kolosov, M. S., Kubin, A., Loew, H. G., & Moan, J. 2003, "Photodynamic effect of hypericin and a water-soluble derivative on isolated crayfish neuron and surrounding glial cells", *J.Photochem.Photobiol.B*, vol. 72, no. 1-3, pp. 27-33.

Uzdensky, A. B., Ma, L. W., Iani, V., Hjortland, G. O., Steen, H. B., & Moan, J. 2001, "Intracellular localisation of hypericin in human glioblastoma and carcinoma cell lines", *Lasers Med.Sci.*, vol. 16, no. 4, pp. 276-283.

11

Diagnostic Evaluation of Diffuse Gliomas

Jens Schittenhelm
Department of Neuropathology, Institute of Pathology and Neuropathology
University of Tübingen,
Germany

1. Introduction

Diffuse gliomas are preferentially located in the subcortical or deep white matter of the cerebral hemispheres and are the most frequent CNS neoplasms accounting for approximately 60 per cent of all CNS tumors (CBTRUS 2011). This definition excludes the circumscribed and biological different pilocytic astrocytoma and pilomyxoid astrocytoma which are covered in a separate chapter in this book. Other rare distinct glial neoplasms with a favourable prognosis such as the subependymal giant cell astrocytoma of lateral ventricles and the pleomorphic xanthoastrocytoma of children and young adults also do not belong into the group of diffuse gliomas. Ependymomas indeed are diffuse growing glial neoplasms but are biologically different. Moreover they appear in a different population as astrocytic and oligodendroglial neoplasms. Because of space limitations the current chapter deals only with astrocytomas, oligodendrogliomas, oligoastrocytomas and glioblastomas. These tumors are grouped here under the umbrella term "diffuse gliomas". They have a predilection for frontal and temporal lobes accounting together for more than two third of all cases. However diffuse astrocytomas may be seen in any other region of the brain including cerebellum and spinal cord (Louis et al., 2007a).
Although serious advances in neuroimaging of these brain tumors have been made in the past, histopathologic evaluation of neurosurgically removed tumor specimens is still required for definite diagnosis of diffuse gliomas. These CNS tumors show an extensive variety of histologcial and cytological appearance making diagnosis somewhat difficult for those who are not familiar in working with brain tumors. The current chapter focuses on neuropathological features of the different types of diffusely infiltrating gliomas based on the latest World Health Organization (WHO) classification of tumors of the nervous system. Core features and distinct pattern and variants are also introduced and illustrated. Immunohistochemistry and molecular biology have contributed to an improved classification and shown in some cases to be of prognostic value. The advantages and limitations of the most commonly used antibodies such as GFAP, WT1, MAP2, MIB-1, P53, IDH1R132H; NOGO-A are discussed in the current chapter. Molecular analysis of 1p19q codeletion, MGMT promoter methylation, Tp53 and isocitrate dehydrogenase mutations are presented in detail and their implications are discussed.

2. Incidence and overview

Regional incidences vary with generally higher number in developed countries and are estimated between 2.2 per million people for low-grade lesions (i.e. WHO grade II

neoplasms) and up to 4.6 per 100.000 people for glioblastoma (Ohgaki et al., 2005a). There is a strong correlation between age of presentation and histological tumor grade. The mean age of diagnosis for diffuse astrocytoma grade II WHO is 39 years, for anaplastic astrocytomas grade III WHO is 45 years and 61 years for glioblastoma grade IV WHO. The mean age for oligodendroglioma is 43 years, for anaplastic oligodendrogliomas grade III it is 47 years. Mean age for oligoastrocytomas is 40 years, for anaplastic oligoastrocytomas is 44 years (Louis et al., 2007a). A similar age distribution has been observed in our institution. Less than 10% of astrocytic and less than 2% of oligodendroglial tumors develop in the pediatric age group. Thus, the pathologist should always take patients age into mind when considering possible differential diagnoses. There is a slight predominance of males (Ohgaki et al., 2005b) but in contrast to meningiomas or germ cell tumors this is not of diagnostic relevance. Higher socioeconomic status is also a risk factor.
The histologic subtypes are not evenly distributed. Diffuse astrocytomas represent 5-10%, anaplastic astrocytomas approximately 10% and glioblastomas between 75-85 per cent of all astrocytic neoplasms (CBTRUS, 2011). This can be explained by the fact that glioblastomas are a heterogenous group of tumors with distinct genetic features but similar morphology. Diffuse astrocytomas show a tendency to progress to a more malignant phenotype during disease progression within 6-8 years, ending finally as secondary glioblastomas, (10-15% of all glioblastomas). However there is no biomarker that can predict the time to progression in individual patients. The majority of glioblastomas develop without a precursor lesion ("de novo") and are genetically distinct from the secondary glioblastomas (Ohgaki et al, 2007). In primary glioblastomas several activated oncogenic pathways are known, but all share a similiar dismal prognosis. Oligodendroglial tumors account for 5-6% of all gliomas and in this group 70% are diagnosed as grade II oligodendrogliomas and 30% as grade III anaplastic oligodendrogliomas (CBTRUS, 2011). While there is no doubt that oligodendroglioma undergo a similar malignant tumor progression as astrocytic neoplasms, there is still debate about how much of these truly develop into glioblastomas. Because of divergent classification criteria true estimates for mixed gliomas vary between 1 and 10% of all gliomas. According to the more stringent CBTRUS criteria, only 2% of all gliomas meet the criteria for a mixed oligodendroglial - astrocytic neoplasm (CBTRUS, 2011).

2.1 General grading of diffuse gliomas

In 1979 the World Health Organization issued a publication for classification of tumors of the central nervous system which has been updated lastly in 2007. This included a grading scheme based on malignancy behaviour of the tumors. Grading of diffuse gliomas is performed in a four-tiered score ranging from grade I to grade IV, the latter bearing the worst prognosis. Histological factors that influence grading are nuclear atypia, cellularity, mitosis, necrosis and endothelial proliferations. Among diffuse gliomas grade II is assigned to diffuse astrocytoma, oligodendroglioma and oligoastrocytoma. Grade III neoplasms include anaplastic astrocytoma, anaplastic oligodendroglioma and anaplastic oligoastrocytoma. Grade IV is reserved for glioblastoma. This score is used to separate the histologic continuum of diffuse gliomas.

3. Astrocytoma

3.1 Macroscopy

The invaded CNS tissue is usually enlarged, but main anatomical structures remain relatively intact. The overlying cerebral cortex might be affected with a blurred gray-white junctional zone. Tissue from this area instead of the deeper white matter might be not diagnostic or carries the risk of undergrading the tumor. The fixated tissue appears yellowish to gray and may be of varying texture, either softer or firmer than the surrounding normal appearing brain. Larger cysts are uncommon but when present are usually filled with a clear fluid. In cases with extensive microcystic formations of the tumor, a gelatinous appearance is present. Calcifications within the tumor is not the role. In spinal cord, cystic lesions may extend from the tumor poles.

3.2 Histology

Astrocytomas might display a wide range of cytologic and histologic features so that some autors even state that "astrocytomas are best defined as infiltrating gliomas that cannot be classified as oligodendrogliomas" (Burger & Scheithauer 2007). One important diagnostic marker is the hypercellularity of the CNS tissue. The number of tumor cells is usually slightly increased with a cellularity of two to five times than normal and the distribution of cells is irregular. Neoplastic astrocytes usually exhibit irregular elongated, hyperchromatic nuclei lacking a perinuclear halo with often minimal fibrillar cytoplasm ("naked nuclei"). The tumor cells lie between myelinated axons which can be visualized with luxol fast blue stains. In some cases there is a prominent pink cytoplasm with short stout processes and eccentrically placed nuclei, a so called "gemistocytic appearance". These tumors are prone to perivascular lymphocytic cuffs which are also seen in glioneuronal tumors (Takeuchi et al., 1976). Nuclei in gemistocytic variants are more rounded and less irregular and might show micronucleoli. Since almost all astrocytomas exhibit some gemistocytic tumor cells, a cut off of more than 20% gemistocytes has been proposed for the gemistocytic variant of astrocytoma (Tihan et al., 2006). Tumor margins in astrocytomas are rarely discernible. The neoplastic astrocytes rest on a fibrillary background which often shows some microcystic changes and increased density of cellular processes. These microcavities are usually absent in reactive gliosis. Cases with extensive mucoid degeneration and rarity of glial processes are designated as protoplasmatic astrocytomas. All three morphologies fibrillar, gemistocytic and protoplasmatic are considered histological variants of diffuse astrocytomas. Since a different clinical outcome for these is not firmly established some authors rather consider these as divergent patterns of differentiation (Louis et al., 2007b).
Compared to diffuse astrocytomas, anaplastic astrocytomas exhibit increased cellularity, distinct nuclear atypia and mitotic activity but lack the micovascular proliferation and necrosis of glioblastomas. Multinucleated tumor cells are often diagnostic for a grade III lesion but not required for their diagnosis. One should also be aware of possible previous radiation therapy of the tumor leading to an increase of cell pleomorphism together with a decrease of mitotic activity (Gerstner 1977).
The original St. Anne-Mayo grade system did not allow mitoses in a low-grade lesion. Current criteria suggest that presence of zero or one mitosis do not alter survival and thus is still compatible with a WHO grade II neoplasm (Giannini et al., 1999). Unfortunately the WHO classification allows for a broad range of interobserver variability in borderline cases of low-grade gliomas, as presence of mitotic activity has to be interpreted in regard to the total sample size (Louis et al., 2007). In small specimens such as stereotactic biopsies a single mitosis suggests at least a grade III lesion but in larger specimens the presence of a single mitosis is not sufficient (Giannini et al., 1999). Cases with low cellularity of astrocytic tumor cells but exhibiting several mitoses should be considered as grade III or IV lesions. Diffuse

astrocytomas (WHO grade II) have normal appearing vessels and a vessel density that is only slightly greater than in normal human brain. Compared to grade II lesions the vessel density increases further in grade III astrocytomas (Brat et al., 2001).

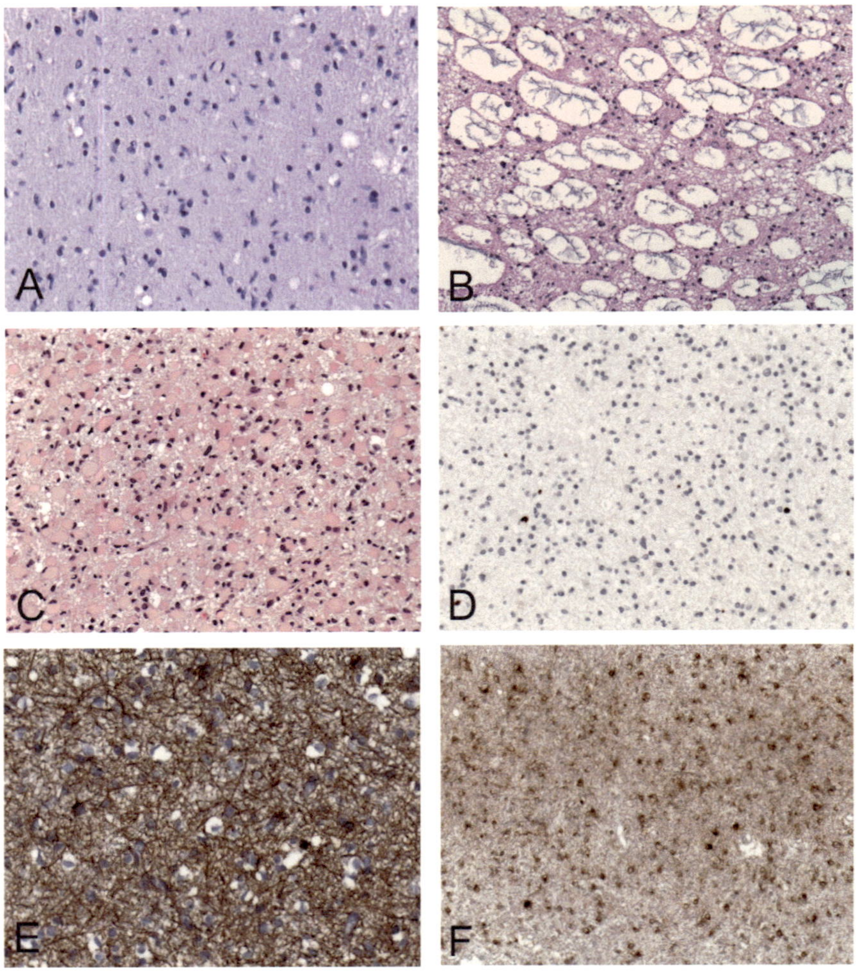

Fig. 1. Histology of **diffuse astrocytoma**: HE stains of (A) fibrillary astrocytoma, (B) protoplasmatic astrocytoma and (C) gemistocytic astrocytoma. The proliferation in these tumors, as determined by MIB-1 nuclear immunoreactivity (D) is low (1-2%). Strong, consistent GFAP expression in neoplastic astrocytes (E). IDH1 mutations are found in up to 70% of these tumors, the most common R132H mutation can be detected immunohistochemically (F).

Differential diagnosis also includes reactive changes of the CNS. In astrocytic neoplasm, tumor cells are morphologically similar but less evenly distributed than reactive cells which are in different stages of activation. In addition reactive astrocytes show longer stellate processes. It is also important to recognize entrapped neurons and differentiate these from the more pleomorphic or even multinucleated neuronal tumor cells of a ganglioglioma.

Ventricular tumors with bizarre giant cells but low mitotic activity are often subependymal giant cell astrocytomas (WHO grade I).

3.3 Immunohistochemistry

Astrocytomas show an expression of glial fibrillary acidic protein in tumor cells (Yung et al,. 1985). Especially the gemistocytic tumor cell cytoplasm and rare interdispersed Rosenthal fibers show a strong immunoreactivity for GFAP (Tascos et al., 1982). In addition the fibrillary neuropil displays almost always shows a diffusely positive background. Fibrillary astrocytes often show a small perinucelar rim, while interdispersed small round cells might be GFAP-negative. In independent studies all examined diffuse astrocytomas, were at least focally positive for GFAP (Cosgrove et al., 1986, Waidelich et al., 2010). Astrocytomas also express consistently S-100 and vimentin (Tabuchi et al., 1982, Yung et al., 1985). While S-100 is also present in the nuclei, Vimentin is often absent in distant cell processes. The malignancy-associated expression of WT1 is less intense than in high-grade astrocytic lesions (Hashiba et al., 2007, Rushing et al., 2010) but usually more prominent as in reactive lesions or oligodendrogliomas. WT1 is expressed in 52% of all diffuse astrocytomas, but tumors with more than 75% positive WT1 cells should prompt the diagnosis of a high grade glioma (Schittenhelm et al., 2009). A single study demonstrated that oligodendroglia-associated marker Nogo-a is absent in grade II and III astrocytomas (Kuhlmann et al., 2008). Caution should be employed when using epithelial antigens, such as cytokeratins and epithelial membrane antigen for differential diagnosis of carcinomas, as variable expression of these markers have been observed in astrocytomas (Franke et al.,1991; Ng et al.,1989). A bcl-2 expression in diffuse astrocytomas is more prominent than in reactive lesions and frequently seen in gemistocytic tumor cells (Hussein et al., 2006).

The microtubuli-associated protein 2 which has once been considered as a neuronal marker is expressed in 92-97% of astrocytomas (Wharton et al., 2002). Cytoplasmic staining is preferentially seen in the larger, more pleomorphic, tumour cells and expression is generally more intense in high-grade lesions than in astrocytomas grade II. Some authors propose, that presence of MAP2-positive ramifying cytoplasmic processes aids in differentiating astrocytomas from oligodendogliomas where MAP2 is expressed in a capped fashion highlighting the rounded cells (Blümcke et al., 2004). MAP2 might also help to distinguish astrocytic tumors from ependymal neoplasms which show usually only solitary MAP2-positive cells in one third of cases examined.

Expression of p53 is seen in 72% of diffuse astrocytomas and more prominent in gemistocytic tumor cells and younger patients (Vital et al., 1998). However we have observed p53 in up to 63% of reactive lesions. The phospho-histone H3 marker might be useful to detect mitoses in tumor specimens with a proposed cutoff of 4/1000 between grade II and grade III astrocytomas (Colman et al., 2006). MIB-1 tumor proliferation is usually between 2-3%, rarely exceeding 4% (Sallinen et al., 1994). In protoplasmatic variants the MIB-1 proliferation index is usually lower than in other tumor variants (Prayson et al., 1996). The MIB-1 proliferative activity of astrocytomas grade III usually ranges between 5-10% and there is an overlap on both sides to grade II and grade IV lesions. Rare astrocytoma cases may show focal islands of small oligodendrocyte-like cells with immunoreactivity for synaptophysin and NeuN between conventional glial tumor cells (Barbashina et al., 2007).

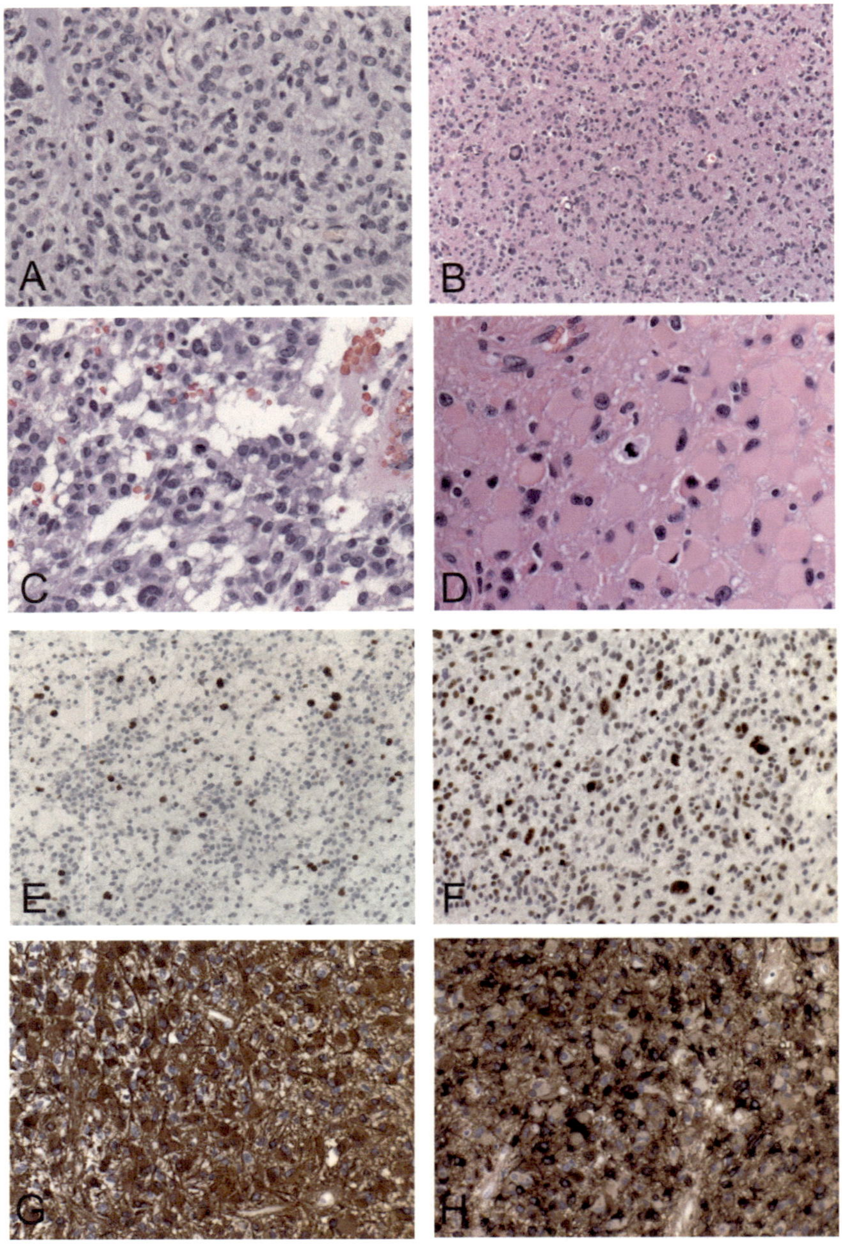

Fig. 2. **Anaplastic astrocytomas** are histologically characterized by (A) increased cellularity, (B) nuclear pleomorphism, (C) presence of several mitoses. Gemistocytic tumors (D) are prone to undergo a more rapid tumor progression. Immunohistochemistry shows increased MIB-1 prolifation index (E). Extensive p53 nuclear immunoreactivity (F) is more frequent in astrocytomas than oligodendrogliomas or glioblastomas. GFAP (G) also marks the elongated tumor cell processes. Anaplastic astrocytomas have a considerably higher presence of MAP2 positive tumor cells (H) than grade II astrocytomas.

3.4 Electron microscopy

Utrastructurally astrocytomas contain abundant 7 to 11nm sized not always parallel aligned intermediate filaments independent of fibrillary, gemistocytic or protoplasmic phenotype of the tumor cells (Duffell 1963). Cells contain dilated cisterns of endoplasmatic reticulum, lysosomes and lipid deposits. Eosinophilic granular bodies display as dense osmiophilic masses between intermediate fibrils. The ultrastructural picture of glioblastomas is similar.

4. Glioblastoma

4.1 Macroscopy

The most malignant astrocytic glioma widely known by its acronym "GBM" was orginally designated as "glioblastoma multiforme" because of extensive variability of tumor histologies. However, individual tumors can also appear quite monorpous on histology. For this reason the "multiforme" is no longer used by the current WHO classification (Burger & Scheithauer, 2007). In our institution we prefer to use the term "multicentric" for single tumors with radiologically or macroscopically separate lesions and the term "multifocal" for true multiple lesions for which no histological continuum between the tumor centers exists. Common tumor spreading routes include fornix, corpus callosum, anterior comissure and radiation optica because of the high affinity of tumor cells for myelinated structures (Burger et al., 1983). Tumors that reach the dura show often marked desmoplasia leading to a firm texture resembling gliosarcoma or meningioma (Stavrinou et al., 2010).

The necrotic center of the tumor is often surrounded by a gray rim and varying yellowish-grayish texture of the surrounding white matter. Black hemorrhagic streaks and thrombosed veins are typically for a grade IV lesion. Symmetric tumors spreading over the corpus callosum are called "butterfly gliomas". Glioblastoma tumor borders are usually diffuse but rare cases (especially giant cell pseudoepithelial glioblastomas) can be very circumscribed mimicking a carcinoma metastasis.

4.2 Histology

The prominent eosinophilic cytoplasm of pleomorphic tumor cells with small fibrillary zones indicates astrocytic heritage of the glioblastoma but this is not the rule for all tumors. Marked nuclear atypia and elevated mitotic activity is common. Either microvascular proliferations or necrosis or both are required to secure the diagnosis. Tumor appearance can be so heterogenous that diagnosis is often based on tissue patterns rather than individual tumor cell morphology. Occasionally perinuclear halos may resemble oligoendrogliomas, however glioblastoma tumor nuclei lack the monotony roundness of true oligodendrogliomas. Small cells with little cytoplasm can appear so monomorphous that small cell glioblastomas mimic anaplastic oligodendrogliomas. Small undifferentiated tumor cells intermingled with gemistocytes are more likely seen in secondary glioblastomas developing from gemistocytic astrocytomas. Some tumors may show prominent perivascular rosettes resembling anaplastic ependymomas but usually lack the more uniform roundness of ependymal tumor cells. Tumor cells can be elongated and arranged in fascicles so that at the first view sarcoma comes into mind.

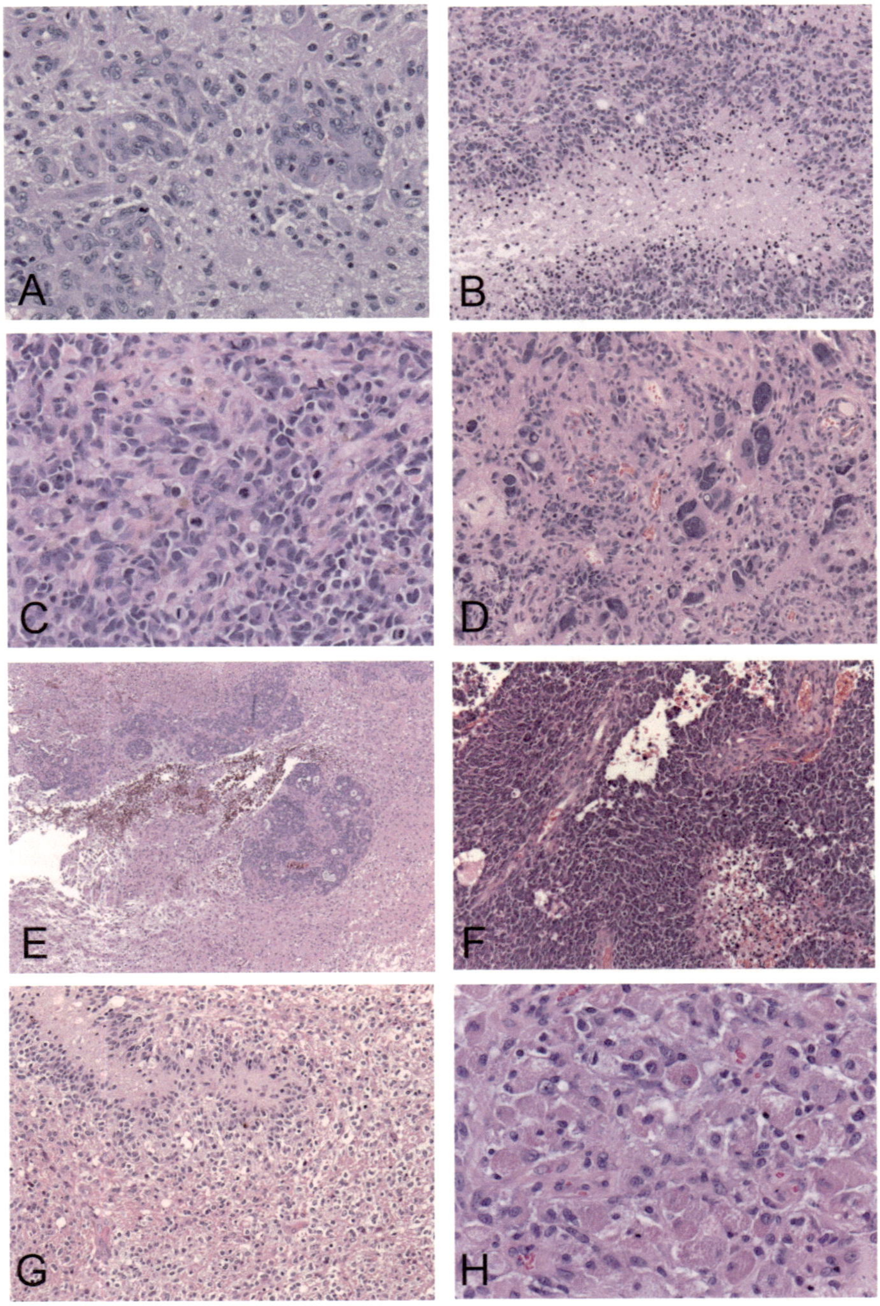

Fig. 3. **Glioblastomas** are defined through microvascular proliferations (A) and pesudopalisading necroses (B). The tumor is mitotically active (C) and may show a high degree of anaplasia (D). Glioblastoma cell composition can be so heterogenous with adenoid epithelial metaplasia (E), small cell component (F), focal oligodendroglial differentiation (G) or granular cells (H) in some cases.

Morphologic variants include granular cell astrocytoma which is characterized by large, PAS-positive cells with a degenerative granular lysosomal content. These look similar to the benign granular cell tumor of the pituitary stalk (Schittenhelm et al., 2010). Another variant is the often subcortical located giant cell glioblastoma showing multinucleated giant cells in more than 50% of tumor cells that can be associated with reticulin deposits (Palma et al., 1989). These tumors need to be distinguished from the more benign subependymal giant cell astrocytomas or pleomorphic xanthoastrocytoma. Another variant contains a biphasic pattern of alternating reticulin-free glial and reticulin-containing mesenchymal deposits and are aptly named gliosarcomas (Louis et al., 2007a). These tumors account for 2% of all glioblastomas (Meis 1991). Metaplastic transformation can be so extensive that chondroid and osseous formations in gliomas are possible (Schittenhelm et al., 2007). Furthermore gliomas can show focal areas of epithelial differentiation that ranges from positive immunreactivity of epithelial antigens to adenoid or squamous formations leading to misdiagnosis of carcinoma (Rodriguez et al., 2008). Rare cases may show a melanotic differentiation (Jaiswal et al., 2010).

In average 3 pseuopalisading necroses are present in a glioblastoma specimen (Brat et al., 2004). Pseudopalisading cells are usually less proliferative and exhibit higher rates of apoptosis due to hypoxic conditions but are usually without a prominent inflammatory infiltrate. More than half of the palisades show a central vascular lumen, in about twenty percent intravascular thrombosis is also seen (Brat et al., 2004). Vascular proliferations may be present throughout the tumor but there is a tendency for these structures to accumulate in the peripheral region of high cellularity corresponding to the contrast-enhancing ring seen in radiological images (Louis et al., 2007a). Tumor vessels in glioblastoma have an increased density and show hyperplasia (Brat et al., 2001). Tumor vessel arrangement in a garland-like fashion is not uncommon. Vascular proliferation in form of glomeruloid bodies in glioblastomas is more frequently than in tumors from any other organ system (Plate et al., 1999).

Infiltrative growth is mostly characterized by small undifferentiated cells growing along axonal structures in the white matter or along the brain surface and blood vessels. These are designated as 'secondary structures of Scherer' (Scherer, 1938). In the spinal cord, tumor cells might extend into the subarachnoid space (Burger & Scheithauer, 2007). Apoptosis of tumor cells is not a major feature but most prominent in areas of pseudopalisading necrosis.

4.3 Immunohistochemistry

The immunoprofile of glioblastomas is in many ways similar to astrocytomas. The vast majority of glioblastomas express the glial markers GFAP and EAAT1 (Waidelich et al., 2010) but these antigens may occasionally lacking (especially in small glioblastomas). S-100 immunostaining is then helpful to indicate a glial origin of the neoplastic cells. Strong MAP2 immunoreactivity is seen in 90% of glioblastomas (Blümcke et al., 2004). Vimentin immunoreactivity is very unspecific. Diffuse growth of gliomas can be supported by identifying axons with neurofilament stains within the tumor, but extensive neurofilament immunoreactivity of the tumor should prompt the diagnosis of an (anaplastic) ganglioglioma. In gliosarcomas, GFAP is lacking in sarcomatous areas. A complementary reticulin staining pattern in these tumors is diagnostic. The proliferation varies greatly, usually 15-25% of the nuclei are MIB-1 positive, but tumors with small cell morphology can show up to 90% proliferating cells. Tumors with previous radiation or gemistocytic morphology may show little proliferating activity. Because of inconsistent laboratory techniques and varying evaluation methods, MIB-1 immunoreactivity has no established cutoffs between low-grade and high-grade lesions. WT1 expression is consistently expressed in glioblastomas (Schittenhelm et al., 2009). In our experience expression is similar in primary and secondary tumors but expression can be reduced in recurrent tumors. In addition there is evidence that tumors that contain a Tp53 mutation show reduced WT1 levels compared to Tp53 wild type glioblastomas (Clark et al., 2007). IDH1 R132H antibody expression is found in 4% of primary and in 71% of secondary glioblastoma (Capper et al., 2010). Tp53 immunoreactivity is less present than in astrocytomas but can be considerably high in giant cell glioblastomas. Microglial markers such as CD68 are regularly found in glioblastomas and can be very extensive in tumors with granular cell component and need to be distinguished from demyelinating lesions. Cytokeratin expression in glioblastomas (especially in giant cell glioblastomas and glioblastomas with true epithelial metaplasia) is an important diagnostic pitfall (Rodriguez et al., 2008). Dot-like EMA immunoreactivity is less frequently observed in glioblastomas than in ependymomas, where usually more than 5 EMA-positive dots per high-power field are seen (Hasselblatt & Paulus 2003). Immunohistochemistry of EGFR wild type protein is more prominent in primary glioblastomas as in grade II or III gliomas (Simmons et al. 2001).

5. Oligodendroglioma

5.1 Macroscopy

Like all other diffuse growing tumors, oligodendroglioms show diffuse borders. The tumors are usually soft and have a grey to pink color. They may appear hemorrhagic and / or calcified but this is not a specific feature for oligodendrogliomas Superficial growth can expand the cortical grey matter. The anaplastic forms lack a central necrosis typically for glioblastoma but may show focally smaller necroses. Rare disseminating cases may grow as superficial gelatinous mass extending along the spinal cord (Mittelbronn et al., 2005).

5.2 Histology

In contrast to astrocytomas, oligodendrogliomas are dominated by histologic monotony of the round to oval shaped tumor cells which are best seen in smears. Nuclei have a bland chromatin and prominent nucleoli. The very characteristic perinuclear halo - a fixation artefact resulting from autolytic water absorption - is absent in frozen sections or specimens that have been quickly processed resulting from a short fixation time. Delicate branching capillaries and tumor calcifications that also may affect tumor vessels are more frequent in oligodendrogliomas than in other CNS tumors. Overun cortical areas show a perineuronal satellitosis of the tumor cells and tumor cells may concentrate along subpial structures. In addition cortical structures show often smaller microcystic changes.

Anaplastic oligodendrogliomas show increased nuclear pleomorphism that is mostly restricted to focal areas and increased mitotic activity compared to grade II lesions. Some authors prefer a mitotic cutoff of 6 mitoses per 10 high power fields to discriminate between grade II and grade III lesions (Giannini et al., 2001). Focal elevated cellular areas as nodules do not warrant tumor designation as a grade III lesion in absence of other anaplastic features. In contrast to astrocytomas where endothelial proliferations lead to the diagnosis of glioblastoma, vascular proliferations or extended vascular hyperplasia are typical for anaplastic oligodendroglioma grade III. In addition smaller areas of necrosis may be

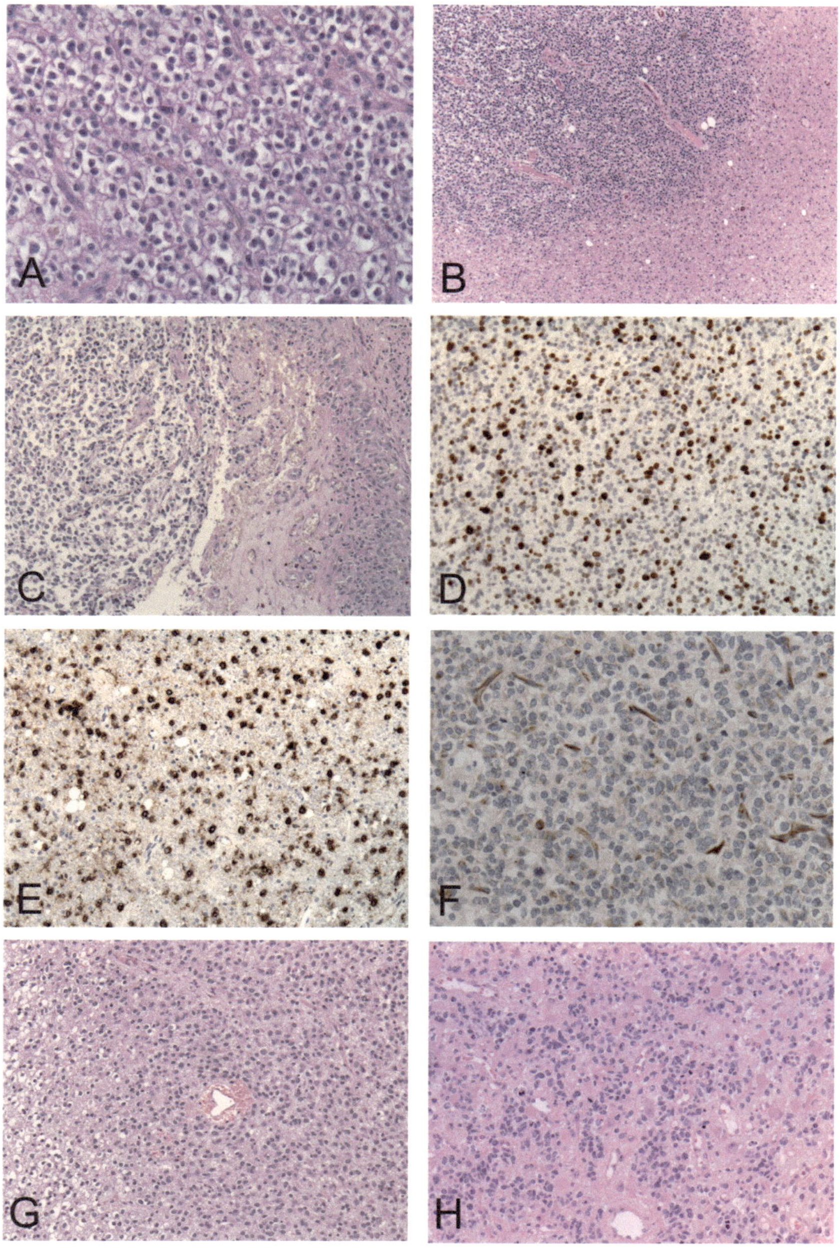

Fig. 4. **Oligodendrogliomas** show a typical honeycomb pattern (A). Tumor borders can be discrete infiltrative (B). Anaplastic oligodendroglioma with endothelial proliferations (C) and increased MIB-1 proliferation index (D). Oligodendroglial tumors typically exhibit a marked perinuclear MAP2 immunoreactivity (E) and show far less WT1 immunopositive cells (F) than astrocytomas. **Mixed oligodendroglioma-astrocytoma** can present either as true biphasic tumors (G) or as strongly intermixed (H) as in this anaplastic oligoastrocytoma with extensive mitotic activity.

present but not typically in the pseudopalisading forms of glioblastoma. The current WHO classification however explicitly allows presence of pseudopalisading necroses in anaplastic oligendrogliomas and thus weakens a sufficient discrimination to glioblastomas with oligodendroglial differentiation. Anaplastic oligodendrogliomas may contain smaller cells with pink cytoplasm and eccentric placed nuclei, so called minigemistocytes and areas with increased fibrillar background and plump process-bearing gliofibrillary oligoendrocytes. These eosionophilic cells are seen more often in grade III than grade II oligodendrogliomas. Finally some oligodendroglioma tumor cells may have sharp delineated borders resembling epitheloid differentiation. In the tumor edges severeal astrocytic cells might be present but unless clearly neoplastic in nature their presence does not warrant the diagnosis of mixed oligoastrocytoma. Focally parallel tumor cell growth may resemble polar spongioblastomas (Louis et al., 2007). Rare cases of oligodendrogliomas may show focally neuopil islands that have to be distinguished from neurocytomas. Tumor cells with signet-ring cell morphology have also been described in oligodendrogliomas (Kros et al., 1997).

5.3 Immunohistochemistry

There is no distinct single antibody availabe to discriminate reliably between oligodendroglial and astrocytic neoplasms. It is adviseable to use a panel of different antibodies for which expression patterns in these neoplasms has been extensively studied. In our institution we stain routinely gliomas for MIB1, GFAP, MAP2, WT1 and IDH1 R132H. Expression of GFAP is usually absent in tumor cytoplasm of oligodendroglia, however in our daily practice sometime there is ample overlapping of GFAP-positive fibrillary neuropil background. In addition minigemistocytes and gliofibrillar oligodendrocytes are usually positive for GFAP. MAP2 is constantly expressed in oligodendrogliomas, but also found in 92% of astrocytomas and glioblastomas (Blümcke et al., 2004). A perinuclear "capped" expression pattern is more typical for oligodendrogliomas, while in astrocytomas the elongated cell processes are also immunoreactive for MAP2. WT1 in oligodendrogliomas is usually restricted to single WT1-positive tumour cells or completely absent while WT1 is strongly expressed in 83-92% of high grade astrocytic lesions (Schittenhelm et al., 2009). Therefore, in our experience, expression of WT1 in more than 50% of tumor cells indicates either astrocytoma or oligoastrocytoma rather than oligodendroglioma. Nogo-A is found in 71% oligodendrogliomas and 24% glioblastomas but is absent in astrocytomas (Kuhlmann et al., 2008). While Olig2 immunoreactivity is slightly stronger in oligodendrogliomas is also constantly seen in other glial neoplasms (Ligon et al., 2004). Alpha internexin is found in 45-59% of oligodendrogliomas ans seems to be associated with an 1p19q codeletion (Ducray et al., 2011). Positive IDH1-R132H immunoreactivity is so frequent in oligodendroglial tumors (up to 91% in grade II and 94% in grade III lesions) that this marker is very useful to discriminate oligodendrogliomas from other brain tumors with oligodendroglial morphology (Capper et al., 2011). Diffuse immunoreactivity of p53 is uncommon in oligodendroglial tumors but when present indicates an intact chromosomal 1p arm (Hirose et al., 2010). Oligodendrogliomas with neurocytic differentiation may show synaptophysin-positive neuropil islands and rosettes but usually lack the NeuN nuclear immunoreactivity of neurocytomas. In addition presence of IDH1 or IDH2 mutation strongly favors diagnosis of oligodendroglioma over neurocytoma (Capper et al., 2011).

5.4 Electron microscopy

The short tumor cell processes contain microtubuli and ocassionally pericellular spiral laminations but usually lack the abundant intermediate filament of astrocytic tumor cells (Min et al., 1994). Electron microscopy is not used in regular routine practice as combined data from histology, immunistochemistry and molecular pathology is usually sufficient enough do diagnose an oligodendroglioma or mixed glioma.

6. Oligoastrocytoma

Criteria for mixed astrocytomas / oligodendrogliomas are weakly defined. Not surprisingly interobserver variaibility is great ranging from 9-80% as seen in a study on 155 tumors that were initially classified as oligoastrocytomas (Fuller et al., 2003). Macoscopically these tumors are similar to other diffuse grade II or grade III lesions. Histological diagnosis of oligoastrocytoma requires that both astrocytic and oligodendrogial neoplastic tumor cells are present in the same tumor. These may appear biphasic as two distinct tumor areas or more commonly as intermingled tumor. The minimal amount to which one tumor component has to be present is unfortunately not properly defined. Some authors are satisfied when one single high power field has either astrocytic or oligodendroglial tumor cells, other authors request at least a minimum of 50% neoplastic astrocytes. Separation of astrocytes and oligodendrocytes is not always possible. Every pathologist has seen tumor cells that have features of both lineages. It is important however to distinguish minigemistocytes and gliofibrillar oligodendrocytes in oligodendrogliomas from astrocytes, as they do not warrant the diagnosis of oligoastrocytoma. Single mitoses are compatible with a grade II oligoastrocytoma, however in our institution we have an relaxed approach, when mitoses are increased in a distinct oligodendroglial compartment only. Anaplastic oligoastrocytomas show increased nuclear atypia, elevated cellularity and abundant mitoses. Microvascular proliferations are frequent in grade III oligoastrocytomas. Discrimination of anaplastic oligoastrocytoma from glioblastomas with oligodendroglial differentiation is especially difficult, as WHO criteria allows pseudopalisading necroses to be present in oligoastrocytic tumors. In our institution decision is based on whether necroses are present in astrocytic tumor parts indicating a glioblastoma or is limited to oligodendroglial tumor parts indicating anaplastic oligoastrocytoma. Like histology, immunhistochemistry results are very mixed and represent the immunophenotype of neoplastic astrocytes or oligodendrogytes as discussed in their sections. Grade II tumors have a MIB-1 proliferation index usually less than 6% (Deckert et al., 1989).

7. Molecular biology

Because of their favourable prognostic value 1p19q codeletion, MGMT promoter methylation and isocitrate dehydrogenase mutations are considered important clinical biomarkers for diffuse gliomas. In addition p53 is useful for diagnostic purposes. These markers are requested with increasing frequency and are discussed in detail below. Even when the diagnosis of a specific glioma type is readily apparent in histological stains, pathologist need to take care, that sufficient tissue is available for future molecular analysis.

7.1 Tumor protein 53 mutations

Since Tp53 mutations are broadly distributed, exons 5-8 need to be screened by single-strand conformational polymorphism analysis followed by direct sanger sequencing of samples exhibiting mobility shifts. In unremarkable cases, sequencing analysis is usually extended to exons 4, 9 and 10. Because of these efforts, Tp53 molecular analysis is not part of routine diagnosis unlike p53 immunostaining. A Tp53 mutation in diffuse astrocytomas grade II WHO is observed in 52-60% of the tumors, while Tp53 mutations are present in 35-44% of oligoastrocytomas and in 10% oligodendrogliomas (Okamoto et al., 2004, Kim et al., 2010). Especially astrocytomas with gemistocytic tumor cell morphology may contain Tp53 mutations in up to 82% of tumors (Watanabe et al., 1998). Since Tp53 mutations are acquired early, their frequency does not increase much further during tumor progression (Watanabe 1997). In pediatric glioblastomas, Tp53 mutations were found in 60% of tumors examined (Srivastava et al., 2010). Grade II WHO diffuse astrocytomas may show in 49% a combined TP53 mutation and IDH1 or IDH2 mutation (Kim et al., 2010). A Tp53 mutation without associated IDH1/2 mutation is rare (3%), thus indicating that IDH mutations occur at an earlier stage of tumorgenesis.

7.2 Isocitrate dehydrogenase mutations

The NADP-dependent enzymes IDH1 and IDH2 catalyze the conversion from isocitrate in alpha-ketoglutarate. Mutations of the catalytic center in gliomas result in accumulation of the oncogenic metabolite D-2-hydroxyglutarate (Dang et al., 2009). It is thought that the reduced NADPH levels in IDH mutated gliomas could sensitize tumors to radiation and chemotherapy (Bleeker et al., 2010). The frequency of IDH mutations is high in diffuse astrocytomas, anaplastic astrocytomas and secondary glioblastomas evolving from these precursor lesions, while presence of IDH mutations is seen in only 3-7% primary glioblastomas (Hartmann et al., 2009). The vast majority of IDH1 mutations are point mutations leading to a distinct amino acid substitution on codon 132 (Arg132His) for which an specific antibody has been developed (Capper et al., 2010). The other amino exchange mutations can be detected either by direct sanger sequencing or restriction-endonuclease based PCR (Meyer et al., 2010).

IDH1 mutations are found in 59-88% diffuse astrocytomas, 50-78% anaplastic astrocytomas and 50-88% secondary glioblastomas, IDH2 mutations are present in 1-7% diffuse astrocytomas, 1-4% anaplastic astrocytomas and seem to be absent in secondary glioblastomas (Bourne et al., 2010). The rate of IDH2 mutations in oligodendrogliomas is higher as in astrocytomas (4-8% in oligodendrogliomas grade II and grade III, 1-6% of oligoastrocytomas grade II and grade III) but still lower than number of IDH1 mutations (68-82% oligoadendrogliomas grade II, 49-75% anaplastic oligodendrogliomas grade III, 50-100% oligoastrocytomas, 63-100% anaplastic oligoastrocytomas grade III) (Bourne et al., 2010). In addition the IDH1 R132C mutation is strongly associated with an astrocytoma phenotype (Hartmann et al., 2009).

7.3 MGMT methylation status

The DNA repair enzyme O-methylguanine-DNA methyltransferase (MGMT) removes alkyl groups from the O^6 position resulting in an increased tumor resistance to alkylating agents therapy. Methylation of the MGMT promotor region results in decreased MGMT activity which in turn increases glioblastoma tumor cell sensivity to therapy with temozolomide and is therefore a predictive molecular marker (Hegi et al., 2005). MGMT expression in tumor cells of astrocytomas and glioblastomas can be determined by nuclear immunoreactivity of tumor cells (Capper et al., 2008). Together with other sophisticated methods such as realtime RT-PCR or methylation-specific pyrosequencing, they lack a valid definition for clinically relevant cut-off values (von Deimling et al., 2010). Usually MGMT is determined in formalin-fixated paraffin-embedded specimens through methylation-specific PCR, yet reliability and reproducibility are still limited in the current standard method (Preusser, et al., 2008b, Elezi et al., 2008). Not only is MGMT protein expression within tumors heterogenous, but also highly dependent on the method used and changes during therapy (Jung et al., 2010, Preusser et al., 2008a, Janzer et al., 2008). Thus reports on MGMT methylation range from 93% in frozen tissue sections in diffuse astrocytoma grade II (Everhard et al., 2006) to 30-35% in glioblastoma paraffin blocks (Tabatabai et al., 2010). In pediatric glioblastomas approximately half of the tumors are methylated (Srivastava et al., 2010). Despite these shortcomings MGMT analysis is essential for almost all clinical studies and one of the most requested molecular analysis in neuropathology routine practice.

7.4 Loss of 1p/19q

A loss of heterozygosity is usually assessed though use of microsatellite marker PCR. This method requires corresponding blood samples to determine allele status. Therefore use of fluorescent in situ hybridisation is preferred by some laboratories but carries the risk of misdiagnosing cases with only partial loss. This risk can be covered by additional PCR that contains several loci along the chromosomal arms (Riemenschneider et al. 2010).

Loss of heterozygosity in 1p and 19q are found in 78% of oligodendrogliomas grade II, 44% of oligoastrocytomas and 17% of diffuse astrocytomas grade II WHO. Therefore 1p19q codeletion is strongly associated with a oligodendroglial tumor morphology and often used as a diagnostic marker. In addition in oligodendrogliomas up to 73% of codeleted tumors also show either additional IDH1 or IDH2 mutations (Kim et al., 2010). Not surprisingly journal reviewers often require 1p19q deletions in oligodendrogliomas for sample homogeneity.

8. Prognostic implications

8.1 Immunohistochemistry

Generally, tumor grade increases with age and younger age of onset is one of the strongest predictive factor of prolonged survival (Kita et al., 2009) and thus heavily influences all other markers found. Despite this fact, many publications do not take patients age into account when analyzing biomarkers on patient survival. In astrocytomas, MIB-1 proliferation values above 5% are considered to be associated with a shorter survival (Jaros et al., 1992). Because of study population heterogeneity, predictive data on Tp53 mutations are limited. Some authors see p53 immunoreactivity to be associated with a shorter survival or shorter time to malignant progression (Jaros et al., 1992, Ständer et al., 2004). It is noteworthy, that not all p53 immunoreactive tumors contain mutations in the TP53 gene (Kösel et al., 2001). Further contrasting to immunohistochemistry data, a molecular study on 159 grade II astrocytomas and oligoastrocytomas did not found an influence on overall survival, but reported a significant shorter progression-free survival (Peraud et al., 2002). In glioblastomas p53 mutation status does not correlate with patients outome (Weller et al., 2009). Thus, p53 is only useful as a diagnostic marker but not prognostic.

8.2 Molecular biology

Patients with IDH1/2 mutations in anaplastic astrocytomas and glioblastomas are usually younger than those lacking a IDH mutation (Nobusawa et al., 2009, Hartmann et al., 2009). In addition IDH1 mutations are a prognostic marker of favorable outcome in grade III and IV tumors (Yan et al., 2009, Nobusawa et al., 2009, Sanson et al., 2009). There is even a study demonstrating that IDH1-positive glioblastomas WHO grade IV have a better prognosis than IDH1-negative anaplastic astrocytomas WHO grade III (Hartmann et al., 2010). In contrast patients with IDH1 mutations in diffuse astrocytomas grade II WHO are older (Kim et al., 2010) or show at least a similar age distribution (Balss et al., 2008). The prognostic role of IDH1 in grade II diffuse astrocytomas is still to be determined. Sanson and colleagues found IDH1 to be an independent prognostic factor for longer survival in 100 samples (Sanson et al., 2009), while Kim et al. in 174 grade II tumors did not observe a more favorable outcome (Kim et al., 2010). So far IDH tumor status has not been incorporated into any current therapeutic trials but is likely to be included in the future.

Analysis of low-grade astrocytomas did not found any association with MGMT promoter methylation and overall survival (Komine et al., 2003). In anaplastic gliomas, MGMT promoter hypermethylation is associated with longer progression free survival (Wick et al., 2009). In glioblastomas, MGMT methylation status in addition as a marker of prolonged survival is a predictor to therapy response (Hegi et al., 2005). In oligodendroglial tumors there is a strong association between MGMT promoter methylation and 1p19q codeletion the latter also contributing to the improved survival of patients with MGMT methylation (Levin et al., 2006; Kesari et al., 2009). MGMT alone is useful as a prognostic marker but not useful to predict outcome of adjuvant treatment in oligodendrogliomas (van den Bent et al., 2009).

In oligodendrogliomas 1p19q codeletion is associated with improved survival (Jeon et al., 2007, McLendon et al., 2005). Presence of oligodendroglial histopathology and 1p19q deletetion shows a better overall survival for anaplastic oligodendrogliomas treated with radiation and PCV chemotherapeutic regimen (Giannini et al., 2008). The same study also demonstrated that 1p19q deletion alone is associated with a longer progression-free survival but that this effect is independent of initial treatment of oligodendrogliomas and mixed oligoastrocytomas (van den Bent et al., 2006). There is an inverse correlation with p53 mutation and codeletion of chromosomal arms 1p and 19q in oligodendrogliomas implicating that oligodendrogliomas harbouring a Tp53 mutation have a reduced overall survival (Jeon et al., 2006, McLendon et al., 2005).

In 9% of astrocytomas grade II WHO no common genetic alterations are detected (Kim et al., 2010). In small biopsy specimen these tumors may enter the differential diagnosis of pilocytic astrocytoma. The latter often show BRAF abnormalities, wich drive MAPK pathway activation (Cin et al., 2011) but are absent in diffuse astrocytoma (Korshunov et al., 2009). Another possible differential diagnosis to low-grade diffuse astrocytoma is ganglioglioma and pleomorphic xanthoastrocytoma which in addition to their unique histological properties also exhibit BRAF V600E mutations, at present not known to be in diffuse astrocytomas (Schindler et al., 2011).

9. Conclusion

Histological classification of diffuse gliomas based on the WHO grading scheme is a prerequisite to optimal patient treatment decisions. Clinicians need to be aware that diffuse gliomas form a histological continuum and that the four-tiered scores introduces a somewhat artificial separation. Tumors on the edge between grade II and III lesions behave different than tumors showing beginning endothelial proliferations indicating close progression to grade IV. A panel of different antibodies is very helpful to secure the diagnosis and avoids potential differential diagnosis pitfalls. Immunohistochemistry has also shown that several antibodies show divergent expression patterns. Researchers therefore should strive to clearly delineate between astrocytomas, oligodendrogliomas and oligoastrocytomas, when examining new biomarkers. Primary and secondary glioblastomas are another example of "convergent evolution showing a similar phenotype of genotypically different tumor cells" (Basanta et al., 2011). The distinction of primary and secondary glioblastomas does not immediately influence management decisions, but because of their different genetic profile, it is expected that they may also differ in response to experimental therapies. Recent years have seen a progress in supplementing histological diagnosis of diffuse gliomas with an increasing spectrum of molecular markers. The utility of MGMT and 1p/19q in predicting response to therapy has led to their inclusion in current clinical trials. Implementation of these markers into routine diagnostic setting is expected after further successful results. Especially in oligoastrocytomas they complement histological results and provide a more objective classification. However clear cut-off levels for each assay is needed to guarantee interlaboratory compatibility. Histological control of the tissue used for molecular neuroonclogy through (neuro)pathologists is indispensable to avoid false-negative test results. Determining IDH1 status in diffuse gliomas is of diagnostic and clinical relevance. Not only indicates equal presence of IDH mutations a likely common origin of astrocytomas and oligodendrogliomas, but also the strong prognostic role in high-grade gliomas is likely to be included in future revisions of the current WHO classification.

10. Acknowledgment

The author thanks his colleagues at the Department of Neuropathology for valuable feedback in discussion rounds, the laboratory technicians for excellent stains and Petra Stauder-Simmons for proofreading.

11. References

Barbashina V.; Salazar P.; Ladanyi M.; Rosenblum M.K. & Edgar M.A. (2007). Glioneuronal tumor with neuropil-like islands (GTNI): a report of 8 cases with chromosome 1p/19q deletion analysis. *Am J Surg Pathol*. Vol. 31, No.8, pp 1196-1202.

Balss J.; Meyer J.; Mueller W.; Korshunov A.; Hartmann C. & von Deimling A. (2008). Analysis of the IDH1 codon 132 mutation in brain tumors. *Acta Neuropathol*. Vol.116, No.6, pp 597-602.

Basanta D.; Scott JG.; Rockne R.; Swanson K.R. & Anderson A.R. (2011). The role of IDH1 mutated tumour cells in secondary glioblastomas: an evolutionary game theoretical view. *Phys Biol*. Vol.8, No.1, p 015016.

Bleeker F.E.; Atai N.A.; Lamba S.; Jonker A.; Rijkeboer D.; Bosch K.S.; Tigchelaar W.; Troost D.; Vandertop W.P.; Bardelli A. & Van Noorden C.J. (2010). The prognostic IDH1(

R132) mutation is associated with reduced NADP+-dependent IDH activity in glioblastoma. *Acta Neuropathol*. Vol.119, No.4, pp 487-494.

Blümcke I.; Müller S.; Buslei R.; Riederer B.M & Wiestler O.D. (2004). Microtubule-associated protein-2 immunoreactivity: a useful tool in the differential diagnosis of low-grade neuroepithelial tumors. *Acta Neuropathol*. Vol.108, No.2, pp 89-96.

Bourne T.D. & Schiff D. (2010). Update on molecular findings, management and outcome in low-grade gliomas. *Nat Rev Neurol*. Vol.6, No.12, pp 695-701.

Brat D.J. & Van Meir E.G. (2001). Glomeruloid microvascular proliferation orchestrated by VPF/VEGF: a new world of angiogenesis research. *Am J Pathol*. Vol.158, No.3, pp 789-796.

Brat D.J., Castellano-Sanchez A.A.; Hunter S.B.; Pecot M.; Cohen C.; Hammond E.H.; Devi S.N.; Kaur B & Van Meir E.G. (2004). Pseudopalisades in glioblastoma are hypoxic, express extracellular matrix proteases, and are formed by an actively migrating cell population. *Cancer Res*. Vol.64, No.3, pp 920-927.

Burger P.C.; Dubois P.J; Schold S.C.; Smith K.R.; Odom G.L.; Crafts D.C. & Giangaspero F. (1983). Computerized tomographic and pathologic studies of the untreated, quiescent, and recurrent glioblastoma multiforme. *J Neurosurg* Vol. 58 pp 159–169.

Burger P.C. & Scheithauer B.W. (2007). *Tumors of the Central Nervous System.; AFIP Atlas of Tumor Pathology Series 4,* ARP Press, ISBN 978-953-7619-34-3, Washington, USA

Capper D.; Mittelbronn M.; Meyermann R & Schittenhelm J. (2008). Pitfalls in the assessment of MGMT expression and in its correlation with survival in diffuse astrocytomas: proposal of a feasible immunohistochemical approach. Acta Neuropathol. Vol.115, No.2, pp 249-259.

Capper D.; Weissert S.; Balss J.; Habel A.; Meyer J.; Jäger D.; Ackermann U.; Tessmer C.; Korshunov A.; Zentgraf H.; Hartmann C. & von Deimling A. (2010). Characterization of R132H mutation-specific IDH1 antibody binding in brain tumors. Brain Pathol. Vol.20, No.1, pp 245-254.

Capper D.; Reuss D.; Schittenhelm J.; Hartmann C.; Bremer J.; Sahm F.; Harter P.N.; Jeibmann A.; von Deimling A. (2011). Mutation-specific IDH1 antibody differentiates oligodendrogliomas and oligoastrocytomas from other brain tumors with oligodendroglioma-like morphology. Acta Neuropathol. Vol.121, No.2, pp 241-252.

CBTRUS Central brain tumor registry of United States. Statistical report table (2011): accessed:
http://www.cbtrus.org/2011-NPCR-SEER/WEB-0407-Report-3-3-2011.pdf

Cin H.; Meyer C.; Herr R.; Janzarik W.G.; Lambert S.; Jones D.T.; Jacob K.; Benner A.; Witt H.; Remke M.; Bender S.; Falkenstein F.; Van Anh T.N.; Olbrich H.; von Deimling A.; Pekrun A.; Kulozik A.E.; Gnekow A.; Scheurlen W.; Witt O.; Omran H.; Jabado N.; Collins V.P.; Brummer T.; Marschalek R.; Lichter P.; Korshunov A. & Pfister S.M. (2011). Oncogenic FAM131B-BRAF fusion resulting from 7q34 deletion comprises an alternative mechanism of MAPK pathway activation in pilocytic astrocytoma. Acta Neuropathol. Vol. 121, No.6, pp 763-774.

Clark AJ.; Santos WG.; McCready J.; Chen MY.; Van Meter TE.; Ware JL.; Wolber SB.; Fillmore H. & Broaddus WC. (2007). Wilms tumor 1 expression in malignant gliomas and correlation of +KTS isoforms with p53 status. J Neurosurg. Vol.107, No.3, pp 586-592.

Colman H.; Giannini C.; Huang L.; Gonzalez J.; Hess K.; Bruner J.; Fuller G.; Langford L.; Pelloski C.; Aaron J.; Burger P. & Aldape K. (2006). Assessment and prognostic significance of mitotic index using the mitosis marker phospho-histone H3 in low and intermediate-grade infiltrating astrocytomas. Am J Surg Pathol. Vol.30,No.5, pp 657-664.

Cosgrove M.; Fitzgibbons P.L.; Sherrod A.; Chandrasoma P.T.& Martin S.E. (1989). Intermediate filament expression in astrocytic neoplasms. Am J Surg Pathol. Vol.13, No.2, pp 141-145.

Dang L.; White D.W.; Gross S.; Bennett B.D.; Bittinger M.A.; Driggers E.M.; Fantin V.R.; Jang H.G.; Jin S.; Keenan M.C.; Marks K.M.; Prins R.M.; Ward P.S.; Yen K.E.; Liau L.M.; Rabinowitz J.D.; Cantley L.C.; Thompson C.B.; Vander Heiden M.G. & Su SM. (2010). Cancer-associated IDH1 mutations produce 2-hydroxyglutarate. Nature. Vol.462, No.7273, pp 739-744.

Deckert M.; Reifenberger G. & Wechsler W. (1989). Determination of the proliferative potential of human brain tumors using the monoclonal antibody Ki-67. J Cancer Res Clin Oncol. Vol.115, No.2, pp 179-188.

Ducray F.; Mokhtari K.; Crinière E.; Idbaih A.; Marie Y.; Dehais C.; Paris S.; Carpentier C.; Dieme M.J.; Adam C.; Hoang-Xuan K.; Duyckaerts C.; Delattre J.Y. & Sanson M. (2011). Diagnostic and prognostic value of alpha internexin expression in a series of 409 gliomas. Eur J Cancer. Vol.47, No.5, pp 802-808.

Duffell D.; Farber L.; Chou S.; Hartmann J.F &; Nelson E. (1963). Electron Microscopic Observations on Astrocytomas. (1963) Am J Pathol. Vol.43, pp 539-545.

Everhard S.; Kaloshi G.; Crinière E.; Benouaich-Amiel A.; Lejeune J.; Marie Y.; Sanson M.; Kujas M.; Mokhtari K.; Hoang-Xuan K.; Delattre J.Y. & Thillet J. (2006). MGMT methylation: a marker of response to temozolomide in low-grade gliomas. Ann Neurol. Vol.60, No.6, pp 740-743.

Franke F.E.; Schachenmayr W.; Osborn M. & Altmannsberger M. (1991). Unexpected immunoreactivities of intermediate filament antibodies in human brain and brain tumours. Am J Pathol Vol. 139 pp 67-79.

Fuller C.E.; Schmidt R.E.; Roth K.A.; Burger P.C.; Scheithauer B.W.; Banerjee R.; Trinkaus K.; Lytle R. & Perry A. (2003). Clinical utility of fluorescence in situ hybridization (FISH) in morphologically ambiguous gliomas with hybrid oligodendroglial/astrocytic features. J Neuropathol Exp Neurol. Vol.62, No.11, pp 1118-1128.

Gerstner L.; Jellinger K.; Heiss W.D.& Wöber G. (1977). Morphological changes in anaplastic gliomas treated with radiation and chemotherapy. Acta Neurochir (Wien). Vol.36, No.1-2, pp 117-138.

Giannini C.; Scheithauer B.W.; Burger P.C.; Christensen M.R.; Wollan P.C.; Sebo T.J.; Forsyth P.A.; Hayostek C.J. (1999). Cellular proliferation in pilocytic and diffuse astrocytomas. J Neuropathol Exp Neurol. Vol.58, No.1, pp 46-53.

Giannini C.; Scheithauer B.W.; Weaver A.L.; Burger P.C.; Kros J.M.; Mork S.; Graeber M.B.; Bauserman S.; Buckner J.C.; Burton J.; Riepe R.; Tazelaar H.D.; Nascimento A.G.; Crotty T.; Keeney G.L.; Pernicone P. & Altermatt H. (2001). Oligodendrogliomas: reproducibility and prognostic value of histologic diagnosis and grading. J Neuropathol Exp Neurol. Vol.60, No.3, pp 248-262.

Giannini C.; Burger P.C.; Berkey B.A.; Cairncross J.G.; Jenkins R.B.; Mehta M.; Curran W.J. & Aldape K. (2008). Anaplastic oligodendroglial tumors: refining the correlation among histopathology: 1p 19q deletion and clinical outcome in Intergroup Radiation Therapy Oncology Group Trial 9402. Brain Pathol. Vol.18, No.3, pp 360-369.

Hartmann C.; Meyer J.; Balss J.; Capper D.; Mueller W.; Christians A.; Felsberg J.; Wolter M.; Mawrin C.; Wick W.; Weller M.; Herold-Mende C.; Unterberg A.; Jeuken J.W.; Wesseling P.; Reifenberger G.; von Deimling A. (2009). Type and frequency of IDH1 and IDH2 mutations are related to astrocytic and oligodendroglial differentiation and age: a study of 1.010 diffuse gliomas. Acta Neuropathol. Vol.118,No.4, pp 469-474.

Hartmann C.; Hentschel B.; Wick W.; Capper D.; Felsberg J.; Simon M.; Westphal M.; Schackert G.; Meyermann R.; Pietsch T.; Reifenberger G.; Weller M.; Loeffler M. & von Deimling A. (2010). Patients with IDH1 wild type anaplastic astrocytomas exhibit worse prognosis than IDH1-mutated glioblastomas, and IDH1 mutation status accounts for the unfavorable prognostic effect of higher age: implications for classification of gliomas. Acta Neuropathol. Vol.120, No.6, pp 707-718.

Hashiba T.; Izumoto S.; Kagawa N.; Suzuki T.; Hashimoto N.; Maruno M. & Yoshimine T. (2007). Expression of WT1 protein and correlation with cellular proliferation in glial tumors. Neurol Med Chir (Tokyo). Vol.47, No.4, pp 165-170.

Hasselblatt M. & Paulus W. (2003). Sensitivity and specificity of epithelial membrane antigen staining patterns in ependymomas. Acta Neuropathol. Vol.106, No.4, pp 385-388.

Hegi M.E.; Diserens A.C.; Gorlia T.; Hamou M.F.; de Tribolet N.; Weller M.; Kros J.M.; Hainfellner J.A.; Mason W.; Mariani L.; Bromberg J.E.; Hau P.; Mirimanoff R.O.; Cairncross J.G.; Janzer R.C.& Stupp R. (2005). MGMT gene silencing and benefit from temozolomide in glioblastoma. N Engl J Med. Vol.352, No.10, pp 997-1003.

Hirose T.; Ishizawa K. & Shimada S. (2010). Utility of in situ demonstration of 1p loss and p53 overexpression in pathologic diagnosis of oligodendroglial tumors. Neuropathology. Vol.30, No.6, pp 586-596.

Hussein M.R.; El-Ghorori R.M. & El-Rahman Y.G. (2006). Alterations of p53, BCL-2 and hMSH2 protein expression in the normal brain tissues, gliosis and gliomas. Int J Exp Pathol. Vol.87, No.4, pp 297-306.

Jaiswal S.; Agrawal V.; Vij M.; Sahu R.N.; Jaiswal A.K. & Behari S. (2010) Glioblastoma with melanotic differentiation. Clin Neuropathol. Vol. 29, No.5, pp 330-333.

Jaros E.; Perry R.H.; Adam L.; Kelly P.J.; Crawford P.J.; Kalbag R.M.; Mendelow A.D.; Sengupta R.P. & Pearson AD. (1992). Prognostic implications of p53 protein.; epidermal growth factor receptor.; and Ki-67 labelling in brain tumours. Br J Cancer. Vol.66, No.2, pp 373-385.

Jeon Y.K.; Park K.; Park C.K.; Paek S.H.; Jung H.W.; Park S.H. (2007). Chromosome 1p and 19q status and p53 and p16 expression patterns as prognostic indicators of oligodendroglial tumors: a clinicopathological study using fluorescence in situ hybridization. Neuropathology. Vol.27, No.1, pp 10-20.

Jung T.Y.; Jung S.; Moon K.S.; Kim I.Y.; Kang S.S.; Kim Y.H.; Park C.S. & Lee K.H. (2010). Changes of the O6-methylguanine-DNA methyltransferase promoter methylation and MGMT protein expression after adjuvant treatment in glioblastoma. Oncol Rep. Vol.23, No.5, pp 1269-1276.

Kesari S.; Schiff D.; Drappatz J.; LaFrankie D.; Doherty L.; Macklin E.A.; Muzikansky A.; Santagata S.; Ligon K.L.; Norden A.D.; Ciampa A.; Bradshaw J.; Levy B.; Radakovic G.; Ramakrishna N.; Black P.M. & Wen P.Y. (2009). Phase II study of protracted daily temozolomide for low-grade gliomas in adults. Clin Cancer Res. Vol.15, No.1, pp 330-337.

Kim Y.H.; Nobusawa S.; Mittelbronn M.; Paulus W.; Brokinkel B.; Keyvani K.; Sure U.; Wrede K.; Nakazato Y.; Tanaka Y.; Vital A.; Mariani L.; Stawski R.; Watanabe T.; De Girolami U.; Kleihues P. & Ohgaki H. (2010). Molecular classification of low-grade diffuse gliomas. Am J Pathol. Vol.177, No.6, pp 2708-2714.

Kita D.; Ciernik I.F.; Vaccarella S.; Franceschi S.; Kleihues P.; Lütolf U.M. & Ohgaki H. (2009). Age as a predictive factor in glioblastomas: population-based study. Neuroepidemiology. Vol.33, No.1, pp 17-22.

Komine C.; Watanabe T.; Katayama Y.; Yoshino A.; Yokoyama T. & Fukushima T (2003). Promoter hypermethylation of the DNA repair gene O6-methylguanine-DNA methyltransferase is an independent predictor of shortened progression free survival in patients with low-grade diffuse astrocytomas. Brain Pathol Vol.13, pp 176–184.

Korshunov A.; Meyer J.; Capper D.; Christians A.; Remke M.; Witt H.; Pfister S.; von Deimling A. & Hartmann C. (2009). Combined molecular analysis of BRAF and IDH1 distinguishes pilocytic astrocytoma from diffuse astrocytoma. Acta Neuropathol. Vol.118, No.3, pp 401-405.

Kösel S.; Scheithauer B.W. & Graeber M.B. (2001). Genotype-phenotype correlation in gemistocytic astrocytomas. Neurosurgery. Vol.48, No.1, pp 187-193.

Kros J.M.; van den Brink W.A.; van Loon-van Luyt J.J. & Stefanko S.Z. (1997). Signet-ring cell oligodendroglioma--report of two cases and discussion of the differential diagnosis. Acta Neuropathol. Vol.93, No.6, pp 638-643.

Kuhlmann T.; Gutenberg A.; Schulten HJ.; Paulus W.; Rohde V. & Bruck W. (2008). Nogo-a expression in glial CNS tumors: a tool to differentiate between oligodendrogliomas and other gliomas? Am J Surg Pathol. Vol. 32, No.10, pp 1444-1453.

Levin N.; Lavon I.; Zelikovitsh B.; Fuchs D.; Bokstein F.; Fellig Y. & Siegal T. (2006). Progressive low-grade oligodendrogliomas: response to temozolomide and correlation between genetic profile and O6-methylguanine DNA methyltransferase protein expression. Cancer. Vol. 106, No.8, pp 1759-1765.

Ligon K.L.; Alberta J.A.; Kho A.T.; Weiss J.; Kwaan M.R.; Nutt CL.; Louis D.N.; Stiles C.D. & Rowitch D.H. (2004). The oligodendroglial lineage marker OLIG2 is universally expressed in diffuse gliomas. J Neuropathol Exp Neurol. Vol. 63, No.5, pp 499-509.

Louis DN.; Ohgaki H.; Wiestler OD. & Cavenee WK. WHO Classification of Tumours of The Central Nervous system IARC Press Lyon 2007

Louis D.N.; Ohgaki H.; Wiestler O.D.; Cavenee W.K.; Burger P.C.; Jouvet A.; Scheithauer B.W & Kleihues P. (2007). The 2007 WHO Classification of Tumours of the Central Nervous System. Acta Neuropathol. Vol.114, No.2, pp 97–109.

McLendon R.E.; Herndon J.E 2nd.; West B.; Reardon D.; Wiltshire R.; Rasheed B.K.; Quinn J.; Friedman H.S.; Friedman A.H.; Bigner D.D. (2005) Survival analysis of presumptive prognostic markers among oligodendrogliomas. Cancer. Vol.104, No.8, pp 1693-1699.

Meis J.M.; Martz K.L. & Nelson J.S. (1991). Mixed glioblastoma multiforme and sarcoma. A clinicopathologic study of 26 radiation therapy oncology group cases. Cancer. Vol.67, No.9, pp 2342-2349.

Meyer J.; Pusch S.; Balss J.; Capper D.; Mueller W.; Christians A.; Hartmann C. & von Deimling A. (2010). PCR- and restriction endonuclease-based detection of IDH1 mutations. Brain Pathol. Vol.20, No.2, pp 298-300.

Min K.W. & Scheithauer BW. (1994). Oligodendroglioma: the ultrastructural spectrum. Ultrastruct Pathol. Vol.18, No.1-2, pp 47-56.

Mittelbronn M.; Wolff M.; Bültmann E.; Nägele T.; Capper D.; Beck R.; Meyermann R. & Beschorner R. (2005). Disseminating anaplastic brainstem oligodendroglioma associated with allelic loss in the tumor suppressor candidate region D19S246 of chromosome 19 mimicking an inflammatory central nervous system disease in a 9-year-old boy. Hum Pathol. Vol.36, No.7, pp 854-857.

Ng H.K. & Lo S.T.H. (1989). Cytokeratin immunoreactivity in gliomas. Histopathol 1989; Vol. 14, pp 359-368.

Nobusawa S.; Watanabe T.; Kleihues P. & Ohgaki H. (2009). IDH1 mutations as molecular signature and predictive factor of secondary glioblastomas. Clin Cancer Res. Vol.15, No.19, pp 6002-6007.

Ohgaki H & Kleihues P. (2005). Population-based studies on incidence, survival rates and genetic alterations in astrocytic and oligodendroglial gliomas. J Neuropathol Exp Neurol. Vol.64, No.6, pp 479-489.

Ohgaki H & Kleihues P. (2005). Epidemiology and etiology of gliomas. Acta Neuropathol. Vol.109, No.1, pp 93-108.

Ohgaki H & Kleihues P. (2007). Genetic pathways to primary and secondary glioblastoma. Am J Pathol. Vol.170, No.5, pp 1445-1453.

Okamoto Y.; Di Patre P.L.; Burkhard C.; Horstmann S.; Jourde B.; Fahey M.; Schüler D.; Probst-Hensch N.M.; Yasargil M.G.; Yonekawa Y.; Lütolf U.M.; Kleihues P. & Ohgaki H. (2004). Population-based study on incidence.; survival rates.; and genetic alterations of low-grade diffuse astrocytomas and oligodendrogliomas. Acta Neuropathol. Vol.108, No.1, pp 49-56.

Palma L.; Celli P.; Maleci A.; Di Lorenzo N. & Cantore G. (1989). Malignant monstrocellular brain tumours. A study of 42 surgically treated cases. Acta Neurochir (Wien). Vol.97, No.1-2, pp 17-25.

Peraud A.; Kreth F.W.; Wiestler O.D.; Kleihues P. & Reulen H.J. (2002). Prognostic impact of TP53 mutations and P53 protein overexpression in supratentorial WHO grade II astrocytomas and oligoastrocytomas. Clin Cancer Res. Vol.8, No.5, pp 1117-1124.

Plate KH. (1999). Mechanisms of angiogenesis in the brain. J Neuropathol Exp Neurol. Vol.58, No.4, pp 313-320.

Prayson R.A. & Estes M.L. (1996). MIB1 and p53 immunoreactivity in protoplasmic astrocytomas. Pathol Int. Vol.46, No.11, pp 862-866.

Preusser M.; Janzer C.R.; Felsberg J.; Reifenberger G.; Hamou M.F.; Diserens A.C.; Stupp R.; Gorlia T.; Marosi C.; Heinzl H.; Hainfellner J.A. & Hegi M. (2008). Anti-O6-methylguanine-methyltransferase (MGMT) immunohistochemistry in glioblastoma multiforme: observer variability and lack of association with patient survival impede its use as clinical biomarker. Brain Pathol. Vol.18, No.4, pp 520-532.

Preusser M.; Elezi L. & Hainfellner J.A. (2008). Reliability and reproducibility of PCR-based testing of O6-methylguanine-DNA methyltransferase gene (MGMT) promoter methylation status in formalin-fixed and paraffin-embedded neurosurgical biopsy specimens. Clin Neuropathol. Vol.27, No.6, pp 388-390.

Riemenschneider M.J.; Jeuken J.W.; Wesseling P & Reifenberger G. (2010). Molecular diagnostics of gliomas: state of the art. Acta Neuropathol. 2010 Vol.120, No.5, pp 567-584.

Rodriguez F.J.; Scheithauer B.W.; Giannini C.; Bryant S.C. & Jenkins R.B. (2008). Epithelial and pseudoepithelial differentiation in glioblastoma and gliosarcoma: a comparative morphologic and molecular genetic study. Cancer. Vol.113, No.10, pp 2779-2789.

Rushing E.J.; Sandberg G.D. & Horkayne-Szakaly I. (2010). High-grade astrocytomas show increased Nestin and Wilms's tumor gene No.WT1) protein expression. Int J Surg Pathol. Vol.18, No.4, pp 255-259.

Sallinen P.K.; Haapasalo H.K.; Visakorpi T.; Helén P.T.; Rantala I.S.; Isola J.J. & Helin H.J. (1994). Prognostication of astrocytoma patient survival by Ki-67 (MIB-1), PCNA and S-phase fraction using archival paraffin-embedded samples. J Pathol. Vol.174, No.4, pp 275-282.

Sanson M.; Marie Y.; Paris S.; Idbaih A.; Laffaire J.; Ducray F.; El Hallani S.; Boisselier B.; Mokhtari K.; Hoang-Xuan K. & Delattre J.Y. (2009). Isocitrate dehydrogenase 1 codon 132 mutation is an important prognostic biomarker in gliomas. J Clin Oncol. Vol.27, No.25, pp 4150-4154.

Scherer HJ. (1983). Structural development in gliomas. Am J Cancer 1938; 34: 333–351.

Schindler G.; Capper D.; Meyer J.; Janzarik W.; Omran H.; Herold-Mende C.; Schmieder K.; Wesseling P.; Mawrin C.; Hasselblatt M.; Louis D.N.; Korshunov A.; Pfister S.; Hartmann C.; Paulus W.; Reifenberger G. & von Deimling A. (2011). Analysis of BRAF V600E mutation in 1.;320 nervous system tumors reveals high mutation frequencies in pleomorphic xanthoastrocytoma, ganglioglioma and extra-cerebellar pilocytic astrocytoma. Acta Neuropathol. Vol.121, No.3, pp 397-405.

Schittenhelm J.; Erdmann T.; Maennlin S.; Will B.E.; Beschorner R.; Bornemann A.; Meyermann R. & Mittelbronn M. (2007). Gliosarcoma with chondroid and osseous differentiation. Neuropathology. Vol.27, No.1, pp 90-94.

Schittenhelm J.; Beschorner R.; Simon P.; Tabatabai G.; Herrmann C.; Schlaszus H.; Capper D.; Weller M.; Meyermann R.; Mittelbronn M. (2009). Diagnostic value of WT1 in neuroepithelial tumours. Neuropathol Appl Neurobiol. Vol.35, No.1, pp 69-81.

Schittenhelm J. & Psaras T. (2010). Glioblastoma with granular cell astrocytoma features: a case report and literature review. Clin Neuropathol. Vol.29, No.5, pp 323-329.

Simmons M.L.; Lamborn K.R.; Takahashi M.; Chen P.; Israel M.A.; Berger M.S.; Godfrey T.; Nigro J.; Prados M.; Chang S-; Barker F.G. 2nd & Aldape K. (2001). Analysis of complex relationships between age, p53, epidermal growth factor receptor, and survival in glioblastoma patients. Cancer Res. Vol. 61, pp 1122–1128.

Srivastava A.; Jain A.; Jha P.; Suri V.; Sharma M.C.; Mallick S.; Puri T.; Gupta D.K.; Gupta A.; Sarkar C. (2010). MGMT gene promoter methylation in pediatric glioblastomas. Childs Nerv Syst. Vol.26, No.11, pp 1613-1618.

Ständer M.; Peraud A.; Leroch B. & Kreth FW. (2004). Prognostic impact of TP53 mutation status for adult patients with supratentorial World Health Organization Grade II astrocytoma or oligoastrocytoma: a long-term analysis. Cancer. Vol.101, No.5, pp 1028-1035.

Stavrinou P.; Magras I.; Stavrinou L.C.; Zaraboukas T.; Polyzoidis K.S. & Selviaridis P. (2010). Primary extracerebral meningeal glioblastoma: clinical and pathological analysis. Cen Eur Neurosurg. Vol.71, No.1, pp 46-49.

Tabatabai G.; Stupp R.; van den Bent M.J.; Hegi M.E.; Tonn J.C.; Wick W. & Weller M. (2010). Molecular diagnostics of gliomas: the clinical perspective. Acta Neuropathol. Vol.120, No.5, pp 585-592.

Tabuchi K.; Moriya Y.; Furuta T.; Ohnishi R & Nishimoto A. (1982). S-100 protein in human glial tumours. Qualitative and quantitative studies. Acta Neurochir (Wien). Vol.65, No.3-4, pp 239-251.

Takeuchi J. & Barnard R.O. (1976). Perivascular lymphocytic cuffing in astrocytomas. Acta Neuropathol. Vol.35, No.3, pp 265-271.

Tascos N.A.; Parr J. & Gonatas N.K. (1982). Immunocytochemical study of the glial fibrillary acidic protein in human neoplasms of the central nervous system. Hum Pathol. 1982 May;13No.5, pp 454-8.

Tihan T.; Vohra P.; Berger M.S. & Keles G.E. (2006). Definition and diagnostic implications of gemistocytic astrocytomas: a pathological perspective. J Neurooncol. Vol.76, No.2, pp 175-183.

Waidelich J.; Schittenhelm J.; Allmendinger O.; Meyermann R & Beschorner R (2010). Glutamate transporters in diagnostic neurooncology. Brain Pathology Vol. 20, (Suppl. 1), pp 1–99.

Wharton SB.; Chan KK. & Whittle I.R. (2002). Microtubule-associated protein 2 (MAP-2) is expressed in low and high grade diffuse astrocytomas. J Clin Neurosci. Vol.9, No.2, pp 165-169.

Wick W.; Hartmann C.; Engel C.; Stoffels M.; Felsberg J.; Stockhammer F Sabel MC, Koeppen S, Ketter R, Meyermann R, Rapp M, Meisner C, Kortmann R.D, Pietsch T, Wiestler O.D, Ernemann U, Bamberg M, Reifenberger G, von Deimling A & Weller M. (2009). NOA-04 randomized phase III trial of sequential radiochemotherapy of anaplastic glioma with procarbazine, lomustine and vincristine or temozolomide. J Clin Oncol. Vol.27, pp 5874–5880.

van den Bent MJ.; Dubbink H.J.; Sanson M.; van der Lee-Haarloo C.R.; Hegi M.; Jeuken J.W.; Ibdaih A.; Brandes A.A.; Taphoorn M.J.; Frenay M.; Lacombe D.; Gorlia T.; Dinjens W.N. & Kros J.M. (2009). MGMT promoter methylation is prognostic but not predictive for outcome to adjuvant PCV chemotherapy in anaplastic oligodendroglial tumors: a report from EORTC Brain Tumor Group Study 26951. J Clin Oncol. Vol.27, No.35, pp 5881-5886.

van den Bent M.J.; Carpentier A.F.; Brandes A.A.; Sanson M.; Taphoorn M.J.; Bernsen H.J.; Frenay M.; Tijssen C.C.; Grisold W.; Sipos L.; Haaxma-Reiche H.; Kros J.M.; van Kouwenhoven M.C.; Vecht C.J.; Allgeier A.; Lacombe D. & Gorlia T. (2006). Adjuvant procarbazine, lomustine and vincristine improves progression-free survival but not overall survival in newly diagnosed anaplastic oligodendrogliomas and oligoastrocytomas: a randomized European Organisation for Research and Treatment of Cancer phase III trial. J Clin Oncol. Vol.24, No.18, pp 2715-2722.

von Deimling A.; Korshunov A. & Hartmann C. (2011). The next generation of glioma biomarkers: MGMT methylation.; BRAF fusions and IDH1 mutations. Brain Pathol. 2011 Vol.21, No.1, pp 74-87.

Vital A.; Loiseau H.; Kantor G.; Daucourt V.; Chene G.; Cohadon F.; Rougier A.; Rivel J. & Vital C. (1998). p53 protein expression in grade II astrocytomas: immunohistochemical study of 100 cases with long-term follow-up. Pathol Res Pract. Vol.194, No.12, pp 831-836.

Watanabe K.; Sato K.; Biernat W.; Tachibana O.; von Ammon K.; Ogata N.; Yonekawa Y.; Kleihues P. & Ohgaki H. (1997). Incidence and timing of p53 mutations during astrocytoma progression in patients with multiple biopsies. Clin Cancer Res. Vol.3, No.4, pp 523-530.

Watanabe K.; Peraud A.; Gratas C.; Wakai S.; Kleihues P. & Ohgaki H. (1998). p53 and PTEN gene mutations in gemistocytic astrocytomas. Acta Neuropathol. Vol.95, No.6, pp 559-564.

Weller M.; Felsberg J.; Hartmann C.; Berger H.; Steinbach J.P.; Schramm J.; Westphal M.; Schackert G.; Simon M.; Tonn JC.; Heese O.; Krex D.; Nikkhah G.; Pietsch T.; Wiestler O.; Reifenberger G.; von Deimling A. & Loeffler M. (2009). Molecular predictors of progression-free and overall survival in patients with newly diagnosed glioblastoma: a prospective translational study of the German Glioma Network. J Clin Oncol. Vol.27, No.34, pp 5743-5750.

Yan H.; Parsons DW.; Jin G.; McLendon R.; Rasheed BA.; Yuan W.; Kos I.; Batinic-Haberle I.; Jones S.; Riggins GJ.; Friedman H.; Friedman A.; Reardon D.; Herndon J.; Kinzler K.W.; Velculescu V.E.; Vogelstein B & Bigner D.D. (2009). IDH1 and IDH2 mutations in gliomas. N Engl J Med. Vol.360, No.8, pp 765-773.

Yung WK.; Luna M. & Borit A (1985). Vimentin and glial fibrillary acidic protein in human brain tumors. J Neurooncol. Vol.3, No.1, pp 35-38.

12

Magnetic Resonance Imaging of Gliomas

Pilar López-Larrubia, Eva Cañadillas-Cárdenas,
Ana M. Metelo, Nuria Arias, Miguel Martínez-Maestro,
Aire Salguero and Sebastián Cerdán
Instituto de Investigaciones Biomédicas "Alberto Sols", CSIC-UAM
Spain

1. Introduction

Brain cancer is a life threatening neurological disorder in which malignant cells, grow, proliferate and invade the original cerebral structures of the host, hampering seriously adequate brain function. Malignant cells generate eventually a dedifferentiated tumoral mass that interferes with vital brain functions as sensory and motor activations, memory and perception and neuroendocrine regulation, among others. The fully developed tumoral mass consumes a significant part of cerebral volume resulting in cerebral compression and serious neurological impairments, such as vision or hearing disturbances and eventually lethal cerebrovascular complications. Most brain tumors remain asymptomatic during early development, revealing their symptoms and lethal nature only at later stages. Therapy is facilitated many times by an early finding, a circumstance making the neuroimaging approaches particularly useful in the detection and handling of these lesions.

In the last decades, Magnetic Resonance Imaging (MRI) approaches have evolved into the most powerful and versatile imaging tool for brain tumor diagnosis, prognosis, therapy evaluation, monitoring of disease progression and planning of neurosurgical strategies. MRI methods enable the non invasive assessment of glioma morphology and functionality providing a point of likeness into histopathological grading of the tumor and helping in this way a more successful patient management. This impressive evolution is based not only for the high resolution and quality of the anatomical images obtained, but on the additional possibilities to achieve quantitative functional information on tumoral physiopathology and its repercussions in the sensorial, motor and integrative functions through the brain. The use of conventional paramagnetic or superparamagnetic contrast media allows for the identification of areas with blood-brain barrier (BBB) disruption and the recent molecular imaging approaches enable researchers to visualize molecular events associated to tumor proliferation and invasion, bringing the potentials of diagnostic imaging to the cellular and molecular aspects of tumor biology. Moreover, functional MRI approaches as performed in the clinic are endowed with the potential to detect and characterize the earliest neoangiogenic, metabolic and hemodynamic alterations induced by the neoplasm.

Several advanced magnetic resonance (MR) methodologies have been proposed in the last years to assess the functional competence in healthy and pathologic brain tissue. Diffusion and perfusion MRI are probably the two main approaches that have reached a relevant clinical role in brain oncology, particularly in neovascular imaging (Calli, Kitis et al. 2006). The diffusion approaches investigate the thermally induced random molecular motions of water molecules in tissues. The perfusion phenomenon describes and quantifies the microvascular blood flow which feeds a volume element of an organ or tissue. At a first glance these two phenomena seem to be very different, however a closer look identifies they both concerned with underlying molecular motions. Moreover, the random distribution of capillaries in tissues such as brain, provides tissue perfusion with some of the characteristic features of diffusive motion.

This chapter will summarize the arsenal of MRI approaches providing functional information on gliomas based on diffusion and perfusion MRI methods. We begin with a description of the pathological classification of gliomas and its implications for MRI diagnosis, continuing with the applications of diffusion weighted imaging (DWI), diffusion tensor imaging (DTI) and tractography to the characterization of these brain tumors. We conclude showing the MRI methodologies available for the evaluation of cerebral and tumoral perfusion, addressing the use of Dynamic Susceptibility Contrast (DSC), Dynamic Contrast Enhanced (DCE) MR images and Arterial Spin Labelling (ASL). Our review focuses mainly in the clinical applications of these methodologies, providing a brief introduction into the physical principles of each one. For interested readers, the following review articles provide more detailed descriptions of the corresponding physical principles of diffusion weighted (DW) MRI (Mori and Barker 1999), DTI (Basser and Jones 2002) and Tractography (Mori and van Zijl 2002) or the different approaches to investigate microvascular perfusion (Ostergaard 2005; Detre, Wang et al. 2009; Larsson, Courivaud et al. 2009).

2. Histological classification of gliomas. Implications in MRI diagnosis

Glioma is a non-specific term, broadly suggesting that the observed tumor originates from glial cells. These tumors account for more than 85% of primary brain neoplasms classified histologically, immunohistochemically and structurally as astrocytomas, ologodendrogliomas or oligoastrocytomas, depending on their morphological, immunochemical or molecular features. Gliomas are assigned a grade depending on their histolopathological properties (figure 1). The grade provides insight into the growth rate of the tumor. According to the classification of the World Health Organization (WHO), tumors in grade I depict the lowest malignancy, their cells look nearly normal and the tumor grows slowly. Grade II tumors are also slow growing, but show a slightly abnormal microscopic appearance. Grade III tumors are malignant by definition. Their cells look very different from the original neural cells and are actively proliferating. Grade IV is the most malignant and aggressive, defined by galloping genetic instability, complete morphological and metabolic reprogramming, fast and uncontrolled proliferation, intense resistance to apoptosis, diffuse infiltration, robust angiogenesis and propensity to necrosis. From this group Glioblastoma multiforme (GBM) is the most frequent, aggressive and lethal intracranial tumor, reaching approximately 50% of all astrocytomas (Furnari, Fenton et al. 2007). Despite decades of intensive research, high-grade gliomas (WHO grade III and IV) are currently estimated incurable with a poor or very poor survival, up to one year in glioblastoma and from two to three years in anaplastic astrocytomas (Reardon, Rich et al. 2006).

The tumor grade determines the most appropriate chemotherapeutic or surgical treatment, but histology, requiring a tumor biopsy, remains currently the only method able to yield unambiguously this information. In spite of this, many of the histopathological features of gliomas are amenable to MRI explorations. In particular, the growth rate and the appearance of necrotic zones may be followed by sequential morphological MRI examinations, the cellularity and tumor microstucture investigated by diffusion weighted MRI, the compression effects of the tumor on surrounding neuronal tracts of the white matter may be examined by MRI tractography from DTI approaches and the development of the neoangiogenic vasculature characterized by perfusion imaging. These properties entail the MRI method with unprecedented capabilities to asses non invasively glioma grade and its potential repercussions. In the following sections we shall provide a description of main physical principles underlying these methodologies and provide illustrative examples on their applications.

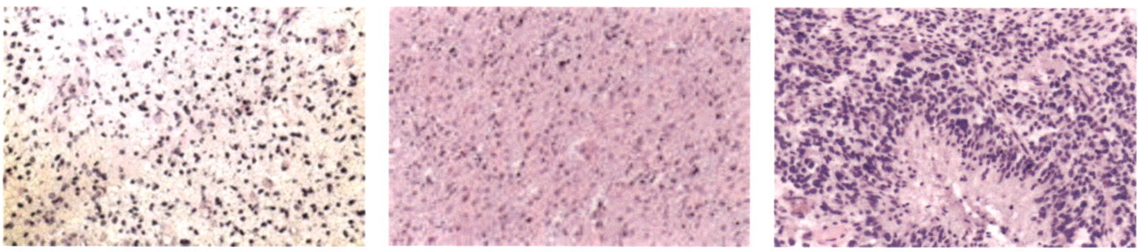

(a) (b) (c)

Fig. 1. Histopathological features from gliomas of increasing grade as revealed by haematoxylin/eosin staning. (a) WHO grade II astrocitoma , (b) WHO grade III anaplastic astrocytoma and (c) WHO grade IV glioblastoma multiforme

3. Diffusion magnetic resonance imaging

The diffusion phenomenon describes quantitatively the random (Brownian) molecular motion translations of water molecules originating ultimately from thermal energy. In a tissue, like the brain, the mechanism of diffusion involves mainly the motion of water molecules on a scale of 5 to 15 micrometers over the approximate 40 ms of measurement time. It is described by an Apparent Diffusion Coefficient (ADC), representing the average translational displacement of a water molecule during a time unit. The diffusion process has a vectorial nature, involving magnitude and direction. Its magnitude and direction in vivo depend on a variety of factors including permeability barriers and their spacing, microviscosity of the intracellular milieu, molecular obstructions to water displacements, duration of the diffusion measurement and, eventually the bulk flow within capillaries and water active transporters in tissue. These circumstances make the interpretation of diffusion measurements complex, but at the same time highly informative on all the aspects influencing it.

In vivo Diffusion Weighted Imaging (DWI) provides images with an inherent contrast different from that obtained by conventional structural MR techniques. In this sense, DWI gives unique information about the microstructure and viability of brain tissue, with the signal intensity of the image depending on the average translational motion of water molecules, an aspect known to be appreciably modified in cerebral tumors (Schaefer, Grant et al. 2000).

3.1 Apparent Diffusion Coefficient

The first description of a diffusion study was provided by Stejskal and Tanner, who used a spin-echo acquisition protocol in which two gradient pulses equal in magnitude but opposite in directions (figure 2) were intercalated before and after the 180 degrees refocusing pulse, thus allowing the measurement of molecular water motions in the direction of the applied gradient (Stejskal and Tanner 1965).

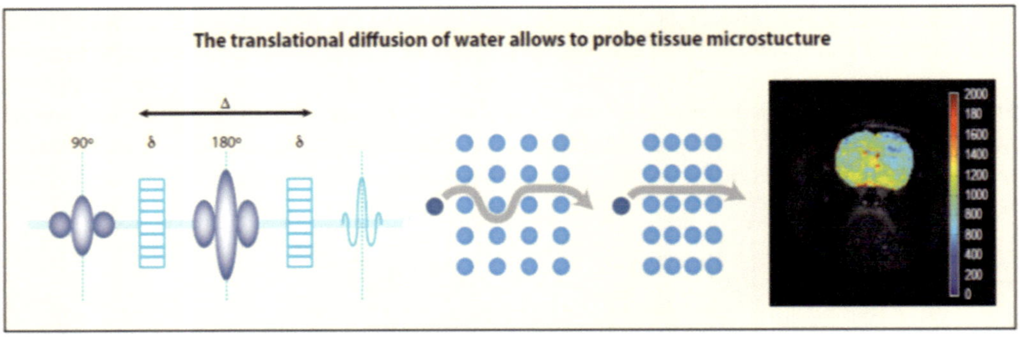

Fig. 2. Diffusion Weighted MR Imaging. Left: The Stejskal-Tanner pulse sequence. The basic spin-echo sequence is sensitized to diffusion using two phase gradients of duration δ, separated by the diffusional time Δ, located symmetrically before and after the 180 pulse. Center: Influence of cellularity on the translational diffusion measurements. Note that in the same time, a water molecule will move translationally a shorter path in an increased cellular density and molecularly more crowded medium. A representative image of the ADC measured in the normal rat brain (Pacheco-Torres, Calle et al.). Reproduced with permission

Because of the same magnitude and the opposite directions of these two gradients, the MR signal of water molecules without net motion will be identical to its intensity as obtained without diffusion gradients in the same cerebral location. However, for locations showing net translational motion of water molecules in the direction of the applied gradient, the opposing effects of the two gradients will not be cancelled, and the resulting image will depict lower intensity in these regions. Signal intensity will be smaller, the faster the average movement of water molecules or the larger ADC. This leads to a DW image depicting hypointensity in the tissue voxels containing faster moving water molecules and hiperintensity in those with slower water displacements.

Under these conditions, the MR signal loss is related to: (i) the diffusion coefficient of the water and (ii) the duration and strength of the magnetic field gradients used in the measurement. The following equation applies:

$$SI = SI_0 \times \exp(-b \times ADC) \quad (1)$$

where; SI_0 represents the signal intensity for each pixel in the absence of gradient pulses, b is an experimentally modifiable parameter including the duration δ, intensity and delay separation Δ of the applied magnetic field gradients and ADC is the apparent diffusion coefficient of the water in the investigated tissue voxel. Using images acquired with increasing b values and thus, increasingly sensitized to diffusion, a parametric map can be calculated by plotting for every pixel the linear relationship between the natural logarithm of the relative signal loss (SI/SI_0) versus b. This affords the calculation of the corresponding ADC on a pixel-by-pixel base, representing then every pixel value in the resulting ADC map.

In vivo measurements of ADC in the human brain by using MRI are well documented both in physiological and physiopathological conditions (Le Bihan, Breton et al. 1986; Thomsen, Henriksen et al. 1987; Chien, Buxton et al. 1990; Hajnal, Doran et al. 1991; Schaefer, Grant et al. 2000). Regions of increased or decreased diffusion due to pathology can be clearly identified in a diffusion weighted MRI study by the corresponding changes in intensity, either in the diffusion weighted images or in fitted ADC maps.

3.2 Diffusion weighted imaging of gliomas

Although DWI studies were initially focused on stroke (Warach, Chien et al. 1992), multiple sclerosis (Larsson, Thomsen et al. 1992) and hydrocephalus (Gideon, Thomsen et al. 1994), an increasing number of diffusion studies on brain is being performed.

In 1994 Tien et al. acquired diffusion images in patients with high-grade gliomas using Echo Planar Imaging (EPI) techniques to measure ADC along cephalocaudal axis, comparing the obtained results with those found by using conventional (SE) or fast spin-echo (FSE) MRI (Tien, Felsberg et al. 1994). The ADC images enabled these authors to differentiate various regions within the tumor, concluding that echo-plannar DWI appeared a more powerful tool in the characterization of brain neoplasm than conventional techniques.

In 1995 Brunberg et al. reported their study performed with a motion-insensitive spin-echo sequence measuring ADC along three orthogonal axes (Brunberg, Chenevert et al. 1995). They aimed to determine if there was a relationship between water diffusion coefficients or its anisotropy in MR-defined regions of normal and abnormal parenchyma in patients with cerebral gliomas. They were able to distinguish between normal white matter, cystic or necrotic areas, regions of edema and solid enhancing tumor by comparing anisotropic ADC values in those regions.

In 1997 Krabbe et al. measured ADC in different regions of patients with brain tumors (Krabbe, Gideon et al. 1997). They reported diffusion values in contrast-enhancing tumor, non-enhancing tumor, cyst or necrosis, edema and cerebro-spinal fluid (CSF) for malignant gliomas, low–grade gliomas, metastases, meningiomas and cerebral abscess. They found that mean ADC in contrast-enhancing tumor was significantly higher in metastases than in high-grade gliomas, while no significant differences were found between ADC in contrast-enhancing tissue in meningiomas and metastases or high-grade gliomas. The highest ADC was always found in CSF. ADC in edema was higher than in contrast-enhancing tumor, and in edema around cerebral metastases was significantly higher than those around high-grade gliomas. These findings could help to distinguish on this basis high-grade gliomas and metastases prior to the surgery.

After these initial reports, a large number of results have been published demonstrating the vast possibilities of diffusion MRI in brain oncology. These cover the applications of DWI from glioma characterization and evaluation to the identification of patients with poor treatment response or tumor recurrence (Provenzale, Mukundan et al. 2006; Hamstra, Rehemtulla et al. 2007; Hamstra, Galban et al. 2008). In addition, DWI imaging may allow the non invasive grading of tumor cellularity since cells constitute barriers that restrict microscopically the motion of the water molecules within the tissue. In this sense, the diffusion of water molecules across the tumor as compared to the diffusion in normal brain tissue is expected be different, depicting different diffusivity and ADC depending on the tumor cellularity and grade. As cells constitute a barrier to water motion, tumors with higher cellularity are expected to show lower ADC values than less cellularly crowded tumors (Sugahara, Korogi et al. 1999; Gauvain, McKinstry et al. 2001). On the other hand, an increase in ADCs usually is correlated with decreased cellularity, revealing successful therapy and/or induced necrosis (Lyng, Haraldseth et al. 2000). Although some authors have reported lower diffusivity of water in high-grade than in low grade gliomas (Bulakbasi, Kocaoglu et al. 2003), it should be mentioned that there is a considerable overlap between ADCs in both types of neoplasm (Kono, Inoue et al. 2001). Even so, there is clearly an inverse correlation between tumor cellularity and ADC values measured in brain tumors allowing to distinguish these from other intracranial lesions. Figure 3 illustrates the important differences found in ADC of intratumoral and extratumoral regions, in two different neoplasm types. Images (c) depict ADC maps in two patients with different brain tumor types. Upper panel shows a high average ADC in the patient with partially resected GBM, while in lower pannel reveals a low average ADC in a patient with a primary CNS lymphoma. Regions of white matter edema distal to enhancing tumor margins usually show diffusion coefficient values significantly different from normal white and grey matter, and from areas of tumor cyst or necrosis, respectively. Notably, there are not appreciable differences between these ADCs from edema regions and those from enhancing tumor.

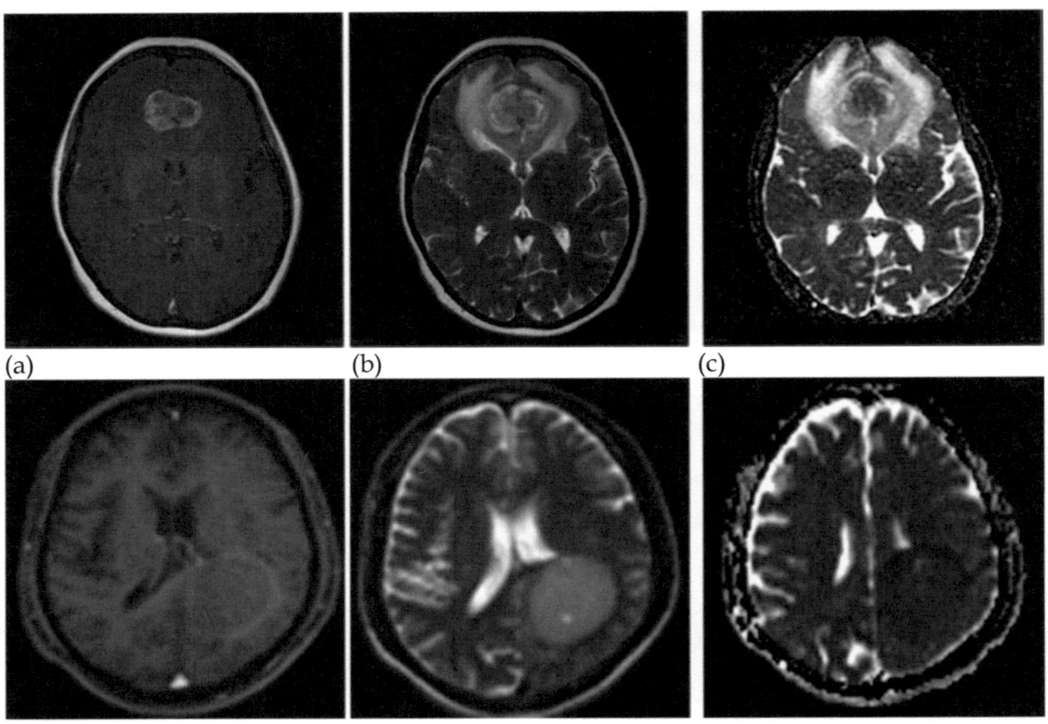

Fig. 3. *Upper panels*: A patient with GBM and high ADC values. (a) Axial contrast-enhanced T1W image shows a mass; (b) T2W image shows lesion and edema; (c) ADC map shows that mean ADC in tumor is much higher than in normal brain. *Lower panels*: A patient with primary CNS lymphoma and low ADC values. (a) Axial contrast-enhanced T1W image shows non enhancing lesion; (b) T2W image shows signal intensity in tumor darker than gray matter; (c) ADC map shows mean ADC in tumor is lower than in normal tissue. (http://radiopaedia.org/encyclopaedia/cases) Reproduced with permission.

This is probably related with the fact that there is an increase in intracellular water in edematous white matter as well as within the tumor. Although this is true for almost all gliomas, its important to consider here, that interpretation of diffusion images and ADC values for diagnostic and prognostic purposes may be tumor type and individual-dependent.

3.3 Diffusion Tensor Imaging

Water molecules are not able to diffuse with equal freedom in all directions through the brain, as surrounding cellular membranes and tissue structures limit to different extents their translational mobility in different directions. As a result, the ADC values measured in different directions are not equal and cerebral diffusion becomes anisotropic. This occurs mainly in white matter since molecular diffusion is relatively unrestricted along the trajectory of the neuronal axons and nerve fibres, but significantly more restricted in the perpendicular plane. The ADC in the grey matter, containing mainly neuronal bodies is more isotropic, with similar restrictions in all directions (Hajnal, Doran et al. 1991). This anisotropic behaviour of the molecular motions of water molecules in the brain can be observed by MRI obtaining images with the diffusion gradients applied in different spatial directions. The dominant direction and magnitude of water diffusion in every pixel is then obtained by calculating the resulting tensor from the ADC vectors measured in all investigated directions. This methodology is known as Diffusion Tensor Imaging (DTI), a method requiring the sampling of the ADC in six or more directions (Nucifora, Verma et al. 2007). This relatively complex mathematical modelling approach allows the preparation of three-dimensional ADC anisotropy maps, a very potent tool in the examination of the brain microstructure, inaccessible to other neuroimaging modalities. Using DTI sequences, it is possible to explore the integrity of white matter structures and detect abnormalities not visible in the conventional MRI acquisitions. DTI also allows to calculate tractography maps, revealing white matter fiber tracts, very useful to determine the infiltration or degeneration of the original fiber tracts by invading tumors (Mori and van Zijl 2002; Witwer, Moftakhar et al. 2002).

3.3.1 Fractional Anisotropy and Mean Diffusivity

Diffusion properties assessed by DTI, such as the fractional anisotropy (FA) and average of diffusion coefficient or mean diffusivity (MD), have become nowadays the most frequently used parametric images in neuro-oncology. Such images are correlated with cellular physiology and tissue microstructure, being extensively used to delineate glioma grades. MD measurements allow differentiation of necrotic areas within a high-grade gliomas and peritumoral edema from adjacent white matter; but they are not able to assess tumor infiltration adequately (Tropine, Vucurevic et al. 2004). On the other hand, FA values can be associated to functional tumoral characteristics, including WHO grade. So, combination of DTI related parameters in a multiparametric approach may facilitate glioma characterization and classification. In this respect, several reports aimed, at the precise elucidation of individual anisotropy patterns of brain water diffusivity which can reflect histopathological features used to graded gliomas (Jakab, Molnar et al.). Jakab et al. reported that these parameters can be used as indicators of glioma classification types and tumor physiopathology features like proliferation, metabolism or blood flow. These authors proved a consistent relationship between DTI-related information and histopathological data obtained from biopsies.

FA and MD are very sensitive indicators of white matter integrity also. Some clear examples of color-based images obtained from DTI acquisition are shown in figure 4 and 5, where not only edema region can be clearly distinguished from solid tumor by MD and FA color-based maps (figure 4), but also anisotropic directional maps depict those regions of fiber tract degeneration.

The diffusion MRI study of a brain tumor patient may show a lack of a significant difference in mean diffusion anisotropy between cerebral cortex and solid tumor reflecting the disruption of myelinated fiber orientation by the pathology. In cystic or necrotic regions there is not anisotropy in diffusion. However, the mass effect of a tumor can induce a displacement or distortion of fiber tracts, by mechanical compression, yielding a decrease in mean ADC values and an increase in diffusion anisotropy relative to white matter in health hemisphere as it is shown in figure 5. Moreover, a significant difference in diffusion anisotropy appears between regions of white matter edema and tumor, enhancing or not. This difference is related to the existence of intact myelin membranes within the edema region and the loss of that integrity in areas of active tumor cell proliferation. This promises useful applications in diagnosis and preoperative planning since ADC values alone do not allow the distinction between enhancing central tumor and surrounding tissue.

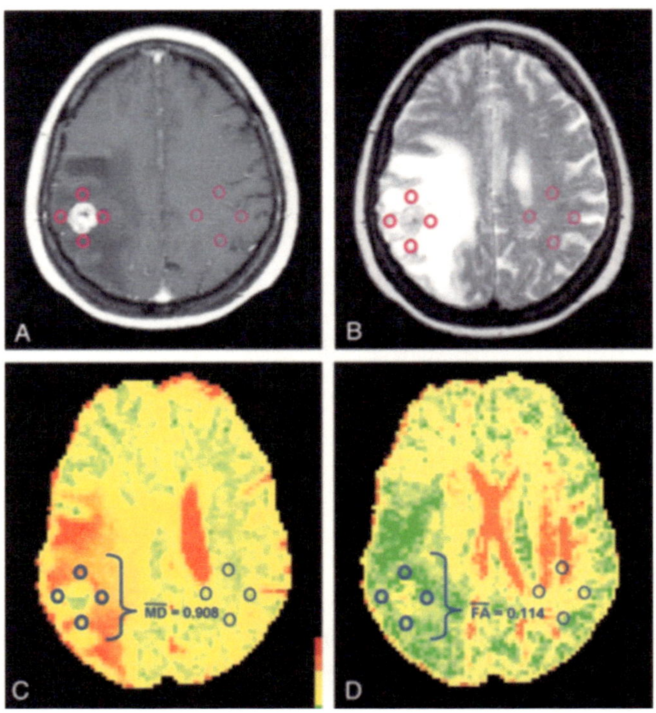

Fig. 4. Metastatic brain tumor. A: T1W image; B: T2W image; C and D show MD and FA overlay maps respectively, and mean values from peritumoral edema. (Lu, Ahn et al. 2003; Kinoshita, Yamada et al. 2005). Reproduced with permission

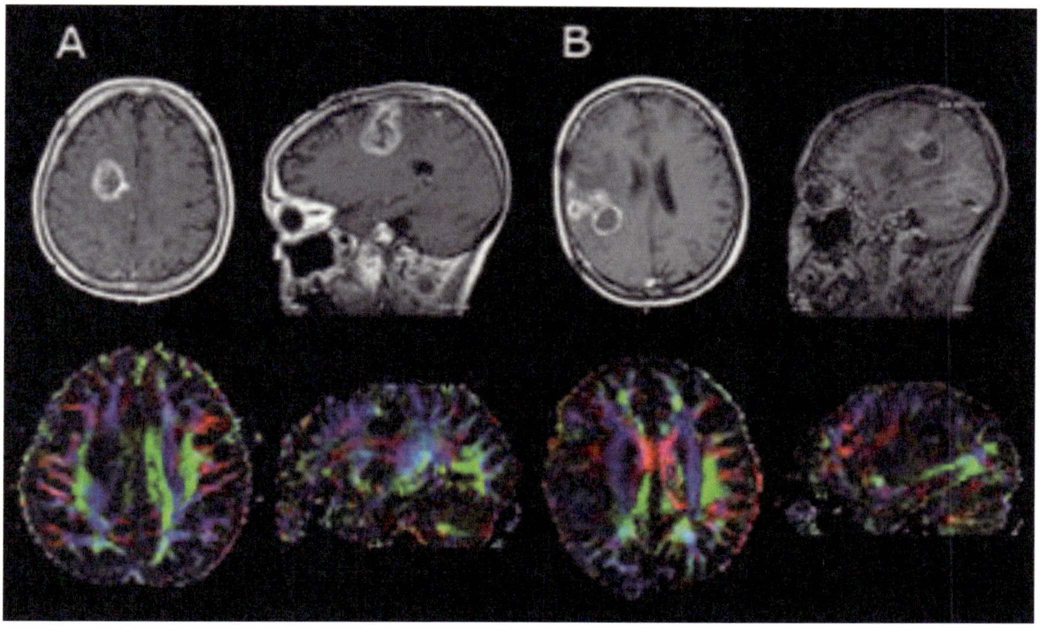

Fig. 5. T1W (upper) and relative anisotropy maps (lower). Each color indicates the principal eigenvector. Color intensity correlates with anisotropy grade. A: right frontal brain tumor; B: anaplastic ependymoma. In lower panels is clearly detected the loss of white matter integrity in both cases. (Lu, Ahn et al. 2003; Kinoshita, Yamada et al. 2005). Reproduced with permission

3.3.2 Tractography

Gliomas are infiltrating tumors in which the tumor cells may invade cerebral structures following the path of normal fiber tracts, making it difficult to differentiate tumoral from healthy tissue and detect the extension of white matter infiltration. Although several approaches from DTI have been reported to make the detection and reliable quantification of this diffuse tumor infiltration (Price, Burnet et al. 2003; Tropine, Vucurevic et al. 2004), this aspect still represents a very challenging question. One of the best developments to improve this situation is based in the visualization of diffusion tensor field by ellipsoids and colour coding of the main diffusion orientations (MDO) that allows the assessment of fibre bundles infiltration more reliably (Schluter, Stieltjes et al. 2005). The color maps and diffusion ellipsoids permit the identification of the particular fibre tracts bundles leading to the periphery of glioma by a reduced FA. Obviously, this approach is helping to improve therapeutic decisions and to minimize interventional risk. Additionally, it has been found that tumor recurrence has the tendency to occur along directions where the region of abnormal isotropic diffusion spreads beyond the region of abnormal anisotropic diffusion. On these grounds, it is eventually possible to predict regions of potential tumor infiltration and/or recidive by detecting abnormalities with high spatial resolution by using DTI. An aspect of increasing interest is the development of new applications that allow obtaining not only presurgical but also postsurgical information related to the tumor affected tissue for a more accurate postoperative prognosis.

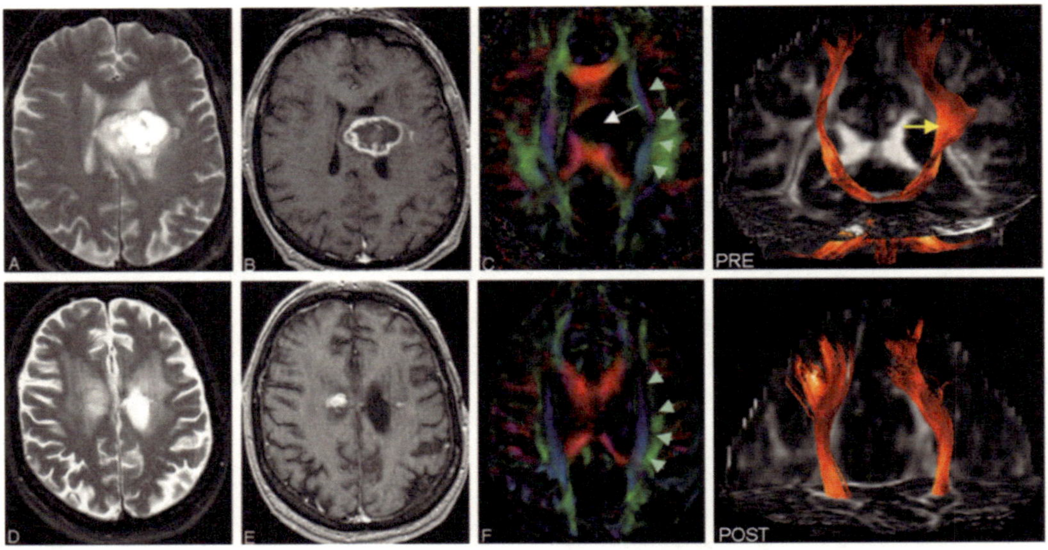

Fig. 6. MR images of a grade III glioma in the superior medial region of the left frontal lobe of a patient before (upper panels) and after (lower panels) surgery. A, D: T2W images, B, E: Gd-enhanced T1W images, C, F: anisotropy weighted color maps allow differentiation of WM fiber tracts (green arrows) located in the tumor (white arrow) vicinity, PRE, POST: tractograms of the cortico-spinal tract. Yellow arrow signals deviation and deformation of the tract in the tumor proximity. (Lazar, Alexander et al. 2006). Reproduced with permission.

As shown in figure 6, DTI is probably one of the most useful clinical applications in this direction, but one of the major obstacles for accurate reconstruction of white matter trajectories is the use of an adequate and suitable tracking algorithm. Simple tracking algorithms are not appropriate in anatomically complex fascicular pathways often leading to incorrect directional information. To solve this, sophisticated algorithms have been developed to improve reconstruction of fiber tracts in these complex areas. Even more, one of the main challenges in DTI fiber tractography studies is to have the skill to reconstruct white matter tracts related to a specific network. This becomes even more complicated in the presence of a tumor where functionally relevant regions are displaced or infiltrated in the surrounding tissue. That goal has encouraged some authors to develop strategies by combining functional MRI and DTI (fMRI-guided DTI) to define related structures based on functional anatomy for subsequent fiber tracking (Kleiser, Staempfli et al.). Obviously, the ability to extract the most useful information from DTI acquisition in diagnosis, prognosis and therapy validation of gliomas is an active and challenging area of interest in clinic and research.

3.4 Assessment of treatment response with diffusion MRI

Since ADC measurements are able to monitor cancer progression, they may be also sensitive to assess the effectiveness to therapy. An increase in the translational motion of water molecules is expected when there are physiological responses like a loss of membrane integrity, a decrease in cellularity, changes in cellular size, extracellular volume or membrane permeability (Hamstra, Rehemtulla et al. 2007). Even more, changes in ADC have been reported to be dose dependent either on chemotherapy or radiotherapy in human brain tumors (Chenevert, Stegman et al. 2000). Concluding, by carrying out DWI studies and determining diffusion coefficients in glioma patients it is possible to distinguish different regions within the tumor, not accessible to conventional MRI techniques as well as to obtain an early prediction of the therapeutic efficacy.

3.4.1 Functional Diffusion Maps

More recently Functional Diffusion Maps (fDMs) were developed as a new application of DWI that can be used as a surrogate biomarker for brain tumor cellularity (Ellingson, Malkin et al. ; Moffat, Chenevert et al. 2005). fDMs obtained computationally allow establishing the correlation between water diffusivity and cellularity mainly to predict the effectiveness of tumor treatment on a voxel-by-voxel pixel analysis. These color based maps are obtained by comparing diffusion MR images at two time points, before and after therapy, to evaluate quantitatively the therapeutic-induced changes in ADC values of the tumor. These maps are depicted in three colors by segmenting the tumor in different regions depending on the magnitude and directions of the ADC changes, allowing the use of this computational analysis as a surrogate marker of the early tumor response to the treatment as depicted in figure 7.

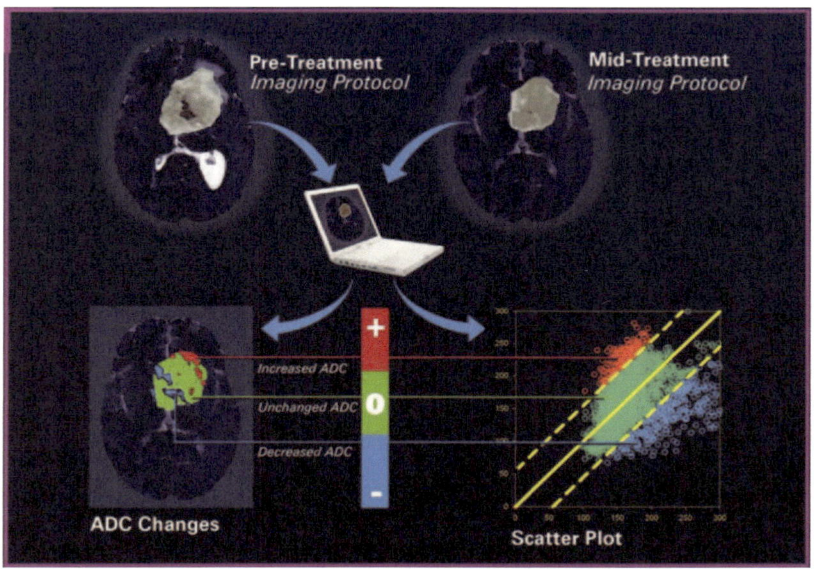

Fig. 7. fMD map involving coregistration of images before and after the treatment. A three-color overlay of postprocessed and analyzed maps show ADC values in the tumor that are unchanged (green), significantly increased (red), or significantly decreased (blue). These regions may be associated to unresponsive (green) or responsive (red, blue) regions. Data can be also represented in a scatter plot allowing quantitative assessment of ADCs changes (Moffat, Chenevert et al. 2006). Reproduced with permission.

Some authors have concluded that fDMs as obtained from the analysis of longitudinal diffusion images appear as a potent tool to detect the therapeutic response of tumors through the early detection of induced changes in their morphology (Moffat, Chenevert et al. 2006; Hamstra, Galban et al. 2008). A patient with a brain tumor that shows significant changes in its ADC values after treatment is supposed to be responsive to therapy. There is the hypothesis that the water liberated by cell necrosis as induced by therapy is the major mechanism for the induced ADC increase. So, the magnitude of change in tumor water diffusion as detected by MRI is related to the quantity of cells killed by therapy and hence, to its efficacy. These changes precede the volume changes in the tumor by several weeks, providing the main justification for DWI as an early predictor of treatment response in individual patients. Even more, no changes in diffusion coefficient indicate a therapeutically unresponsive tumor suggesting the prescription of an alternative therapeutic option.

4. Perfusion magnetic resonance imaging

Clinical perfusion MRI measurements are currently recognized as one of the most powerful tools to assess tumor vascularisation and responses to treatment through the evaluation of hemodynamic parameters. MRI approaches to measure perfusion, can be divided in two broad classes: those monitoring tissue signal changes using an exogenous relaxation contrast agent and those that use endogenous contrast. MR perfusion weighted imaging (PWI) allows for the noninvasive estimation of tumor grade preoperatively. This can help by directing the surgeon to biopsy the most aggressive portions of the neoplasm. In addition, perfusion MR provides an exquisite delineation of tumor margins and it is useful in the follow-up of brain tumor patients after treatment by allowing differentiation between radiation effects and recurrent tumor zones. Looking into the future, perfusion changes in brain tissues hold promise as surrogate markers of response to therapy in clinical trials of new antiangiogenic drugs.

4.1 Physiological principles

Histopathology as gold standard of tumor grading suffers of several limitations. Mainly, since just a few samples of tissue are obtained after biopsy, the most malignant regions may be missed. Neovascularization is one of the most important criteria of malignancy for glioma grading. Malignant astrocytomas recruit existing vessels in the microenvironment and lead to form new vascular networks to supply the nutrients and oxygen required for tumor growth and proliferation. Hence, it is widely accepted nowadays the importance of neoangiogenic pathways in the treatment of brain tumors, since tumor growth of a few millimeters, involves the development of sufficiently competent networks of vascular supplies (Folkman 1971). The net result is a complex system of abnormal vessels in the peritumoral space, characterized by abnormal blood flow and increased permeability to macromolecules, both factors being potentially used as biomarkers for the evaluation of tumor growth. Concomitantly, tumor vessels are more tortuous than the healthy brain, increasing the distance that blood must travel as it moves through the tumor. Perfusion abnormalities are therefore detected not only because the increased number of vessels in gliomas but also for the aberrant reaction of those vessels to the environment. Under these circumstances, disruption of angiogenesis plays an important role in established therapies of gliomas and in the development of new ones.

4.2 Techniques and methods

Currently, there are three principal methods to measure hemodynamic perfusion parameters by using MRI: T2*-weighted DSC, ASL, and T1-weighted DCE acquisitions, respectively. Any of them involves the serial acquisition of images through the brain as magnetically labelled blood passes through it. The labelling procedure can be either based on an exogenous contrast material, typically a paramagnetic complex of gadolinimum (Gd), or on an endogenous magnetic label. Among them, T2*W dynamic susceptibility imaging is probably the most consolidated method to carry out MR perfusion in clinical environments not only in brain oncology but also in many other pathologies, mainly neurodegenerative diseases.

4.2.1 Dynamic Susceptibility Contrast

Nowadays, PWI employing DSC techniques is one of the most relevant procedures of functional MRI with an increasing number of clinical applications depending on software and hardware availability. DSC enhanced images allow for the evaluation of regional cerebral hemodynamics by analyzing changes in the intensity of the MR signal during the first pass (and often second) of a narrow and concentrated bolus of an exogenous CA, through the brain microvascular bed. This technique is often called *bolus tracking* and performs perfusion measurements employing very rapid imaging to capture the first pass of a rapidly injected intravenous contrast material (Rosen, Belliveau et al. 1990), exploiting the T2* susceptibility effects induced by the large local concentrations of the agent rather than the T1 shortening effects routinely used in contrast enhancement by conventional MRI. For accurate assessment of the circulation it is necessary to measure signal drop during the passage of the bolus with sequences endowed with high sensitivity and temporal resolution to the magnetic susceptibility changes occurring in the tissue during the pass of the agent. One approach is to use EPI sequences enabling acquisition times of less than one second because the whole raw data set of an image is acquired after a single spin excitation. EPI is merely a read-out technique and can be combined with any technique of spin excitation (such as spin-echo or gradient echo). Due to the special readout scheme of EPI, and because major parts of k-space are affected by T2*, each EPI sequence is inherently T2* sensitive.

In the brain, the first-pass extraction of the agent is zero when the blood-brain barrier (BBB) is intact, and the complete intravascular compartmentalization of the contrast creates strong, microscopic magnetic susceptibility gradients. These gradients cause dephasing of spins as the spins diffuse through the vessel. In general, pulse sequences without complete refocusing of static field inhomogeneities, as such gradient-echo (GE) will suffer a general signal loss due to the presence of microscopic field disturbances in the vessels. In terms of relaxivity, the shortening of T1 values affects only those protons near the unpaired electron clouds of the agent. This is a short-range effect. A distinct feature of the signal loss on T2*W images is that all protons near the CA are affected because the magnetic susceptibility effect spreads far beyond the immediate vicinity of the agent. This is considered a long-range effect. However, direct damage of the BBB in a tumor may cause a disruption in it and a leakage of contrast material, a circumstance indicating that the factors responsible of the observed MR signal may be more complex.

Experimentally, the contrast medium at high concentrations (narrow bolus), induces T2* shortening yielding firstly a signal loss, followed by a recovery as the agent is diluted in tissues (i.e. healthy brain and tumor). So, the bolus can be tracked by the acquisition of a multislice series of T2*-sensitive images from which a graph of relative signal intensity against time can be composed showing the pixel by pixel effects of the CA transit in the image. There is an approximate linear relationship between tissue contrast agent concentration and change in T2* relaxation rate, and from the signal-time course, the concentration-time course of the contrast medium can be calculated with the expression:

$$Ct\ (t) = -1/TE\ [\ln\ (St-S_0)] \qquad (2)$$

where Ct(t) is the concentration of the agent, St is the signal intensity at any time point, S_0 is the basal signal intensity before the CA injection and TE the echo time. The concentration of contrast medium is linearly proportional to changes in rate of relaxation T2* (R2*). MR data can then be converted to $\Delta R2^*$ versus time evolution and these values can be fitted to a gamma variate function to correct for tracer recirculation. Assuming uniform arterial concentration profiles in all arterial inputs, relative cerebral blood volume (CBV) measurements are determined simply by integrating the area under the concentration time curve (figure 8). The peak integral (that is, the peak area under the curve) is taken as the relative CBV because this represents the volume of the effect. Other parameters of interest that can be measure in the curve are the time to peak (TTP) and the mean transit time (MTT), although the true MTT requires knowledge of the input function of the bolus. Figure 8 depicts a simulation of the process.

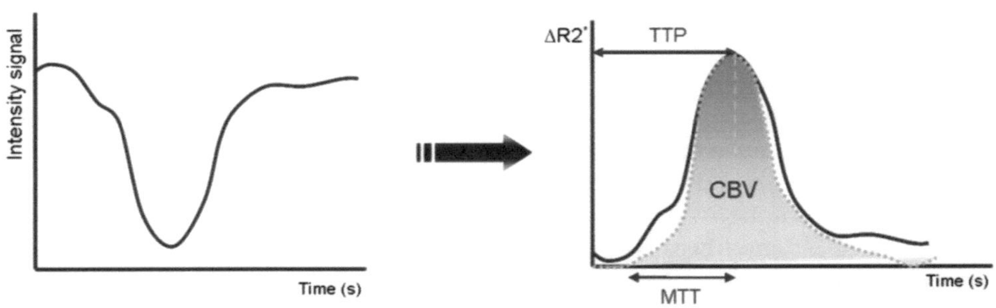

Fig. 8. Schematic behaviour of MR signal intensity as CA passes across the imagin plain in brain tissue

In this way, post-processing of DSC enhanced MR images allows mapping CBV, cerebral blood flow (CBF) and MTT by using singular value decomposition and deconvolution (Ostergaard, Weisskoff et al. 1996). Regional CBV (rCBV) is defined as the total volume of blood traversing a given brain region, measured in milliliters of blood per gram of brain tissue (mL/g). Regional CBF (rCBF) is defined as the net volume of blood traversing a given brain region per unit time, measured in milliliters of blood per gram of brain tissue per minute (mL/g/min). The definition of regional MTT is more complex, but it can be described as the average amount of time it takes any water molecule or particle of CA to pass through the capillary bed, that is, to transverse between arterial inflow and venous outflow measured in seconds (s) (Covarrubias, Rosen et al. 2004). rMTT is equal to the ratio rCBV/rCBF and although CBV may be measured with other methods, MTT measurements necessarily rely on techniques sensitive to motion.

The higher vascularity of gliomas is usually assessed with PWI methods by measuring CBV in the tumor. A potential problem with the use of these techniques arises in regions of severe BBB disruptions as it happens in high-grade gliomas. The leakage of the contrast medium into the extravascular space during its first passage across the tumor capillary bed, increases signals above baseline due to the T1 shortening effect of the paramagnetic label used. Since the algorithm used to calculate CBV assumes a constant baseline, this signal increasing relies in an area above the concentration curve of CA versus time (left panel in figure 8) interpreted as a negative blood volume. This may yield a significant underestimation of CBV in gliomas (Aronen and Perkio 2002). Several improvements and multiple methods have been proposed to address this problem. One of the most extensively used in clinical settings is the presaturation of the extravascular extracellular space in the lesion with the preinjection of a low dose of CA (0.05 mmol/Kg) before starting perfusion MR acquisition with a normal dose of Gd (typically 0.2 mmol/Kg) intravenously injected at a high rate. Another approach consists in using a dysprosium (Dy) based contrast medium as a paramagnetic metal with stronger T2* effects than Gd but only slight capability in T1 shortening (Vander Elst, Roch et al. 2002). A third option to reduce T1 effects goes through increasing the repetition time (TR) which reduces T1 effects but increases total acquisition time, thus reducing temporal resolution.

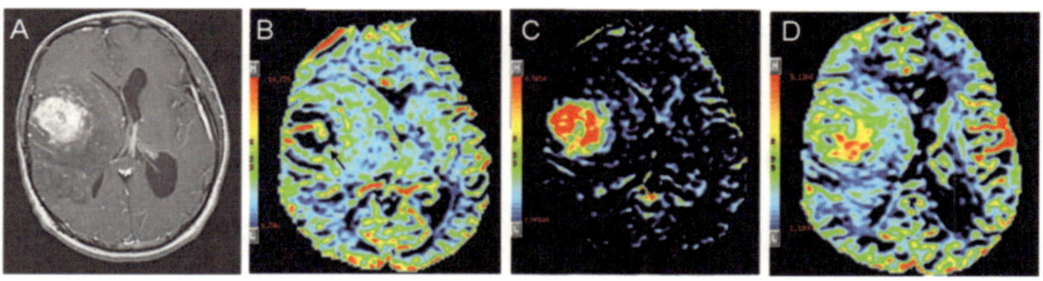

Fig. 9. Correction of CBV underestimation in a high-grade glioma. A: T1W image (Gd 0.2 mmol/Kg) shows an enhanced mass. B: Uncorrected CBV map shows low CBV within the lesion (black arrow). C: K2 first-pass permeability map shows increased permeability within the lesion, consistent with severe BBB breakdown. D: Corrected CBV map shows increased CBV within the lesion, as expected for a high-grade neoplasm (Covarrubias, Rosen et al. 2004) Reproduced with permission.

In addition, different computational approaches have been reported to avoid the CBV underestimation. In these methods, the images are mathematically corrected to account for extravasation of contrast material in regions of BBB breakdown under the premise that the observed Gd concentration can be divided in intra- and extravascular components (Aronen and Perkio 2002; Provenzale, Wang et al. 2002). With these methods, based in a two-compartmental model, permeability can be estimated in regions of BBB disruption by generation of permeability (K2) maps that can be used to correct CBV as shown in figure 9.

Although DSC has the potential to allow quantitative imaging of perfusion parameters at a high signal to noise ratio in a short scan time, quantification of MTT and CBF depends critically on accurate and precise measurement of an arterial input function (AIF). The AIF relies on the measurement of the signal response in the artery or arteries that feed the tissue of interest. This is one factor that limits the ability to quantitate hemodynamic parameters from DSC studies. To measure AIF the imaging planes through the brain have to be chosen to contain a major intracranial artery feeding the tissue, typically one paraclinoid internal carotid artery or the middle cerebral artery (Covarrubias, Rosen et al. 2004). Then, a deconvolution algorithm is used to post-process the data and generate CBF and MTT maps. However, the absolute determination of hemodynamic parameters in not a crucial factor in grading human gliomas, the resulting ratios being equally valid for this purposes since they incorporate the measurement errors from both values.

4.2.2 Dynamic Contrast Enhancement

Dynamic contrast-enhanced T1W MRI (DCE-MRI) was developed in the 1990s for estimating BBB leakage (Tofts and Kermode 1991). It is entirely an approach to measure perfusion based on the T1 shortening caused by the infusion of a paramagnetic contrast media. The main objective of this technique is to measure tumor permeability by dynamic T1W imaging after the intravenous administration of a contrast medium. Typically, a single lower dose (0.1 mmol/Kg) and a lower rate than in DSC studies is injected to the patient followed by repetitive image acquisitions (every 15-30 seconds) through the tumor up to 5-10 minutes rather than the first pass of the bolus. The method is focussed in allowing the leakage of the CA into the extravascular space and coming into equilibrium after several passes of the bolus through the microvascular tumor bed.

In this sense, one of the main advantages of this method is that the extravasation of the contrast material through the BBB is not an artefact to be corrected. Dynamic T1W MRI acquisitions afford better visualization of tumoral heterogeneity in gliomas, improving the accuracy of the technique to detect tumor staging, tumor recurrence and follow-up response to therapies.

Appropriate information from DCE images requires measuring the real T1 values of the tissues to take them as a baseline to perform an accurate pharmacokinetic analysis (Evelhoch 1999). To get an optimal temporal resolution, three dimensional imaging schemes are typically used obtaining the arterial input function in the centre of the acquisition volumes. Hence, data acquisition parameters may influence data analysis and it is necessary to optimize them. Several post-processing methods have been developed to measure perfusion in gliomas using DCE approaches. M. Pauliah et al. described an improved procedure to perform cerebral perfusion maps using a spoiled gradient-recalled echo sequence and reporting not only morphological but also functional information in a single imaging acquisition (Pauliah, Saxena et al. 2007). Authors estimate a quantitative evaluation of both regional CBV and CBF using singular value decomposition (SVD)-based deconvolution techniques in which the concentration of contrast material passing through a given voxel can be expressed as a convolution of the AIF with the residue function tissue concentration (Ostergaard, Sorensen et al. 1996; Ostergaard, Weisskoff et al. 1996). Figure 10 shows one particular case from this study.

In summary, DCE is a powerful tool capable of providing quantitative assessment of contrast uptake and characterization of microvascular structure in human gliomas. Even more, several comparative studies have reported that DCE MRI studies of tumour enhancement in glioma patients can be used for repeated studies with reasonable reproducibility (Jackson, Jayson et al. 2003).

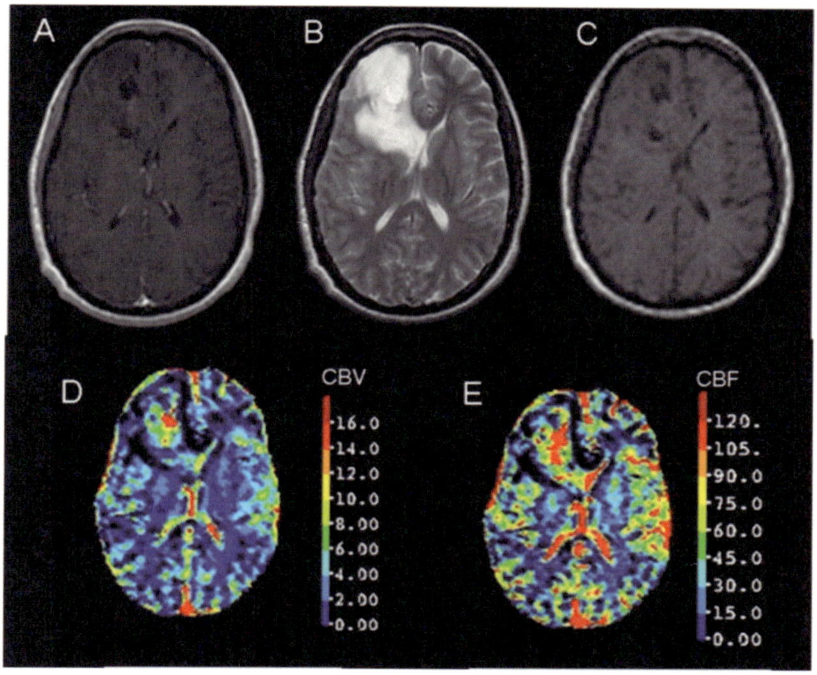

Fig. 10. DCE images of a patient with histologycally proved astrocytoma grade III. A: Post Gd-injection T1W image. B: T2W image. D: T1W image (without CA administration). C: CBV and E: CBF maps generated

4.2.3 Arterial Spin Labelling

ASL perfusion imaging in the brain adds a new functional dimension to non invasive evaluation of the brain functionality with MRI. It is the only method that yields quantitative monitoring of cerebral perfusion over a period of several hours. Its non invasive nature allows an unlimited number of repeated measurements to be made with a high temporal resolution. ASL uses spatially selective inversion of the inflowing arterial blood magnetization as a method to label water molecules in blood. So, in a typical experiment the arterial blood is tagged and after a given delay, this tagged blood arrives at the imaging plane and an image is acquired. The MRI signal from inverted magnetization is made negative relative to uninverted one. When the labelled blood reaches the tissue, it attenuates the pre-existing signal from the image of that tissue. Therefore, a control measurement is required without tagging the arterial blood. The difference in signal intensity between both images is proportional to rCBF, through a calibration factor that depends primarily on global properties of blood. A schematic diagram of the process is shown in figure 11. This difference signal measures how much of the original arterial magnetization created by the inversion pulse has been delivered to the voxel and survives to the time of measurement. The magnetization difference (control minus taged) carried out into the voxel can be conceptually similar to a contrast material delivered to it by CBF. Under this assumption the same kinetic modelling arguments used in bolus tracking or DSC studies can be applied to ASL (Buxton, Frank et al. 1998). Nevertheless, several premises remain to be taken into account for an accurate quantification of CBF by using ASL. The method necessarily has to: i) perform an accurate control measurement; ii) create a well-defined tagged bolus of arterial blood, waiting sufficiently long for the bolus to be delivered to the imaging plane; and iii) account for relaxation of the magnetization label (Buxton 2005).

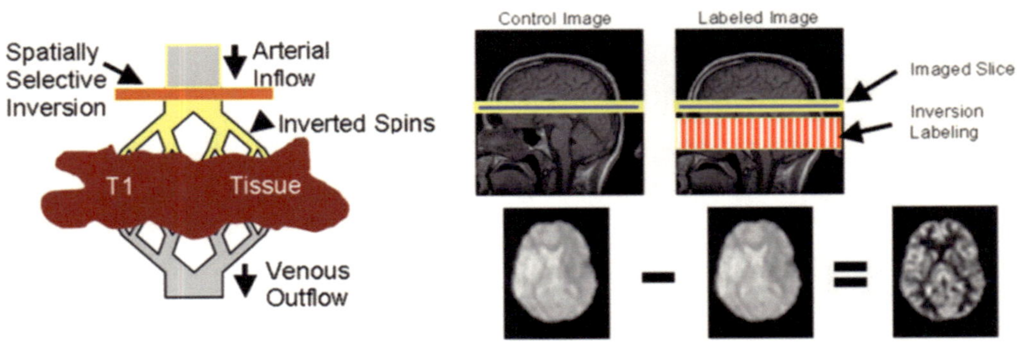

Fig. 11. Fundamentals of the ASL method: Arterial blood is tagged by inverting the magnetization and, after a delay, it arrives to imaging plane decreasing its intensity in manner proportional to blood flow (taken from "ASL Perfusion Imaging: Concepts and Applications", David C. Alsop., ISMRM-2006). Reproduced with permission.

ASL is an attractive and ingenious method for clinical applications because it does not use an intravenous contrast agent, but merely a manipulation of the proton spin of water molecules within the vasculature, that has the potential to provide a robust estimation of CBF. Hence, the agent used in ASL for assessing perfusion is labelled water and not a paramagnetic or superparamagnetic contrast medium, potentially affecting the physical, chemical or physiological properties of the blood. Another advantage of this approach is that it is independent of tumor permeability, without the need to perform additional corrections in the post-processing of the data. The perfusion map obtained by difference of images is available just after acquisition with minimal post-processing, representing a clear benefit in routine clinical settings. On the other hand, ASL leads reliable absolute quantification of CBF that is not affected by BBB damages.

The ASL methods apply a powerful magnetic gradient to invert the inflowing blood magnetization tagging it as it flows upstream. ASL techniques can be divided in two main classes, depending on how the tag is applied: continuous (CASL) or pulsed (PASL). In CASL the inflowing arterial blood is continuously labelled bellow the slab to be imaged until the tissue magnetization gets a steady state (Petersen, Zimine et al. 2006). In PASL the spin inversion is achieved using short inversion pulses in a thick slab located next to the slice of interest. This method is easier to implement and has less practical problems as compared with CASL (Petersen, Zimine et al. 2006). Interestingly, PASL does not suffer as many magnetization transfer effects as CASL methods, and the selective inversion applied is closer to the image slices yielding smaller signal attenuation because of the reduced transit delay and a better inversion efficiency. Even more, short inversion pulses minimize problems of energy deposition in humans at high fields.

ASL has been also used as a functional method to detect CBF changes in local CBF during task activation as a surrogate marker or neuronal activity. This can be very helpful in the assessment of gliomas. To investigate if ASL methodologies contribute measurements that can be used as reliable markers of tumor grade, several studies have compared the perfusion results obtained by MRI with histological data in glioma patients (Warmuth, Gunther et al. 2003; Wolf, Wang et al. 2005). As perfusion MR leads to images of the entire neoplasm, these can help in characterizing the malignancy in gliomas overcoming some of the limitations of histopathology sampling. In this line, ASL perfusion images allow delineating tumor heterogeneity and this can be used to guide biopsy towards the most malignant region of the tumor. Some examples of perfusion maps obtained from ASL acquisitions in gliomas are shown in Figure 12.

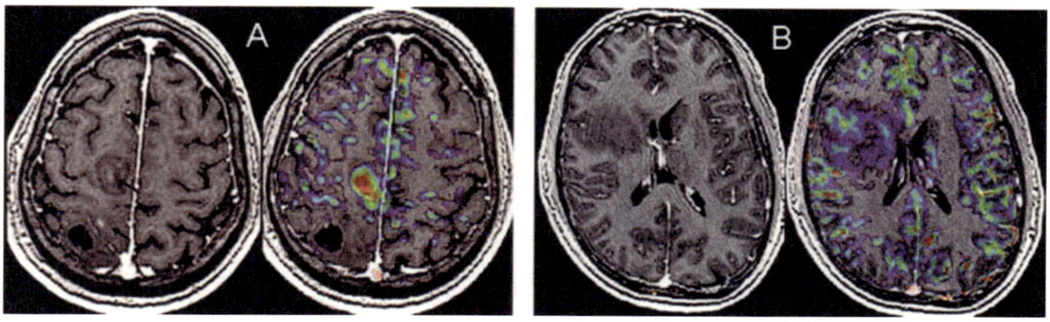

Fig. 12. Differential diagnosis of gliomas using ASL perfusion. A: Giant cells glioblastoma. B: Anaplastic astrocytomas. In both, left: post-contrast T1W; right: perfusion map from PASL (Tourdias, Rodrigo et al. 2008). Reproduced with permission.

A close relationship has been established between ASL and bolus tracking methods in determining CBF in brain tumors, been both approaches able to differentiate between high-grade and low-grade gliomas. Probably, the main limitation of using ASL sequences is that they only allow for the calculation of CBF, whereas MR perfusion measurements based on the administration of a contrast material can provide additionally, CBV and MTT values by using DSC methods (T2*W based images), and permeability values by DCE sequences (T1W based images). This additional information may contribute appreciably to the characterization and grading of gliomas. On the other hand, comparative studies in glioma patients have shown that the ASL technique is more suitable than exogenous contrast-based perfusion analysis for assessing hypervascularized lesions, whereas it has a bigger error rate in the assessment of hypovascularized ones (Warmuth, Gunther et al. 2003).

4.3 Tumor grading by perfusion MRI

Current methods to grade gliomas have inherent limitations, the infiltrative proliferation as an intrinsic feature of the tumor becoming a significant problem. Conventional MR images with CA provide important information regarding Gd-based enhancement that is useful in characterizing tumor grade. The most malignant enhancing brain tumors include

high-grade gliomas, metastases, and lymphomas. These methods assign the most aggressive and malignant grade to the most enhanced tumors, but regarding the gliomas, this is not always reliable. A high-grade glioma may be often mistaken for a low-grade one when images show minimal edema, no gadolinium enhancement, no necrosis and no mass effect. Equally, low-grade gliomas can depict sometimes peritumoral edema, contrast enhancement, necrosis and mass effect leading to a high-grade false diagnosis (Law, Yang et al. 2003). In histopathology grading of gliomas, tumor cellularity and vascularity are the major factors to be taken into account. This information is accessible by the advanced functional MRI methodologies detailed in this chapter and can help in brain tumor grading. As regarding perfusion-based maps it is widely accepted that high regional CBV is more likely in high-grade gliomas. This parameter can reflect tumor vascularity and be used as an indicator of histological grade. In fact, many groups have shown the ability of DSC MRI for estimating the histopathological glioma grade. Several studies reported rCBV values measured in a large number of brain tumor patients suggesting that this parameter can improve distinction between high-grade and low-grade gliomas (Aronen, Gazit et al. 1994; Calli, Kitis et al. 2006) with a high true-positive rate and a very low false-negative rate. On the other hand, gliomas have a great histopathological variability and in this sense, perfusion maps allow also for the localization of foci with very high rCBV values within the tumor. PWI can thus be very helpful not only for a valuable preoperative grading, but also for guiding the surgeon to the most appropriate site to obtain a representative biopsy of the most malignant portion.
Although CBV is the most commonly used hemodynamic parameter in glioma grading, the largest limitation, entailing special clinical relevance, is the lack of discrimination between anaplastic gliomas and glioblastoma multiforme, the two most aggressive tumors of the high-grade glioma group. Perfusion MRI studies report no significant difference in rCBV for both of them (Covarrubias, Rosen et al. 2004).

4.4 Assessment of permeability with perfusion MRI

A link between permeability, angiogenesis and malignancy in gliomas is normally assumed. Several perfusion MRI studies suggest a correlation between permeability and malignancy, but they do not establish a link between angiogenesis and permeability or angiogenesis and malignancy. What is widely accepted is that high permeability to macromolecules, due to the presence of endothelial gaps in tumor vasculature, is an important mediator of tumor growth and a pathognomonic feature for malignancy. Permeability studies are typically based in the determination of the transfer constant of contrast between the plasma and the extravascular extracellular space (K^{trans}). Measurements of K^{trans} are increasingly popular as a method for the quantification of contrast enhancement since they are designed to describe the distribution of contrast agent, free from scanning and machine dependant variables, which allow comparison of results from different studies and imaging centers. Nowadays, perfusion MRI parameters such as K^{trans} and CBV can be directly correlated with histopathological changes in the brain.
T1W dynamic contrast MRI is probably the preferred method to analyze vascular permeability in gliomas and for mapping tumor angiogenesis. There are important studies showing a strong correlation between tumor grade and microvascular permeability by using DCE imaging methods (Roberts, Roberts et al. 2002). The net result is that blood vessel

permeability in gliomas can be used as a non invasive surrogate marker able to provide information related to rate of angiogenesis in the tumor. High-grade gliomas depict high vascular permeability, a consequence of the massive BBB disruption leading to extravasation of contrast material into the extravascular space that becomes detectable in MR images.

Although studies in humans have been typically carried out with DCE methods, it is also possible to perform and compare permeability measurements in grading gliomas employing T2* DSC techniques, within certain limitations (Provenzale, Wang et al. 2002). In this case, the K^{trans} maps can be generated by employing a calculation that allows the separation of T1 effects from the analysis. The advantage of using this method is that it is possible to obtain CBV and permeability maps from the same data set, providing simultaneously, two types of valuable information.

4.5 Assessment of treatment response with perfusion MRI

At present, the predominant method to assess tumor response to treatment is to measure the size of the lesion by using conventional, paramagnetically enhanced MRI. However, tumor size is not always specific of tumor behaviour and neoplastic features associated with aggressiveness of the tumor may vary without changes in the tumor size. On the other hand, since angiogenesis plays a critical role not only in the development of brain tumors but also in the malignant transformation, many of the novel therapies currently investigated are focused on antiangiogenic strategies. Monitoring the success of such therapeutic methods relies on the ability to quantify tumor vascularization through the measurements of hemodynamic parameters. It is widely accepted now that the use of quantitative measurements of tissue enhancement characteristics provides a more valuable indicator to monitor the therapeutic response of tumours to novel antiangiogenic drugs in the treatment of gliomas. For example, rCBV is supposed to reflect microvessel density, an early response in this parameter to antiangiogenic therapies should show a decrease, thus providing the potential to predict growth or regression.

Figure 13 shows a clear example of this behaviour. While T1W images show tumor growth even 6 weeks after initiating the treatment, rCBV maps from PWI depict a much earlier drop in tumor perfusion. This demonstrates that tumor size and perfusion may lead opposite conclusions because they represent indeed, different tumor features.

Because the increase in endothelial permeability is a primary effect of vascular endothelial growth factor (VEGF) and other angiogenic cytokines, changes in the capillary leakage of contrast media may offer a predictable response to anti-angiogenic therapies. Quantification of the enhancement effect is therefore a good candidate as a potential biomarker of drug activity. Changes in permeability occur rapidly in response to VEGF inhibitions, so assessment of these changes either by DSC or DCE can be used as a marker of antiangiogenic therapy responses. Although quantification of permeability would be an optimal strategy, this is in fact, extremely difficult to achieve. Along these lines, several pharmacokinetic models to analyze dynamic enhancement data have been developed to estimate K^{trans} and used it as an therapeutic indicator (Jackson, Jayson et al. 2003). Now, it is accepted and recommended the use of perfusion MRI to monitor tumor angiogenesis and evaluate the response to antiangiogenic therapies, a subject that has gained considerable clinical and research efforts, even leading to published recommendations concerning this important capacity of MRI (Brasch, Li et al. 2000).

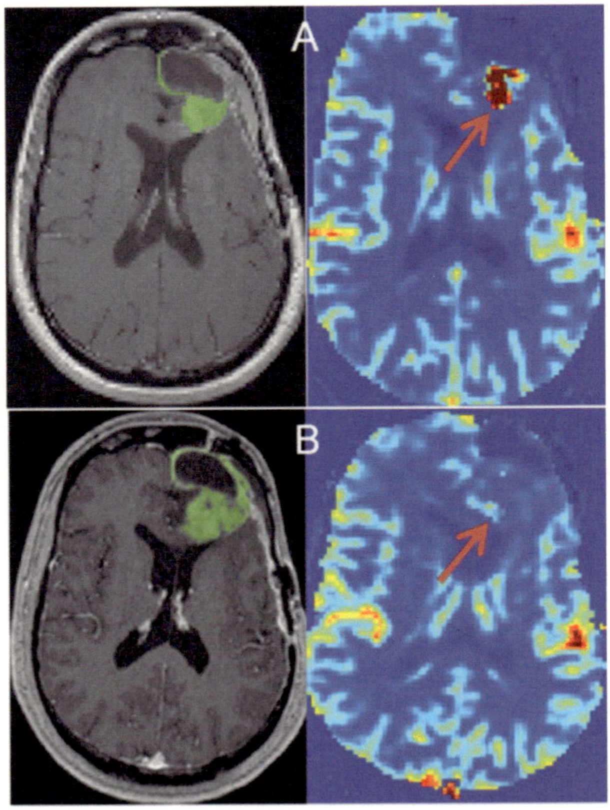

Fig. 13. Change in perfusion in a pathologically confirmed GMB case before (A) and after (B) the initiation of anti-angiogenic chemotherapy. Left images in both panels show contrast enhanced T1W images used to measure tumor volume (green). Right images depict CA leakage corrected rCBV maps showing tumor perfusion (red arrow) (Sawlani, Raizer et al.) Reproduced with permission.

5. Concludig remarks and future perspectives

In summary, we presented an overview of the fundamentals and clinical applications of advanced Magnetic Resonance Imaging protocols providing in situ information on water diffusion and blood perfusion in gliomas. These methodologies have shown considerable ability to provide functional information on the malignancy of these lesions as well as in its response to therapy. Together, they allow for a more adequate patient management based fully in non invasive non destructive examinations. These MRI approaches have been, however, applied independently in most cases. The future use of combinations of these two strategies may offer the possibility to compensate the limitations of one technology with the strengths of the other, still maintaining their non invasive character. In this sense, combined diffusion-perfusion methodologies may provide in the future significant advances, becoming even more effective in clinic for the diagnosis, prognosis and therapy assessment of gliomas.

6. Acknowledgements

This work was supported in part by grants CTQ2010-20960-C02-02 to P.L.L. and grant SAF2008-01327 to S.C. A.M.M. held an Erasmus Fellowship from Coimbra University and E.C.C. a predoctoral CSIC contract. The valuable contribution of Mr. Javier Perez drafting the illustrations is gratefully acknowledged.

7. References

Aronen, H. J., I. E. Gazit, et al. (1994). "Cerebral blood volume maps of gliomas: comparison with tumor grade and histologic findings." Radiology 191(1): 41-51.

Aronen, H. J. and J. Perkio (2002). "Dynamic susceptibility contrast MRI of gliomas." Neuroimaging Clin N Am 12(4): 501-23.

Basser, P. J. and D. K. Jones (2002). "Diffusion-tensor MRI: theory, experimental design and data analysis - a technical review." NMR Biomed 15(7-8): 456-67.

Brasch, R. C., K. C. Li, et al. (2000). "In vivo monitoring of tumor angiogenesis with MR imaging." Acad Radiol 7(10): 812-23.

Brunberg, J. A., T. L. Chenevert, et al. (1995). "In vivo MR determination of water diffusion coefficients and diffusion anisotropy: correlation with structural alteration in gliomas of the cerebral hemispheres." AJNR Am J Neuroradiol 16(2): 361-71.

Bulakbasi, N., M. Kocaoglu, et al. (2003). "Combination of single-voxel proton MR spectroscopy and apparent diffusion coefficient calculation in the evaluation of common brain tumors." AJNR Am J Neuroradiol 24(2): 225-33.

Buxton, R. B. (2005). "Quantifying CBF with arterial spin labeling." J Magn Reson Imaging 22(6): 723-6.

Buxton, R. B., L. R. Frank, et al. (1998). "A general kinetic model for quantitative perfusion imaging with arterial spin labeling." Magn Reson Med 40(3): 383-96.

Calli, C., O. Kitis, et al. (2006). "Perfusion and diffusion MR imaging in enhancing malignant cerebral tumors." Eur J Radiol 58(3): 394-403.

Covarrubias, D. J., B. R. Rosen, et al. (2004). "Dynamic magnetic resonance perfusion imaging of brain tumors." Oncologist 9(5): 528-37.

Chenevert, T. L., L. D. Stegman, et al. (2000). "Diffusion magnetic resonance imaging: an early surrogate marker of therapeutic efficacy in brain tumors." J Natl Cancer Inst 92(24): 2029-36.

Chien, D., R. B. Buxton, et al. (1990). "MR diffusion imaging of the human brain." J Comput Assist Tomogr 14(4): 514-20.

Detre, J. A., J. Wang, et al. (2009). "Arterial spin-labeled perfusion MRI in basic and clinical neuroscience." Curr Opin Neurol 22(4): 348-55.

Ellingson, B. M., M. G. Malkin, et al. "Validation of functional diffusion maps (fDMs) as a biomarker for human glioma cellularity." J Magn Reson Imaging 31(3): 538-48.

Evelhoch, J. L. (1999). "Key factors in the acquisition of contrast kinetic data for oncology." J Magn Reson Imaging 10(3): 254-9.

Folkman, J. (1971). "Tumor angiogenesis: therapeutic implications." N Engl J Med 285(21): 1182-6.

Furnari, F. B., T. Fenton, et al. (2007). "Malignant astrocytic glioma: genetics, biology, and paths to treatment." Genes Dev 21(21): 2683-710.

Gauvain, K. M., R. C. McKinstry, et al. (2001). "Evaluating pediatric brain tumor cellularity with diffusion-tensor imaging." AJR Am J Roentgenol 177(2): 449-54.

Gideon, P., C. Thomsen, et al. (1994). "Increased self-diffusion of brain water in hydrocephalus measured by MR imaging." Acta Radiol 35(6): 514-9.

Hajnal, J. V., M. Doran, et al. (1991). "MR imaging of anisotropically restricted diffusion of water in the nervous system: technical, anatomic, and pathologic considerations." J Comput Assist Tomogr 15(1): 1-18.

Hamstra, D. A., C. J. Galban, et al. (2008). "Functional diffusion map as an early imaging biomarker for high-grade glioma: correlation with conventional radiologic response and overall survival." J Clin Oncol 26(20): 3387-94.

Hamstra, D. A., A. Rehemtulla, et al. (2007). "Diffusion magnetic resonance imaging: a biomarker for treatment response in oncology." J Clin Oncol 25(26): 4104-9.

Jackson, A., G. C. Jayson, et al. (2003). "Reproducibility of quantitative dynamic contrast-enhanced MRI in newly presenting glioma." Br J Radiol 76(903): 153-62.

Jakab, A., P. Molnar, et al. "Glioma grade assessment by using histogram analysis of diffusion tensor imaging-derived maps." Neuroradiology.

Jenkinson, M. D., D. G. Du Plessis, et al. (2007). "Advanced MRI in the management of adult gliomas." Br J Neurosurg 21(6): 550-61.

Kinoshita, M., K. Yamada, et al. (2005). "Fiber-tracking does not accurately estimate size of fiber bundle in pathological condition: initial neurosurgical experience using neuronavigation and subcortical white matter stimulation." Neuroimage 25(2): 424-9.

Kleiser, R., P. Staempfli, et al. "Impact of fMRI-guided advanced DTI fiber tracking techniques on their clinical applications in patients with brain tumors." Neuroradiology 52(1): 37-46.

Kono, K., Y. Inoue, et al. (2001). "The role of diffusion-weighted imaging in patients with brain tumors." AJNR Am J Neuroradiol 22(6): 1081-8.

Krabbe, K., P. Gideon, et al. (1997). "MR diffusion imaging of human intracranial tumours." Neuroradiology 39(7): 483-9.

Larsson, H. B., F. Courivaud, et al. (2009). "Measurement of brain perfusion, blood volume, and blood-brain barrier permeability, using dynamic contrast-enhanced T(1)-weighted MRI at 3 tesla." Magn Reson Med 62(5): 1270-81.

Larsson, H. B., C. Thomsen, et al. (1992). "In vivo magnetic resonance diffusion measurement in the brain of patients with multiple sclerosis." Magn Reson Imaging 10(1): 7-12.

Law, M., S. Yang, et al. (2003). "Glioma grading: sensitivity, specificity, and predictive values of perfusion MR imaging and proton MR spectroscopic imaging compared with conventional MR imaging." AJNR Am J Neuroradiol 24(10): 1989-98.

Lazar, M., A. L. Alexander, et al. (2006). "White matter reorganization after surgical resection of brain tumors and vascular malformations." AJNR Am J Neuroradiol 27(6): 1258-71.

Le Bihan, D., E. Breton, et al. (1986). "MR imaging of intravoxel incoherent motions: application to diffusion and perfusion in neurologic disorders." Radiology 161(2): 401-7.

Lu, S., D. Ahn, et al. (2003). "Peritumoral diffusion tensor imaging of high-grade gliomas and metastatic brain tumors." AJNR Am J Neuroradiol 24(5): 937-41.

Lyng, H., O. Haraldseth, et al. (2000). "Measurement of cell density and necrotic fraction in human melanoma xenografts by diffusion weighted magnetic resonance imaging." Magn Reson Med 43(6): 828-36.

Moffat, B. A., T. L. Chenevert, et al. (2005). "Functional diffusion map: a noninvasive MRI biomarker for early stratification of clinical brain tumor response." Proc Natl Acad Sci U S A 102(15): 5524-9.

Moffat, B. A., T. L. Chenevert, et al. (2006). "The functional diffusion map: an imaging biomarker for the early prediction of cancer treatment outcome." Neoplasia 8(4): 259-67.

Mori, S. and P. B. Barker (1999). "Diffusion magnetic resonance imaging: its principle and applications." Anat Rec 257(3): 102-9.

Mori, S. and P. C. van Zijl (2002). "Fiber tracking: principles and strategies - a technical review." NMR Biomed 15(7-8): 468-80.

Nucifora, P. G., R. Verma, et al. (2007). "Diffusion-tensor MR imaging and tractography: exploring brain microstructure and connectivity." Radiology 245(2): 367-84.

Ostergaard, L. (2005). "Principles of cerebral perfusion imaging by bolus tracking." J Magn Reson Imaging 22(6): 710-7.

Ostergaard, L., A. G. Sorensen, et al. (1996). "High resolution measurement of cerebral blood flow using intravascular tracer bolus passages. Part II: Experimental comparison and preliminary results." Magn Reson Med 36(5): 726-36.

Ostergaard, L., R. M. Weisskoff, et al. (1996). "High resolution measurement of cerebral blood flow using intravascular tracer bolus passages. Part I: Mathematical approach and statistical analysis." Magn Reson Med 36(5): 715-25.

Pacheco-Torres, J., D. Calle, et al. "Environmentally sensitive paramagnetic and diamagnetic contrast agents for nuclear magnetic resonance imaging and spectroscopy." Curr Top Med Chem 11(1): 115-30.

Pauliah, M., V. Saxena, et al. (2007). "Improved T(1)-weighted dynamic contrast-enhanced MRI to probe microvascularity and heterogeneity of human glioma." Magn Reson Imaging 25(9): 1292-9.

Petersen, E. T., I. Zimine, et al. (2006). "Non-invasive measurement of perfusion: a critical review of arterial spin labelling techniques." Br J Radiol 79(944): 688-701.

Price, S. J., N. G. Burnet, et al. (2003). "Diffusion tensor imaging of brain tumours at 3T: a potential tool for assessing white matter tract invasion?" Clin Radiol 58(6): 455-62.

Provenzale, J. M., S. Mukundan, et al. (2006). "Diffusion-weighted and perfusion MR imaging for brain tumor characterization and assessment of treatment response." Radiology 239(3): 632-49.

Provenzale, J. M., G. R. Wang, et al. (2002). "Comparison of permeability in high-grade and low-grade brain tumors using dynamic susceptibility contrast MR imaging." AJR Am J Roentgenol 178(3): 711-6.

Reardon, D. A., J. N. Rich, et al. (2006). "Recent advances in the treatment of malignant astrocytoma." J Clin Oncol 24(8): 1253-65.

Roberts, H. C., T. P. Roberts, et al. (2002). "Quantitative estimation of microvascular permeability in human brain tumors: correlation of dynamic Gd-DTPA-enhanced MR imaging with histopathologic grading." Acad Radiol 9 Suppl 1: S151-5.

Rosen, B. R., J. W. Belliveau, et al. (1990). "Perfusion imaging with NMR contrast agents." Magn Reson Med 14(2): 249-65.

Sawlani, R. N., J. Raizer, et al. "Glioblastoma: a method for predicting response to antiangiogenic chemotherapy by using MR perfusion imaging--pilot study." Radiology 255(2): 622-8.

Schaefer, P. W., P. E. Grant, et al. (2000). "Diffusion-weighted MR imaging of the brain." Radiology 217(2): 331-45.

Schluter, M., B. Stieltjes, et al. (2005). "Detection of tumour infiltration in axonal fibre bundles using diffusion tensor imaging." Int J Med Robot 1(3): 80-6.

Stejskal, E. O. and J. E. Tanner (1965). "Spin Diffusion Measurements: Spin Echoes in the Presence of a Time-Dependent Field Gradient." The Journal of Chemical Physics 42(1): 288-292.

Sugahara, T., Y. Korogi, et al. (1999). "Usefulness of diffusion-weighted MRI with echo-planar technique in the evaluation of cellularity in gliomas." J Magn Reson Imaging 9(1): 53-60.

Thomsen, C., O. Henriksen, et al. (1987). "In vivo measurement of water self diffusion in the human brain by magnetic resonance imaging." Acta Radiol 28(3): 353-61.

Tien, R. D., G. J. Felsberg, et al. (1994). "MR imaging of high-grade cerebral gliomas: value of diffusion-weighted echoplanar pulse sequences." AJR Am J Roentgenol 162(3): 671-7.

Tofts, P. S. and A. G. Kermode (1991). "Measurement of the blood-brain barrier permeability and leakage space using dynamic MR imaging. 1. Fundamental concepts." Magn Reson Med 17(2): 357-67.

Tourdias, T., S. Rodrigo, et al. (2008). "Pulsed arterial spin labeling applications in brain tumors: practical review." J Neuroradiol 35(2): 79-89.

Tropine, A., G. Vucurevic, et al. (2004). "Contribution of diffusion tensor imaging to delineation of gliomas and glioblastomas." J Magn Reson Imaging 20(6): 905-12.

Vander Elst, L., A. Roch, et al. (2002). "Dy-DTPA derivatives as relaxation agents for very high field MRI: the beneficial effect of slow water exchange on the transverse relaxivities." Magn Reson Med 47(6): 1121-30.

Warach, S., D. Chien, et al. (1992). "Fast magnetic resonance diffusion-weighted imaging of acute human stroke." Neurology 42(9): 1717-23.

Warmuth, C., M. Gunther, et al. (2003). "Quantification of blood flow in brain tumors: comparison of arterial spin labeling and dynamic susceptibility-weighted contrast-enhanced MR imaging." Radiology 228(2): 523-32.

Witwer, B. P., R. Moftakhar, et al. (2002). "Diffusion-tensor imaging of white matter tracts in patients with cerebral neoplasm." J Neurosurg 97(3): 568-75.

Wolf, R. L., J. Wang, et al. (2005). "Grading of CNS neoplasms using continuous arterial spin labeled perfusion MR imaging at 3 Tesla." J Magn Reson Imaging 22(4): 475-82.

13

Assessment of Rodent Glioma Models Using Magnetic Resonance Imaging Techniques

Rheal A. Towner, Ting He, Sabrina Doblas and Nataliya Smith
Advanced Magnetic Resonance Center, Oklahoma Medical Research Foundation
Oklahoma City
U.S.A.

1. Introduction

There is a strong need to obtain precise surrogate biomarkers to improve the accuracy of diagnosis for gliomas, and to effectively evaluate therapeutic response. Often pre-clinical models of disease are used to develop diagnostic procedures and assess the effectiveness of a potential therapy. For gliomas, there are a variety of rodent models that have been investigated by numerous investigators over the past few decades, ranging from intracranial rodent glioma cell implantation models, intracranial human glioma xenografts, orthotopic implantation of human glioma stem cells, multipotent human glioblastoma stem-like neurosphere lines, transgenic mouse models, to viral-induced progenitor or stem cell derived glioma models. Tumor grades in these models vary from low to high grade tumors, with many of the high-grade glioma models sharing some of the characteristics of human grade IV glioblastoma multiforme (GBM). Many of the characteristic features of gliomas can be assessed diagnostically with *in vivo* imaging techniques such as magnetic resonance imaging (MRI). MRI has the capability of obtaining morphological/anatomical, functional, biophysical, molecular and metabolic information of a disease at various pathological stages of development. Tumor characteristics often associated with aggressive gliomas include an invasive growth pattern, angiogenesis, necrosis, hypoxia, edema, and alterations in major metabolic pathways. Morphological features, such as tumor size and position, infiltrative growth, hemorrhaging, necrotic lesions, edema, mass effect, heterogeneity, and cyst formation, can be followed using standard contrast-enhanced T_1-weighted MR imaging or non-contrast T_2-weighted imaging.

Although conventional MRI provides us with some indication about the nature of the lesion or tumor, it has limited sensitivity and specificity in determining histological type and grade, delineating margins and differentiating edema, as well as effectively evaluating therapeutic effects or side-effects. Incorporating some advanced MR techniques, such as MR angiography (MRA), perfusion-weighted MR imaging (PWI), diffusion-weighted MR imaging (DWI), MR spectroscopy (MRS), and molecular MRI (mMRI), may help to overcome some of those limitations. Angiogenesis associated with major blood vessels can be assessed using MR angiography, whereas perfusion-weighted imaging can be used to monitor angiogenesis associated with capillary vessels in tumors. Biophysical parameters such as water diffusion, as measured by diffusion-weighted imaging, have also provided information regarding alterations in tissue structure associated with glioma tumors. An extension of the diffusion-weighted imaging technique is diffusion tensor imaging (DTI), which can provide information on white matter neuronal fiber tractography. MR spectroscopy can be used to assess alterations in tumor metabolites associated with glucose, bioenergetics, amino acid or lipid metabolism, for example. Many of these advanced MR techniques are used in a clinical setting. More recently, molecular MRI (mMRI) which incorporates a MRI contrast agent as a signaling molecule and an affinity component that targets specific tumor markers associated with tumor growth, angiogenesis, cell invasion, inflammation, or apoptosis, can be used to characterize *in vivo* molecular events associated with gliomas.

This review will focus on various glioma models that have been studied *in vivo*, with particular emphasis on MR image and/or spectroscopy evaluation of these models, and the use of MR image criteria (morphological, biophysical, molecular and metabolic) to evaluate therapeutic treatments. The aims are to: (1) provide an overview on current rodent glioma models being studied; (2) provide an overview regarding currently used MR methods, including advanced MR techniques (e.g. MRA, DWI, PWI, MRS and mMRI), relevant to glioma research; and (3) summarize studies that have used MR methods to evaluate therapeutic response in pre-clinical models for gliomas.

2. Human gliomas

Gliomas represent 40% of all primary central nervous system (CNS) tumors diagnosed. Among them, glioblastomas (GBM) are the most malignant, with a very poor survival time of about 15 months for most patients diagnosed with this grade IV brain tumor (CBTRUS 2011). High grade gliomas are the most common primary brain tumors in adults, and their malignant nature ranks them as the fourth largest cause of cancer death (Niclou *et al.*, 2010). There are four tumor grades for gliomas: Grade I which is a non-malignant, fairly circumscribed astrocytoma that is rare and appears in young adults; Grade II which are a more common diffusely infiltrating astrocytoma; Grade III which is an anaplastic astrocytoma; and Grade IV which is a glioblastoma multiforme (Niclou *et al.*, 2010). Grades II-IV gliomas generally are found in the adult population, and often recur following current treatment options (including surgical resection, radiotherapy, and chemotherapy) (Niclou *et al.*, 2010).

Grading and identification criteria that can be used to provide information regarding tumor behavior are cell proliferation (cellularity and mitotic activity), nuclear atypia, neovascularization and the presence of necrosis and/or apoptotic regions (Gudinaviciene *et al.*, 2004). Grade II gliomas (also referred to as diffuse astrocytomas) and grade III gliomas (also referred to as anaplastic astrocytomas) only differ based on their mitotic activity, and this difference accounts for a substantial decrease in the 5-year survival for patients, from 47% to 29% (from grade II to III, respectively) (CBTRUS 2011). Grade IV gliomas (GBM) are often characterized by the presence of large necrotic areas (Gudinaviciene *et al.*, 2004) and generally have a 3% 5-year survival (CBTRUS 2011).

3. Rodent models of gliomas

Animal models are often used when researching a disease and trying to understand how a particular pathological process occurs, as well as a means of studying the efficacy of potential new therapies. This review will provide examples of commonly used and new experimental animal models for gliomas, which make up a large portion of primary brain tumors. The majority of models involve intracerebral implantation of rodent (rat or mouse) or human glioma cells into synergetic rats or mice, or immunocompromised rodents (e.g. nude or athymic rats or mice). There are also a limited number of transgenic mouse models for gliomas. One approach to better simulate a human tumor is to obtain human glioma neurospheres from patients during tumor resection, and then culture the cells prior to intracerebral implantation into immunocompromised rodents. Another recent approach is to implant non-replicating viruses that can stimulate neuronal stem cells to turn into glioma cells which develop into diffuse tumors similar to those found in high-grade or malignant gliomas called, glioblastoma multiforme (or GBM).

3.1 Intracerebral cell implantation models

Glioma cells (rat, mouse or human origin) are injected into the cerebral cortex of rats or mice (synergetic if cells are transplanted into the same species and strain that they were obtained from, or immune-compromised rats or mice if human cells are used) using a stereotaxic device for precise implantation into a brain region. As tumors grow over a period of 1-2 months, this model is considered a short-term model. Different cell lines varying in their degree of malignancy, such as rat C6, 9L/LacZ, F98 and RG2 cells, mouse GL261 cells and human U87 cells, provide a range of gliomas from moderately aggressive to GBM-like.

Many of these models have some characteristics associated with human gliomas, such as aggressive tumor growth, angiogenesis, and tumor necrosis (in a few models), however the diffuse nature of high-grade gliomas, glioblastoma multiforme (GBM), is not well represented. In many instances the intracerebrally-implanted rodent tumors have defined tumor boundaries, which do not represent the infiltrative nature of GBMs well. A comprehensive review that discusses the advantages and disadvantages of rat brain tumor models, most of them involving intracerebral implantation of rat glioma cells, is discussed in a paper by Barth and Kaur (2009).

The rat C6 cell line produces diffusively invasive astrocytomas (Barth, 1998; Barth and Kaur, 2009), which have been found to be similar to human glioma cells regarding the expression of genes mainly involved in tumor progression (Sibenaller *et al.*, 2005). C6 gliomas were induced in an outbred Wistar rat strain repeatedly injected with methylnitrosourea (MNU), which makes it non-syngeneic in inbred strains, and increases its potential to evoke an alloimmune response (Barth and Kaur, 2009). As a result of some genetic similarities to human gliomas, the C6 model has been widely used as a GBM model for a number of years (Grobben *et al.*, 2002; Barth and Kaur, 2009). The 9L/LacZ-derived tumors are aggressive and infiltrative, and are angiogenic (Plate *et al.*, 1993), which are some of the characteristics associated with human GBM (Weizsaecker *et al.*, 1981). Although the aggressive 9L/LacZ gliomas are highly invasive (Szatmori *et al.*, 2006) and have extensive neovascularization (Plate *et al.*, 1993), due to their pronounced immunogenicity (Barth, 1998) and the fact that they are classified as gliosarcomas (Sibenaller *et al.*, 2005), makes these cells a poor choice for glioma studies. F98 gliomas are classified as anaplastic malignant tumors, which have an infiltrative pattern of growth, and also have attributes associated with human GBM (Barth, 1998; Barth and Kaur, 2009). The aggressive and invasive nature (Barth, 1998; Barth and Kaur, 2009) of RG2 tumors (Groothuis *et al.*, 1983), as well as the highly tumorigenic human glioblastoma U87 MG cell line *(Martens et al.*, 2006; Cheng *et al.*, 1996), both mimics human high-grade gliomas via inducing vascular alterations. U87 pcDNA3 and U87 IRE1 DN human glioma cells were selected as malignant glioma models that form highly versus poorly vascularized tumors, respectively (Drogat *et al.*, 2007; Wehbe *et al.*, 2010). GL261 cells give rise to quickly growing, and diffusively invasive intracranial tumors in C57BL/6 mice (Szatmori *et al.*, 2006). RG2 and F98 glioma cell lines were both obtained from chemical induction as a result of administering ethylnitrosourea (ENU) to pregnant rats, where the progeny developed brain tumors that were isolated, and propagated and cloned in cell culture (Barth and Kaur, 2009). Human U87 cells are of high interest for angiogenesis studies (Cheng *et al.*, 1996). The immunogenicity issue of the 9L/Lacz model can be resolved by using non-immunogenic models (e.g. RG2).

Xenograft models, induced by orthotopic (into native tumor sites) injection of primary tumor cells or tumor cell lines, represent the most frequently used *in vivo* cancer model systems for glioma research (Waerzeggers *et al.*, 2010). Both cell culture and xenograft model systems lack the stepwise genetic alterations that are thought to occur during tumor progression, and often do not represent the genetic and cellular heterogeneity of primary tumors, as well as the complex tumor-stroma interaction (Waerzeggers *et al.*, 2010). Genetically engineered mouse models (discussed below in the "Transgenic Mouse Models" section) better represent the causal genetic events and subsequent *in situ* molecular evolution, the tumor-stroma interactions, and consist of cellular subpopulations such as cancer stem cells (discussed further in the "Human Glioma Neurospheres" and "Viral-Induced Glioma Models" sections below), that occur in native tumors (Waerzeggers *et al.*, 2010).

3.2 Chemical-induced model

Slow-growing, low- and high-grade, spontaneous gliomas can be generated with a chemically-induced model from the administration of ENU (Kish *et al.*, 2001; Koestner, 1990). Transplacental ENU exposure of a pregnant female a day before gestation, results in the formation of low-grade oligodendrogliomas and mixed gliomas, with a tumor incidence approaching 100%, in rat pups at approximately 3-6 months of age (Koestner, 1990). In addition to oligodendrogliomas and mixed gliomas, unfortunately the ENU-induced model also results in the formation of meningiomas (Koestner *et al.*, 1971), spinal cord tumors (Koestner *et al.*, 1971) and other primitive neuroectodermal tumors (Vaquero *et al.*, 1992), decreasing its potential as a reproducible model. In addition to the isolation of RG2 and F98 rat glioma cells from ENU induction, A15A5 neoplastic astrocytes have also been cloned (Davaki and Lantos, 1980).

3.3 Transgenic mouse models

As we are beginning to understand the genetic mutations associated with gliomas, it is possible to generate transgenic mouse models that have these genetic mutations. Recent findings suggest that brain tumors originate from neural stem or progenitor cells. Some examples of transgenic mutations include deletions of gene combinations, such as Rb/p53, Rb/p53/PTEN or PTEN/p53 (Jacques *et al.*, 2010). pRb is a retinoblastoma protein, which is a tumor suppressor protein that is dysfunctional in many cancers. Rb controls excessive cell growth by inhibiting cell cycle progression until the cell is ready to divide (Chinnam and Goodrich, 2011; Lohmann, 2010). p53 which is also known as protein 53 is a tumor suppressor protein responsible for regulating the cell cycle (Kim et al., 2011; Maclaine and

Hupp, 2011; Muller et al., 2011). PTEN, which stands for phosphatase and tensin homolog, is a tumor suppressor gene also involved in the regulation of the cell cycle (Natsume et al., 2011; Alexiou and Voulgaris, 2010). Rb/p53 mice developed malignant tumors in approximately 9 months (Jacques *et al.*, 2010). PTEN/Rb/p53 tumors had an appearance that was similar to the Rb/p53 tumors (Jacques *et al.*, 2010). Deletion of Rb/p53 or Rb/p53/PTEN resulted in the formation of primitive neuroectodermal tumors (PNET), which alludes to the role of an initial Rb loss involved in driving the PNET phenotype (Jacques *et al.*, 2010). It was found that targeted deletion of PTEN and p53 in subventricular zone (SVZ) stem cells resulted in glioma formation with a latency period of approximately 7-8 months (Jacques *et al.*, 2010). The tumors from the recombination of PTEN/p53 were histologically infiltrative, diffuse, necrotic and had signs of micro-vascular proliferation, which are all characteristics of human high-grade gliomas (Jacques *et al.*, 2010).
Another successful transgenic mouse model involves the deletion of the *TP53* (tumor protein 53) gene (*Trp53 null* background), and over-expressing human PDGF (platelet-derived growth factor) under the control of the GFAP (glial fibrillary acidic protein) promoter, which developed tumors with human glioblastoma-like features and with the integrated development of PDGFRα^+ tumor cells and PDGFRβ^+ Nestin$^+$ vasculature in 2-6 months (Hede *et al.*, 2009). The tumor suppressor gene *TP53* is either lost or commonly mutated in astrocytic brain tumors, and these *TP53* alterations are often combined with excessive growth factor signaling via the PDGF/PDGFRα complex (Hede *et al.*, 2009). PDGF is one of many growth factors that regulate cell growth and division, and has been found to be widely associated with malignant gliomas (Calzolari and Malatesta, 2010; Shih and Holland, 2006).

4. Human glioma neurospheres

GBM cancer-initiating cells have been found to mediate resistance to chemotherapy and radiation treatment, both used as follow-up therapies following surgical resection of the main tumor mass (Wei *et al.*, 2010). Cells isolated from GBM that possess the capacity for self-renewal following radiation and chemotherapy, can form neurospheres when cultured *in vitro* (Wei *et al.*, 2010). The glioma-associated cancer-initiating cells were found to express MHC-I (major histocompatibility I) but not MHC-II, CD-40 or CD80, which induces T-cell immune deficiency, and express the costimulatory inhibitory molecule, B7-H1, which plays a role in mediating immune resistance in gliomas and induces T-cell apoptosis (Wei *et al.*, 2010). These neurospheres can be intracerebrally implanted into immune-compromised rodents to develop tumors *in vivo,* and therefore provide an experimental model that more closely resembles recurrent human GBM (radiation and chemotherapeutic resistant and induce immunosuppression) to evaluate new therapies. Another approach that takes into consideration the role of tumor-initiating stem cells, is to orthotopically implant tiny fragments of surgically-resected tumors, containing brain tumor stem cells within the glioblastoma tissue, into immunocompromised mice (xenograft model) brains with the use of a trocar system (Fei *et al.*, 2010).

4.1 Viral-induced glioma models

Glial progenitor cells in the white matter and subventricular zone within the central nervous system were recently found to be the likely candidates for glioma-initiating cells (Assanah *et al.*, 2006, 2009; Masui *et al.*, 2010). Intracerebral implantation of PDGFB-green fluorescent protein (GFP)-expressing retroviruses into rodents were found to induce tumors that closely resembled diffuse human malignant gliomas which have been challenging to treat (Assanah *et al.*, 2006; Masui *et al.*, 2010). This model involves the use of a viral vector that stimulates neuronal stem cells to become glioma cells by expressing PDGF, which is involved in generating tumor cells (Masui *et al.*, 2010). These studies demonstrate that both adult white matter and glial progenitors generate gliomas, as well as recruit resident progenitors to proliferate within the mitogenic environment of a tumor, and therefore contributing to the heterogeneous mass of cells that make up a malignant glioma (Assanah *et al.*, 2006; Masui *et al.*, 2010). It was previously demonstrated that PDGF-B could play a dose-dependent role in glial tumorigenesis, where PDGFR (PDGF receptor) signaling via elevating levels of PDGF-B chain expression quantitatively regulates tumor grade, and that PDGF-B expression is required to sustain high-grade oligodendrogliomas (Shih *et al.*, 2004). PDGF-B expression in tumor cells was elevated by removing inhibitory regulatory elements in the *PDGFB* mRNA and a retroviral delivery system (Shih *et al.*, 2004). To generate tumors, DF1 cells transfected with RCAS (repeat with splice acceptor) retroviral vectors, generating a culture of virus-producing cells, were injected intracranially into N-tva transgenic mice (Shih *et al.*, 2004). By inhibiting PDGFR activity, it was possible to convert tumors from high to low grade (Shih *et al.*, 2004).

Another recent study involved intracranial injection of lentiviral vectors with GFAP (glial fibrially acidic protein) or CMV (cytomegalovirus) vectors into compound *LoxP*-conditional mice, which resulted in K-Ras^{v12} expression and loss of p16^{Ink4a}/p19^{Arf}, with or without concomitant loss of p53 or Pten (de Vries *et al.*, 2010). Like GFAP, CMV is a promoter (de Vries *et al.*, 2010). CMV-Cre injection into *p53;Ink4a/Arf;K-Ras*^{v12} mice was particularly found to result in the formation of high-grade gliomas within 2-3 weeks that had invasiveness and blood-brain barrier functionality characteristics that are found in human high-grade gliomas (de Vries *et al.*, 2010).

5. MRI methods to detect gliomas

Magnetic resonance imaging (MRI) techniques are becoming more commonly used to provide information on brain tumor growth, vasculature, biochemical metabolism, and molecular changes in preclinical models, as MRI is the optimal imaging tool as part of the diagnostic process for human gliomas. Conventional MRI techniques, such as T_1- and T_2-weighted imaging, contrast-enhanced T_1-weighted imaging, dynamic contrast enhanced (DCE) imaging, and diffusion-weighted imaging (DWI) methods can provide useful information on tumor location and extent of growth, blood-brain barrier (BBB) disruption, brain invasiveness, regional blood flow and blood volume, and tumor cellularity, all of which are characteristics associated with glioma grade and prognosis in a clinical setting (Waerzeggers *et al.*, 2010).

Morphological MRI (T_2-weighted or T_1-weighted contrast-enhanced imaging) is used to provide information on tumor volumes and growth rates, which can be used to distinguish between tumor grades. Contrast-enhanced imaging can be used to assesses BBB disruption, however this feature can be absent in diffuse infiltrative tumor regions or when assessing therapeutic treatment (Waerzeggers *et al.*, 2010). DCE imaging can be used to follow tumor angiogenesis by measuring changes in tumor vascular permeability, vascular density and vessel morphology (Waerzeggers *et al.*, 2010), particularly regarding the capillary bed. Magnetic resonance angiography (MRA) is also used to provide information on tumor vasculature associated with angiogenesis, however it tends to be restricted to major blood vessels >50 microns in diameter (Doblas *et al.*, 2010). DWI has been used in cancer imaging to evaluate tumor cellularity and infiltration, as well as monitor therapeutic response (Kauppinen, 2002). Metabolic information can be obtained by monitoring tumor metabolites by a method called MR spectroscopy (MRS), or variations thereof, such as MR spectroscopic imaging (MRSI) or chemical shift imaging (CSI). Molecular alterations can be assessed with the use of targeting MR contrast agents which can specifically indicate levels of cancer biomarkers that may be elevated in malignant tumors. The development of targeted imaging ligands attached to MRI contrast agents allows the *in vivo* evaluation of tumor biology, such as tumor cell apoptosis, angiogenic blood vessels or the expression of specific tumor antigens or signaling pathways (Waerzeggers *et al.*, 2010).

5.1 Tumor morphology

MRI is obtained on small animal MR imaging systems (7 - 11.7 Tesla), that can accommodate rodents such as mice and rats. MR images are obtained in multiple slices (0.5-1 mm thick) to visualize an entire tumor (Gartesier *et al.*, 2010). Examples of rodent tumor models for gliomas (e.g. rat C6 and RG2 models, and mouse GL261 model) are shown in Figure 1, depicting heterogeneous tumors (right cerebral cortex, upper regions) following intracerebral (orthotopic) implantation of rat or mouse glioma cells (Doblas *et al.*, 2010).

From the multiple image slices through a tumor, tumor volumes can be measured, and the growth rate can be calculated from multiple imaging sessions over several days, weeks or months (as shown in Figure 2). Tumor areas are traced in multiple slices to calculate tumor volumes, which can be used to determine tumor growth and doubling times (Doblas *et al.*, 2008, 2010; Garteiser *et al.*, 2010). Robust tumor volume determinations can be made by using manual or automated segmentation techniques, which can be used to delineate tumor margins on the basis of signal intensity differences from surrounding brain tissue (Waldman *et al.*, 2009).

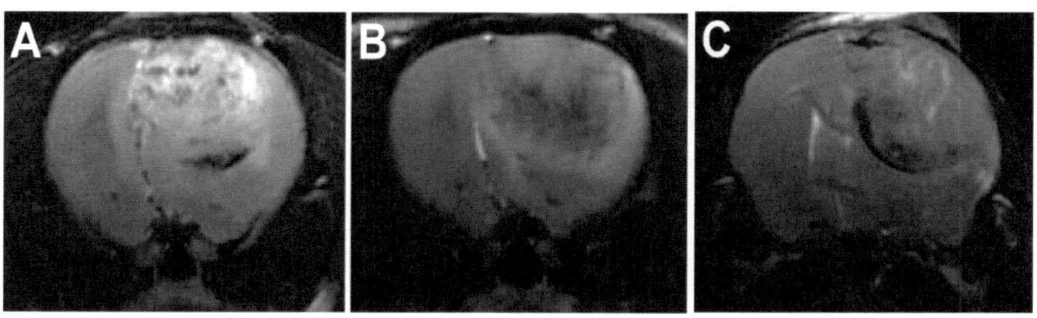

Fig. 1. MR images of rodent gliomas. T_2-weighted images of the rat C6 (A; 18 days following intracerebral implantation of cells) and RG2 (B; 13 days following cell implantation), and the mouse GL261 (C; 26 days following cell implantation) glioma models. Tumors appear as heterogeneous regions in the upper right area of the cerebral cortex regions.

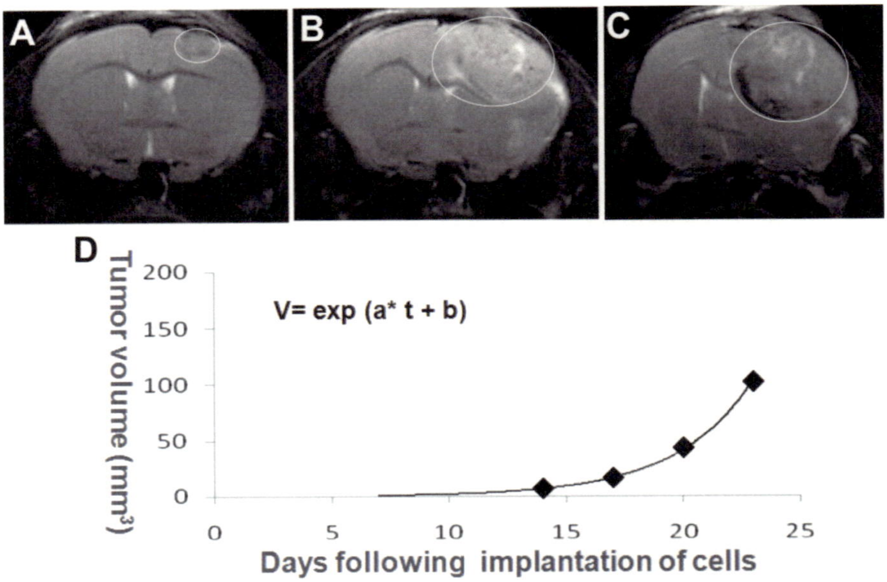

Fig. 2. MR images used to calculate tumor volumes and tumor growth. T_2-weighted images of a mouse GL261 glioma at 14 (A), 23 (B) and 26 days (C) following intracerebral implantation of cells. Tumors are outlined (white ellipses). (D) Calculated GL261 tumor volumes which follow an exponential increase over time.

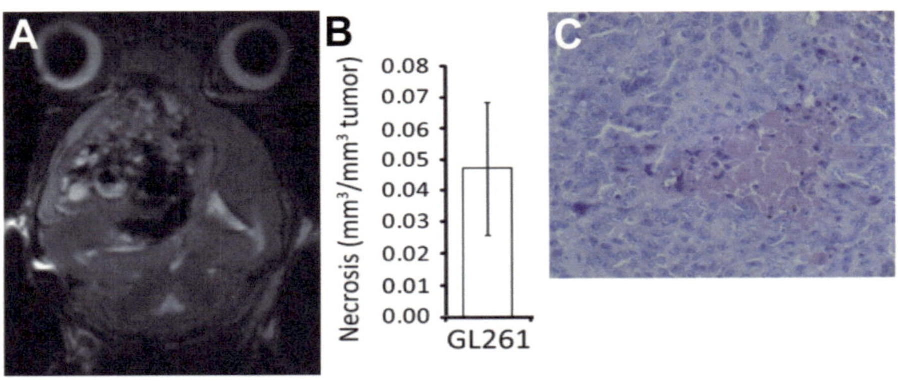

Fig. 3. Determination of necrotic volumes from MR image-observed tumors. (A) T_2-weighted MR image of a GL261 mouse glioma at 23 days following intracerebral implantation of cells. Note dark void regions in the heterogeneous tumor which are necrotic lesions. (B) Necrotic volumes from tumors can be measured (n=5; mean±S.D.). (C) Corresponding histological slide depicting necrosis in a GL261 tumor.

Tumor morphology can also provide information on tumor invasiveness and necrotic lesions. Necrotic lesions are depicted as dark void regions in a tumor (as shown in Fig. 3A), of which volumes (e.g. Fig. 3B) can be measured from multiple slices (Towner *et al.*, 2010a). A comparison between the orthotopic rat glioma models, C6 and RG2, and the chemical

ENU-induced model, indicated that percent necrosis was highest in the ENU model, compared to RG2, and least in the C6 model (Towner *et al.*, 2010a). Although the ENU-induced model is used to generate low-grade gliomas, it generates a heterogeneous population of glioma cells ranging from low- to high-grade, which contributes to the high incidence of necrotic lesions (Towner *et al.*, 2010a). RG2 gliomas are known to be more aggressive, invasive and infiltrative than C6 gliomas (Groothuis *et al.*, 1983). It has also been shown that RG2 gliomas have more diffuse margins at the interface to adjacent brain tissue, whereas C6 gliomas are less infiltrative with a distinct peritumoral region at the margin of the tumor (Doblas *et al.*, 2010).

5.2 Tumor vasculature and ultrastructure

MR angiography can provide information on new blood vessels formed in tumors, a process known as angiogenesis which is required to maintain tumor growth. On small animal imaging MRI systems, the image in-plane resolution is >50 μm, which allows visualization of major blood vessels, arterioles and venules (Doblas *et al.*, 2008, 2010). Quantitation of brain and tumor blood vessels can also be obtained, as well as measurements on blood vessel diameters and lengths (Doblas *et al.*, 2008, 2010). An increase in total brain tumor blood volume was found to directly correlate with increasing tumor volumes during tumor growth (Doblas *et al.*, 2010).

Quantification of the Brownian motion of water or diffusion within tissues can be measured through the apparent diffusion coefficient (ADC) which is obtained from diffusion-weighted imaging datasets. DWI yields ultrastructural information on cellular density and the extracellular matrix (Waldman *et al.*, 2009; Sadeghi *et al.*, 2003). Figure 5 shows an example of an ADC (Fig. 5 b) map in a C6 glioma-bearing rat brain, indicating higher ADC values in tumor tissue compared to contralateral 'normal' brain tissue (Garteiser *et al.*, 2010).

Temporal diffusion spectroscopy based on oscillating gradient spin-echo (OGSE) MRI was used to detect microscopic structural variations at the subcellular scale in C6 rat gliomas

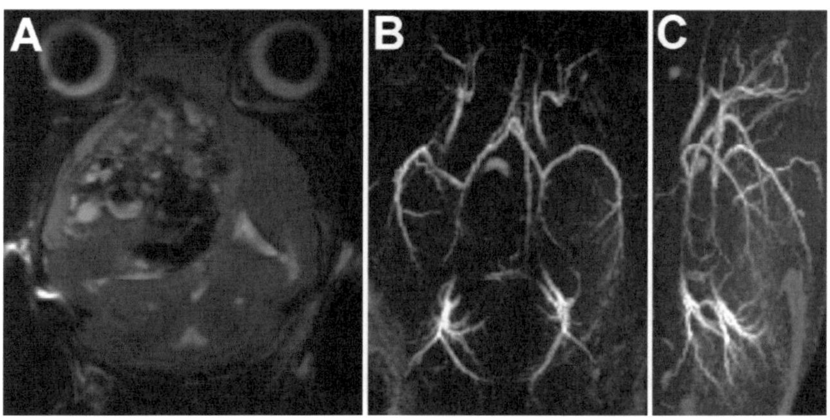

Fig. 4. MR angiography of a GL261 mouse glioma. (A) T_2-weighted MR image of a GL261 glioma-bearing mouse brain (23 days following intracerebral implantation of cells.) (B) and (C), 3 dimensional angiograms of mouse brain blood vessels of a GL261 glioma-bearing mouse. Note altered vasculature on left-hand side in image B, as well as increased blood vessels (middle cerebral artery; depicted in left-mid-region of image C) in the tumor region.

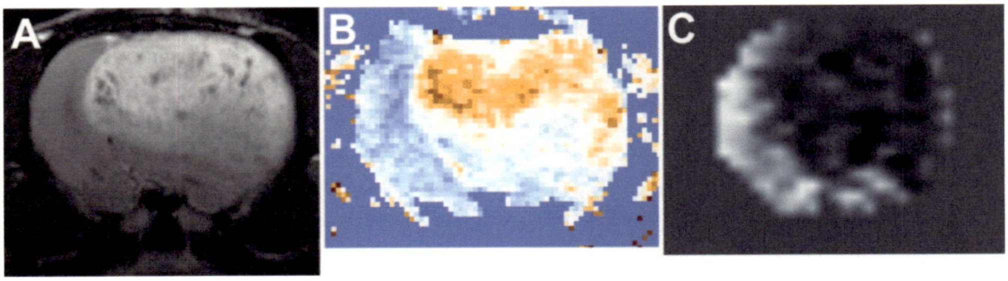

Fig. 5. Diffusion- and perfusion-weighted imaging of a rat C6 glioma. (A) T_2-weighted MR image of a C6 glioma-bearing rat brain (20 days following intracerebral implantation of cells). (B) ADC map (1×10^{-4} mm^2/s) of a C6 glioma. Note higher ADC values in the tumor compared to 'normal' brain tissue. (C) Perfusion map (ml/(100g×min)) in a C6 glioma. Note decreased perfusion values in tumor tissue, compared to 'normal' brain tissue.

(Colvin *et al.*, 2008). An extension of DWI is diffusion tensor imaging (DTI) which obtains multidirectional images that can be used to obtain diffusional directionality information quantified as fractional anisotropy and displayed as dominant white fiber tract maps (tractography) ((Waldman *et al.*, 2009). DTI was used to differentiate between two rat glioma models, which observed C6 glioma-induced ischemia of tumor-surrounding tissues, compared to the more infiltrative nature of F98 gliomas that penetrated into the corpus callosum (Asanuma *et al.*, 2008a, 2008b).

Arterial spin labeling (ASL), a perfusion-weighted MRI method, uses a MR image signal based on the influx of magnetically labeled water into blood, as a means of quantifying absolute levels of cerebral blood flow (CBF) (Waldman *et al.*, 2009). Another widely used perfusion method is dynamic susceptibility contrast MRI (DSC-MRI), which can be used to measure relative cerebral blood volume, relative cerebral blood flow (rCBF) and mean transit time from the kinetics resulting from a change in signal intensity following the bolus administration of a gadolinium (Gd)-based contrast agent (Waldman *et al.*, 2009). Steady-state susceptibility contrast (SSC) images were used to obtain MRI vessel caliber index (VCI) measurements in a xenograft orthotopic U87 mouse brain tumor model, and were found to correlate closely with intravital optical microscopy (IVM) measurements (Farrar *et al.*, 2010). Dynamic contrast-enhanced MRI (DCE-MRI) is commonly used to measure the permeability of the blood-brain-barrier (BBB). The transfer coefficient, K^{trans} is associated with endothelial permeability, vascular surface area and blood flow ((Waldman *et al.*, 2009). DCE-MRI revealed a significant change in tumor vessel permeability that was dependent on tumor progression and size in a GL26 orthotopic mouse glioblastoma model (Veeravagu *et al.*, 2008). Fig. 5C depicts decreased perfusion values in a C6 glioma, compared to contralateral 'normal' brain tissue, obtained using the ASL method. Perfusion values were found to be increased in the more aggressive RG2 rat glioma compared to C6 (Towner *et al.*, 2010a), which is associated with increased vascular proliferation in this model. The increased perfusion in the RG2 model was also correlated with increased capillary vascularity visualized in 3D confocal microscopy fluorescence images, as well as more diffuse and smaller blood vessels observed by MRA, compared to the C6 model (Towner *et al.*, 2010a). A study by Valable *et al.* demonstrated that there was a slight reduction in vessel density in the tumor center within RG2 gliomas compared to a more increased reduction in vessel density within C6 gliomas, which was characterized by an increased blood volume fraction, and a smaller relative increase in vessel size index in the RG2 tumor (Valable *et al.*, 2008). The vessel density eventually decreased with increasing tumor cell proliferation (Valable *et al.*, 2008). It was thought that early expression of Ang-2, MMP-2 and MMP-9, which has been found in C6 gliomas, could account for the destabilization of vessel walls and a reduction in vessel density during C6 tumor growth (Valable *et al.*, 2008).

5.3 Tumor metabolism

Magnetic resonance spectroscopy (MRS) is an MR method that allows regional metabolite levels to be measured in tumors compared to surrounding non-tumor tissue. Important metabolites that can be assessed by ^{1}H-MRS in brain tumors include N-acetyl aspartate (NAA), total creatine (tCr), total choline (tCho), lactate, *myo*-inositol and mobile lipids associated with necrosis. Metabolite levels can be quantified as metabolite ratios or absolute concentrations, or analyzed using pattern recognition (Waldman *et al.*, 2009). Figure 6 depicts an example of regional MR spectra obtained in a rat C6 glioma within tumor and contralateral 'normal' brain tissues. Glioma tissue has characteristic increased mobile lipid signals at 1.3 and 0.9 ppm, as well as decreased NAA, tCr and tCho, compared to surrounding 'normal' brain tissue. Metabolites measured by MRS can provide information on brain tissue status, such as (1) NAA being a marker of healthy neuronal integrity, which is compromised within brain tumors, (2) choline-containing compounds being associated with cell membrane turnover, (3) creatine-containing compounds being associated with the cellular energy status, (4) lactate being linked to anaerobic respiration, and (5) mobile lipids resulting from intracellular lipid droplets and necrosis (Waldman *et al.*, 2009). Spatially resolved ^{1}H-MRS was used to reveal significantly decreased levels of NAA and tCr and increased lactate (or lipids) in intracerebral rat C6 gliomas, compared to the contralateral hemisphere (Ross *et al.*, 1992; Terpstra *et al.*, 1996). In F98 rat gliomas there were detected increases in tCho, *myo*-inositol and lipids, as well as the absence of a NAA signal (Gyngell *et al.*, 1994).

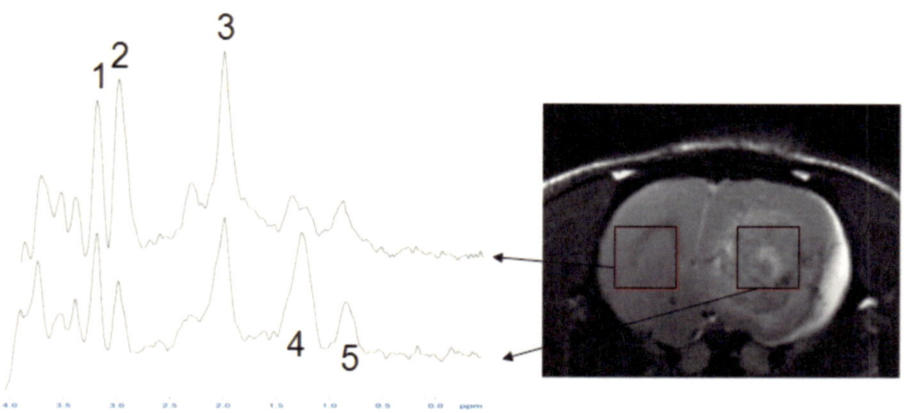

Fig. 6. MR spectroscopy of a rat C6 glioma. Regional (PRESS; point-resolved spectroscopy; 3×3×3 mm^3 or 27 μl volume) was obtained in tumor (right region in T_2-weighted; bottom spectrum) and 'normal' (left region; top spectrum) brain tissues (19 days post-intracerebral implantation of C6 cells). Peak assignments: (1) tCho (total choline), (2) tCr (total creatine), (3) NAA (N-acetyl aspartate), (4) methylene $(-CH_2-)_n$ lipid hydrogens, and (5) methyl $(-CH_3)$ lipid hydrogens.

Other atomic nuclei, other than ^{1}H, have also been used to assess ^{13}C and ^{19}F containing compounds in rodent gliomas. Hyperpolarized ^{13}C MR metabolic imaging was used to follow the metabolism of hyperpolarized [1-(13)C]-pyruvate to lactate in rats with human glioblastoma xenografts (U-251 MG and U-87 MG), indicating higher levels in tumor versus normal brain tissue, and variations between tumor models (Park *et al.*, 2010). Rat 9L glioma cells labeled with perfluoro-15-crown-5-ether *ex vivo* and implanted into rat striatum was used to measure intracellular partial pressure of oxygen (pO_2) (oximetry) in tumors (Kadayakkara *et al.*, 2010).

5.4 Molecular imaging

The concept used in molecular imaging is to couple a targeting moiety (antibody or peptide targeted to a protein of interest) to a reporter molecule, such as a MRI contrast agent. Two commonly used MRI contrast agents are gadolinium (Gd)-based compounds, or iron oxide-based nanoparticles. The targeted MR probes are often injected via a tail-vein in rats or mice. The expression of cell adhesion molecules, such as integrins, has been found to be up-regulated during tumor growth and angiogenesis, and $\alpha_V\beta_3$ expression which has been correlated with tumor aggressiveness, can be measured by MRI with targeted paramagnetic-labeled cyclic arginine-glycine-aspartic acid (RGD) peptides (Sipkins *et al.*, 1998; Waerzeggers *et al.*, 2010). Within U87MG xenograft tumors in nude mice, RGD-labeled ultrasmall superparamagnetic iron oxide (USPIO) probes were found to accumulate only within the neovasculature associated with tumors, but not within tumor cells (Kiessling *et al.*, 2009). Tumor angiogenesis was also monitored via the expression of CD105 in F98 tumor-bearing rats with the use of Gd-DTPA liposomes targeted to CD105 (CD105-Gd-SLs) and MR imaging (Zhang *et al.*, 2009). Combined MRI-coupled fluorescence tomography was used to assess epidermal growth factor receptor (EGFR) status in high- and low-EGFR expression tumor cells injected into nude mice by measuring the levels of a near-infrared fluorophore bound to a EGF ligand (Davis *et al.*, 2010).

MR imaging probes have also been developed to monitor *in vivo* levels of other angiogenic proteins known to be over-expressed in malignant brain tumors, such as VEGF-R2 (vascular endothelial growth factor receptor 2) (He *et al.*, 2010; Towner *et al.*, 2010b); a tumor cell migration/invasion marker, such as c-Met, a tyrosine kinase receptor for the scatter factor (also known as the hepatocyte growth factor) (Towner *et al.*, 2008, 2010c); and the inflammatory marker, inducible nitric oxide synthase (iNOS) (Towner *et al.*, 2010a). With the use of a Gd-DTPA-albumin-anti-VEGFR2-biotin probe, regional differences in VEGFR2 levels were detected by MRI *in vivo* in a C6 glioma model, and probe-specificity for glioma tissue, particularly in the peri-tumor and peri-necrotic regions, was confirmed by tagging the biotin moiety of the probe in excised tissues with streptavidin-Cy3 (He *et al.*, 2010). The control non-specific probe had rat IgG conjugated to the albumin, instead of the VEGFR2 antibody. A similar result was obtained when an aminated dextran-coated iron-oxide nanoparticles conjugated with a VEGFR2 antibody was used in a C6 glioma model, where distribution of the probe was mainly in the peri-tumor and peri-necrotic regions of the tumor (He *et al.*, 2010). Confirmation of the presence of the nanoprobes was obtained by using Prussian blue stain for the VEGFR2-targeting iron oxide nanoparticles in excised tumor tissues (He *et al.*, 2010).

Both Gd- and iron oxide-based probes were also developed to characterize c-Met levels in C6 gliomas. c-Met is a tumor marker that is over-expressed in many malignant cancers, indicative of the invasive nature of a tumor. The distribution of c-Met was found to be more widely dispersed, but mainly concentrated in peri-tumor regions (Towner *et al.*, 2008, 2010c). Figure 7A depicts the contrast-enhancement in a C6 glioma 3 hours following i.v. administration of a Gd-DTPA-albumin-anti-c-Met-biotin probe, and the corresponding perfusion map showing the increased uptake of the anti-c-Met probe in the peri-tumor regions (Towner *et al.*, 2008).

iNOS levels were found to vary in different rat glioma models, as detected with a Gd-DTPA-albumin-anti-iNOS-biotin (anti-iNOS) probe, where percent MRI signal intensity changes were highest in the C6 tumor, compared to the RG2 and ENU-induced tumors (Towner *et al.*, 2010a). Dynamic kinetic monitoring of the anti-iNOS probe indicated sustained uptake over 3 hours within tumor tissue regions, and no specific uptake of a control Gd-DTPA-albumin-IgG-biotin contrast agent within tumors (Towner *et al.*, 2010a). Fluorescence imaging of the anti-iNOS probe by targeting the biotin moiety with streptavidin-Cy3, verified higher levels of probe uptake in C6 tumors versus RG2 gliomas, despite the increased perfusion and micro-vascularity detected in the RG2 tumors (Towner *et al.*, 2010a). Confirmation of the presence of iNOS in glioma cell membrane, but not in normal astrocytes, was obtained by transmission electron microscopy of gold-labeled anti-iNOS antibodies (Towner *et al.*, 2010a).

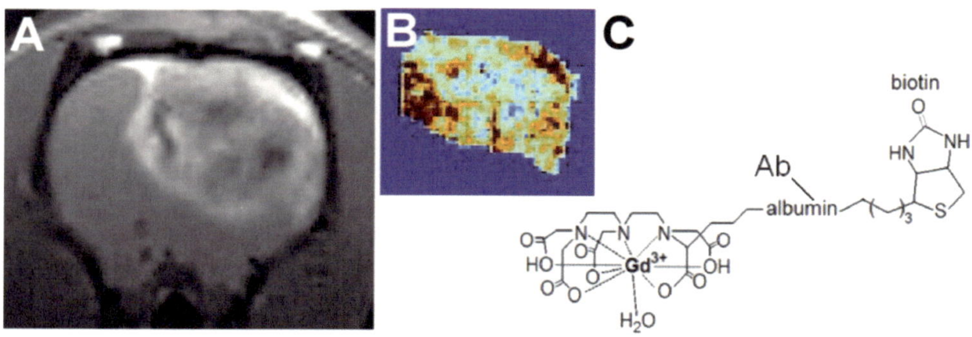

Fig. 7. Molecular MR imaging of c-Met levels in a rat C6 glioma. (A) T_1-weighted MR image 3 hours following i.v. administration of a Gd-DTPA-albumin-anti-c-Met-biotin probe. Note contrast enhancement in peri-tumor regions. (B) Perfusion map depicting distribution of the anti-c-Met probe. (C) Illustration of the Gd-DTPA-albumin-anti-c-Met-biotin probe, with the antibody (Ab) conjugated to albumin.

6. MRI evaluation of therapeutics against gliomas

Clinically, therapeutic response to surgical resection of gliomas, followed by radiation and chemotherapy, can be assessed by dynamic contrast-enhanced morphological MRI, increases in ADC values detected by DWI (Waerzeggers *et al.*, 2010), decreases in the fractional tumor volume with a corresponding low relative cerebral blood volume detected by perfusion imaging, and/or reduced choline levels detected by MRS (Waldman *et al.*, 2009). DCE-MRI was used to establish reduced Gd enhancement consistent with decreased vascular permeability following i.v. bevacizumab and carboplatin therapy in a human glioma (UW28) nude rat model (Jahnke *et al.*, 2009). DCE-MRI using a high molecular weight contrast agent, albumin-Gd-DTPA, showed significantly increased K^{trans} at the rim of a VEGFR tyrosine kinase inhibitor (Vetanalib, PTK787) (anti-angiogenic) treated U251 gliomas in rats (Ali *et al.*, 2010). Low-molecular-weight (Gd-DOTA; gadoterate meglumine) and macromolecular (P846, 3.5 kDa) MR contrast-enhanced imaging was used to assess the therapeutic effect of an anti-angiogenic compound, sorafenic, and microbeam radiation therapy in a 9L gliosarcoma model, finding that anti-angiogenic therapy decreased tumor vessel permeability to the macromolecular contrast agent (Lemasson *et al.*, 2010). Dynamic perfusion MRI using iron oxide nanoparticles (ferumoxytol) was used to assess the vascular effects of an anti-angiogenic agent versus corticosteroid (dexamethasone) treatment in a U87MG human glioma model in athymic rats, which found that bevacizumab significantly decreased the tumor blood volume and decreased permeability as determined by an increased time-to-peak enhancement (Varallyay *et al.*, 2009).

Morphological MRI, MR angiography and perfusion imaging were used to assess the therapeutic efficacy of nitrone-based compounds as anti-glioma agents in a rat C6 glioma model. It was demonstrated that the nitrone, α-phenyl-*tert*-butyl nitrone (PBN) was able to prevent and/or decrease tumor volumes (by ~60-fold, with significance, $p<0.001$), increase animal survival (>90%), and decrease total tumor blood volumes (by ~20%), in comparison to non-treated rats bearing C6 gliomas (Doblas *et al.*, 2008). Another cohort of rats were intracerebrally implanted with C6 glioma cells, monitored for tumor growth, and when tumors reached a volume of ~50 mm^3 (approximately at 15 days post-intracerebral implantation of C6 glioma cells), PBN was administered (drinking water, 0.065% w/v) for a period of 25 days (Doblas *et al.*, 2008). In the post-tumor treatment group, PBN was found to increase survival (40% of the treated rats, $p<0.05$), and decrease tumor volumes by ~2-fold, but was found to be non-significant (Doblas *et al.*, 2008). Regarding post-tumor treatment, PBN was also found to not significantly affect blood tumor volumes, compared to non-treated rats (Doblas *et al.*, 2008). It was concluded from these studies that PBN, when administered prophylactically, may have an effect on angiogenesis (Doblas *et al.*, 2008).

Conversely, rats post-tumor treated with a PBN-derivative, OKN-007, were found to have significantly decreased tumor volumes (~3-fold, $p<0.05$), decreased the apparent diffusion coefficients (ADC) (~20%, $p<0.05$), and increased tissue perfusion rates (~60%, $p<0.05$) in tumors, compared to non-treated rats (Garteiser et al., 2010). OKN-007 was administered in the drinking water at 10 mg/kg/day starting when tumors had reached ~50 mm^3 in volume (about day 15 following intracerebral implantation of rat C6 glioma cells), and continued for a total of 10 days (Garteiser *et al.*, 2010). One group of rats was euthanized after the 10 day treatment period, and a second group was monitored for an additional 25 days following the treatment period (Garteiser *et al.*, 2010). In the cohort of animals that were treated for 10 days and then euthanized, percent survival was 100% ($p<0.0001$), whereas for the rats that were monitored for an additional 25 days the percent survival was greater than 80% ($p<0.001$) (Garteiser *et al.*, 2010). Morphological MRI was used to calculate tumor volumes; diffusion-weighted imaging (DWI) was used to measure ADC, which assesses changes in water diffusion due to tissue structural alterations; and perfusion-weighted MRI (pMRI) was used to characterize tissue perfusion rates, which can provide information on alterations in the vascular capillary bed. Currently, the known pharmacological effects of the nitrones are primarily anti-inflammatory in nature. The parent nitrone compound, PBN, is known to inhibit (1) cyclooxygenase-2 (COX-2), (2) inducible nitric oxide synthase (iNOS), and (3) nuclear factor kappaB (NF-κB) (Floyd *et al.*, 2008).

ADC values have been found to increase particularly in the early phase of anticancer therapies (Waerzeggers *et al.*, 2010). Increases in ADC were found to be a time and dose sensitive marker of tumor (mouse xenografts) response to radiation therapy (Larocque *et al.*, 2009). Contrast-enhanced MRI and DWI were used to characterize the vascular and cellular responses of GL261 and U87 gliomas to the tumor-vascular disrupting agent (VDA) 5,6-dimethylxanthenone-4-acetic acid (DMXAA), which indicated significantly increased ADC values and the accumulation of contrast agent in treated tumors (Seshadri and Ciesielski, 2009). ADC and 3D T_2*-weighted MRI measurements were used to validate ZD6474 (tyrosine kinase receptor inhibitor) inhibition on tumor growth and angiogenesis in EGFRvIII-expressing GBM8 gliomas (Yiin *et al.*, 2010).
In a gene therapy-induced apoptosis (ganciclovir-treated herpes simplex thymidine kinase (HSV-tk) gene-transfected BT4C gliomas) study, combined DWI and ^{1}H-MRS assessment was used to find interconnecting trends following therapeutic response in water diffusion and water-referenced concentrations of mobile lipids (Liimatainen *et al.*, 2009). It is thought that apoptosis leads to an increase in ^{1}H-MRS detectable mobile cholesterol compounds and unsaturated lipids resulting from the gene therapy-induced apoptosis (Hakumäki et al., 1999; Liimatainen *et al.*, 2006, 2009). Amide proton transfer (APT) MRI was recently used to differentiate between different glioma models (SF188/V$^+$ glioma and 9L gliosarcoma) and radiation-induced necrosis, where viable glioma tissue was hyperintense and radiation necrosis was hypointense to isointense (Zhou *et al.*, 2011).
Iron oxide-based nanoparticles have recently been used as cell tracking agents, or non-targeted or targeted drug delivery. Magnetically-labeled cytotoxic T-cells were used as cellular probes and tracked by T_2- and T_2*-weighted MRI to differentiate glioma tissue from focal radiation necrosis in U-251 glioma-bearing rodents (Arbab *et al.*, 2010). Focused ultrasound, which was used to permeabilize the blood-brain barrier and increase passive diffusion, was found to increase the delivery of drug (1,3-bis(2-chloroethyl)-1-nitrosourea and iron oxide nanoparticles that can be monitored with MRI, in a rat C6 glioma model (Chen *et al.*, 2010). EGFRvIII antibody-conjugated iron oxide nanoparticles were used for convection-enhanced delivery and targeted therapy in glioblastoma mouse xenografts (U87DeltaEGFRvIII), and assessed by T_2-weighted MRI (Hadjipanayis *et al.*, 2010).

7. Conclusions

There are several orthotopic rodent glioma models that have been used for several decades, and more recent transgenic, orthotopic xenograft neurosphere- or PDGFB-expressing virus-induced models that better reflect the genetic and stem-cell involvement in glia tumorigenesis. It is important that appropriate glioma models are used that best represent our current knowledge of malignant glioblastomas in humans. Ideally the more recent models should be used if possible, however if an orthotopic syngeneic model is required, then the rat F98 or RG2, and mouse GL26(1) models seem to have some characteristics that resemble aspects of human glioblastomas, such as vascular proliferation, and aggressive and infiltrative tumor growth. The human U87 MG glioma cell xenograft model in athymic rodents also has beneficial characteristics resembling some aspects of human GBM. Choosing an appropriate model is particularly important when evaluating new anti-glioma therapies, as these models need to consider recurrent gliomas, possibly derived from cancer stem cells, which are radiation- and chemotherapy-resistant, and currently reflect the poor prognosis of high-grade gliomas in humans.

The evaluation of critical changes during tumorigenesis, as well as monitoring therapeutic responses, requires the use of appropriate imaging technologies. The focus of this review has been on the use of MR imaging and spectroscopy methodologies in pre-clinical rodent models for gliomas, many of which translate to clinical applications. DCE-MRI and ASL perfusion imaging, and MRA, can provide valuable information regarding morphological and dynamic alterations associated with tumor vasculature or angiogenesis. The ADC, as measured by DWI, and DTI, can assess tissue structural and organizational changes that occur during tumor formation. MR spectroscopy provides metabolic markers, such as NAA, tCr, tCho, lactate, and mobile lipids that undergo significant changes in concentrations during glial tumorigenesis, as a result of neuronal degradation (NAA), cell proliferation (tCho), anaerobic respiration (lactate), and necrosis (mobile lipids). These MRI-observable changes, such as tumor ADC, rCBF, K^{trans}, cerebral blood volume, and ^{1}H-MRS detectable metabolites, can all be important criteria to assess therapeutic efficacy. Molecular MRI (mMRI) is a targeted approach that can be used to assess specific tumor molecular markers associated with angiogenesis, apoptosis, cell migration/invasion, metastasis, proliferation, or inflammation. Targeted probes can also be used to deliver therapeutic compounds to tumors that express high levels of a specific molecular marker, and if these probes have a Gd-, manganese (Mn)- or iron oxide-based construct, then they can be monitored by MRI.

8. References

Alexiou, G.A. & Voulgaris S. (2010) The role of the PTEN gene in malignant gliomas. *Neurol. Neurochir. Pol.*, 44(1): 80-6. ISSN:0028-3843

Ali, M.M., Janic, B., Babajani-Feremi, A., Varma, N.R., Iskander, A.S., Anagli, J. & Arbab, A.S. (2010) Changes in vascular permeability and expression of different angiogenic factors following anti-angiogenic treatment in rat glioma. *PLoS One*, 15;5(1):e8727. ISSN:1932-6203

Arbab, A.S., Janic, B., Jafari-Khouzani, K., Iskander, A.S., Kumar, S., Varma, N.R., Knight, R.A., Soltanian-Zadeh, H., Brown, S.L. & Frank, J.A. (2010) Differentiation of glioma and radiation injury in rats using *in vitro* produce magnetically labeled cytotoxic T-cells and MRI. *PLoS One*, 26;5(2):e9365. ISSN:1932-6203

Asanuma, T., Doblas, S., Tesiram, Y.A., Saunders, D., Cranford, R., Pearson, J., Abbott, A., Smith, N. & Towner, R.A. (2008a) Diffusion tensor imaging and fiber tractography of C6 rat glioma. *J. Magn. Reson. Imaging*, 28(3): 566-573. ISSN:1053-1807

Asanuma, T., Doblas, S., Tesiram, Y.A., Saunders, D., Cranford, R., Yasui, H., Inanami, O., Smith, N., Floyd, R.A., Kotake, Y. & Towner, R.A. (2008b) Visualization of the protective ability of a free radical trapping compound against rat C6 and F98 gliomas with diffusion tensor fiber tractography. *J. Magn. Reson. Imaging*, 28(3): 574-587. ISSN:1053-1807

Assanah, M., Lochhead, R., Ogden, A., Bruce, J., Goldman, J. & Canoll, P. (2006) Glial progenitors in adult white matter are driven to form malignant gliomas by platelet-deived growth factor-expressing retroviruses. *J. Neurosci.*, 26(25): 6781-6790. ISSN:0270-6474

Assanah, M.C., Bruce, J.N., Suzuki, S.O., Chen, A., Goldman, J.E. & Canoll, P. (2009) PDGF stimulates the massive expansion of glial progenitors in the neonatal forebrain. *Glia*, 57(16): 1835-1847. ISSN:0894-1491

Barth, R.F. (1998) Rat brain tumor models in experimental neuro-oncology: the 9L, C6, T9, F98, RG2 (D74), RT-2 and CNS-1 gliomas. *J Neurooncol.,* 36(1): 91-102. ISSN:0167-594X

Barth, R.F. & Kaur, B. (2009) Rat brain tumor models in experimental neuro-oncology: the C6, 9L, T9, RG2, F98, BT4C, RT-2 and CNS-1 gliomas. *J. Neurooncol.,* 94(3): 299-312. ISSN:0167-594X

Calzolari, F. & Malatesta, P. (2010) Recent insights into PDGF-induced gliomagenesis. *Brain Pathol.,* 20(3): 527-38. ISSN:1015-6305

Central Brain Tumor Registry of the United States (CBTRUS). 2011 CBTRUS Statistical Report: Primary Brain and Central Nervous System Tumors Diagnosed in the United States in 2004-2007. http://www.cbtrus.org/2011-NPCR-SEER/WEB-0407-Report-3-3-2011.pdf. pp. 54-57.

Chen, P.Y., Liu, H.L., Hua, M.Y., Yang, H.W., Huang, C.Y., Chu, P.C., Lyu, L.A., Tseng, I.C., Feng, L.Y., Tsai, H.C., Chen, S.M., Lu, Y.J., Wang, J.J., Yen, T.C., Ma, Y.H., Wu, T., Chen, J.P., Chuang, J.I., Shin, J.W., Hsueh, C. & Wei, K.C. (2010) Novel magnetic/ultrasound focusing system enhances nanoparticles drug delivery for glioma treatment. *Neuro. Oncol.,* 12(10): 1050-60. ISSN:1522-8517

Cheng, S.Y., Huang, H.J., Nagane, M., Ji, X.D., Wang, D., Shih, C.C., Arap, W., Huang, C.M. & Cavenee, W.K. (1996) Suppression of Glioblastoma Angiogenicity and Tumorigenicity by Inhibition of Endogenous Expression of Vascular Endothelial Growth Factor. *Proc. Natl. Acad. Sci. U. S. A.,* 93(16): 8502-8507. ISSN:0027-8424

Chinnam, M. & Goodrich, D.W. (2011) RB1, development, and cancer. *Curr. Top. Dev. Biol.,* 94: 129-69. ISSN:0070-2153

Colvin, D.C., Yankeelov, T.E., Does, M.D., Yue, Z., Quarles, C. & Gore, J.C. (2008) New insights into tumor microstructure using temporal diffusion spectroscopy. *Cancer Res.,* 68 (14): 5941-7. ISSN:0008-5472

Davaki, P. & Lantos, P.L. (1980) Morphological analysis of malignancy: a comparative study of transplanted brain tumors. *Br. J. Exp. Pathol.,* 61(6): 655-60. ISSN:0007-1021

Davis, S.C., Samkoe, K.S., O'Hara, J.A., Gibbs-Strauss, S.L., Payne, H.L., Hoopes, P.J., Paulsen, K.D. & Pogue, B.W. (2010) MRI-coupled fluorescence tomography quantifies EGFR activity in brain tumors. *Acad. Radiol.* 17 (3): 271-6. ISSN:1076-6332

De Vries, N.A., Bruggeman, S.W., Hulsman, D., de Vries, H.I., Zevenhoven, J., Buckle, T., Hamans, B.C., Leenders, W.P., Beijnen, J.H., van Lohuizen, M., Berns, A.J.M. & van Tellingen, O. (2010) Rapid and robust transgenic high-grade glioma mouse models for therapy intervention studies. *Clin. Cancer Res.,* 16(13): 3431-3441. ISSN:1078-0432

Doblas, S., Saunders, D., Kshirsagar, P., Pye, Q., Oblander, J., Gordon, B., Kosanke, S., Floyd, R.A. & Towner, R.A. (2008) Phentyl-tert-butyl nitrone induces tumor regression and decreases angiogenesis in a C6 rat glioma model. *Free Radical Biology & Medicine,* 44(1): 63-72. ISSN:0891-5849

Doblas, S., He, T., Saunders, D., Pearson, J., Hoyle, J., Smith, N., Lerner, M. & Towner, R.A. (2010) Glioma morphology and tumor-induced vascular alterations revealed in seven glioma models by in vivo magnetic resonance imaging and angiography. *J. Magn. Reson. Imaging,* 32(2): 267-275. ISSN:1053-1807

Drogat, B., Auguste, P., Nguyen, D.T., Bouchecareilh, M., Pineau, R., Nalbantoglu, J., Kaufman, R.J., Chevert, E., Bikfalvi, A. & Moenner, M. (2007) IRE1 signaling is essential for ischemia-induced vascular endothelial growth factor-A expression and contributes to angiogenesis and tumor growth *in vivo*. *Cancer Res.*, 67(14): 6700-07. ISSN:0008-5472

Farrar, C.T., Kamoun, W.S., Ley, C.D., Kim, Y.R., Kwon, S.J., Dai, G., Rosen, B.R., di Tomaso, E., Jain, R.K. & Sorensen, A.G. (2010) In vivo validation of MRI vessel caliber index measurement methods with intravital optical microscopy in a U87 mouse brain tumor model. *Neuro. Oncol.*, 12 (4): 341-50. ISSN:1522-8517

Fei, X.F., Zhang, Q.B., Dong, J., Diao, Y., Wang, Z.M., Li, R.J., Wu, Z.C., Wang, A.D., Lan, Q., Zhang, S.M. & Huang, Q. (2010) Development of clinically relevant orthotopic xenograft mouse model of metastatic lung cancer and glioblastoma through surgical tumor tissues injection with trocar. *J. Exp. Clin. Cancer Res.*, 29: 84. ISSN:0392-9078

Floyd, R.A., Kopke, R.D., Choi, C.-H., Foster, S.B., Doblas, S. & Towner, R.A. (2008) Nitrones as therapeutics. *Free Radical Biology & Medicine*, 45(10): 1361-1374. ISSN:0891-5849

Garteiser, P., Doblas, S., Watanabe, Y., Saunders, D., Hoyle, J., Lerner, M., He, T., Floyd, R.A. & Towner, R.A. (2010) Multiparametric assessment of the anti-glioma properties of OKN007 by magnetic resonance imaging. *J. Magnetic Resonance Imaging*, 31(4): 796-806. ISSN:1053-1807

Grobben, B., De Deyn, P.P. & Slegers, H. (2002) Rat C6 glioma as experimental model system for the study of glioblastoma growth and invasion. *Cell Tissue Res.*, 310(3): 257-270. ISSN:0302-766X

Groothuis, D.R., Fischer, J.M., Pasternak, J.F., Blasberg, R.G., Vick, N.A. & Bigner, D.D. (1983) Regional measurements of blood-to-tissue transport in experimental RG-2 rat gliomas. *Cancer Res.*, 43(7): 3368-3373. ISSN:0008-5472

Gudinaviciene, I., Pranys, D. & Juozaityte, E. (2004) Impact of morphology and biology on the prognosis of patients with gliomas. *Medicina (Kaunas)*, 40(2): 112-120. ISSN:1010-660X

Gyngell, M.L., Hoehn-Berlage, M. & Hossmann, K.A. (1994) Proton MR spectroscopy of experimental brain tumors *in vivo*. *Acta Neurochir. Suppl. (Wien)*, 60: 350-2. ISSN:0065-1419

Hadjipanayis, C.G., Machaidze, R., Kaluzova, M., Wang, L., Schuette, A.J., Chen, H., Wu, X. & Mao, H. (2010) EGFRvIII antibody-conjugated iron oxide nanoparticles for magnetic resonance imaging-guided convection-enhanced delivery and targeted therapy of glioblastoma. *Cancer Res.*, 70(15):6303-12. ISSN:0008-5472

Hakumäki, J., Poptani, H., Sandmair, A.-M., Ylä-Herttuala, S. & Kauppinen, R.A. (1999) 1H MRS detects polyunsaturated fatty acid accumulation during gene therapy of glioma: implications for the in vivo detection of apoptosis. *Nature Medicine*, 5 (11) 1323-1327. ISSN:1078-8956

He, T., Smith, N., Saunders, D., Doblas, S., Watanabe, Y., Hoyle, J., Silasi-Mansat, R., Lupu, F., Lerner, M., Brackett, D.J. & Towner, R.A. (2010) Molecular MRI assessment of vascular endothelial growth factor receptor-2 in rat C6 gliomas. *J. Cell. Mol. Med.* In press. 1582-4934

Hede, S.-M., Hansson, I., Afink, G.B., Eriksson, A., Nazarenko, I., Andrae, J., Genove, G., Westermark, B. & Nister, M. (2009) GFAP promoter driven transgenic expression of PDGFB in the mouse brain leads to glioblastoma in a Trp53 null background. *Glia*, 57(11): 1143-1153. ISSN:0894-1491

Jacques, T.S., Swales, A., Brzozowski, M.J., Henriquez, N.V., Linehan, J.M., Mirzadeh, Z., O'Malley, C., Naumann, H., Alvarez-Buylla, A. & Brandner, S. (2010) Combinations of genetic mutations in the adult neural stem cell compartment determine brain tumor phenotypes. *The EMBO Journal*, 29(1): 222-235. ISSN:0261-4189

Jahnke, K., Muldoon, L.L., Varallyay, C.G., Lewin, S.J., Kraemer, D.F. & Neuwelt, E.A. (2009) Bevacizumab and carboplatin increase survival and asymptomatic tumor volume in a glioma model. *Neuro. Oncol.*, 11 (2): 142-50. ISSN:1522-8517

Kadayakkara, D.K., Janjic, J.M., Pusateri, L.K., Young, W.B. & Ahrens, E.T. (2010) In vivo observation of intracellular oximetry in perfluorocarbon-labeled glioma cells and chemotherapeutic response in the CNS using fluorine-19 MRI. *Magn. Reson. Med.*, 64 (5): 1252-9. ISSN:0740-3194

Kauppinen, R.A. (2002) Monitoring cytotoxic tumor treatment response by diffusion magnetic resonance imaging and proton spectroscopy. *NMR Biomed.*, 15 (1): 6-17. ISSN:0952-3480

Kiessling, F., Huppert, J., Zhang, C., Jayapaul, J., Zwick, S., Woenne, E.C., Mueller, M.M., Zentgraf, H., Eisenhut, M., Addadi, Y., Neeman, M. & Semmler, W. (2009) RGD-labeled USPIO inhibits adhesion and endocytototic activity of alpha v beta3-integrin-expressing glioma cells and only accumulates in the vascular tumor compartment. *Radiology*, 253 (2): 462-9. ISSN:0033-8419

Kim, D.H., Kundu, J.K. & Surh, Y.J .(2011) Redox modulation of p53: Mechanisms and functional significance. *Mol. Carcinog.*, 50(4): 222-34. ISSN:0899-1987

Kish, P.E., Blaivas, M., Strawderman, M., Muraszko, K.M., Ross, D.A., Ross, B.D. & McMahon, G. (2001) Magnetic resonance imaging of ethyl-nitrosourea-induced rat gliomas: a model for experimental therapeutics of low-grade gliomas. *J. Neurooncol.*, 53(3): 243-257. ISSN:0167-594X

Koestner, A., Swenberg, J.A. & Wechsler, W. (1971) Transplacental production with ethylnitrosourea of neoplasms of the nervous system in Sprague-Dawley rats. *Am. J. Pathol.*, 63(1):37-56. ISSN:0002-9440

Koestner, A. (1990) Characterization of N-nitrosourea-induced tumors of the nervous system; their prospective value for studies of neurocarcinogenesis and brain tumor therapy. *Toxicologic pathology*, 18(1 Pt 2): 186-192. ISSN:0192-6233

Larocque, M.P., Syme, A., Yahya, A., Wachowicz, K., Allaunis-Turner, J. & Fallone, B.G. (2009) Temporal and dose dependence of T2 and ADC at 9.4 T in a mouse model following single fraction radiation therapy. *Med. Phys.*, 36 (7): 2948-54.
ISSN:0094-2405

Lemasson, B., Serduc, R., Maisin, C., Bouchet, A., Coquery, N., Robert, P., Le Duc, G., Troprès, I., Rémy, C. & Barbier, E.L. (2010) Monitoring blood-brain barrier status in a rat model of glioma receiving therapy: dual injection of low-molecular-weight and macromolecular MR contrast media. *Radiology*, 257 (2): 342-52. ISSN: 0033-8419

Liimatainen, T., Lehtimäki, K., Ala-Korpela, M. & Hakumäki, J. (2006) Identification of mobile cholesterol compounds in experimental gliomas by 1H MRS in vivo: effects of ganciclovir-induced apoptosis on lipids. *FEBS Letters*, 580(19): 4746-50. ISSN:0014-5793

Liimatainen, T., Hakumäki, J.M., Kauppinen, R.A. & Ala-Korpela, M. (2009) Monitoring of gliomas in vivo by diffusion MRI and (1)H MRS during gene therapy-induced apoptosis: interrelationships between water diffusion and mobile lipids. *NMR Biomed.*, 22 (3): 272-9. ISSN:0952-3480

Lohmann ,D. (2010) Retinoblastoma. *Adv. Exp. Med. Biol.* 685: 220-7. ISSN:0065-2598

Maclaine, N.J. & Hupp, T.R. (2011) How phosphorylation controls p53. *Cell Cycle*, Mar 15; 10(6). ISSN:1538-4101

Martens, T., Schmidt, N.O., Eckerich, C., Fillbrandt, R., Merchant, M., Schwall, R., Westphal, M. & Lamszus, K. (2006) A novel one-armed anti-c-Met antibody inhibits glioblastoma growth in vivo. *Clin. Cancer Res.*,12(20 Pt 1): 6144-6152.ISSN:1078-0432

Masui, K., Suzuki, S.O., Torisu, R., Goldman, J.E., Canoll, P. & Iwaki, T. (2010) Glial progenitors in the brainstem give rise to malignant gliomas by platelet-derived growth factor stimulation. *Glia*, 58(9): 1050-1065. ISSN:0894-1491

Muller, P.A., Vousden, K.H. & Norman, J.C. (2011) p53 and its mutants in tumor cell migration and invasion. *J. Cell Biol.* 192(2): 209-18. ISSN:0021-9525

Natsume, A., Kinjo, S., Yuki, K., Kato, T., Ohno, M., Motomura, K., Iwami, K. & Wakabayashi, T. (2011) Glioma-initiating cells and molecular pathology: implications for therapy. *Brain Tumor Pathol.* 28(1): 1-12. ISSN:1433-7398

Niclou, S.P., Fack, F. & Rajcevic, U. (2010) Glioma proteomics: status and perspectives. *J. Proteomics* 73(10): 1823-1838. ISSN:1874-3919

Park, I., Larson, P.E., Zierhut, M.L., Hu, S., Bok, R., Ozawa, T., Kurhanewicz, J., Vigneron, D.B., Vandenberg, S.R., James, C.D. & Nelson, S.J. (2010) Hyperpolarized 13C magnetic resonance metabolic imaging: application to brain tumors. *Neuro. Oncol.*, 12 (2): 133-44. ISSN:1522-8517

Plate, K.H., Breier, G., Millauer, B., Ullrich, A. & Risau, W. (1993) Up-Regulation of Vascular Endothelial Growth Factor and its Cognate Receptors in a Rat Glioma Model of Tumor Angiogenesis. *Cancer Res.*, 53(23): 5822-5827. ISSN:0008-5472

Ross, B.D., Merkle, H., Hendrich, K., Staewen, R.S. & Garwood, M. (1992) Spatially localized *in vivo* ^{1}H magnetic resonance spectroscopy of an intracerebral rat glioma. *Magn. Reson. Med.*, 23 (1): 96-108. ISSN:0740-3194

Sadeghi, N., Camby, I., Goldman, S., Gabius, H.J., Baleriaux, D., Salmon, I., Decaesteckere, C., Kiss, R. & Metens, T. (2003) Effect of hydrophilic components of the extracellular matrix on quantifiable diffusion-weighted imaging of human gliomas: preliminary results of correlating apparent diffusion coefficient values and hyaluronan expression level. *Am. J. Roentgenol.*, 181 (1): 235-41. ISSN:0361-803X

Seshadri, M. & Ciesielski, M.J. (2009) MRI-based characterization of vascular disruption by 5,6-dimethylxanthenone-acetic acid in gliomas. *J. Cereb. Blood Flow Metab.*, 29 (8): 1373-82. ISSN:0271-678X

Shih, A.H., Dai, C., Hu, X., Rosenblum, M.K., Koutcher, J.A. & Holland, E.C. (2004) Dose-dependent effects of platelet-derived growth factor-B on glial tumorigenesis. *Cancer Res.*, 64(14): 4783-4789. ISSN:0008-5472

Shih, A.H. & Holland, E.C. (2006) Platelet-derived growth factor (PDGF) and glial tumorigenesis. *Cancer Lett.*, 232(2): 139-47. ISSN:0304-3835

Sibenaller, Z.A., Etame, A.B., Ali, M.M., Barua, M., Braun, T.A., Casavant, T.L. & Ryken, T.C. (2005) Genetic characterization of commonly used glioma cell lines in the rat animal model system. *Neurosurg. Focus*, 19(4): E1-E9. ISSN:1092-0684 (Electronic)

Sipkins, D.A., Cheresh, D.A., Kazemi, M.R., Nevin, L/M., Bednarski, M.D. & Li, K.C. (1998) Detection of tumor angiogenesis *in vivo* by alphaVnbeta3-targeted magnetic resonance imaging. *Nat. Med.*, 4 (5): 623-626. ISSN:1078-8956

Szatmari, T., Lumniczky, K., Desaknai, S., Trajcevski, S., Hidvegi, E.J., Hamada, H. & Safrany, G. (2006) Detailed characterization of the mouse glioma 261 tumor model for experimental glioblastoma therapy. *Cancer Science,* 97(6): 546-553. ISSN:1347-9032

Terpstra, M., High, W.B., Luo, Y., de Graaf, R.A., Merkle, H. & Garwood, M. (1996) Relationship among lactate concentration, blood flow and histopathologic profiles in rat C6 glioma. *NMR Biomed.*, 9 (5): 185-94. ISSN:0952-3480

Towner, R.A., Smith, N., Doblas, S., Tesiram, Y., Garteiser, P., Saunders, D., Cranford, R., Silasi-Mansat, R., Herlea, O., Ivanciu, L., Wu, D. & Lupu, F. (2008) *In vivo* detection of c-Met expression in a rat C6 glioma model. *J. Cell. Mol. Med.* 12(1): 174-186. ISSN:1582-1838

Towner, R.A., Smith, N., Doblas, S., Garteiser, P., Watanabe, Y., He, T., Saunders, D., Herlea, O., Silasi-Mansat, R. & Lupu, F. (2010a) In vivo detection of inducible nitric oxide synthase in rodent gliomas. *Free Radic. Biol. Med.*, 48(5): 691-703. ISSN:0891-5849

Towner, R.A., Smith, N., Asanao, Y., He, T., Doblas, S., Saunders, D., Silasi-Mansat, R., Lupu, F. & Seeney, C.E. (2010b) Molecular magnetic resonance imaging approaches used to aid in the understanding of angiogenesis *in vivo*: implications for tissue engineering. *Tissue Engineering Part A*, 16 (2) : 357-364). ISSN:1937-3341

Towner, R.A., Smith, N., Asano, Y., Doblas, S., Saunders, D., Silasi-Mansat, R., & Lupu, F. (2010c) Molecular magnetic resonance imaging approaches used to aid in the understanding of the tissue regeneration marker Met *in vivo*: implications for tissue engineering. *Tissue Engineering Part A*, 16 (2) 365-371. ISSN:1937-3341

Valable, S., Lemasson, B., Farion, R, Beaumont, M., Segebarth, C., Remy, C. & Barbier, E.L. (2008) Assessment of blood volume, vessel size, and the expression of angiogenic factors in two rat glioma models : a longitudinal in vivo and ex vivo study. *NMR Biomed.*, 21(10): 1043-56. ISSN:0952-3480

Vaquero, J., Coca, S., Zurita, M. , Oya, S., Arias, A., Moreno, M. & Morales, C. (1992) Synaptophysin expression in "ependymal tumors" induced by ethyl-nitrosourea in rats. *Am. J. Pathol.*, 141(5):1037-1041. ISSN:0002-9440

Varallyay, C.G., Muldoon, L.L., Gahramanov, S., Wu, Y.J., Goodman, J.A., Li, X., Pike, M.M. & Neuwelt, E.A. (2009) Dynamic MRI using iron oxide nanoparticles to assess early vascular effects of antiangiogenic versus corticosteroid treatment in a glioma model. *J. Cereb. Blood Flow Metab.*, 29 (4): 853-60. ISSN:0271-678X

Veeravagu, A., Hou, L.C., Hsu, A.R., Cai, W., Greve, J.M., Chen, X. & Tse, V. (2008) The temporal correlation of dynamic contrast-enhanced magnetic resonance imaging with tumor angiogenesis in a murine glioblastoma model. *Neurol. Res.*, 30 (9): 952-9. ISSN:0161-6412

Waerzeggers, Y., Monfared, P., Viel, T., Winkeler, A. & Jacobs, A.H. (2010) Mouse models in neurological disorders: Applications of non-invasive imaging. *Biochimica et Biophysica Acta*, 1802(10): 819-839. ISSN:0006-3002

Waldman, A.D., Jackson, A., Price, S.J., Clark, C.A., Booth, T.C., Auer, D.P., Tofts, P.S., Collins, D.J., Leach, M.O. & Rees, J.H. (2009) Quantitative imaging biomarkers in neuro-oncology. *Nature Reviews Clin. Oncol.*, 6(8): 445-454. ISSN:1759-4774

Wehbe, K., Pineau, R., Eimer, S., Vital, A., Loiseau, H. & Deleris, G. (2010) Differentiation between normal and tumor vasculature of animal and human glioma by FTIR imaging. *Analyst*, 135(12): 3052-9. ISSN:0003-2654

Wei, J., Barr, J., Kong, L.-Y., Wang, Y., Wu, A., Sharma, A.K., Gumin, J., Henry, V., Colman, H., Sawaya, R., Lang, F.F. & Heimberger, A.B. (2010) Glioma-associated cancer-initiating cells induce immunosuppression. *Clin. Cancer Res.*, 16(2): 461-473. ISSN:1078-0432

Weizsaecker, M., Deen, D.F., Rosenblum, M.L., Hoshino, T., Gutin, P.H. & Barker, M. (1981) The 9L Rat Brain Tumor: Description and Application of an Animal Model. *J. Neurol.*, 224(3): 183-192. ISSN:0340-5354

Yiin, J.J., Schornack, P.A., Sengar, R.S., Liu, K.W., Feng, H., Lieberman, F.S., Chiou, S.H., Sarkaria, J.N., Wiener, E.C., Ma, H.I. & Cheng, S.Y. (2010) ZD6474, a multitargeted inhibitor for receptor tyrosine kinases, suppresses growth of gliomas expressing an epidermal growth factor receptor mutant, EGFRvIII, in the brain. *Mol. Cancer Ther.*, 9 (4): 929-41. ISSN:1535-7163

Zhang, D., Feng, X.Y., Henning, T.D., Wen, L., Lu, W.Y., Pan, H., Wu, X. & Zou, L.G. (2009) MR imaging of tumor angiogenesis using sterically stabilized Gd-DTPA liposomes targeted to CD105. *Eur. J. Radiol.*, 70 (1): 180-9. ISSN:0720-048X

Zhou, J., Tryggestad, E., Wen, Z., Lai, B., Zhou, T., Grossman, R., Wang, S., Yan, K., Fu, D.X., Ford, E., Tyler, B., Blakeley, J., Laterra, J. & van Zijl, P.C. (2011) Differentiation between glioma and radiation necrosis using molecular magnetic resonance imaging of endogeneous proteins and peptides. *Nature Medicine*, 17(1): 130-4. ISSN:1078-8956

Part 3

Therapeutic Advances

14

Stereotactic Radiosurgery for Gliomas

Mehmet Tönge and Gökhan Kurt
Gazi University, Department of Neurosurgery
Turkey

1. Introduction

The idea of stereotactic radiosurgery (SRS) was first conceived in 1951 by Swedish neurosurgeon Lars Leksell. Focus of his idea was to destroy the surgically inaccessible intracranial tissues or lesions with single fraction high-dose radiation obtained from multiple radiation beams directed to target by stereotactic instruments. He designed the first prototype of gamma knife with Larsson in the light of this idea and performed on his first patient in a nuclear building in 1967. Device was installed at Sophiahemmet hospital in Karolinska - Sweden in the following year. Although only a limited number of patients were treated with gamma knife until 80's, the technique became more popular afterwards and pervaded all around the world. By the time, different radiosurgical devices were developed (Pollock & Brown, 2005; Stieber & Ellis, 2005).

SRS was also used in the management of gliomas as well as many other intracranial lesions for years. Some data acquired despite the lack of reported large case series and long term follow up results. Gliomas are believed to arise from neuroglial cells which encounter the most frequent intracranial tumors in different series, constitute 45-60% of all intracranial tumors. Gliomas have astrocytic, oligodendroglial, ependymal and mixed subtypes. They are also graded I to IV according to histological and clinical behavior. Whereas the grade I and II are accepted as "low grade", the grade III and IV are "high grade" gliomas (Louis et al., 2007). However a portion of low grade gliomas (LGG) are curable by means of current multimodal treatment techniques, the main goal in high grade gliomas (HGG) is the prolongation of survival with a high quality of life as much as possible. Besides, the malignant transformation of LGGs is a well-known issue. Extensive surgical resection followed by radiation therapy (RT) and chemotherapy is the golden standard within most of the treatment protocols; particularly for HGGs. Currently, there are many ongoing clinical studies focused on the role of SRS in the management of gliomas. In most cases, the treatment protocols should be individualized.

1.1 Radiotherapy versus radiosurgery

The term "radiotherapy" refers to the treatment of malignant neoplasms and some benign situations by ionizing radiation. The history of RT goes back almost to the exploration of radiation. Many techniques have been developed for performing RT over time which made the RT more accurate and lesion targeted. Recently, techniques such as 3D conformal RT provided by multileaf-collimators and intensity modulated RT are available in addition to conventional RT. External beam radiotherapy (EBRT) is frequently performed in multiple low-dose fractions for post-surgical residuals or recurrences in the management of gliomas.

A typical RT session is performed with approximately 30 day fractions by a cumulative ~60 Gy dose except the hypofractioned RT for HGGs. Radiation has prominent effects on tumor tissue like cytotoxicity via early and late DNA damage; inflammatory reactions and edema. Radiosensitivity of the tissue is substantially related with the tissue's proliferation index. Because the normal brain cells are more constant than the tumor cells, the radiation doses between specific ranges tend to effect more on tumor cells. Currently, more conformal and intensity modulated irradiation is preferred to whole brain irradiation in RT protocols.

SRS efforts to effect only to the target lesion while protecting surrounding tissues in a single fractioned high-dose radiation. In contrast to conventional RT, radiosurgery doesn't rely on the increased radiation sensitivity of the target compared with the normal brain. One of the key elements in stereotactic radiosurgery is the use of many radiation fields distributed over space all focusing on a target. This feature minimizes the effect to surrounding normal tissue. Besides, the applied re-irradiation dose and cumulative normalized total doses increase with a change in irradiation technique from conventional RT to radiosurgery re-treatment without increasing the probability of normal brain necrosis (Mayer & Sminia, 2008; Niyazi et al., 2011). The goal of radiosurgery is to arrest the cell division capability of target cells, regardless of the individual cell's mitotic activity and radiosensitivity. Radiosurgery also allows for delayed intratumoral vascular obliteration (Hadjipanayis et al., 2002a). Mechanisms of cell damage are sudden cell death via apoptosis in acute stage; and endothelial proliferation, luminal narrowing and thrombosis in the late stage (Witham et al., 2005). Deliverance of radiation dose in single fraction increases the biological effect of the radiation 2.5 to 3 times compared with multi-fractioned RT which allows decreasing the total treatment dose (Crowley et al., 2006). This means a radiation dose of 15 Gy has similar biological efficacy with approximately 40-45 Gy dose delivered by fractioned RT. However, the edema and radionecrosis caused by irradiation is more relevant in high-dose single fraction deliverance. For that reason, it's not applicable on large intracranial volumes. SRS is almost always a one-day treatment protocol. However SRS has different application protocols, basic steps are the same:

- Establishment of a fiducial system for targeting
- Stereotactic imaging
- Dosimetric planning
- Irradiation

Main differences between conventional RT and SRS are shown in table 1.

	RT	SRS
Radiation beam	X ray	X ray, gamma ray or charged particles
Tissue selectivity	Regarding mitotic activity and radiosensitivity of the tissue	Regardless of the mitotic activity and radiosensitivity of the tissue
Total dose of the treatment	High (45-70 Gy)	Low (10-20 Gy)
Fractions	Multiple	Single or few
Duration of the treatment	Weeks	Single day or few days
Tumor size	Not a criteria	<3-3.5 cm in diameter

Table 1. Differences between conventional RT and SRS.

1.2 Radiosurgical devices

Radiosurgical devices may be divided into two main groups according to working principles: a) Photon based systems b) Particle based systems. X or gamma rays are used in photon based systems which are substantially capable to penetrate sufficiently into cranium and to generate energy deposition. While X rays are obtained from crashing accelerated electrons on a metallic surface, the gamma rays occur during subatomic particle interactions. They are commonly obtained by courtesy of the natural decay of $cobalt^{60}$ to $nickel^{60}$. Techniques like unifying multiple beams at a target point or intensity modulation are performed to achieve the maximal effect on target due to the potential of these beams to affect the normal tissues on their way.

1.2.1 Gamma knife

Main components of a gamma knife are; a gamma knife device with a Co^{60} source, a stereotactic head frame and a software to make calculations of dose planning. Technology of the device has been developed concurrent with the developments in neuroimaging and computer technology since its first introduction in 1968. In current version of gamma knife, patient undergoes brain imaging following the fixation of a stereotactic head frame onto head. Then, the images are processed with the software and dose planning is performed. Finally, the patient is irradiated by the device. Radiation originating from Co^{60} source is divided into 201 beams through a hemispheric helmet and targeted into lesion. Beams can be shaped into 4, 8, 14 or 18 mm in diameter radiation balls by using different helmets. Also the shape of the radiation shots can be modified through plugging and shielding techniques thus the eloquent structures like cornea, optic nerves and brainstem can be prevented against adverse radiation effects. Rigid fixation of the head frame by four screws into the outer table of calvarium results in high accuracy with less than 1 mm deviation at dose planning. Automatic positioning system (APS) enables the computer controlled treatment session without interruption (Pollock & Brown, 2005). Furthermore, the superimposition of CT, MR, functional MR, MR tractography, PET scan and angiography images increases the accuracy and efficacy of dose planning (Pantelis et al., 2010). A commonly used term for dose planning is the "marginal dose" which refers to dosage of the radiation measured at peripheral margin of the lesion. For example, the marginal dose of 12 Gy within 50% isodose means the central dose lesion received is 24 Gy. A dose planning image is shown in figure 1.

1.2.2 Linear accelerator (LINAC)

However the LINAC based RT has been used since 1950s; LINAC was applied to radiosurgery in 80s. Typical current version of a LINAC device consists of a stereotactic head frame, floor stand, 6 megavolts linear accelerator, collimators and high precision attachments. A stream of electrons is accelerated almost to light speed and crash onto a metallic surface which results in production of mainly heat and lesser X rays. These rays are transferred to target point following modulation by multileaf collimators. Multileaf collimators allow to integration of multiple rays coming from different directions at a definite target point (Pollock & Brown, 2005).

1.2.3 CyberKnife

CyberKnife® technology (Accuray, Sunnyvale, CA) was developed by Adler & colleagues, and was approved by FDA (Food and Drug Administration) for radiation treatment in 2001

(Adler et al., 1999). CyberKnife system consists of a lightweight LINAC device mounted on an industrial robotic arm and computer software. This structure provides multiaxial movement capability to the device. Real time X ray motion detector cameras monitor the patient's movements during treatment session which minimizes probable accuracy problems. Patient comfort and convenience are served by eliminating invasive frame replacement. In addition, because imaging and planning can occur any time before the radiosurgery procedure, the coordination of radiological resources, physician schedules and patient needs is simplified. Most patients undergo convenient outpatient treatment sessions that are completed within 1 hour, and they complete a treatment plan of two to five fractions in the same number of days (Kuo et al., 2003).

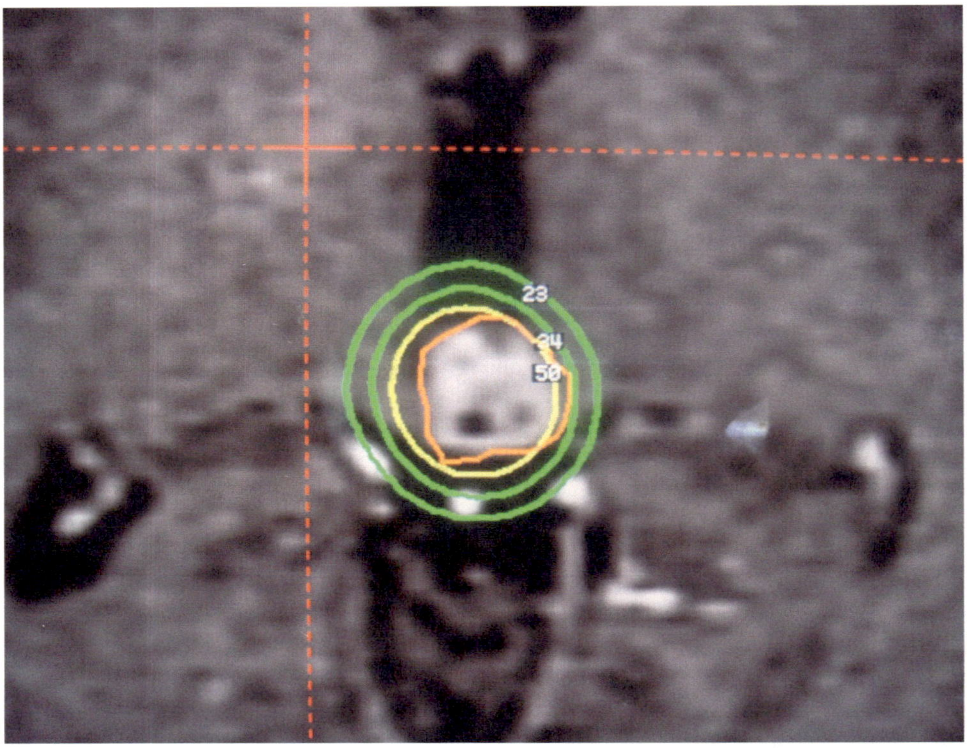

Fig. 1. Snapshot view of gamma knife dose planning on MRI. Orange circle indicates the borders of the tumor, yellow circle indicates the treatment dose of 15 Gy shot isocenter (within 50% isodose) and peripheral two green circles indicate 12 and 8 Gy isodose fields.

1.2.4 Charged particle beam therapy

Proton based SRS was pioneered by Kjellberg & colleagues in the 1960s. This discipline uses either charged protons or helium ions instead of photons. Protons are generated by stripping an atom of its electron and accelerating the residual proton in the magnetic field of a cyclotron or a synch-cyclotron. It's also known as "hadron therapy". A phenomenon called "Bragg peak effect" is very important for a better understanding of fundamentals of proton beam therapy. The pattern of energy distribution of a proton beam consists of an entrance region of a slowly rising dose, a rapid rise to a maximum (Bragg peak) and a rapid fall to near zero. This feature provides a moderate entrance dose on the surface structures; a uniform high dose within the target point; and a zero dose beyond the target. A single monoenergetic proton beam irradiates a volume of approximately 1 cc. superimposing of multiple beams allows to irradiation of larger lesions. The proton therapy is tended to be performed for larger and more complex lesions in comparison with photon therapy.

Because the relatively longer planning procedure, patient undergoes imaging and treatment on separate days. Beads are implanted into the outer table of the patient's skull and the head of the patient is fixed by a rigid head frame prior to treatment (Chen et al., 2007). Proton beam therapy is performed by only limited number of centers around the world because of the complexity of particle-beam treatment planning, the need for a cyclotron to generate the protons and the expense of these units (Pollock & Brown, 2005).

2. Current SRS approaches for glioma

However the SRS is a relatively young treatment modality, over 400.000 patients were treated with gamma knife all around the world. Currently, there are sufficient data proving the efficacy of SRS on lesions such as arterio-venous malformations, acoustic schwannomas, trigeminal neuralgia and skull base meningiomas. Indications for SRS in gliomas are not definite yet because of the lack of large randomized clinical trials, and multiplicity of gliomas subtypes despite the widespread use (Rejis, 2009).

2.1 High grade astrocytoma

High grade astrocytoma (HGA) includes anaplastic astrocytoma (AA), glioblastome multiforme (GBM), giant cell GBM and gliosarcoma according to WHO (World Health Organization) classification system (Louis et al., 2007). Whilst AA is grade III, rests are grade IV tumors. AA and GBM account for 60-65% of all gliomas (Sloan et al., 2005). The overall survival for untreated GBM is only 2-3 months which increases to mean 9-12 months with addition of gross total resection and RT. Addition of chemotherapy to this modality brings approximately 5 more months. Currently, overall survival for GBM following surgical resection and RT increased to 14-19 months by addition of a latterly popularized chemotherapeutic agent temazolamide (Combs et al, 2005). Median survival for AA is about 2-3 years with surgical resection, RT and chemotherapy. 5 years survival rate for AA is reported 18%. Most of the AA cases transform into GBM during the course of disease. The treatment approaches for HGA remains palliative, not curative. There is a general consensus for a classification system for evaluating the response of the tumor to SRS treatment (Table 2).

Terminology	Description
Complete response (CR)	Complete disappearance of enhancing or non-enhancing tumor
Partial response (PR)	>50% shrinkage of the tumor
No change (NC)	Less than 50% reduction or 25% increase in tumor volume (stable disease)
Progressive disease (PD)	>25% increase in volume of the enhancing or non-enhancing tumor

(CR+PR+NC = Tumor Control Rate (TCR), CR+PR = Effectiveness)

Table 2. Classification of responsiveness of the tumor to SRS treatment.

A review by Yoshikawa et al on malignant glioma included seven clinical studies of RT plus SRS comparing with four clinical studies of RT only showed 20.2 and 11.1 months median overall survivals, respectively. Also the progression free survival (PFS) is found a median 281 days for SRS and 130 days for RT group (Yoshikawa et al., 2006). (Table 3).

Group	First author, year	Pathology	Number of patients	SRS modality	Median survival after diagnosis (months)	Mean survival of the group (months)
SRS	Masciopinto, 1995	GBM	31	LINAC	9.5	20.2
	Gannett, 1995	Malignant glioma	30	LINAC	13.9	
	Kondziolka, 1997	GBM	64	Gamma knife	26	
	Shrieve, 1999	GBM	78	LINAC	19.9	
	Nwokedi, 2002	GBM	31	Gamma knife	25	
	Prisco, 2002	Malignant glioma	15	Gamma knife	21.4	
	Yoshikawa, 2006	GBM	18	CyberKnife	20.7	
RT	Curran, 1993	Malignant glioma	1578	NA*	11.3	11.1
	Nwokedi, 2002	GBM	33	NA	13	
	Prisco, 2002	Malignant glioma	17	NA	11.6	
	Laws, 2003	GBM	413	NA	10.2	

Table 3. Review of studies comparing SRS with conventional RT by means of survival rates. *(NA*: Not available)*

Current multimodal treatment regimen for HGA includes a diagnostic or cytoreductive surgery followed by boost RT. For that reason, it's not so possible to meet with cases only treated with SRS without RT. Preliminary results of cases treated only with SRS for HGA suggested poor outcomes (Crowley et al., 2006). Certain indications and guidelines for patient selection criteria is not established yet on SRS for HGA. However long term outcome results of randomized controlled trials for SRS in HGA is not well reported yet, some helpful criteria standing out are described below.

2.1.1 Timing of SRS

Timing of SRS for HGAs is controversial. While some of the authors have performed SRS for residual disease following surgical resection as a boost or in combination with RT, others have tended to perform as salvage for recurrence following RT. ASTRO (The American Society for Therapeutic Radiology and Oncology) has reported a comprehensive evidence-based review on SRS for HGA in 2005. They found level I-III evidence that the use of radiosurgery boost followed by RT and BCNU doesn't confer benefit in terms of overall survival, local tumor control or quality of life as compared with RT and BCNU.

Furthermore, they pointed that the boost radiosurgery is associated with increased long term toxicity. They also reported that there is not sufficient evidence yet to show the effectiveness of SRS on recurrent or progressive malignant glioma (Anker et al., 2010; Tsao et al., 2005).
A multicentric study including 46 patients on CyberKnife comparing the use as a boost with salvage reported median overall survival of 11.5 and 21 months for GBM respectively. This study also suggested no significant difference of survival between boost SRS and not to perform SRS (Villavicencio et al., 2009). In another study including 48 GBM patients, the use of SRS as boost or salvage was related with median survival of 15.1 and 17.1 months respectively. Difference in survivals was also statistically significant in this study (Pouratian et al., 2009). Contrarily, median survivals for GBM was found 10 and 16.7 months with boost and salvage SRS respectively in another study including 51 GBM patients in which the difference was statistically not meaningful (Hsieh et al., 2005). A study including 32 recurrent GBM patients treated with LINAC radiosurgery following conventional approach (surgery + RT) reported median 10 months of PFS following initial conventional treatment. SRS has contributed an additional 5 months of PFS to patients and a median 22 months of overall survival has been achieved. Survival rates of the study for 1st, 2nd and 3rd years are 88%, 41% and 19%, respectively (Combs et al., 2005). Besides, current studies on efficacy of repetitive SRS for multiple recurrences suggest no benefit on overall survival (Yoshikawa et al., 2006).

2.1.2 Tumor volume

Increased tumor volume is associated with increased complication rates in SRS. Treatment dose should be decreased while tumor volume increases to avoid the complications such as radionecrosis and edema; which weakens the effectiveness of the treatment (Combs et al., 2007; Niyazi et al., 2011). Despite the lack of a definite threshold, SRS is not recommended for lesions larger than 3 cm diameter. Kong et al have reported the <10 ml tumor volume as the most important prognostic factor for SRS for malignant glioma in a series of 114 patients (Tsao et al., 2005). While adverse radiation effects occur rarely for tumors under 10 ml volume, Cho et al reported a high late complication rate of 30% for treatment of mean 30 ml tumors with mean 17 Gy (Cho et al., 1999).

2.1.3 Histological grade

HGAs are classified as grade III and IV tumors. Various studies suggested the significant effect of histological grade on SRS treatment outcome. Yoshikawa et al reported an effectiveness rate and TCR of 27.2% and 63.3% for GBM respectively at least four weeks after SRS. Nevertheless, they found 18.2% and 45.5% for AA. Another study reported by Kong et al suggested a significant increase in overall median survival rate with SRS for GBM group and no difference in AA group as compared with control group (Kong et al., 2008). These results suggest that SRS may have a potential benefit on grade IV HGA.

2.1.4 Tumor location and extent of surgical resection

Extent of surgical resection and effective post-operative RT are important prognostic factors for HGA. However, extensive surgical resection is not always possible particularly for tumors located in eloquent areas as optic nerves, brainstem and midbrain. Surgical approach generally remains limited with biopsy for these locations. While the median survival is only 6 months in HGA patients who underwent biopsy followed by RT and SRS. The survival rises up to 21 months in patients who undergo gross total resection in anytime during the course of disease (Villavicencio et al., 2009). Pouratian et al reported more favorable overall survival rates following SRS in RTOG (Radiation Therapy Oncology Group) Class-III patients (patients who underwent extensive surgical resection and without need for steroids at the time of SRS). Adjuvant treatments like RT and chemotherapy come forward when the surgical resection is not feasible. Different biological structures have different radiation limits. For example, the calculated cumulative radiation maximum point dose limits for lens is 10 Gy, retina 50 Gy and optic nerve, chiasm and brainstem is 55 Gy. Biological equivalents of these limits are lesser for SRS (lens: 1-2 Gy, optic nerve & chiasm: 8-10 Gy and brainstem: 12 Gy) (Sharma et al. 2008). Unfortunately, a cumulative dose of >60 Gy is required for effective irradiation HGA. This requirement let the physicians to combine lower dose RT with SRS to achieve an effective treatment. A median 18 months survival was achieved for GBM patients within eloquent locations with combination of 50 Gy RT, 10 Gy SRS and temazolamide following biopsy (Oermann et al., 2010). Contrarily, no significant difference was observed by means of overall survival rates in another study comparing RT only with RT plus gamma knife following biopsy for unresectable GBMs (Kong et al., 2006). Interestingly, the Karnofsky performance scores (KPS) of RT+SRS group has been found to be significantly higher than the RT only group in first 3 months follow-ups.

2.1.5 Tumor control and functional outcome

Because the recurrences typically occur within 2-3 cm of the tumor resection bed in 63-90% of the patients, local control of the tumor has a particular importance in the management of HGA. Preliminary results for HGA suggest that SRS increases local tumor control rate, progression free and overall survival, and quality of life (Blomquist et al., 2005; Gerosa et al., 2003). It's shown that the SRS delays neurological deterioration in HGA and provides better KPS during the course of the disease (Jagannathan et al., 2004). Pre-SRS >90 KPS is also associated with better overall survival.

2.1.6 Other aspects of SRS for HGA

SRS is preferable for patients with progressive or recurrent disease following initial surgical resection and RT if re-resection is not feasible. However, a significant difference has been shown on median survival between patients responsive to initial RT and irresponsive (15.8 vs. 7.3 months, respectively) (Patel et al., 2009). There are not definite evidences for the role of age and gender as prognostic factors.

Current treatment modality for HGA includes surgical resection as extensive as possible, post-operative RT and administration of temazolamide (Sathornsumetee & Rich, 2008). SRS is considerable only for a limited number of patients with particularly WHO grade IV, recurrent, well circumscribed and small lesions as a palliative.

2.2 Low grade astrocytoma

Low grade astrocytoma (LGA) includes grade I (subependymal giant cell astrocytoma and pilocytic astrocytoma) and grade II (pilomyxoid, diffuse astrocytoma and pleomorphic xanthoastrocytoma) tumors according to WHO classification system (Louis et al., 2007).

LGA accounts for 15% of all primary CNS tumors in adult (Heppner et al., 2005). However the peak age for LGA is 35; the pilocytic astrocytoma is more frequent in pediatric population. Gross total resection is the golden standard in the treatment of LGA. RT is especially preferred in older patients underwent subtotal resection (Morantz, 2001). Survival rate for LGA is inversely correlated with histologic grade and age. While the 10 year median survival for pilocytic astrocytoma in pediatric age is above 90%, it's about 7% for diffuse astrocytoma patients in sixth decade (Henderson et al. 2009). A brief review of available studies on effectiveness of SRS for LGA is given below (Table 4).

First author / Year	Number of patients	Tumor type	Med age	Med target volume (ml)	Med dose (Gy)	Med follow up (mns)	PFS or PFS rate	TCR
Hadjipanayis, 2002a	12	Fibrillary astrocytoma	25	4.6	15	52	67% for 52 mns	NA
Hadyipanayis, 2002b	37	Grade I	14	3	15	28	NA	68%
Boethius, 2002	19	Grade I	10.6	2.2	10	56.4	NA	94.7%
Hadjipanayis, 2003	49	PA (n:37), Grade II (n:12)	14 (PA), 25 (Grade II)	3.3	15	32	NA	67%
Heppner, 2005	49	Grade I and II	27	2.4	15	63	44 mns	NA
Wang, 2006	21	Grade I and II	20	2.4	14.5	67	65% (10 year)	NA
Yen, 2007	20	PA (n:5), Non-PA (n:5), NHP* (n:10)	19.1	2.5	12.8	78	NA	80%
Kano, 2009a	14	Grade I	32.3	4.7	13.3	36.3	89.3%, 31.5% and 31.5% for 1,3 and 5 years	NA
Kano, 2009b	50	Grade I	10.5	2.1	14.5	55.5	91.7%, 82.8% and 70.8% for 1,5 and 10 years	NA
Henderson, 2009	12	Grade I and II	17.4	4.4	13	48.2	75% for 48 mns	NA
Park, 2011	6	SEGA**	16.5	2.75	14	73	NA	67%

Table 4. Review of available literature on SRS treatment for LGA. *(NHP*: Not histologically proven, SEGA**: Subependymal giant cell astrocytoma, NA: Not available, PA: Pilocytic astrocytoma, TCR: Tumor control rate.)*

2.2.1 Timing of SRS

SRS may either be performed alone or as a boost in combination with RT for residual tumor in early post-operative period; or as salvage treatment at the time of recurrence. Whether or not to perform and when to perform is the moot point. Boost SRS concurrent with RT was found to cause more adverse radiation effect in comparison with salvage (adjuvant) SRS (Wang et al., 2006). 10 year median survival rate was found 88.9% for PA patients underwent partially resection or biopsy followed by SRS alone as the principal treatment. The ratio was also found 44.5% for PA patients received delayed SRS for recurrent disease. Delayed SRS for recurrent tumor seems to be associated with poor PFS (Kano et al., 2009b). On the other hand, it doesn't seem so reasonable to make a generalization for timing of SRS because the tumors highly tended to recur already have poor prognosis. Another study reported TCR of 56.3 months for boost SRS versus 44.4% for late SRS. However, this difference was not statistically significant (Park et al., 2010). The beginning of shrinkage following SRS occurs between a median 13-16 months (range; 3-92.4) for LGA (Yen et al., 2007; Kano et al. 2009a & 2009b). In case of progression, the mean time from SRS to the beginning of progression has been found about 23 months (Hadjipanayis et al., 2002a). That's why the patients should be periodically followed-up in a long time period. Despite the lack of large series on effectiveness of repetitive SRS for recurrent LGA; achievement of effective tumor control has been reported for sporadic cases. More studies are needed intended to timing of SRS for LGAs. Available literature suggests better tumor control for residual PA with early SRS.

2.2.2 Tumor location and pattern

Even though the primary treatment for LGA is the surgical resection, SRS following pathological diagnosis serves as an option for tumors located in eloquent areas and for unresectable tumors. However, the treatment dose should be diminished to avoid damage to surrounding tissues for tumors in close proximity to eloquent tissues, which results in reduction of effectiveness of the treatment. SRS is preferable instead of whole brain irradiation for LGA because of the locally invasive nature of these tumors.

Brainstem gliomas account for less than 2% of adult and 10-20% of pediatric age glial tumors. Although 52-69% of brainstem gliomas are low grade, they carry greater potential for malignant transformation with respect to other locations (Bricolo, 2009). 80% TCR during 78 month follow-up was reported in a series of 20 unresectable focal brainstem gliomas with gamma knife with mean 12.8 Gy doses (Yen et al., 2007). Another study comparing TCR for LGA between brainstem and other locations reported 59% and 67% TCR, respectively (Hadjipanayis et al., 2003). Progression rate following SRS was also found 45% for brainstem versus 10% for other locations. Major reasons for lower success rate of SRS for brainstem gliomas are the more aggressive nature of tumor at this location and the requirement of dose reduction. Unresectable low grade optic glioma may also benefit from fractionated SRS. Effective TCR and prevention of progressive visual symptoms were reported for optic gliomas (Kurt et al., 2010).

LGAs may include solid or cystic components. Better response to the SRS for solid LGA was reported in various series. Furthermore, half of the progressive patients have only cyst enlargement without solid enlargement. TCR for pure solid tumors was 84% in a study including both solid and cystic tumors with overall 68% TCR (Hadjipanayis et al., 2002a). 1,

3 and 5 year PFS rates were found 75%, 50% and 50% for solid, and 88.9%, 17.8% and 0% for mixed solid-cystic tumors respectively in a study (Kano et al, 2009a). Another study reported 3, 5 and 10 year PFS rates of 100%, 94.4% and 85% for solid, and 53.1%, 21.3% and 0% for mixed solid-cystic tumors respectively (Kano et al., 2009b). Peripheral contrast enhancement and cystic changes on MRI are related with poor prognosis (Park et al., 2010). SRS may also be performed for multicentric LGA, but the prognosis of multicentric tumors is poorer than the solitary tumors (Hadjipanayis et al., 2002a).

2.2.3 Tumor volume and radiation dose

Administration of maximal dose to a minimum volume without damaging normal tissue is one of the major goals of SRS. The probability of direct and indirect surrounding tissue damage due to radionecrosis and edema increases in proportion to the tumor volume and radiation dose. However the SRS dose above 15Gy is known as a good prognostic criterion for LGA, high TCR rate (94.7%) with low dose SRS for PA has also been reported (Boethius et al., 2002). Tumor volume less than 6-8 cc is significantly related with better prognosis (Park et al, 2010). Despite the lack of a definite dose range for LGA, doses ranging between 10-15 Gy are currently used. Dose modification or reduction should be considered for patients who have undergone fractionated cranial RT before SRS (Wang et al., 2006).

2.2.4 Histological grade and age

Pilocytic astrocytoma has a better prognosis than grade II astrocytomas. Grade II astrocytoma carries a potential to transform into malignant glioma. Pilocytic astrocytoma also has better prognosis in children than in adults. Median 1, 3 and 5 year PFS rates are 91.7%, 82.8% and 70.8% for pediatric PA; and 83.8%, 31.5% and 31.5 for adult PA respectively (Kano et al., 2009a, 2009b). SRS as an alternate to RT has been found very effective for PA patients in whom the re-resection is not feasible or with early recurrence. But the place of SRS in multimodal treatment of grade II astrocytoma is controversial. 91.3%, 54.1% and 37.1% PFS rates for 1, 5 and 10 years respectively has been reported for radiosurgical treatment of residual or recurrent grade II astrocytomas (Park et al, 2010). More studies are needed for determining definite indications and criteria of SRS for LGA. Prognostic factors of SRS for LGA are listed below (Table 5).

Good prognosis	Poor prognosis
Pilocytic astrocytoma	Grade II astrocytoma
Solid, well circumscribed tumors	Cystic tumors
Volume < 6-8 cc	Larger volume
Teenagers	Age <10 year or >70 year
Solitary tumors	Multicentric tumors
History of long term effective RT	History of unsuccessful RT
Effective SRS dose	Lower SRS dose
No contrast enhancement on MRI	Peripheral contrast enhancement

Table 5. Prognostic factors of SRS for LGA

Finally, the best candidates for SRS treatment are the pilocytic astrocytomas if previously resected, well circumscribed, and located in critical or deep areas or re-resection is not feasible, or if there is an early recurrence.

2.3 Ependymoma

While ependymomas are classified as grade II in WHO grading system, the anaplastic ependymomas are grade III tumors. However the local tumor control has a great importance for ependymoma management, high propensity of seeding through ventricular system and central canal serves as a problem. The most prominent poor diagnostic factor is the spinal metastasis for ependymomas. Current treatment modality includes surgical resection followed by RT. Chemotherapy is also indicated for anaplastic ependymomas. Better local tumor control for ependymomas with SRS has been reported in limited number of preliminary studies. Results with boost SRS + RT are better than SRS for late recurrences conversely to other gliomas. There is a proportion between time to recurrence and success rate for adjuvant SRS. 100% TCR was found at a mean 21 months follow up in a series of 22 anaplastic ependymoma patients following adjuvant SRS (Jawahar et al., 1999). But 44% patients recurred at a distant site of the CNS in further follow ups. Definite predictors of better prognosis for SRS treatment for ependymomas are; (Kano et al., 2009d, 2010)

- Absence of spinal metastasis
- Lower tumor volume
- Time interval between RT and recurrence > 18 months
- Homogeneous contrast enhancement on MRI for low grade ependymomas

Interestingly, no significant relation was found between the grade of the tumor and PFS. SRS seems a valuable treatment option for local control of recurrent or residual ependymomas. On the other hand, the distant seeding and recurrences of the tumor is a pain in the neck (Krieger & McComb, 2009; Lo et al., 2006a, 2006b).

2.4 Oligodendroglioma and mixed oligoastrocytoma

Only seldom studies are available regarding to the effectiveness of SRS for oligodendroglioma and oligoastrocytoma in current literature. A study on SRS for oligodendroglioma reported 5 and 10 year overall survival rates of 90.9% and 68.2% for grade II, and 52.1% and 26.1% for grade III oligodendroglioma, respectively (Kano et al., 2009c). Tumor volume less than 15 cc and patients with 1p19q gene deletion are related with better outcome. Another study on SRS including oligodendroglioma and oligoastrocytoma patients suggested that the younger age is also associated with better outcome (Sarkar et al., 2002). Further studies are needed to assess the effectiveness of SRS for these entities.

3. Complications of SRS

Adverse radiation effects due to SRS include focal edema and radionecrosis. These effects correspondingly intensify with the tumor volume and radiation dose and found more frequently in patients who received boost SRS concurrently with RT. Frequency of adverse radiation effects range between 0 to 40% in different series, albeit it's uncommonly more than 5%. These effects are usually completely reversible with anti-edema medications and rarely results in permanent neurological complications. Previous irradiation history should

be considered particularly for lesions located in eloquent areas and dose should be reduced. Aggressive irradiation might result in excessive edema and radionecrosis requiring additional procedures such as emergent decompression or shunting (Smith et al., 2008).
Radiation induced tumors is another potential complication of SRS. Several sporadic reports of GBM formation in long term following high dose SRS are already present. However long term follow up is needed to assess this potential, incidence seems less than 1:100.000 for now (Berman et al., 2007; Salvati et al., 2003).

4. Case illustrations

Case 1. 25 years old male presented with progressive headache. Cranial MRI showed an intraxial mass lesion in close proximity to pineal region. Patient refused biopsy and considered for gamma knife. Mass disappeared at 6th month post-SRS and didn't recur during 6 year follow ups. (Figure 2)

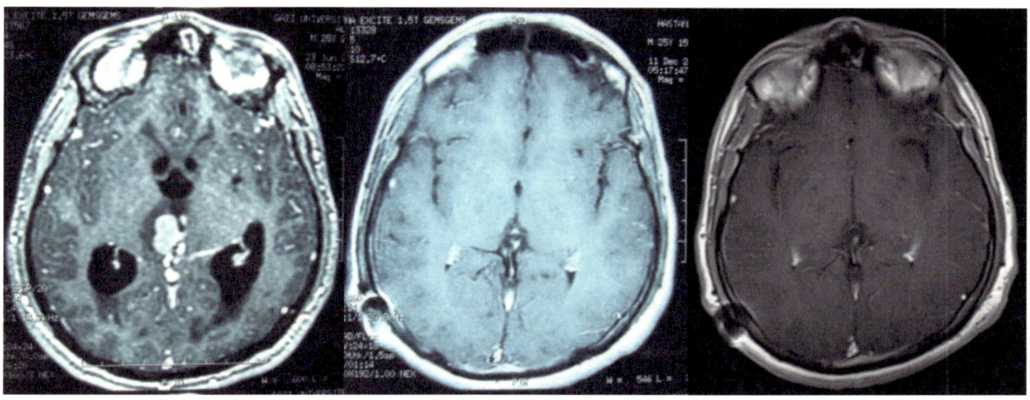

Fig. 2. Left: pre-SRS axial contrast enhanced MRI view. Middle: 6 months after SRS. Right: 6 years after SRS.

Case 2. 37 years old male presented with complete loss of vision at the right eye and progressive loss of vision on the left eye for months. MRI scan revealed an optic glioma located on the right half of the chiasm. Patient underwent low dose fractionated SRS to avoid the damage to the chiasm and optic nerve. (Figure 3) Patient was followed up 66 months following SRS, and neither tumor progression, nor visual deterioration was seen. (Figure 4)

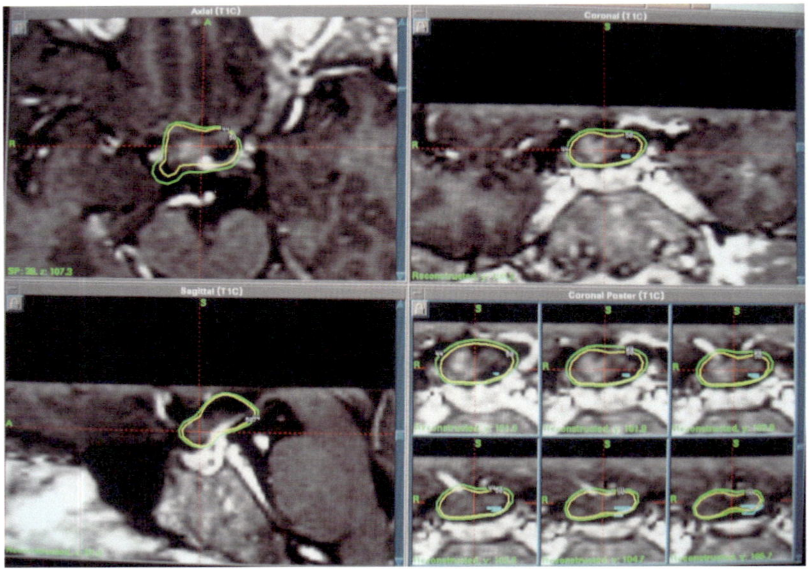

Fig. 3. Gamma knife dose planning.

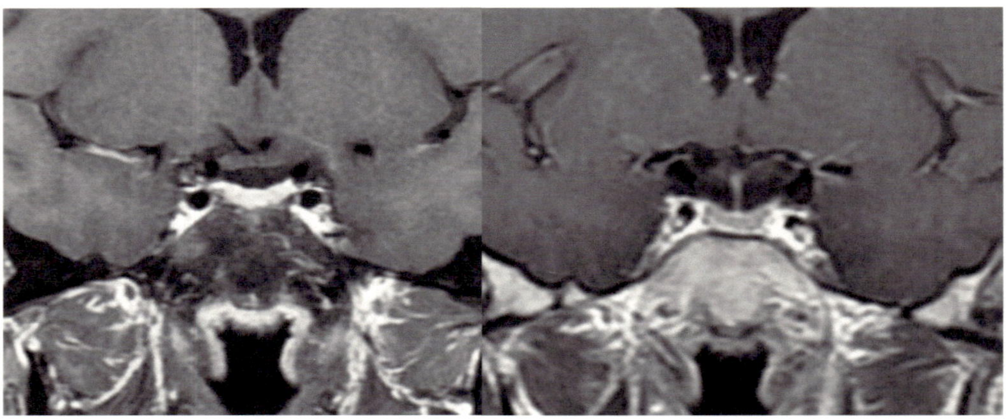

Fig. 4. 39 *(left)* and 66 *(right)* months after SRS; complete disappearance of the tumor.

Case 3. 52 years old male presented with slight right hemiparesis, numbness and progressive headache. Multiple intracranial lesions were detected on MRI scan. Stereotactic biopsy of the tumor revealed GBM. Patient received conventional RT followed by temazolamide immediately after pathologic diagnosis. Regression in two of three tumors and progression in one tumor located at the left trigonal region was found 6 months after diagnosis. Thereupon, adjuvant SRS was performed to the progressive tumor. Nevertheless, tumor kept progressing and required decompressive resection 6 months after SRS. (Figure 5)

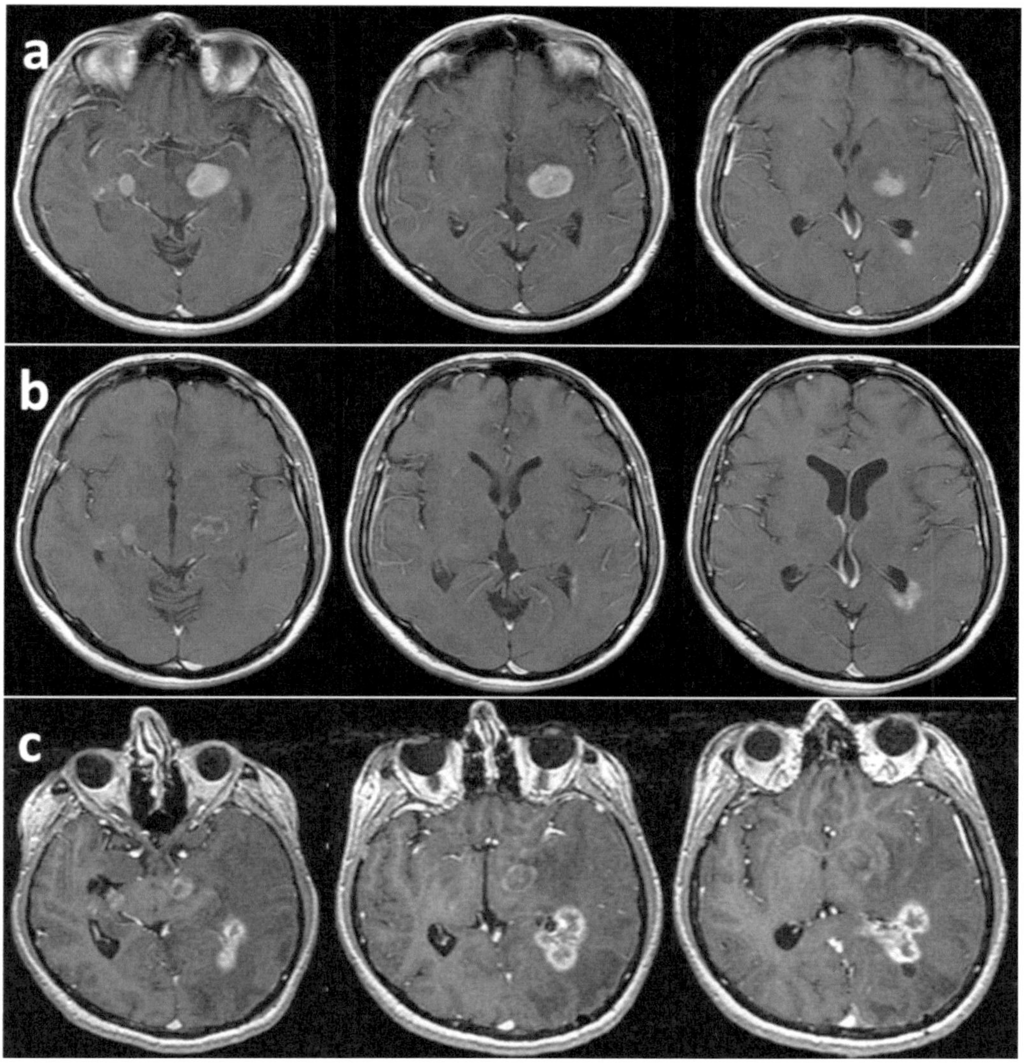

Fig. 5. a) MRI scans of the patient at the time of initial diagnosis. b) Pre-SRS MRI scan of the patient following stereotactic biopsy, RT and temazolamide. c) 6 months after SRS; progressive tumor is visible at the left trigon

5. Conclusion

Although the guideline indications of SRS in the management of gliomas are not definite yet, favorable results are being reported especially for pilocytic astrocytoma and ependymoma. SRS also makes significant contributions to multimodal treatment modality of GBM as an adjuvant, as well. SRS might safely be used for carefully selected patients with low complication rates and high efficacy. Many prudential studies are also conducted in this growing field of neurosurgery. Successful results were reported for combination of SRS with agents like thalidomide, marimastat and gefitinib, hyperbaric oxygen therapy or with genetic treatment modalities like adenoviral or herpetic viral vectors (Kohshi et al., 2007; Larson et al., 2002; Lee et al., 2006; Niranjan et al., 2000; Schwer et al., 2008; Xu et al., 2006). As a result, the SRS is a promising adjuvant technique for glioma treatment.

6. References

Adler, J.R.; Murphy, M.J.; Chang, S.D. & Hancock, S.L. (1999). Image guided robotic radiosurgery. *Neurosurgery,* 44:1299-1307

Anker, C.J.; Hymas, R.V.; Hazard, L.J.; Boucher, K.M.; Jensen, R.L. & Shrieve, D.C. (2010). Stereotactic radiosurgery eligibility and selection bias in the treatment of glioblastoma multiforme. *J. Neurooncol.,* 98:253-263

Berman, E.L.; Eade, T.N.; Brown, D.; Weaver, M.; Glass, J.; Zorman, G. & Feigenberg, S.J. (2007). Radiation-induced tumor after stereotactic radiosurgery for an arteriovenous malformation: Case report. *Neurosurgery,* 61:E1099

Blomquist, E.; Bjelkengren, G. & Glimelius, B. (2005). The potential of proton beam radiation therapy in intracranial and ocular tumors. *Acta Oncologica,* 44:862-870

Boethius, J.; Ulfarsson, E.; Rahn, T. & Lippitz, B. (2002). Gamma knife radiosurgery for pilocytic astrocytomas. *J. Neurosurg.,* 97:677-680

Bricolo, A. (2009). Brainstem tumors, In: Practical Handbook of Neurosurgery from Leading Neurosurgeons, M. Sindou (ed.), Vol.2:349-372, Springer-Verlag/Wien, ISBN 978-3-211-84819-7, Mörlenbach, Germany

Chen, C.C.; Chapman, P.; Petit, J. & Loeffler, J. (2007). Proton radiosurgery in neurosurgery. *Neurosurg. Focus,* 23 (6):E5

Cho, K.H.; Hall, W.A.; Gerbi, B.J.; Higgins, P.D.; McGuire, W.A. & Clark, H.B. (1999). Single dose versus fractionated stereotactic radiotherapy for recurrent high-grade gliomas. *Int. J. Radiation Oncology Biol. Phys.,* 45:1133-1141

Combs, S.E.; Debus, J. & Schulz-Ertner, D. (2007). Radiotherapeutic alternatives for previously irradiated recurrent gliomas (review). *BMC Cancer,* 7:167

Combs, S.E.; Widmer, V.; Thilmann, C.; Hof, H.; Debus, J. & Schulz-Ertner, D. (2005). Stereotactic radiosurgery (SRS); treatment option for recurrent glioblastoma multiforme (GBM). *Cancer,* 104:2168-2173

Crowley, R.W.; Pouratian, N. & Sheehan, J.P. (2006). Gamma knife surgery for glioblastoma multiforme. *Neurosurg. Focus,* 20 (4):E17

Gerosa, M.; Nicolato, A. & Foroni, R. (2003). The role of gamma knife radiosurgery in the treatment of primary and metastatic brain tumors. *Curr. Opin. Oncol.,* 15:188-196, ISSN 1040-8746

Hadjipanayis, C.G.; Kondziolka, D.; Flickinger, J.C. & Lunsford, L.D. (2003). The role of stereotactic radiosurgery for low-grade astrocytomas. *Neurosurg. Focus,* 14 (5): Article 15

Hadjipanayis, C.G.; Kondziolka, D.; Gardner, P.; Niranjan, A.; Dagam, S.; Flickinger, J.C. & Lunsford, L.D. (2002a). Stereotactic radiosurgery for pilocytic astrocytomas when multimodal therapy is necessary. *J. Neurosurg.,* 97:56-64

Hadjipanayis, C.G.; Niranjan, A.; Tyler-Kabara, E.; Kondziolka, D.; Flickinger, J.C. & Lunsford, L.D. (2002b). Stereotactic radiosurgery for well-circumscribed fibrillary grade II astrocytomas: An initial experience. *Stereotact. Funct. Neurosurg.,* 79:13-24

Henderson, M.A.; Fakiris, A.J.; Timmerman, R.D.; Worth, R.M.; Lo, S.S. & Witt, T.C. (2009). Gamma Knife stereotactic radiosurgery for low-grade astrocytomas. *Stereotact. Funct. Neurosurg.*, 87:161-167

Heppner, P.A.; Sheehan, J.P. & Steiner, L.E. (2005). Gamma Knife surgery for low-grade gliomas. *Neurosurgery*, 57:1132-1139

Hsieh, P.C.; Chandler, J.P.; Bhangoo, S.; Panagiotopoulos, K.; Kalapurakal, J.A.; Marymont, M.H. & al. (2005). Adjuvant gamma knife stereotactic radiosurgery at the time of tumor progression potentially improves survival for patients with glioblastoma multiforme. *Neurosurgery*, 57:684-692

Jagannathan, J.; Petit, J.H.; Balsara, K.; Hudes, R. & Chin, L.S. (2004). Long-term survival after gamma knife radiosurgery for primary and metastatic brain tumors. *Am. J. Clin. Oncol.*, 27:441-444, ISSN 0277-3732/04/2705-0441

Jawahar, A.; Kondziolka, D.; Flickinger, J.C. & Lunsford L.D. (1999). Adjuvant stereotactic radiosurgery for anaplastic ependymoma. *Stereotact. Funct. Neurosurg.*, 73:23-30

Kano, H.; Kondziolka, D.; Niranjan, A.; Flickinger, J.C. & Lunsford, L.D. (2009a). Stereotactic radiosurgery for pilocytic astrocytomas part 1: outcomes in adult patients. *J. Neurooncol.*, 95:211-218

Kano, H.; Niranjan, A.; Khan, A.; Flickinger, J.C.; Kondziolka, D.; Lieberman, F. & Lunsford, L.D. (2009c). Does radiosurgery have a role in the management of oligodendrogliomas? *J. Neurosurg.*, 110:564-571

Kano, H.; Niranjan, A.; Kondziolka, D.; Flickinger, J.C. & Lunsford, L.D. (2009d). Outcome predictors for intracranial ependymoma radiosurgery. *Neurosurgery*, 64:279-288

Kano, H.; Niranjan, A.; Kondziolka, D.; Flickinger, J.C.; Pollack, I.F.; Jakacki, R.L. & Lunsford, L.D. (2009b). Stereotactic radiosurgery for pilocytic astrocytomas part 2: outcomes in pediatric patients. *J. Neurooncol.*, 95:219-229

Kano, H.; Yang, H.C.; Kondziolka, D.; Niranjan, A.; Arai, Y.; Flickinger, J.C. & Lunsford, L.D. (2010). Stereotactic radiosurgery for pediatric recurrent intracranial ependymomas. *J. Neurosurg. Pediatrics*, 6:417-423

Kohshi, K.; Yamamoto, H.; Nakahara, A.; Katoh, T. & Takagi, M. (2007). Fractionated stereotactic radiotherapy using gamma knife unit after hyperbaric oxygenation on recurrent high-grade gliomas. *J. Neurooncol.*, 82:297-303

Kong, D.S.; Lee, J.I.; Park, K.; Kim, J.H.; Lim, D.H. & Nam, D.H. (2008). Efficacy of stereotactic radiosurgery as a salvage treatment for recurrent malignant gliomas. *Cancer*, 112:2046-2051

Kong, D.S.; Nam, D.H.; Lee, J.I.; Park, K. & Kim, J.H. (2006). Preservation of quality of life by preradiotherapy stereotactic radiosurgery for unresectable glioblastoma multiforme. *J. Neurosurg. (Suppl)*, 105:139-143

Krieger, M.D. & McComb, J.G. (2009). The role of stereotactic radiotherapy in the management of ependymomas. *Childs Nerv. Syst.*, 25:1269-1273

Kuo, J.S.; Yu, C.; Petrovich, Z. & Apuzzo, M.L.J. (2003). The cyberknife stereotactic radiosurgery system: Description, installation, and an initial evaluation of use and functionality. *Neurosurgery*, 53:1235-1239

Kurt, G.; Tönge, M.; Borcek, A.O.; Karahacioglu, E.; Gurel, O.; Baykaner, K. & al. (2010). Fractionated gamma knife radiosurgery for optic nerve tumors: A technical report. *Turkish Neurosurgery,* 20 (2):241-246

Larson, D.A.; Prados, M.; Lamborn, K.R.; Smith, V.; Sneed, P.K.; Chang, S. & al. (2002). Phase II study of high central dose gamma knife radiosurgery and marimastat in patients with recurrent malignant glioma. *Int. J. Radiation Oncology Biol. Phys.,* 54:1397-1404

Lee, J.I.; Itasaka, S.; Kim, J.T. & Nam, D.H. (2006). Antiangiogenic agent, thalidomide increases the antitumor effect of single high dose irradiation (gamma knife radiosurgery) in the rat orthotopic glioma model. *Oncology Reports,* 15:1163-1168

Lo, S.S.; Abdulrahman, R.; DesRosiers, P.M.; Fakiris, A.J.; Witt, T.C.; Worth, R.M. & al. (2006a). The role of Gamma Knife radiosurgery in the management of unresectable gross disease or gross residual disease after surgery in ependymoma. *Journal of Neuro-Oncology,* 79:51-56

Lo, S.S.; Chang, E.L. & Sloan, A.E. (2006b). Role of stereotactic radiosurgery and fractionated stereotactic radiotherapy in the management of intracranial ependymoma. *Expert Rev. Neurotherapeutics,* 6 (4):501-507, ISSN 1473-7175

Louis, D.N.; Ohgaki, H.; Wiestler, O.D. & Cavenne, W.K. (Eds.) (2007). *WHO Classification of Tumors of the Central Nervous System.* IARC, ISBN 978-92-832-2430-2, Lyon, France

Mayer, R. & Sminia, P. (2008). Reirradiation tolerance of the human brain. *Int. J. Radiation Oncology. Biol. Phys.,* 70:1350-1360.

Morantz, A.R. (2001). Low grade astrocytomas, In: Brain Tumors; An encyclopedic approach, 2nd ed., A.H. Kaye & E.R. Laws JR (eds.), 467-492, Churchill Livingstone-Harcourt, ISBN 0-433-06426-1, London, United Kingdom

Niranjan, A.; Moriuchi, S.; Lunsford, L.D.; Kondziolka, D.; Flickinger, J.C.; Fellows, W. & al. (2000). Effective treatment of experimental glioblastoma by HSV vector-mediated TNFα and HSV-tk gene transfer in combination with radiosurgery and ganciclovir administration. *Molecular Therapy,* 2:114-120

Niyazi, M.; Siefert, A.; Schwarz, S.B.; Ganswindt, U.; Kreth, F.W.; Tonn, J.C. & Belka, C. (2011). Therapeutic options for recurrent malignant glioma. *Radiotherapy and Oncology,* 98:1-14, ISSN 0167-8140

Oermann, E.; Collins, B.T.; Erickson, K.T.; Yu, X.; Lei, S.; Suy, S. & al. (2010). CyberKnife® enhanced conventionally fractionated chemoradiation for high grade glioma in close proximity to critical structures. *Journal of Hematology and Oncology,* 3:22

Pantelis, E.; Papadakis, N.; Verigos, K.; Stathochristopoulou, I.; Antypas, C.; Lekas, L. & al. (2010). Integration of functional MRI and white matter tractography in stereotactic radiosurgery clinical practice. *Int. J. Radiation Oncology Biol. Phys.,* 78:257-267

Park, K.J.; Kano, H.; Kondziolka, D.; Niranjan, A.; Flickinger, J.C. & Lunsford, L.D. (2010). Early or delayed radiosurgery for WHO grade II astrocytomas. Available from: http://www.springerlink.com/content/1686r1055h613182/ DOI 10.1007/s11060-010-0409-0

Park, K.J.; Kano, H.K.; Kondziolka, D.; Niranjan, A.; Flickinger, J.C. & Lunsford, L.D. (2011). Gamma Knife surgery for subependymal giant cell astrocytomas. *J. Neurosurg.,* 114:808-813

Patel, M.; Siddiqui, F.; Jin, J.Y.; Mikkelsen, T.; Rosenblum, M.; Movsas, B. & Ryu, S. (2009). Salvage reirradiation for recurrent glioblastoma with radiosurgery: radiographic response and improved survival. *J. Neurooncol.*, 92:185-191

Pollock, B.E. & Brown, P.D. (2005). Stereotactic radiosurgery, In: *Principles of Neurosurgery 2nd Ed.*, S.S. Rengachary & R.G. Ellenbogen (eds.), 729-740, Mosby-Elsevier, ISBN 0-7234-3222-8, London, United Kingdom

Pouratian, N.; Crowley, R.W.; Sherman, J.H.; Jagannathan, J. & Sheehan, J.P. (2009). Gamma knife radiosurgery after radiation therapy as an adjunctive treatment for glioblastoma. *J. Neurooncol.*, 94:409-418

Regis, J. (2009). Radiosurgery for intracranial tumors, In: Practical Handbook of Neurosurgery from Leading Neurosurgeons, M. Sindou (ed.), Vol.2:385-404, Springer-Verlag/Wien, ISBN 978-3-211-84819-7, Mörlenbach, Germany

Salvati, M.; Frati, A.; Russo, N.; Caroli, E.; Polli, F.M.; Minniti, G. & Delfini, R. (2003). Radiation-induced gliomas: Report of 10 cases and review of the literature. *Surg. Neurol.*, 60:60-67

Sarkar, A.; Pollock, B.E.; Brown, P.D. & Gorman, D.A. (2002). Evaluation of gamma knife radiosurgery in the treatment of oligodendrogliomas and mixed oligoastrocytomas. *J. Neurosurg.*, 97:653-656

Sathornsumetee, S. & Rich, J.N. (2008). Designer therapies for glioblastoma multiforme. *Ann. N. Y. Acad. Sci.*, 1140:108-132

Schwer, A.L.; Damek, D.M.; Kavanagh, B.D.; Gaspar, L.E.; Lillehei, K.; Stuhr, K. & Chen, C. (2008). A phase I dose-escalation study of fractionated stereotactic radiosurgery in combination with gefitinib in patients with recurrent malignant gliomas. *Int. J. Radiation Oncology. Biol. Phys.*, 70:993-1001

Sharma, M.; Kondziolka, D.; Khan, A.; Kano, H.; Niranjan, A.; Flickinger, J.C. & Lunsford, L.D. (2008). Radiation tolerance limits of the brainstem. *Neurosurgery*, 63:728-733

Sloan, A.E.; Abdolvahavi, R. & Hlatky, R. (2005). Gliomas, In: *Principles of Neurosurgery 2nd Ed.*, S.S. Rengachary & R.G. Ellenbogen (eds.), 451-478, Mosby-Elsevier, ISBN 0-7234-3222-8, London, United Kingdom

Smith, K.A.; Ashby, L.S.; Gonzalez, L.F.; Brachman, D.G.; Thomas, T.; Coons, S.W. & al. (2008). Prospective trial of gross-total resection with gliadel wafers followed by early postoperative Gamma Knife radiosurgery and conformal fractionated radiotherapy as the initial treatment for patients with radiographically suspected, newly diagnosed glioblastoma multiforme. *J. Neurosurgery*, 109:106-117

Stieber, V.W. & Ellis, T.L. (2005). The role of radiosurgery in the management of malignant brain tumors. *Current Treatment Options in Oncology*, 6:501-508, ISSN 1527-2729

Tsao, M.N.; Mehta, M.P.; Whelan, T.J.; Morris, D.E.; Hayman, J.A.; Flickinger, J.C. & al. (2005). The American Society for Therapeutic Radiology and Oncology (ASTRO) evidence-based review of the role of radiosurgery for malignant glioma. *Int. J. Radiation Oncology Biol. Phys.*, 63:47-55

Villavicencio, A.T.; Burneikienė, S.; Romanelli, P.; Fariselli, L.; McNeely, L.; Lipani, J.D. & al. (2009). Survival following stereotactic radiosurgery for newly diagnosed and recurrent glioblastoma multiforme: a multicenter experience. *Neurosurg. Rev.*, 32:417-424

Wang, L.W.; Shiau, C.Y.; Chung, W.Y.; Wu, H.M.; Guo, W.Y.; Liu, K.D. & al. (2006). Gamma Knife surgery for low-grade astrocytomas: evaluation of long-term outcome based on a 10-year experience. *J. Neurosurg.*, 105:127-132

Witham, T.F.; Okada, H.; Fellows, W.; Hamilton, R.L.; Flickinger, J.C.; Chambers, W.H. & al. (2005). The characterization of tumor apoptosis after experimental radiosurgery. *Stereotact. Funct. Neurosurg.*, 83:17-24

Xu, D.; Jia, Q.; Li, Y.; Kang, C. & Pu, P. (2006). Effects of Gamma Knife surgery on C6 glioma in combination with adenoviral p53 in vitro and in vivo. *J. Neurosurg.*, 105:208-213

Yen, C.P.; Sheehan, J.; Steiner, M.; Patterson, G. & Steiner, L. (2007). Gamma Knife surgery for focal brainstem gliomas. *J. Neurosurg.*, 106:8-17

Yoshikawa, K.; Saito, K.; Kajiwara, K.; Nomura, S.; Ishihara, H. & Suzuki, M. (2006). CyberKnife stereotactic radiotherapy for patients with malignant glioma. *Minim. Invas. Neurosurg.*, 49:110-115, ISSN 0946-7211

15

Surgical Treatment of Supratentorial Glioma in Eloquent Areas

Andrea Talacchi[1], Giovanna Maddalena Squintani[2], Barbara Santini[1], Francesca Casagrande[3], Francesco Procaccio[3], Franco Alessandrini[4], Giada Zoccatelli[4], Vincenzo Tramontano[1], Aurel Hasanbelliu[1] and Massimo Gerosa[1]

[1]Institute of Neurosurgery,
[2]Neurological Unit, Department of Neuroscience;
[3]Neurosurgical Intensive Care Unit, Department of Emergency and Intensive Care;
[4]Neuroradiological Unit, Department of Radiology;
University Hospital, Verona,
Italy

1. Introduction

Awake surgery (AS) and cortical mapping have gained wider acceptance for a variety of reasons: new anesthetic agents, improved surgical techniques, increasing use of functional magnetic resonance (fMRI), and growing interest in brain mapping as shown by refinements and upgrading of imaging techniques, such as magnetoencephalography, evoked responses potentials, high density electroencephalography, positron emission tomography (PET), and optical imaging among others (Bookheimer et al., 1997; Nariai et al., 2005; Papanicolau et al., 1999; Pouratian et al., 2002; Ruge et al., 1999; Rutten et al., 1999; Simos et al., 1999). Information technology and image-guided surgery have prompted researchers to compare non-invasive versus invasive mapping while the patient is awake (Hill et al., 2000; Kamada et al., 2007; Rutten et al., 2002). Cortical mapping has rapidly evolved, but the technical characteristics of electrocortical stimulation (ECS) have remained essentially the same since Penfield's time and it is still considered the gold standard for mapping language (Fitzgerald et al., 1997; Pouratian et al., 2004; Weidemayer et al., 2004). During cortical stimulation, task disruption is taken to indicate that the underlying cortex is essential for task performance. What has changed is the increasing feasibility of mapping the brain in vivo in a way that is safe and acceptable for the patient, and the opportunity to use a broad variety of selective tasks in standardized conditions (Bulsara et al., 2005; Serletis & Bernstein, 2007; Sielbergeld et al., 1992). This has stimulated translational research and cooperation between neuroscientists and neurosurgeons from the basic sciences to clinical applications.

1.1 Historical background

Direct ECS has been used in Neurosurgery since 1930, first by Foerster, and then later by Penfield and colleagues (Foerster, 1931; Penfield & Boldrey, 1937; Penfield & Erickson, 1942;

Penfield & Rasmussen, 1950). In recent years, intraoperative ECS has been adopted for the identification and preservation of language function and motor pathways. Of note is that while cortical mapping was originally applied to epilepsy surgery where resection is essentially limited to the cortex, its indications were later extended to tumor surgery which involves the white matter. Whether these differences result in different clinical and operative settings is unclear and there exist mixed situations between the two extremes. The pathology that benefits most from AS is low-grade glioma (LGG). LGGs pose a considerable challenge in that they have characteristics of both epilepsy and tumors, with a long history that could influence neurofunctional anatomy in patients presenting normal neurological findings (Duffau et al., 2005; Duffau, 2005b, 2006a, 2006b, 2007). Importantly, tumor surgery and epilepsy surgery differ as to the aims of treatment: minimizing neurological sequelae is only one aspect, which can be tailored to lesion characteristics, as determined by clinical and instrumental studies. Basically, the two pathologies differ in symptoms and impairment. Improvement of preoperative clinical impairment and radical tumor resection are the end-points for tumor surgery, while improvement of preoperative performance is the end-point in epilepsy treatment (Buckner, 2003; Hamberger et al., 2007). In glioma surgery, the definitive clinical advantages are broader indications for tumor removal, higher rate of radical tumor resection, and lower rate of postoperative impairment (Duffau 2005a,b).

1.2 Aim of brain mapping

In surgical treatment of cerebral gliomas the goals are to obtain complete tumor removal to the extent the nature of the pathology allows and to accomplish this without injuring normal anatomic structures (Yasargil, 1996a). Although LGGs and high-grade gliomas (HGGs) are distinct in biological features, clinical behavior and outcomes, understanding the effect of surgery remains equally important for both. This is especially true for lesions in areas of eloquence, where the proximity of critical pathways can present a significant challenge to standard operative strategies. The concept of eloquent area is evolving and may be potentially extended to all measurable functions. Thanks to collaborative teamwork in neuroscience and neuro-oncology, current neurosurgical innovations aim to improve our anatomical, physiological, and functional understanding of the surgical region of interest with a view to prevent potential morbidity during resection and improve the patient's quality of life (QoL), an essential outcome measure.

2. Requirements and methodological constraints

One of the main requirements for brain mapping is to have a valid, repeatable, sensitive tool to stimulate functional areas while administering an appropriate test. Electrical stimulation parameters and tests may be adapted to the individual patient according to several individual variables. This makes the mapping procedure extremely variable and imposes methodological constraints subject to validation in individual cases. The method involves comparing intraoperative against postoperative findings classified as true positive (with or without intervention), true negative, false positive, false negative (Wiedmayer et al., 2004). Task must be easy to perform and robust, capable to impact postoperative clinical state without limiting surgical resection. Clinical feedback is used to validate the overall intraoperative strategy while considering additional outcome parameters suggested by surgical management guidelines: extent of resection; complications; neurological and neuropsychological state; functional state and survival (Chang et al., 2003). Finally, new mapping techniques, like fMRI and DT imaging-based tractography (DTI), should be compared with ECS to determine their sensitivity and specificity.

2.1.1 Patient cooperation and compliance in awake surgery

Candidates for awake surgery face an unpredictable experience. To date, the choice depends on the patient who will have received a detailed description of the procedure and provided fully informed consent. Although awake craniotomy is generally considered to be well tolerated, complications such as emotional distress and agitation are not uncommon, with loss of control, the need for more sedation and failure of the mapping project. Failure rates due to agitation vary from 2 to 8% but are not systematically reported (Danks et al., 1998; Sahjipaul, 2000; Whittle et al., 2005).

2.1.2 Preoperative clinical assessment

Together with imaging, symptoms and objective findings will guide the surgical strategy. Disturbances in language-related functions, whether transient or progressive, functional or organic, are more indicative of operative risks than the lesion location itself (Benzagmout et al., 2007; Peraud et al.,2004). The standard assessments for dominance are the Edinburgh handness test, the Wada test and/or fMRI with the verb generation task (Duffau et al., 2003a).

The second step in patient assessment is neurological examination. It can reveal motor impairment (Medical Research Council scale, John, 1984) and disturbances in speech and cognition; however, it cannot provide reliable or sufficient information about the type of dysphasia or specific classification nor recognize mild impairments. This is an important drawback, since the rate of patients with mild-moderate deficits undergoing AS for mapping is quite high (26-55%) (Bello et al., 2007; Sanai et al., 2008; Skirboll et al., 1996).

While there is general consensus that mapping requires that patients present no significant disturbance at intraoperative task testing, some authors have underlined the utility of preoperative assessment, showing how sensitive tasks can maximize testing efficiency. The clinical aim is to recognize preserved functions or subprocesses in order to preserve them intraoperatively (Petrovich Brennan et al., 2007; Pouratian et al., 2003). This research can be pursued through consultation with a group of cognition experts during operative planning to develop personalized tests and tasks for a given patient. Specific functions include: spontaneous speech; language fluency; object naming; written/oral comprehension; reading; dictation; and repetition (baseline for French authors). Added to these are tasks involving writing sentences and words, oral controlled association by phonetic cue and semantic cue, famous face naming, action picture naming, transcoding tasks (Bello et al., 2007; Sanai et al., 2008). Nevertheless, evaluation was limited to the naming task before intraoperative assessment in the majority of cases (Haglund et al., 1994; Hamberger et al., 2005; Ojemann, 1989).

Reviewing the literature, the role of the neuropsychologist in AS is seldom defined in relation to treatment and little attention has been paid to the impact of primary brain tumors on QoL (Buckner et al., 2001; Giovagnoli & Boiardi, 1994; Taphoorn et al., 1992, 2005; Weitzner et al., 1996; Weitzner & Meyers, 1997). Differently from other cancer patients, where the burden of the disease is assessed, in brain tumor patients a decrease in cognitive and emotional functioning may be the result of cerebral disease. Subclinical symptoms, personality changes and mood disturbances may prove to be as burdensome to patients, or more so, as certain focal neurological deficits (Giovagnoli et al., 2005; Talacchi et al., 2010b). Often, they go unrecognized at self assessment; judgment requires trained experts, like those cited above, with oncological experience (Pahlson et al., 2003; Taphoorn et al., 2004). Tumors in the dominant hemisphere may profoundly affect a patient's cognitive function well beyond language function. Although some deficits are known to be related to tumor localization, in brain tumor patients, especially in those with a LGG, many studies failed to find deficits restricted to a single cognitive domain (Tucha et al., 2000; Yoshi et al., 2008). This makes the assessment test battery crucial for global evaluation and longitudinal study.

2.1.3 Tasks, functions and circuits

Ojemann attempted to describe a distribution of language functions (Ojemann, 1989, 2003). He reported that naming interferences occur over a wide area of the left lateral cortex, extending beyond the limits of the classical model. He also found substantial variability in individual organization (Ojemann, 1977; Ojemann & Mateer , 1979; Ojeman G.A. et al., 1989; Ojeman, S.G., et al., 2003). Commonly, at least one area was described in the inferior frontal gyrus and one or more areas in the temporo-parietal peri-sylvian cortex. Other studies identified naming locations in specific regions such as the insular lobe, the striatum and opercular region, and the basal temporal language area (Duffau & Fontaine, 2005; Duffau, et al., 2005; Hamberger, et al., 2001; Ilmberger, et al., 2001; Lüders et al, 1988, 1991; Peraud et al 2004). However, even though surgical resection will ordinarily respect positive site margins, patients may still display a postoperative language deficit (Petrovich Brennan et al, 2007).
Single neuron recording provides a very sparse distribution of circuits which can be difficult to study with focal electrical interference (Waydo et al., 2006). Language, whose underlying primary neuronal substrate was termed "module", small areas measuring 1-2 cm^2 with well-defined boundaries, represents a fortunate exception to this observation rather than the rule (Ojemann, G.A. et al., 1989). In addition, many authors showed that naming sites are often in close relationship to specific sites for different language functions, verb generation, reading, counting, comprehension, writing, working memory, and calculation, which justify the terminology adopted for designating them (nodes and shell-core) (Haglund et al., 1994; Schwartz et al., 1999; Schäffler et al., 1996).
Accordingly, the characteristics of the underlying neural circuits differ among functions and are not yet well understood anatomically. This differences may influence the mapping modality, recording the neuronal activity that "participates" in a widely distributed function with some regional differences. This is the case of intraoperative ECS in the right hemisphere for mapping spatial functions where "positive sites" could be removed while monitoring the corresponding partial deficit during tumor resection (Bartolomeo et al., 2007; Gharabaghi et al, 2006; Thiebaut de Schotten et al., 2005).

2.1.4 Item selection

As a standard procedure, an intraoperative task has to be previously verified on each patient before being performed, and those items chosen that patients were able to name during the preoperative testing phase. Items that patients were unable to name at preoperative assessment are deleted (Hamberger et al., 2005; Ojemann, 1989; Roux et al., 2003b). What is not well specified is the cut-off number of items a patient can misname when included in an AS protocol (Roux et al., 2003a; Lubrano et al., 2004). According to Little et al. (Little, et al., 2004), a preoperative object naming error rate greater than 25%

cannot statistically correlate with cortical stimulation and therefore cannot be reliably interpreted as evoked by stimulation.

2.2 Electrical stimulation

Stimulation depolarizes a very focal area of the cortex which, in turn, evokes certain responses. For example, the 50-60 Hz Penfield technique has long been used to elicit motor responses, documented through direct visual observation of contralateral tonic limb movements in the beginning and since the late 1990s through motor evoked potentials (MEP) recordings (Cedzich et al., 1996, 1998; Kombos et al., 2001; Neuloh & Schramm, 2002; Penfield & Boldrey 1937). Although the mechanism of stimulation effects on language are poorly understood, the principle is based on depolarization of local neurons and passing pathways, inducing local excitation or inhibition, as well as possible diffusion to more distant areas by way of orthodromic or antidromic propagation (Ranck, 1975). With the advent of the bipolar probe and electrocorticography (EcoG) for after-discharge (AD) detection as a measure of electrical spreading, avoidance of local diffusion and more precise mapping have been achieved with an accuracy estimated to be ~ 5 mm (Haglund, et al., 1992, 1993).

This diversity among protocols is not trivial because it obviously impacts on the results of stimulation. Therefore, function localization may vary across studies as a result of different stimulation parameters and mapping strategies. Moreover, mapping strategies appear as one of the main variables that may affect the results of stimulation: direct cortical stimulation using the so-called short train technique (5 to 7 stimuli, 0.5 ms duration, ISI 4.0 ms = 250 Hz, with a train repetition rate of 1 or 2 Hz) or the 50-60 Hz Penfield technique (Penfield & Boldrey, 1937); maximizing stimulation currents at each cortical site to ensure the absence of eloquent function according to AD threshold or keeping stimulation intensity constant, while mapping the entire cortex and setting the threshold just below the lowest current observed to induce AD; monopolar or bipolar stimulators; stimulation parameters in subcortical white matter according to cortical response or at the lowest threshold to evoke a response, all these alternatives may be encountered in similar studies.

2.3 Positive sites

Ojemann, using the single sample binomial test to check whether a site is essential for language, examined the accuracy of response during naming (Ojmann & Mateer, 1979; Ojeman, 1989). He gave a nonparametric description to determine if a site can be interpreted as essential: "*a site was determined to be related to language function if the chance probability of errors evoked at that site was less than 0.05 […] evoking errors during two of three stimulations at a site often achieved that level of statistical significance…*". This rate was slightly different in others author's strategies (Hamberger, et al., 2005; Peraud, et al., 2004).

The visual object naming task is easy to apply but is much more difficult to interpret. When classifying the type of errors, the main distinction that needs to be made is between speech arrest, anomia and speech disturbances. Error classification is strongly related to the aim of a study; it can vary from a simple definition of error (every change that occurs during stimulation) to a more articulate definition (Bello et al, 2007; Benzagmout et al, 2007; Duffau et al, 1999, 2003b; Duffau, 2006a).

2.4 The role of imaging in the integrated surgical strategy

Because of the infiltrating nature of gliomas, it is more than likely that a portion of the mass will occupy or be continuous with functional tissue. However, some evidence supports the concept that resection should ideally go beyond the gross tumor margin apparent on preoperative imaging. Therefore, it is not only patients with tumors located within the frontal operculum who may benefit from intraoperative language mapping, but also those with lesions in proximity to this region because of the significant variability in this region's anatomical and functional organization (Edeling et al., 1989; Quiñones-Hinojosa et al., 2003).

Possible causes of damage are: trajectory in subcortical tumors; abnormal anatomy in recurrent tumors; distorted anatomy due to the tumor; tumor infiltrating the functioning brain in LGGs; irregular tumors; and tumor periphery in HGGs. All are known to be crucial factors for surgical outcome, and knowledge of the structural characteristics of eloquent areas may help the surgeon to avoid clinical consequences. Aims may be categorized as linked to: 1) orientation, which is usually not histology-dependent (trajectory, abnormal anatomy, distorted anatomy); and 2) removal, usually used for specific gliomas (low-grade, irregular margins, periphery).

2.4.1 Functional imaging for eloquent tissue localization

Considerable advances in functional imaging have been made in both technology and availability, raising the question of whether it may eventually supplant intraoperative ECS mapping. Devices such as fMRI and PET units may aid in the preoperative planning of resection strategy, but these techniques, while reliable for detecting the motor area, remain too imprecise for complex functions such as language mapping where their sensitivity (PET, 75%; fMRI, 81%) and specificity (PET, 81%; fMI, 53%) are suboptimal. (Fitgerald et al., 1997; Herolz et al., 1996, 1997). These modalities highlight language-associated areas of indeterminate significance, and they do not offer real-time information intraoperatively. To this end, MRI neuronavigational techniques can facilitate not only greater resection, but embedding of DTI can also prevent inadvertent resection of adjacent subcortical pathways (Talos et al., 2007; Wu et al., 2007). Although the use of DTI has not been shown to impact directly on patient survival, its utility resides in maximizing tumor resection while minimizing morbidity. Nevertheless, for the identification of functional language pathways and guidance of safe tumor removal, these diagnostic imaging tools remain supplements to, not substitutes for, direct intraoperative stimulation mapping.

2.4.2 Structural imaging for tumor periphery localization

In glioma surgery, the approach to subcortical diffuse gliomas and the decision to resect the infiltrated brain surrounding the tumor core are the cornerstones of modern, aggressive surgical strategy. This is the rationale for a sound command of knowledge of brain functions at the tumor margin in individual cases. Non-enhancing tumor periphery, pattern (sharp or blurred) and characteristics (edema or infiltrated brain) constitute the challenging part of the operation where most effort is concentrated. MRI, FLAIR and T2-weighted images will visualize structural properties but their priority is controversial. Spectroscopy and DTI have been advocated as promising tools for delineating the extent of tumor infiltration (Price, et al., 2003; Stadbauer, et al., 2004, 2006). In addition, anisotropy measures have attempted to differentiate edema from infiltrated brain (Lu, et al., 2003, 2004). In contrast, perfusion can help to distinguish tumor grading but has not given information about the periphery so far.

3. Intraoperative setting

AS is a challenge for a working team, since it implies substantial modifications in the professional behavior of all physicians involved: for the surgeon working in an uncomfortable situation; the anesthesiologist monitoring the patient continuously; the neuroradiologist awaiting intraoperative confirmation of interpretation of findings; the neuropsychologist making real-time evaluation of scans. AS involves a complex scenario: integration of different types of knowledge, organization of a heterogeneous team, cooperation in different settings (operating room, ward, out-patient clinic), surgical and research protocols to be adopted, technical adjustments to make the research comparable.

3.1 Anesthesiology

Awake surgery is performed as follows. Continuous sedation (Sarang, et al.,2003) was achieved with rapidly acting agents and infiltrative anaesthesia of the scalp. Airway management remains a concern due to the risk of aspiration or oversedation with oxygen saturation <90%. Patients breathe spontaneously during awake surgery. Propofol, fentanyl, remifentanyl and midazolam are commonly used agents. Volatile anaesthetics should not be given because they interfere with electroencephalographic (EEG) recording and cause a dose-dependent distortion on the EEG, with vasodilatation resulting in increased intracranial pressure (ICP) (Himmelseher, et al., 2001). While propofol can also alter the EEG (Herrick, et al., 1997), intravenous drugs are preferable because of their rapid onset and easily manageable duration of action which causes no nausea or vomiting. The sedation level is very important since oversedation results in an uncooperative patient and medical problems (i.e., respiratory depression), whereas undersedation makes the patient uncomfortable and restless. For this purpose, the Modified Observer's Assessment of Alertness/Sedation Scale (Bauerle, et al., 2004) was used.

The feasibility and efficacy of AS have been studied in comparison with general anesthesia (GA). The absolute anesthesiologic exclusion criteria for AS are obstructive sleep apnea and difficult intubation (Picht et al., 2006). Parameters for comparing GA versus AS:

- Duration of surgery: according to Gupta, the mean procedure time was shorter in the GA group than in the AS group (182 min vs. 196 min; p <0,05) (Gupta, et al., 2007). A similar duration was found by Keifer and Taylor (Keifer et al., 2005; Taylor & Bernstein, 1999). Bello reported longer durations: mean 5 h 45 min, longest 6 h 45 min; mean awake time 1 h 45 min (Bello et al., 2007). In Whittle the mean awake duration was 62 min (range 10-105 min) (Whittle et al., 2005).
- Intraoperative medical complications are classified as *anesthetic* (inadequate or excessive sedation, pain, nausea, vomiting); *respiratory* (oxygen saturation <90%, increased CO2, hypoventilation <8/min, airway obstruction); *hemodynamic* (hyper- o hypotension, tachy- or bradycardia); *neurological* (convulsions, brain swelling, new neurological deficit) (Costello et al., 2005; Keifer et al., 2005; Sarang, & Dinsmore, 2003). In a review of the literature, Skucas demonstrated how hyper- and hypotension could be frequent in AS (11 and 56%, respectively) (Skucas, et al., 2006). However, in their study on 332 patients, they observed that airway problems are not so frequent: only 2% of patients developed hypoxemia and only 1.8% required intubation or positioning of respiratory devices. Respiratory issues could arise more frequently in obese patients or those with asthma or chronic obstructive pulmonary disease (COPD). As concerns intractable seizures in unconscious patients, the study reported that seizures occurred in only 3%

of patients, whereas other studies have reported rates as high as 16% (Bello et al., 2007; Petrovich Brennan et al., 2007; Serletis et al., 2007; Taylor & Bernstein, 1999). Some authors advocated the use of propofol to reduce intraoperative seizures (Berkenstadt et al., 2001; Danks et al., 1998; Gignac et al., 1993; Herrick et al., 1997; Huncke et al., 1998; Sarang, & Dinsmore, 2003).

- Blood loss: Gupta observed that blood loss is less in AS than in GA (266 ml vs. 365 ml; $p<0.05$) (Gupta et al., 2007).
- Postoperative local complications: Taylor found a 2.5% wound-complication and postoperative hematoma rate, similar to that described in a large study conducted on 1427 elective supratentorial craniotomies (Taylor et al., 1995; Taylor & Bernstein, 1999).
- Mean postoperative hospital stay and intensive care unit (ICU) stay: these are not significant results (Gupta et al., 2007). An awake craniotomy carries low morbidity and mortality rates and minimizes the need for ICU admission and the total hospital stay.
- Patient age: most authors agree that patients must be older than 11 years (Berger et al., 1989).

3.2 Clinical and imaging recording

Patient response during awake mapping is an important component in the data analysis also after surgery. Published data show different levels of analysis of response depending on the aim of mapping. Specifically, response registrations depend upon the presence of a either professional figure in the operating room for providing a written record of the findings or the use of audiotape or/and videotape recordings to be evaluated by a blinded or multiple postoperative examiners (Corina et al, 2005; Duffau et al., 2006; Haglund 1994; Sanai et al., 2008).

Audio-videotaping the mapping procedures is particularly useful for checking mouth and face muscles in order to classify language disorders and to detect eye movements which, mostly in frontal sites, could interfere with reading (Malow et al., 1996; Milea et al., 2002; Peraud et al., 2004; Roux et al., 2003b; Van Buren & Fedio, 1978). Documentation with pictures or audio-videotape of the brain was systematically obtained during stimulation to match sites with response site by site.

3.3 Positioning

Positioning is a compromise between patient and surgeon comfort. Ideally, positioning attains a head position that should fulfill requisites besides those of the surgeon: patient muscle relaxation; airways accessibility for the anesthesiologist; and the possibility of talking and interacting with the staff including watching the personal computer. For these reasons, the patient is positioned while awake. A rigid headrest with pins is perfectly tolerated by the patient after the administration of a local anesthetic.

3.4 Craniotomy

Language-mapping techniques were historically developed in the context of epilepsy surgery, in which large craniotomies exposed the brain well beyond the region of surgical interest to localize multiple cortical regions containing stimulation-induced language and motor function (i.e., "positive" sites) prior to resection. Recently, with increasing reliance on mapping, craniotomies have gradually been reduced to the size necessary to approach the lesion, thereby allowing for minimal cortical exposure overlying the tumor, less extensive intraoperative mapping, and a more time-efficient neurosurgical procedure (Sanai et al., 2008).

3.5 Surgical instruments

Essential devices for accurate surgical techniques are the intraoperative microscope and the ultrasonic aspirator. The neuronavigator has a multipurpose application: define the cortical boundaries of lesions, especially in LGGs; establish the site of corticectomy and the trajectory to subcortical lesions; provide image-assisted surgery for both fMRI (motor task) and DTI; and establish the distance to anatomical landmarks. These advantages are limited to the first part of the operation prior to brain shift. In this regard, intraoperative MRI is a promising tool for improving accuracy in subcortical mapping of fascicles and functions.

4. Surgical resection strategy

The intraoperative mapping technique involves selecting the tasks in relation to preoperative assessment, the operative tools, the neurophysiologic parameters and the consequent strategy, i.e., the way we combine them in a clinical situation. Taken together, these costly and time consuming procedures point to the importance of methods and surgical strategy.

One substantial limitation to clinical comparative inference is that multiple cortical or subcortical sites are manipulated during an operation making it impossible to relate one event to the manipulation of one site. In other words, when forced to face a number of methodological issues, it is likely that surgical strategy will improve. Choices regarding positioning, surgical technique, tumor definition, clinical and intraoperative information, functional studies, intraoperative tools, all together will favor a good result. In contrast, consideration of only one or a few functional variables may be confounding. This is why research studies should be validated in the clinical setting, taking into account additional variables critical for this purpose (Sawaya et al., 1998). Furthermore, the challenge of AS and cognitive mapping is the working team, i.e., to what extent individual proficiency can contribute to a clinical purpose when working in a group.

4.1 The traditional approach (Yasargil's lesson)

Yasargil lesson's may be summarized as follows: 1) glioma is an infiltrative tumor only in its advanced stages of growth; 2) its growth pattern follows functional pathways and respects compartmental boundaries (neo-archipallial, central nuclei, white matter and ventricles); and 3) tumor debulking starts from the center and proceeds in a circumferential manner till the white matter is exposed ("the deflating ball and one window" techniques) (Yasargil, 1996b, 1996c; Yasargil et al., 2004).

This last point is justified by the risk of damage to adjacent brain areas and forms the basic principle of resection strategy. In light of recent pathological and functional knowledge, however, this defensive strategy for treating both LGGs and HGGs, which seeks foremost to avoid brain injury without considering the infiltrated brain or the functional characteristics of adjacent brain areas, now seems largely unwarranted. Nonetheless, it is not an absolutely safe technique, since HGGs are often highly vascularized tumors and bleeding may mask vascular or parenchymal structures and result in involuntary injury. Moreover, tumor manipulation may induce tissue swelling and physical modifications, altering the typical characteristics of the normal brain, thus confounding the neurosurgeon's judgment, which basically relies on visual inspection.

The simple observation that, as a rule, recurrences originate from the margins of the operative cavity should underline that additional resection is a primary aim of surgery if it does not endanger functions that could impair patient performance, the accurate knowledge of which was the limiting factor of the strategy. Bearing this in mind, the rationale of the current approach becomes readily understandable: attack the tumor at its margins.

4.2 The current approach according to mapping information

As a preliminary consideration, the knowledge how a tumor grows may orientate the cortical approach. As the glioma grows in the gyrus, it infiltrates the short tracts (the u fibers) first and then the longer tracts, rather than the pia. Consequently, a direct or sulcal approach will be unsuitable for diffuse tumors in which resection of the involved gyrus and eventually the adjacent gyrus is preferable (Meyer et al., 2001). Corticectomy at this site, at the tumor margin, is the main surgical innovation of brain mapping. Cortical mapping highlights positive and negative areas before starting resection. This "negative mapping" strategy represents a paradigm shift in language and no-language mapping techniques by eliminating the neurosurgeon's reliance on positive site control in operative exposure, although validation for other related functions is still needed (Berger, 1994; Black et al, 1987; Keles & Berger, 2004; Matz et al., 1999; Sawaya et al., 1999; Toms et al., 1999).

Cortical LGGs may be nearly indistinguishable from normal brain tissue. The neuronavigator is therefore essential for precisely demarcating the superficial limits of the tumor. The arachnoid opening is also useful before deciding on the area of resection. The exact distinction acquired with the neuronavigation system may provide immediate visual feedback during the initial subcortical resection when the resection proceeds between different tissues.

The technique is to start from safe areas and where the vascular supply is expected: following the vessels, skeletonizing and preserving those serving eloquent areas and dividing the others, especially those supplying the tumor, in order to devascularize it. Subcortical pathways perpendicular to positive sites can be followed within the infiltrated brain as far as apparent normal brain is exposed or positive mapping is detected. This is not always possible in language areas, since the closer we come to positive sites, the easier it will be to have intraoperative impairment which will prevent further mapping. Consequently, in language mapping, DTI may be of help in orientating where to map on the tumor periphery in order to stimulate the least possible. DTI may be not considered as more than a imaginary guide.

This strategy may be changed in some situations, for instance, with less cooperative patients and during long operations, by adopting the following sequence: mapping, starting resection close to positive sites and following subcortical pathways, and then approach the vascular supply and safe areas. Repeating the mapping subcortically 2-3 times is usually enough, even when anatomical distortion occurs.

Starting from safe areas enables us to follow the tumor into the transition zone, from the margins to the infiltrated brain till the normal brain. First sight inspection means starting resection from the tumor periphery before causing possible injury, which can alter tissue color. Here, the microscope is essential for magnifying the region in order to differentiate normal brain from infiltrated brain. This major challenge can be successfully addressed only by experienced neurosurgeons. The corridor measures about 1 cm taken mostly from the infiltrated brain and less from the tumor. Since diffuse tumors are heterogeneous, it's better to see the phenotype of the single variant from the beginning and possibly to stay around the tumor, creating a corridor between the infiltrated brain and the normal brain. Starting from the corridor created around the tumor, additional space is obtained by removing or retracting the tumor and leaving the brain untouched. The rule is: expose the normal brain, map and stay away from it. Working very closely to normal brain tissue implies avoiding any pressure and retraction that could cause brain injury. As a rule, use of the self-retaining spatula is unnecessary and dangerous. This strategy provides us with a better anatomical orientation in a context which is still similar to the anatomo-functional picture as acquired preoperatively with MRI.

Following large, randomized prospective studies in Europe, several countries have already approved, and are now using, 5-ALA for improved quality of resection in HGGs, aimed at assisting the surgeon according to the same resection strategy (Stummer et al., 2006).

The standard for subcortical mapping for language is not yet defined: current amplitude, functional significance of fasciculi, safe distance from fasciculi or tolerance of partial injury, tests to be used, false negative stimulation rate, definition of positive sites, method of validation of positive sites. In particular, continuous monitoring is affected by the learning effect, as described by Ojemann (Ojemann J.G., et al., 2002).

The limiting factor to total removal is not always the eloquent areas. In large and diffuse tumors we can state that a strategy aimed at exploring and removing safe areas first is a preliminary condition to continue this aggressive strategy in order to obtain maximal resection which justifies risks in eloquent areas. Safe exposure of deep structures is not always feasible; and facing increasing structural and functional uncertainties is preferable to stopping the operation before taking additional risks in eloquent areas, assuming that the degree of cytoreduction has limited value if total removal cannot be achieved (Lacroix et al., 2001).

Vascular injury may be another limiting factor to tumor removal, especially in insular tumors where transit and terminal arteries, normal and pathological arteries, and venous drainage are ever-present challenges during the operation.

4.2.1 Temporo-insular tumors

The approach to temporal and insular tumors may be trans-cortical or trans-sylvian. When corticectomy is done, the tumor is devascularized by subpial dissection, while trans-sylvian dissection makes it possible to follow the vessels, free the tumor, and then decide which vessels to preserve and which to divide. The lenticulostriate arteries, the parietal trunk of the middle cerebral artery bifurcation on the non-dominant hemisphere and both trunks in the dominant hemisphere and the long perforators running posteriorly are the critical vessels to preserve in order to avoid permanent language and motor deficits. As a rule, vessels smaller than 0.5 mm are pathological. In these tumors, temporal or frontal basal cortical areas are seldom the critical point of resection, and multiple windows can be created between vessels. Accordingly, various sequential options may be weighed in order to start from safe areas and to control arterial vessels (Duffau, 2009; Sanai et al., 2010, Simon et al., 2009).

Mapping techniques allow the neurosurgeon to recognize the internal capsule, which is the critical anatomical point, at least in a non dominant site, while additional information can be obtained from monitoring motor evoked potentials (MEPs) in the course of the operation since insular tumors carry a risk of vascular injury, higher than the risk of direct injury (Figure 1-3). Neuloh and Schramm highlight the semi-quantitative relation between MEP

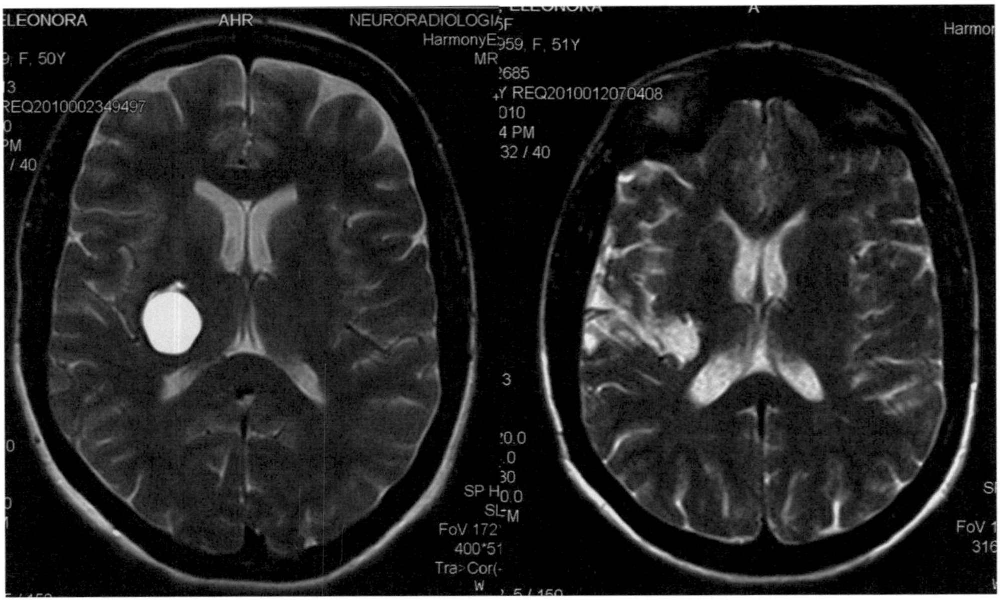

Fig. 1. Pilocytic astrocytoma of the right posterior insula. The tumor was removed via a trans-sylvian approach assisted by intraoperative motor monitoring (preoperative on the left side; postoperative on the right side)

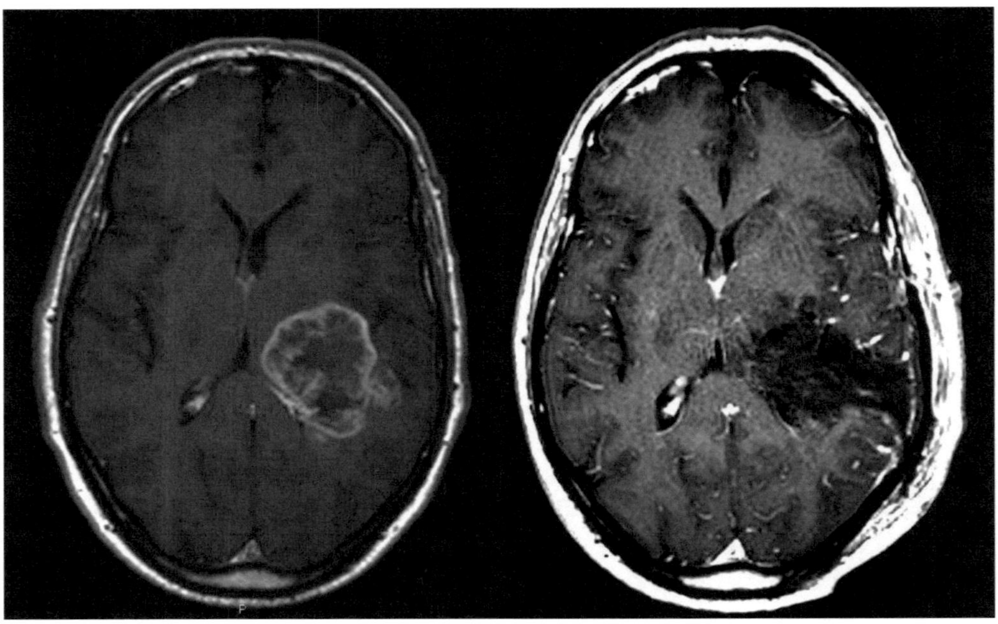

Fig. 2. Left posterior temporo-insular glioblastoma. The tumor was operated on under awake surgery for cortical language mapping and subcortical motor monitoring. Posterior perisylvian cortical sub-cortical approach was used for tumor removal (preoperative on the left side; postoperative on the right side)

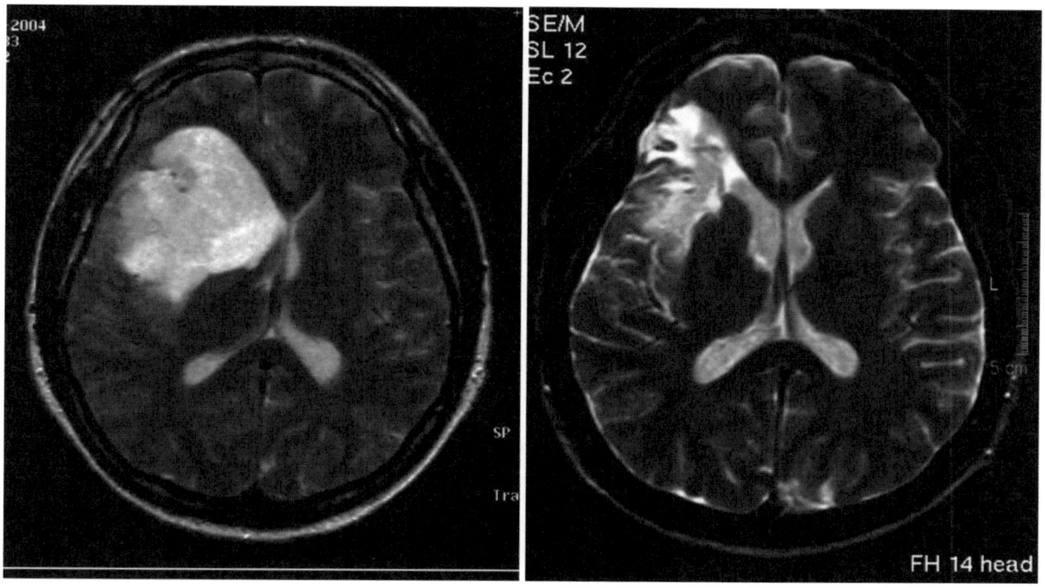

Fig. 3. Right insular fibrillary astrocitoma. Trans-sylvian approach was used and tumor removal was achieved under motor monitoring (preoperative on the left side, postoperative on the right side).

findings and clinical outcome. An amplitude reduction between 25 and 50% increases probability of a postoperative permanent deficit, as well as reversible loss and irreversible loss of MEPs (Neluoh & Schramm, 2004). Typically, MEPs deterioration will allow the neurosurgeon or anesthesiologist to react promptly, with temporary or definitive discontinuation of resection in the critical target area, readjustment or temporary release of retractors if used, application of papaverine to spastic vessels and increased blood pressure.

4.2.2 Rolandic tumors

The well-known corticospinal tract may be difficult to identify in pathological situations where brain distortion alters the normal anatomy. This is the main concern in the surgical approach to fronto-parietal tumors, the supplementary motor area (SMA) being secondary in importance. Image- and neurophysiologic-assisted surgery may be effective as well (Talacchi et al., 2010a). Vascular supply derives from the distal branch of the pericallosal artery and the fronto-parietal distal branches of the middle cerebral artery. Phase reversal, MEPs, cortical and subcortical mapping allow identification of the central sulcus, motor area and descendent pathways, respectively. The closest safe and convenient distance is 5 mA for diffuse tumors and 1-2 mA for circumscribed lesions. This is the site with the best surgical results among eloquent areas (Talacchi et al., 2010a) (Figure 4).

4.2.3 Peri-sylvian dominant tumors

In this area the great advantage of intraoperative mapping was to render tumors operable which were otherwise not amenable to surgery because of an unpredictable risk of aphasia. The language-mapping technique described in detail by Ojemann remains the mainstay of this procedure and may be combined with motor mapping in the fronto-parietal area, for both the periphery in cortical tumors and for trajectory planning in subcortical tumors

(Ojemann G.A. et al., 1989). Methodological validation for subcortical language mapping is still lacking, and landmarks for presumed significant fascicles are not well defined and often altered by anatomical distortion. In awake patients, there is an approximately 10% risk of finding a positive site within the tumor, which remains the main limiting factor to removal (Ojemann G.A. et al.,1989) (Figure 5-6).

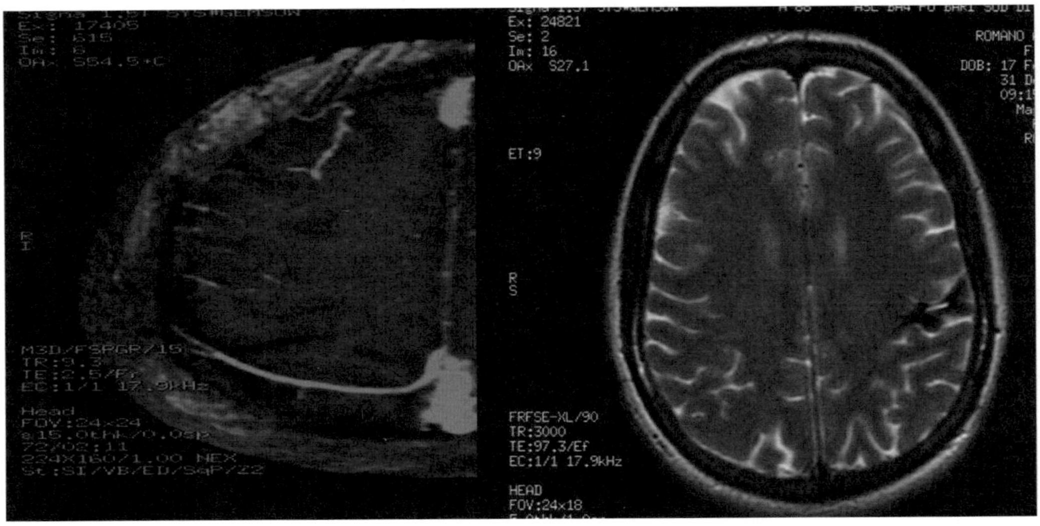

Fig. 4. Left rolandic glioblastoma. The tumor was removed using motor monitoring (preoperative on the left side; postoperative on the right side).

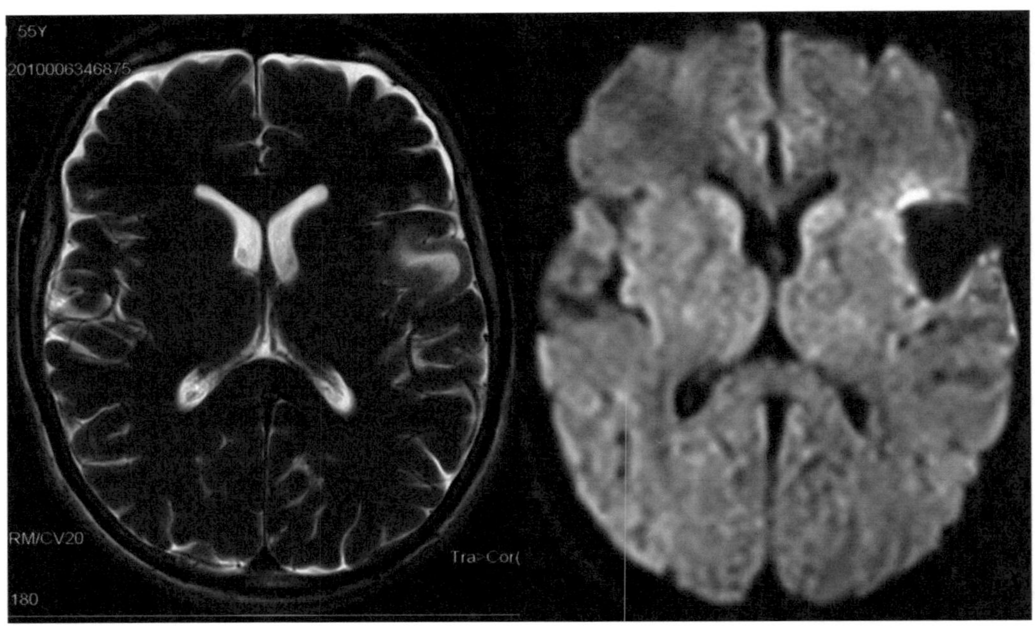

Fig. 5. Left frontal oligodendroglioma in the Broca area. The tumor was removed under awake surgery (preoperative on the left side; postoperative on the right side).

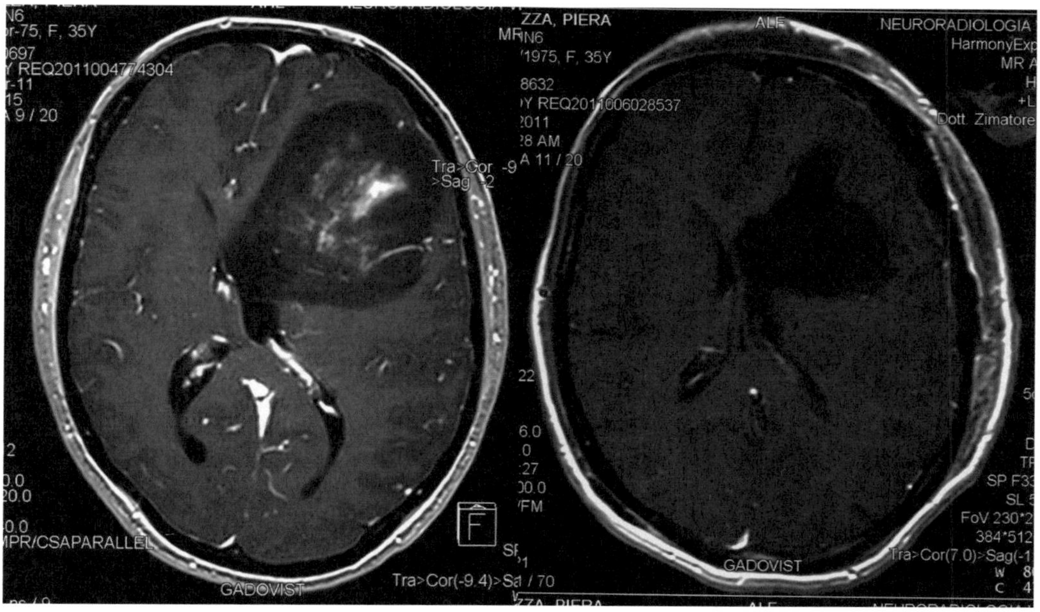

Fig. 6. Huge left frontal oligodendroglioma with intraventricular invasion. Notwithstanding intracranial hypertension awake surgery was used in order to perform a safe perisylvian trans-cortical approach (preoperative on the left side; postoperative on the right side).

5. Outcome assessment

While the initial assumption was that no electrically identified areas should be removed if postsurgical language complications are to be avoided, it was later increasingly assumed that postsurgical language deficits would not occur only if cortex that did not result in language deficits with electrical stimulation was removed (Sanai et al., 2008). This indirect message is gaining strength, although most studies lack pre- and postoperative global assessment and objective determination of cognitive complications. Furthermore, the original assumption that resection of any essential language areas will result in postoperative aphasia has not yet been definitively confirmed nor has the assumption that sparing positive sites for naming task will result in sparing of other language functions (Hamberger, et al., 2005; (Peraud, et al., 2004; Petrovich Brennan, et al., 2007; Seek, et al., 2006; Whittle, et al., 2003, 2005).

Moving from intraoperative naming-assisted surgical resection to other language and cognitive tasks, before relying on new protocols we need a multi-staged system of evidence for the potential and limitations of AS for cognitive mapping, its clinical validity for a single task or battery of tasks and technical standardization (intentionally addressed in the present article). Meanwhile, patient safety must be guaranteed by accurate comparative assessment, which should be discussed and defined (Lacroix et al., 2001; Vives & Piepmeier, 1999).

5.1 The value of glioma extent of resection

Microsurgical resection remains a critical therapeutic modality for all gliomas (Black, 1998; Guthrie & Laws, 1990; Keles et al., 1999; Yasargil et al., 2004). For all gliomas, the identification of universally applicable prognostic factors and treatment options remains a great challenge. Among the many tumor- and treatment-related parameters, only patient age and tumor histological characteristics have been identified as reliable predictors of patient prognosis, although tumor location in an eloquent area and the patient's functional status can also be statistically significant. With significant advances in brain tumor imaging and intraoperative technology during the last 15 years, some reports showed that improved extent of resection has a significant effect on both tumor progression and overall survival (Bauman et al., 1999; McGirt et al., 2008; Sanai et al., 2010; Smith et al., 2008). Although LGGs and HGGs are distinct in their biology, clinical behavior and outcome, understanding the efficacy of surgery remains equally important for both.

As concerns longer overall survival, more aggressive resection for LGGs can also influence the risk of malignant transformation, raising the possibility that surgical intervention can alter the natural history of the disease (Sanai & Berger, 2008). These associations are evident not only in the patient population with hemispheric LGGs but also in those with specific LGGs limited to specific eloquent subregions such as insular LGGs (Chaichana et al., 2010; Sanai et al., 2010; Simon et al., 2009; Smith et al., 2008).

5.2 Clinical outcome

The assumption is that every attempt should be made to preserve neurological functions in order to maintain the preoperative QoL, which is the main clinical outcome. However, postoperative settings vary greatly, often including focal evaluation for the related eloquent area but rarely accounting for complications or a wider battery of cognitive evaluations. Inadequate preoperative assessment can limit postoperative assessment and may lead to overlooking some functions which, though not tested intraoperatively, may still hold prognostic importance.

Interestingly, the peri-operative period, which traditionally lasts for 30 days after surgery, was prolonged in some studies to 3-4 months or up to 12 months, a period conventionally used to define permanent deficits (Duffau et al., 2001; Duffau et al., 2003b; Seitz et al., 1995).

5.2.1 Surgical outcome

The rationale for any treatment is bring about benefit superior to the natural history of the disease and to other treatments. The primary aim is to improve neurological outcome by relieving mass effect on normal brain structures without causing damage. Here, the Glioma Outcome Project deserves mention because it classified postoperative outcome and prospectively provided data for a large number of cases, Class II data, a benchmark for future studies. In this study, the majority of the patients improved (53%), while neurological, regional and systemic complications accounted for 8.1%, 10% and 9.2%, respectively, as observed at 21 days postoperatively. Unfortunately, eloquent areas were not specifically classified (Chang et al., 2003).

5.2.2 Focal outcome

While AS is claimed to decrease postoperative morbidity in eloquent areas, immediate postoperative evaluation showed a high rate of worsening of these functions, usually above 50%, which can be explained by the surgeon's confidence when working with eloquent areas, as demonstrated by progressive improvement within a few weeks (Keles et al., 2004; Talacchi et al., 2010a). At 3 months, this percentage usually decreases to less than 20% and then to 2-10% over the next months (Bello et al., 2008; Duffau 2005; Nariai et al., 2005). The degree of worsening varies substantially depending on the clinical scale used, arbitrarily classified at one level, with a high and low cut-off, which means great differences in deficits, at two levels (mild, moderate-severe) or at three levels (mild, moderate, severe) (Duffau, 2005; Hamberger, 2007; Nariai et al 2005; Seeck et al., 2006; Simos et al., 1999). A few authors used preoperative specific test categories for postoperative evaluation, site by site (Bello et al., 2008; Lucas et al., 2004; Lubrano et al., 2004). Nevertheless, when objective evaluations were adopted, as for motor mapping, the trend was very similar, with lower rates (20%), probably due more reliable testing (Talacchi et al 2010a; Reithmeier et al., 2003; Signorelli et al., 2001).

5.2.3 Functional outcome

Postoperative changes in cognitive functioning depend partly on the patient's level of preoperative abilities, especially in impaired patients (Gupta et al., 2007; Ojemann, 1979, 1983; Ojeman G.A. & Mateer, 1979). This makes the assessment strategy crucial from the beginning, since it can limit interpretations of final results (Hamberger et al., 2003).

Preoperative cognitive assessment is a neglected issue, but of great significance since about 80% of patients present with some degree of impairment (Talacchi et al., 2010b; Tucha et al., 2000). On the other hand, with pre- and intraoperative cognitive assessment, an extended postoperative assessment, including language and other cognitive functions, is required since research is based on the verification of the initial hypothesis and on unexpected results as well as on safety (Vives & Piepmeier, 1999).

Some authors found poor agreement when comparing neuropsychological tests with neurological examination and self-assess, especially in cognition, properly expressed only by neuropsychological testing (Pahlson, et al., 2003). Mental problems proved to have a greater impact on QoL than physical problems, which are specifically expressed by KPS, demonstrating that neuropsychology is a sensitive tool for analyzing brain performance, rather than self-assessment and neurological examination (Giovagnoli et al., 2004; Gustafsson et al., 2006; Påhlson et al., 2003; Taphoorn et al., 1992). In addition, specific cognitive domains such as verbal memory were found to be a better predictor of survival than KPS (Meyers et al., 2000). Accordingly, the main rationale for brain mapping, the preservation of QoL, is still largely biased by inadequate measures whenever they are used.

6. Conclusions

- Some methodological shortcomings derive from the inappropriate transition from epilepsy surgery to tumor surgery.
- Mapping is not a uniform technique, but rather it differs as regards area, function, task, electrical parameters and responses evaluation. Consequently, it requires case-by-case validation.
- The aim is a common methodological framework and personalized intraoperative tasks.
- Mapping the tumor periphery sistematically and mapping impaired patients remain unsolved and difficult tasks.
- Moving from cortical naming-assisted surgical resection to other language and cognitive tasks, poor clinical assessment still limits technical development of tasks and image-guided mapping .

- Through the use of appropriate methods in the clinical setting and in mapping techniques, surgical removal may safely attack the tumor, starting from the margins.
- Visual inspection allows us to "monitor" normal brain tissue which is to be preserved since functional eloquence is far from known in many areas.

7. References

Bartolomeo, P., Thiebaut de Schotten, M. & Duffau, H. (2007) Mapping of visuospatial functions during brain surgery: a new tool to prevent unilateral spatial neglect. *Neurosurgery*, Vol.61, No.6, (December 2007), E1340, ISSN 0148-396X

Bauerle K, Greim CA, Schroth M, Geisselbrecht M, Köbler A, Roewer N. Prediction of depth of sedation and anaesthesia by the Narcotrend EEG monitor. *British Journal of Anaesthesia*, Vol. 92, No. 6, (June 2004), pp.841-845. Epub (April 2004). Erratum in: *British Journal of Anaesthesia*, Vol.92, No.6, (June 2004), pp.912, ISSN 0007-0912

Bauman, G., Pahapill, P., Macdonald, D., Fisher, B., Leighton, C. & Cairncross, G. (1999) Low grade glioma: a measuring radiographic response to radiotherapy. *Canadian Journal of Neurological Sciences*, Vol.26, No.1, (February 1999), pp. 18–22, ISSN: 0317-1671

Bello, L., Gallucci, M., Fava, M., Carrabba, G., Giussani, C., Acerbi, F. et al. (2007) Intraoperative subcortical language tract mapping guides surgical removal of gliomas involving speech areas. *Neurosurgery*, Vol.60, No.1, (January 2007), pp. 67-82, ISSN 0148-396X

Bello, L., Gambini, A., Castellano, A., Carrabba, G., Acerbi, F., Fava, E., Giussani, C., Cadioli, M., Blasi, V., Casarotti, A., Papagno, C., Gupta, AK., Gaini, S., Scotti, G. & Falini, A. (2008) Motor and language DTI Fiber Tracking combined with intraoperative subcortical mapping for surgical removal of gliomas. *Neuroimage*, Vol.39, No.1, (January 2008), pp.369-382, ISSN 1053-8119

Benzagmout, M., Gatignol, P. & Duffau, H. (2007) Resection of World Health Organization Grade II gliomas involving Broca's area: methodological and functional considerations. *Neurosurgery*, Vol.61. No.4, (October 2007), pp. 741-752, ISSN 0148-396X

Berger, M.S., Kincaid, J., Ojemann, G.A. & Lettich, E. (1989) Brain mapping techniques to maximize resection, safety, and seizure control in children with brain tumors. *Neurosurgery*, Vol.25, No.5, (November 1989), pp. 786-792, ISSN 0148-396X

Berger, M.S. (1994) Lesions in functional ("Eloquent") cortex and subcortical white matter. *Clinical Neurosurgery*, Vol.41, pp. 444-463, ISSN 0069-4827, Baltimore

Berkenstadt, H., Perel, A., Hadani, M., Unofrievich, I. & Ram, Z. (2001) Monitored anesthesia care using remifentanil and propofol for awake craniotomy. *Journal of Neurosurgical Anesthesiology*, Vol.13, No.3, (July 2001), pp. 246-249, ISSN 0898-4921

Black, P., McL. & Ronner S.F. (1987) Cortical mapping for defining the limits of tumor resection. *Neurosurgery*, Vol.20, No.6, (June 1987), pp. 914-919, ISSN 0148-396X

Black, P. (1998) Management of malignant glioma: role of surgery in relation to multimodality therapy. *Journal of Neurovirology*, Vol.4, No.2, (April 1998), pp. 227–236, ISSN: 1355-0284

Bookheimer, S.Y., Zeffiro, T.A., Blaxton, T., Malow, B.A., Gaillard WD, Sato S et al. (1997) A direct comparison of PET activation and electrocortical stimulation mapping for language localization. *Neurology*, Vol.48, No.4, (April 1997), pp. 1056-1065, ISSN 0028-3878

Buckner, J.C., Schomberg, P.J., McGinnis, W.L., Cascino, T.L., Scheithauer, B.W., O'Fallon, J.R. et al. (2001) A phase III study of radiation therapy plus carmustine with or without recombinant interferon-alpha in the treatment of patients with newly diagnosed high-grade glioma. *Cancer*, Vol.92, No.2, (July 2001), pp. 420-433, ISSN 0008-543X

Buckner, J.C. (2003) Factors influencing survival in high-grade gliomas. *Seminars in Oncology*, Vol.30, No.6, Suppl.19, (December 2003), pp. 10-14, ISSN 0093-7754

Bulsara, K.R., Johnson, J. & Villavicencio, A.T. (2005) Improvements in brain tumor surgery: the modern history of awake craniotomies. *Neurosurgical Focus*, Vol.18, No.4, E5, (April 2005), pp. 1-3, ISSN: 1092-0684

Cedzich, C., Taniguchi, M., Schäfer, S. & Schramm, J. (1996) Somatosensory evoked potential phase reversal and direct motor cortex stimulation during surgery in and around the central region. Neurosurgery, Vol.38, No.5, (May 1996), pp. 962-970, ISSN 0148-396X

Cedzich, C., Pechstein, U., Schramm, J. & Schafer, S. (1998) Electrophysiological considerations regarding electrical stimulation of motor cortex and brain stem in humans. *Neurosurgery*, Vol.423, No.3, (March 1998), pp. 527-532, ISSN 0148-396X

Chaichana, K.L., McGirt, M.J., Laterra, J., Olivi, A., Quinones- Hiñojosa, A. (2010) Recurrence and malignant degeneration after resection of adult hemispheric low-grade gliomas. *Journal of Neurosurgery*, Vol.112, No.1, (January 2010), pp. 10–17, ISSN 0022-3085

Chang, S.M., Parney, I.F., McDermott, M., Barker, F.G. 2nd, Schmidt, M.H., Huang, W. et al. (2003) Perioperative complications and neurological outcomes at first and second craniotomies among patients enrolled in the Glioma Outcome Project. *Journal of Neurosurgery*, Vol.98, No.6, (June 2003), pp. 1175-1181, ISSN 0022-3085

Corina, D.P., Gibson, E.K., Martin, R., Poliakov, A., Brinkley, J. & Ojemann, G.A. (2005) Dissociation of action and object naming: evidence from cortical stimulation mapping. *Human Brain Mapping*, Vol.24, No.1, (January 2005), pp. 1-10, ISSN 1065-9471

Costello, T.G., Cormack, J.R., Mather, L.E., LaFerlita, B., Murphy, M.A. & Harris, K. (2005) Plasma levobupivacaine concentrations following scalp block in patients undergoing awake craniotomy. *British Journal of Anaesthesia*, Vol.94, No.6, (June 2005), pp. 848-851, ISSN 0007-0912

Danks, R.A., Rogers, M., Aglio, L.S., Gugino, L.D. & Black, P.M. (1998) Patient tolerance of craniotomy performed with the patient under local anaesthesia and monitored conscious sedation. *Neurosurgery*, Vol.42, No.1, (January 1998), pp. 28-36, ISSN 0148-396X

Duffau, H., Capelle, L., Sichez, J-P., Faillot, T., Abdennour, L., Law Koune, J.D. et al. (1999) Intra-operative direct electrical stimulations of the central nervous system: the Salpêtrière experience with 60 patients. *Acta Neurochirurgica (Wien)*, Vol.141, No.11, (November 1999), pp. 1157-1167, ISSN 0001-6268

Duffau, H., Bauchet, L., Lehéricy, S. & Capelle, L. (2001) Functional compensation of the left dominant insula for language. *Neuroreport*, Vol.12, No.10, (July 2001), pp. 2159–2163, ISSN 0959-4965

Duffau, H., Capelle, L., Denvil, D., Sichez, N., Gatignol, P., Taillandier, L. et al. (2003) Usefulness of intraoperative electrical subcortical mapping during surgery for low-grade gliomas located within eloquent brain regions: functional results in a consecutive series of 103 patients. *Journal of Neurosurgery*, Vol.98, No.4, (April 2003), 764-778, ISSN 0022-3085

Duffau, H., Capelle, L., Denvil, D., Sichez, N., Gatignol, P., Lopes, M. et al (2003) Functional recovery after surgical resection of low grade gliomas in eloquent brain: Hypothesis of brain compensation. *Journal of Neurology, Neurosurgery and Psychiatry*, Vol.74, No.7, (July 2003), pp. 901-907

Duffau H & Fontaine D (2005) Successful resection of a left insular cavernous angiomas using neuronavigation and intraoperative language mapping. *Acta Neurochirurgica (Wien)*, Vol.147, No.2, (February 2005), pp. 205-208 ISSN 0001-6268

Duffau, H., Lopes, M., Arthuis, F., Bitar, A., Sichez, J.P., Van Effenterre, R. & Capelle L. (2005) Contribution of intraoperative electrical stimulations in surgery of low grade gliomas: a comparative study between two series without (1985-96) and with (1996-2003) functional mapping in the same institution. *Journal of Neurology, Neurosurgery and Psychiatry*, Vol.76, No.6, (June 2005), pp. 845-851, ISSN 0022-3050

Duffau H. (2005) Intraoperative cortico-subcortical stimulations in surgery of low-grade gliomas. *Expert Review of Neurotherapeutics*, Vol.5, No.4, (July 2005) pp. 473-85, ISSN: 1473-7175

Duffau, H. (2005) Lessons from brain mapping in surgery for low-grade glioma: insights into associations between tumour and brain plasticity. *The Lancet Neurology*, Vol.4, No.8, (August 2005), pp. 476-486, ISSN 1474-4422

Duffau, H. (2006) From intraoperative electrical cortico-subcortical cerebral mapping to research on brain's function and plasticity. *Rivista Medica*, 2006; Vol.12, No.1-2, pp. 15-21, ISSN: 1127-6339

Duffau, H. (2006) New concepts in surgery of WHO grade II glioms: functional brain mapping, connectionism and plasticity. *Journal of Neuro-Oncology*, Vol.79, No.1, (August 2006), pp. 77-115, ISSN 0167-594X

Duffau, H., Taillandier, L., Gatignol, P. & Capelle, L. (2006). The insular lobe and brain plasticity : Lessons from tumor surgery. *Clinical Neurology and Neurosurgery*, Vol.108, No.6, (September 2006), pp. 543-8, ISSN 0303-8467

Duffau, H. (2007) Contribution of cortical and subcortical electrostimulation in brain glioma surgery: methodological and functional considerations. *Neurophysiologie Clinique*, Vol.37, No.6, (December 2007), pp. 373-82, ISSN 0987-7053

Duffau, H. (2009) A personal consecutive series of surgically treated 51 cases of insular WHO Grade II glioma: advances and limitations. *Journal of Neurosurgery*, Vol.110, (April 2009), pp. 696-708, ISSN 0022-3085

Ebeling, U., Steinmetz, H., Huang, Y.X. & Kahn, T. (1989) Topography and identification of the inferior precentral sulcus in MR imaging. *AJR. American Journal of Roentgenology*, Vol.153, No.5, (November 1989), pp. 1051–1056, ISSN 0361-803X

FitzGerald, D.B., Cosgrove, G.R., Ronner, S., Jiang, H., Buchbinder, B.R., Belliveau, J.W. et al. (1997) Location of language in the cortex: a comparison between functional MR imaging and electrocortical stimulation. *AJNR. American Journal of Neuroradiology*, Vol.18, No.8, (September 1997), pp. 1529-1539, ISSN 0195-6108

Foerster, O. (1931) The cerebral cortex in man. *The Lancet*, Vol.218, N.5632, (August 1931), pp. 309–312, ISSN 0140-6736

Gatignol, P., Capelle, L., Le Bihan, R. & Duffau, H. (2004) Double dissociation between picture naming and comprehension: an electrostimulation study. *Neuroreport*, Vol.15, No.1, (January 2004), pp. 191- 195, ISSN 0959-4965

Gharabaghi, A., Fruhmann, B.M., Tatagiba, M. & Karnath, H.O. (2006) The role of the right superior temporal gyrus in visual search – Insights from intraoperative electrical stimulation. *Neuropsychologia*, Vol.44, No.12, 2578-2581, ISSN 0028-3932

Gignac, E., Manninen, P.H. & Gelb, A.W. (1993) Comparison of fentanyl, sufentanil and alfentanil during awake craniotomy for epilepsy. *Canadian Journal of Anaesthesia*, Vol.40, No.5, Pt .1, (May 1993), pp. 421-424, ISSN 0832-610X

Giovagnoli, A.R. & Boiardi, A. (1994) Cognitive impairment and quality of life in long-term survivors of malignant brain tumors. *Italian Journal of Neurological Sciences*, Vol.15, No.9, (December 1994), pp. 481-488, ISSN 0392-0461

Giovagnoli, A.R., Silvani, A., Colombo, E. & Boiardi, A. (2005) Facets and determinants of quality of life in patients with recurrent high grade glioma. *Journal of Neurology, Neurosurgery and Psychiatry*, Vol.76, No.4, (April 2005), pp. 562-568, ISSN 0022-3050

Gupta, D.K., Chandra, P.S., Ojha, B.K., Sharma, B.S., Mahapatra, A.K. & Mehta, V.S. (2007) Awake craniotomy versus surgery under general anesthesia for resection of intrinsic lesions of eloquent cortex- a prospective randomized study. *Clinical Neurology and Neurosurgery*, Vol.109, No.4, (May 2007), pp. 335-343, ISSN 0303-8467

Gustafsson, M., Edvardsson, T. & Ahlstrom, G. (2006) The relationship between function, quality of life and coping in patients with low-grade gliomas. *Supportive Care in Cancer*, Vol.14, No.12, (December 2006), pp. 1205-1212, ISSN 0941-4355

Guthrie, B.L. & Laws, E.R. Jr. (1990) Supratentorial low-grade gliomas. *Neurosurgery Clinics of North America*, January Vol.1, No.1, (January 1990), pp. 37–48, ISSN 1042-3680

Haglund, M.M., Ojemann, G.A. & Hochman, D.W. (1992) Optical imaging of epileptiform and functional activity in human cerebral cortex. *Nature*, Vol.358, No.6388, pp. 668–671, ISSN: 0028-0836

Haglund, M.M., Ojemann, G.A. & Blasdel, G.G. (1993) Optical imaging of bipolar cortical stimulation. *Journal of Neurosurgery*, Vol.78, No.5, (May 1993), pp. 785–793, ISSN 0022-3085

Haglund, M.M., Berger, M.S., Shamseldin, M., Lettich, E. & Ojemann, G.A. (1994) Cortical localization of temporal lobe language sites in patients with gliomas. *Neurosurgery*, Vol.34, No.4, (April 1994), pp. 567-576, ISSN 0148-396X

Hamberger, M.J., Goodman, R.R., Perrine, K. & Tammy, T. (2001) Anatomic Dissociation of Auditory and Visual Naming in the Lateral Temporal Cortex. *Neurology*, Vol.56, No.1, (January 2001), pp.56-61, ISSN 0028-3878

Hamberger, M.J., Seidel, W., Goodman, R.R., Perrine, K. & McKhann, G.M. (2003) Temporal lobe stimulation reveals anatomic distinction between auditory naming processes. *Neurology*, Vol.60, pp. 1478–1483, ISSN 0028-3878

Hamberger, M.J., Seidel, W.T., Mckhann, G.M., Perrine, K. & Goodman, R.R. (2005) Brain stimulation reveals critical auditory naming cortex. *Brain*, Vol.128, No.11, (November 2005), pp. 2742-2749, ISSN 0006-8950

Hamberger, M.J., McClelland, S., McKhann, G.M. II, Williams, A.C. & Goodman, R.R. (2007) Distribution of auditory and visual naming sites in nonlesional temporal lobe epilepsy patients and patients with space-occupying temporal lobe lesions. *Epilepsia*, Vol.48, No.3, (March 2007), pp. 531-538, ISSN 0013-9580

Hamberger, M.J. (2007) Cortical Language Mapping in Epilepsy: A critical Review. *Neuropsychology Review*, Vol.17, No.4, (December 2007), pp. 477-489, ISSN 1040-7308

Herholz, K., Thiel, A., Wienhard, K., Pietrzyk, U., von Stockhausen, H.M., Karbe, H. et al (1996) Individual functional anatomy of verb generation. *Neuroimage*, Vol.3, No.3, (June 1996), pp. 185–194, ISSN 1053-8119

Herholz, K., Reulen, H.J., von Stockhausen, H.M., Thiel, A., Ilmberger, J., Kessler, J. et al (1997) Preoperative activation and intraoperative stimulation of language-related areas in patients with glioma. *Neurosurgery*, Vol.41, No.6, (December 1997), pp. 1253–1262, ISSN 0148-396X

Herrick, I.A., Craen, R.A., Gelb, A.W., Miller, L.A., Kubu, C.S., Girvin, J.P. et al. (1997) Propofol sedation during awake craniotomy for seizures: patient-controlled administration versus neurolept analgesia. *Anesthesia and Analgesia*, Vol.84, No.6, (June 1997), pp. 1285-1291, ISSN 0003-2999

Hill, D.L., Smith, A.D., Simmons, A., Maurer, C.R. Jr., Cox, T.C., Elwes, R. et al. (2000) Sources of error in comparing functional magnetic resonance imaging and invasive electrophysiological recordings. *Journal of Neurosurgery*, Vol.93, No.2, (August 2000), pp. 214-223, ISSN 0022-3085

Himmelseher S, Pfenninger E, Werner C. Intraoperative monitoring in neuroanesthesia: a national comparison between two surveys in Germany in 1991 and 1997. Scientific Neuroanesthesia Research Group of the German Society of Anesthesia and Intensive Care Medicine. *Anesthesia and Analgesia*, Vol.92, No.1, (January 2001), pp.166-171, ISSN 0003-2999

Huncke, K., Van de Wiele, B., Fried, I. & Rubinstein, E.H. (1998) The asleep-awake-asleep anesthetic tecnique for intraoperative language mapping. *Neurosurgery*, Vol.42, No.6, (June 1998),pp. 1312-1316, ISSN 0148-396X

Ilmberger, J., Eisner, W., Schmid, U. & Reulen, H.J. (2001) Performance in picture naming and word comprehension: evidence for common neuronal substrates from intraoperative language mapping. *Brain and Language*, Vol.76, No.2, (February 2001), pp. 111–118, ISSN 0093-934X

John J. (1984) Grading of muscle power: comparison of MRC and analogue scales by physiotherapists. Medical Research Council. *International Journal of Rehabilitation Research*, Vol.7, No.2, (June 1984), pp. 173-181, ISSN: 0342-5282

Kamada, K., Todo, T., Masutani, Y., Aoki, S., Ino, K., Morita, A. & Saito, N. (2007) Visualization of the frontotemporal language fibers by tractography combined with functional magnetic resonance imaging and magnetoencephalography. *Journal of Neurosurgery*, Vol.106, No.1, (January 2007), pp. 90-98, ISSN 0022-3085

Keifer, J.C., Dentchev, D., Little, K., Warner, D.S., Friedman, A.H. & Borel, C.O. (2005) A retrospective analysis of a remifentanil/propofol general anesthetic for craniotomy before awake functional brain mapping. *Anesthesia and Analgesia*, Vol.101, No.2, (August 2005), pp. 502-508, ISSN 0003-2999

Keles, G.E., Anderson, B., Berger, M.S. (1999) The effect of extent of resection on time to tumor progression and survival in patients with glioblastoma multiforme of the cerebral hemisphere. *Surgical Neurology*, Vol.52, No.4, (October 1999), pp. 371–379, ISSN 0090-3019

Keles, G.E., Lundin, D.A., Lamborn, K.R., Chang, E.F., Ojemann, G. & Berger, M.S. (2004) Intraoperative subcortical stimulation mapping for hemispherical perirolandic gliomas located within or adjacent to the descending motor pathways: evaluation of morbidity and assessment of functional outcome in 294 patients. *Journal of Neurosurgery*, Vol.100, No.3, (March 2004), pp. 369-375, ISSN 0022-3085

Keles, G.E. & Berger, M.S. (2004) Advances in neurosurgical technique in the current management of brain tumors. *Seminars in Oncology*, Vol.31, No.5, (October 2004), pp. 659-665, ISSN 0093-7754

Kim, S.S., McCutcheon, I.E., Suki, D., Weinberg, J.S., Sawaya, R., Lang, F.F., Ferson, D., Heimberger, A.B., DeMonte, F. & Prabhu, S.S. (2009) Awake Craniotomy for Brain Tumors Near Eloquent Cortex: Correlation of Intraoperative Cortical Mapping With Neurological Outcomes in 309 Consecutive Patients. *Neurosurgery*, Vol.64, No.5, (May 2009), pp. 836-846, ISSN 0148-396X

Kombos, T., Suess, O., Ciklatekerlio, O. & Brock, M. (2001) Monitoring of intraoperative motor evoked potentials to increase the safety of surgery in and around the motor cortex. *Journal of Neurosurgery*, Vol.95, No.4, (October 2001), pp. 608-614, ISSN 0022-3085

Kurimoto, M., Asahi, T., Shibata, T., Takahashi, C., Nagai, S., Hayashi, N., Matsui, M. & Endo, S. (2006) Safe removal of glioblastoma near the angular gyrus by awake surgery preserving calculation ability. Case Report. *Neurologia Medico-Chirurgica (Tokyo)*, Vol.46, No.1, (January 2006), pp. 46-50, ISSN 0470-8105

Lacroix, M., Abi-Said, D., Fourney, D.R., Gokaslan, Z.L., Shi, W., DeMonte, F. et al. (2001) A multivariate analysis of 416 patients with glioblastoma multiforme: prognosis, extent or resection, and survival. *Journal of Neurosurgery*, Vol.95, No.2, (January 1999), pp. 190-198, ISSN 0022-3085

Little, K. & Friedman, A.H. (2004) Awake craniotomy for malignant glioma resection. *International Congress Series*, Vol.1259, (February 2004), pp. 409- 414, ISSN: 0531-5131

Lu, S., Ahn, D., Johnson, G. & Cha, S. (2003) Peritumoral diffusion tensor imaging of high grade gliomas and metastatic brain tumors. *AJNR. American Journal of Neuroradiology*, Vol.24, No.5, (May 2003), pp. 937-941, ISSN 0195-6108

Lu, S., Ahn, D., Johnson, G., Law, M., Zagzag, D. & Grossman, R.I. (2004) Diffusion-tensor MR imaging of intracranial neoplasia and associated peritumoral edema: introduction of the tumor infiltration index. *Radiology*, Vol.232, No.1, (July 2004), pp. 221-224, ISSN 0033-8419

Lubrano, V., Roux, F.E. & Démonet, J.F. (2004) Writing specific sites in frontal areas: a cortical stimulation study. *Journal of Neurosurgery*, Vol.101, No.5, (November 2004), pp. 787-98, ISSN 0022-3085

Lucas, T.H., McKhann, G.H. & Ojemann, G.A. (2004) Functional separation of languages in the bilingual brain: A comparison of electrical stimulation language mapping in 25 bilingual patients and 117 monolingual control patients. *Journal of Neurosurgery*, Vol.101, No.3, (September 2004), pp. 449–457, ISSN 0022-3085

Lüders, H.O., Lesser, R.P., Dinner, D.S., Morris, H.H., Wyllie, E., Godoy, J. (1988) Localization of cortical function: new information from extraoperative monitoring of patients with epilepsy. *Epilepsia*, Vol.29 , Suppl.2, pp. S56-65, ISSN 0013-9580

Lüders, H.O., Lesser, R.P., Hahn, J., Dinner, D.S., Morris, H.H., Wyllie, E. & Godoy, J. (1991) Basal Temporal Language Area. *Brain*, Vol.114, No.2, (April 1991), pp. 743-754, ISSN 0006-8950

Malow, B.A., Blaxton, T.A., Sato, S., Bookheimer, S.Y., Kufta, C.V., Figlozzi, C.M. & Theodore, W.H. (1996). Cortical stimulation elicits regional distinctions in auditory and visual naming. *Epilepsia*, Vol.37, No.3, (March 1996), pp. 245-52, ISSN 0013-9580

Matz, P.G., Cobbs, C. & Berger, M.S. (1999) Intraoperative cortical mapping as a guide to the surgical resection of gliomas. *Journal of Neuro-Oncology*, Vol.42, No.3, (May 1999), pp. 233-245, ISSN 0167-594X

McGirt, M.J., Chaichana, K.L., Attenello, F.J., Weingart, J.D., Than, K., Burger, P.C. et al. (2008) Extent of surgical resection is independently associated with survival in patients with hemispheric infiltrating low-grade gliomas. *Neurosurgery*, Vol.63, No.4, pp. 700–708, ISSN 0148-396X

Meyer, F.B., Bates, L.M., Goerss, S.J., Friedman, J.A., Windschiti W.L., Duffy, J.R., Perkins W.J. & O'Neill, B.P. (2001) Awake craniotomy for aggressive resection of primary gliomas located in eloquent brain. *Mayo Clinic Proceedings*, Vol.76, No.7, (July 2001), pp. 677-687, ISSN 0025-6196

Meyers, C.A., Hess, K.R., Yung, W.K.A. & Levin, V.A. (2000) Cognitive function as a predictor of survival in patients with recurrent malignant glioma *Journal of Clinical Oncology*, Vol.18, Nr.3, (February 2000), pp. 646-650, ISSN 0732-183X

Milea, D., Lobel, E., Lehéricy, S., Duffau, H., Rivaud-Péchoux, S., Berthoz, A. & Pierrot-Deseilligny, C. (2002) Intraoperative frontal eye field stimulation elicits ocular deviation and saccade suppression. *Neuroreport*, Vol.13, No.10, (July 2002), pp. 1359-1364, ISSN: 0959-4965

Nariai, T., Sato, K., Hirakawa, K., Ohta, Y., Tanaka, Y., Ishiwata, K. et al. (2005) Imaging of somatotopic representation of sensory cortex with intrinsic optical signals as guides for brain tumor surgery. *Journal of Neurosurgery*, Vol.103, No.3, (September 2005), pp. 414-423, ISSN 0022-3085

Neuloh, G. & Schramm, J. (2002) Mapping and monitoring of supratentorial procedures. In: *Neurophysiology in neurosurgery: a modern intraoperative approach*. Deletis V, Shils J (eds), pp 339–404, Academic Press, San Diego

Neuloh, G. & Schramm, J. (2004) Motor evoked potential monitoring for the surgery of brain tumours and vascular malformations. *Advances and Technical Standards in Neurosurgery*, Vol.29, (January 2004), pp. 171-228, ISSN: 0095-4829

Ojemann, G.A. (1977) Language and verbal memory functions during and after human thalamic stimulation. *Neurología, Neurocirugía y Psiquiatría*, Vol.18, Suppl.2-3, pp. 35-45, ISSN 0028-3851

Ojemann, G.A. (1979). Individual variability in cortical localization of language. *Journal of Neurosurgery*, Vol.50, No.2, (February 1979), pp. 164-169, ISSN 0022-3085

Ojemann, G.A. & Mateer, C. (1979) Human language cortex: Localization of memory, syntax, and sequential motor-phoneme identification systems. *Science*, Vol.205, No.4413, (September 1979), pp. 1401-1403, ISSN 0036-8075

Ojemann, G.A. (1983) Brain organization for language from the perspective of electrical stimulation mapping. The Behavioural and Brain Sciences, Vol.6 pp. 189- 230, ISSN 0140-525X

Ojemann, G.A. & Dodrill, C.B. (1985) Verbal memory deficits after left temporal lobectomy for epilepsy. Mechanism and intraoperative prediction. *Journal of Neurosurgery*, Vol.62, No.1, (January 1985), pp. 101-107, ISSN 0022-3085

Ojemann, G.A., Ojemann, J., Lettich, E. & Berger, M. (1989) Cortical language localization in left, dominant hemisphere. An electrical stimulation mapping investigation in 117 patients. *Journal of Neurosurgery*, Vol.71, No.3, (September 1989), pp. 316-326, ISSN 0022-3085

Ojemann, G.A. (1989) Some brain mechanism for reading. *Brain And Reading*, C von Euler (Ed), pp. 47-59, Macmillan, New York

Ojemann, G.A. (2003) The neurobiology of language and verbal memory: observations from awake neurosurgery. *International Journal of Psychophysiology*, Vol.48, No.2, (May 2003), pp. 141–146, ISSN 0167-8760

Ojemann, J.G., Ojemann, G.A. & Lettich, E. (2002) Cortical stimulation mapping of language cortex by using a verb generation task: effects of learning and comparison to mapping based on object naming. *Journal of Neurosurgery*, Vol.97, No.1, (July 2002), pp. 33-38, ISSN: 0022-3085

Ojemann, S.G., Berger, M.S., Lettich, E. & Ojemann, G.A. (2003) Localisation of language function in children: results of electrical stimulation mapping. *Journal of Neurosurgery*, Vol.98, No.3, (March 2003), pp. 465–470, ISSN 0022-3085

Påhlson, A., Ek, L., Ahlström, G. & Smits, A. (2003) Pitfalls in the Assessment of disability in individuals with low-grade gliomas. *Journal of Neuro-Oncology*, Vol.65, No.2, (November 2003), pp. 149-158, ISSN 0167-594X

Papanicolaou, A.C., Simos, P.G., Breier, J.I., Zouridakis, G., Willmore, L.J., Wheless, J.W. et al. (1999) Magnetoencephalographic mapping of the language-specific cortex. *Journal of Neurosurgery*, Vol.90, No.1, (January 1999), pp. 85-93, ISSN 0022-3085

Penfield, W. & Boldrey, E. (1937) Somatic motor and sensory representation in the cerebral cortex of man as studied by electrical stimulation. *Brain*, Vol.60, No.4, (December 1937), pp. 389–443, ISSN 0006-8950

Penfield, W. & Erickson, T.C. (1942) Epilepsy and Cerebral Localization. A Study of the Mechanism, Treatment, and Prevention of Epileptic Seizures. *Archives of Internal Medicine*, Vol.70, No.5, (November 1942), pp. 916-917, ISSN 0003-9926

Penfield, W. & Rasmussen, T. (1950) Secondary sensory and motor representation. In: *The cerebral cortex of man*, pp 109-134, MacMillan, New York

Peraud, A., Ilmberger, J. & Reulen, H-J. (2004) Surgical resection of gliomas WHO grade II and III located in the opercular region. *Acta Neurochirurgica (Wien)*, Vol.146, No.1, (January 2004), pp. 9-18, ISSN 0001-6268

Petrovich Brennan, N.M., Whalen, S., de Morales Branco, D., O'Shea, J.P., Norton, I.H. & Golby, A.J. (2007) Object naming is a more sensitive measure of speech localization than number counting: converging evidence from direct cortical stimulation and fMRI. *NeuroImage*, 2007; Vol.37: Suppl.1, (May 2007), pp. S100–S108, ISSN 1053-8119

Picht, T., Kombos, T., Gramm, H.J., Brock, M. & Suess, O. (2006) Multimodal protocol for awake craniotomy in language cortex tumour surgery. *Acta Neurochirurgica (Wien)*, Vol.148, No.2, (February 2006), pp. 127-137, ISSN 0001-6268

Pouration, N., Bookheimer, S.Y., Rex, D.E., Martin, N.A. & Toga, A.W. (2002) Utility of preoperative functional magnetic resonance imaging for identifying language cortices in patients with vascular malformations. *Journal of Neurosurgery*, Vol.97, No.1, (July 2002), pp. 21-32, ISSN 0022-3085

Pouratian, N., Bookheimer, S.Y., Rubino, G., Martin, N.A. & Toga, A.W. (2003) Category-specific naming deficit identified by intraoperative stimulation mapping and postoperative neuropsychological testing. *Journal of Neurosurgery*, Vol.99, No.1, (July 2003), pp. 170-176, ISSN 0022-3085

Pouratian, N., Cannestra, A.F., Bookheimer, S.Y., Martin, N.A. & Toga, A.W. (2004) Variability of intraoperative electrocortical stimulation mapping parameters across and within individuals. *Journal of Neurosurgery*, Vol.101, No.3, (September 2004), pp. 458-466, ISSN 0022-3085

Price, S.J., Burnet, N.G., Donovan, T., Green, H.A.L., Pena, A., Antoun, N.M. et al. (2003) Diffusion tensor imaging of brain tumors et 3T: a potential tool for assesing whait matter tract invasion? *Clinical Radiology*, 2003; Vol.58, No.6, (June 2003), pp. 455-462, ISSN 0009-9260

Quiñones-Hinojosa, A., Ojemann, S.G., Sanai, N., Dillon, W.P. & Berger, M.S. (2003) Preoperative correlation of intraoperative cortical mapping with magnetic resonance imaging landmarks to predict localization of the Broca area. *Journal of Neurosurgery*, Vol.99, No.2, (August 2003), pp. 311–318, ISSN 0022-3085

Ranck, J.B. Jr. (1975) Which elements are excited in electrical stimulation of mammalian central nervous system: a review. *Brain Research*, Vol.98, No.3, (November 1975), pp. 417–440, ISSN 0006-8993

Reithmeier, T., Krammer, M., Gumprecht, H., Gerstner, W. & Lumenta, C.B. (2003) Neuronavigation combined with electrophysiological monitoring for surgery of lesions in eloquent brain areas in 42 cases: a retrospective comparison of the neurological outcome and the quality of resection with a control group with similar lesions. *Minimally Invasive Neurosurgery*, Vol.46, No.2, (April 2003), pp. 65-71, ISSN 0946-7211

Roux, F-E. & Trémoulet, M. (2002) Organization of language areas in bilingual patients: a cortical stimulation study. *Journal of Neurosurgery*, 2002 Oct; Vol.97, No.4, (October 2002), pp. 857–864, ISSN 0022-3085

Roux, F-E., Boulanouar, K., Lotteri, J.A., Mejdoubi, M., LeSage, J.P. & Berry, I. (2003) Language functional magnetic resonance imaging in preoperative assessment of language areas: correlation with direct cortical stimulation. *Neurosurgery*, Vol.52, No.6, (June 2003), pp. 1335-1347, ISSN 0148-396X

Roux, F-E., Boetto, S., Sacko, O., Chollet, F. & Tremoulet, M. (2003) Writing, calculating and finger recognition in the region of the angular gyrus: a cortical stimulation study of Gerstmann syndrome. *Journal of Neurosurgery*, Vol.99, No.4, (October 2003), pp. 716-727, ISSN 0022-3085

Roux, F-E., Lubrano, V., Lauwers-Cances, V., Trémoulet, M., Mascott, C.R. et al. (2004) Intra-operative mapping of cortical areas involved in reading in mono- and bilingual patients. *Brain*, Vol.127, No.8, (August 2004), pp. 1796–1810, ISSN 0006-8950

Ruge, M.I., Victor, J., Hosain, S., Correa, D.D., Relkin, N.R., Tabar, V., Brennan, C., Gutin, P.H. & Hirsch, J. (1999) Concordance between functional magnetic resonance imaging and intraoperative language mapping. *Stereotactic and Functional Neurosurgery*, Vol.72, No.2-4, (July 1999), pp. 95-102, ISSN 1011-6125

Rutten, G.J., Van Rijen, P.C., Van Veelen, C.W.M. & Ramsey, N.F. Language area localization with three-dimensional functional magnetic resonance imaging matches intrasulcal electrostimulation in Broca's area. *Annals of Neurology*, Vol.46, No.3, (September 1999), pp. 405-408, ISSN 0364-5134

Rutten, G.J., Ramsey, N.F., van Rijen, P.C., Noordmans, H.J. & van Veelen, W.M. (2002) Development of a functional magnetic resonance imaging protocol for intraoperative localization of critical temporoparietal language areas. *Annals of Neurology*, Vol.51, No.3, (March 2002), pp. 350–360, ISSN 0364-5134

Sahjpaul, R.L. (2000) Awake craniotomy: controversies, indication and techniques in the surgical treatment of temporal lobe epilepsy. *Canadian Journal of Neurological Sciences*, Vol.27, Suppl.1, (May 2000), pp. 55-63, discussion pp, 92-96, ISSN 0317-1671

Sanai N, Mirzadeh Z, Berger MS. Functional outcome ater language mapping for glioma resection. *The New England Journal of Medicine*, Vol.358, No.1, (January 2008), pp. 18-27, ISSN 0028-4793

Sanai, N., Polley, M.Y. & Berger, M.S. (2010) Insular glioma resection: assessment of patient morbidity, survival, and tumor progression. Clinical article. *Journal of Neurosurgery*, Vol.112, No.1, (January 2010), pp. 1–9, ISSN 0022-3085

Sarang, A. & Dinsmore, J. Anaesthesia for awake craniotomy - evolution of a technique that facilitates awake neurological testing. *British Journal of Anaesthesia*, Vol.90, No.2, (February 2003), pp. 161-165, ISSN 0007-0912

Sawaya, R., Hammoud, M., Schoppa, D., Hess, K.R., Wu, S.Z., Shi, W-M. & Wuildrick, D.M. (1998) Neurosurgical outcomes in a modern series of 400 craniotomies for treatment of parenchymal tumors. *Neurosurgery*, Vol.42, (May 1998), pp. 1044-1056, ISSN 0148-396X

Sawaya, R., Hammoud, M.A., Ligon, B.E. & Fuller, G.N. (1999) Intraoperative localization of tumor and margins, In: *The Gliomas*, Berger, M.S. & Wilson, C.B. (Ed.), pp. 361-375, Saunders W.B., ISBN-10: 0721648258/ISBN-13: 978-0721648255, Philadelphia

Schäffler, L., Lüders, H.O. & Beck, G.J. (1996) Quantitative comparison of language deficits produced by extraoperative electrical stimulation of Broca's Wernicke's and Basal Temporal Language areas. *Epilepsia*, Vol.37, No.5, (May 1996), pp. 463- 475, ISSN 0013-9580

Schwartz, T.H., Devinsky, O., Doyle, W. & Perrine, K. (1999) Function-Specific high-probability "nodes" identified in posterior language cortex. *Epilepsia*, Vol.40, No.5, (May 1999), pp. 575-583, ISSN 0013-9580

Seeck, M., Pegna ,A.J., Ortigue, S., Spinelli, L., Dessibourg, C.A., Delavelle, J. et al. (2006) Speech arrest with stimulation may not reliably predict language deficit after epilepsy surgery. *Neurology*, 2006 Feb; Vol.66, No.4, (February 2006), pp. 592-594, ISSN 0028-3878

Seitz, R.J., Huang, Y., Knorr, U., Tellmann, L., Herzog, H. & Freund, H.J. (1995) Large-scale plasticity of the human motor cortex. *Neuroreport*, Vol.6, No.5, (March 1995), pp. 742–744, ISSN 0959-4965

Serletis, D. & Bernstein, M. (2007) Prospective study of awake craniotomy used routinely and nonselectively for supratentorial tumors. *Journal of Neurosurgery*, Vol.107, No.1, (July 2007), pp. 1-6, ISSN 0022-3085

Signorelli, F., Guyotat, J., Isnard, J., Schneider, F., Mohammedi, R. & Bret, P. (2001) The value of cortical stimulation applied to the surgery of malignant gliomas in language areas. *Neurological Sciences*, Vol.22, No.1, (April 2001), pp. 3-10, ISSN: 1590-1874

Silbergeld, D.L., Mueller, W.M., Colley, P.S., Ojemann, G.A. & Lettich, E. (1992) Use Propofol (Diprivan) for awake craniotomies: technical note. *Surgical Neurology*, Vol.38, No.4, (October 1992), pp.271-272, ISSN 0090-3019

Simon, M., Neuloh, G., von Lehe, M., Meyer, B., Schramm, J. (2009) Insular gliomas: the case for surgical management. *Journal of Neurosurgery*, Vol.110, No.4, (April 2009), pp. 685–695, ISSN 0022-3085

Simos, P.G., Papanicolaou, A.C., Breier, J.I., Wheless, J.W., Constantinou, J.E.C., Gormley, W.B. & Maggio, W.W. (1999) Localization of language-specific cortex by using magnetic source imaging and electrical stimulation mapping. *Journal of Neurosurgery*, Vol.91, No.5, (November 1999), pp. 787-796, ISSN 0022-3085

Skirboll, S.S., Ojemann, G.A., Berger, M.S., Lettich, E. & Winn, R. (1996) Functional cortex and subcortical white matter located within gliomas. *Neurosurgery*, Vol.38, No.4, (April 1996), pp. 678-684, ISSN 0148-396X

Skucas, A.P. & Artru, A.A. (2006) Anesthetic complications of awake craniotomies for epilepsy surgery. *Anesthesia and Analgesia*, Vol.102, No.3, (March 2006), pp. 882-887, ISSN 0003-2999

Smith, J.S., Chang, E.F., Lamborn, K.R., Chang, S.M., Prados, M.D., Cha, S., et al. (2008) Role of extent of resection in the long-term outcome of low-grade hemispheric gliomas. Journal of Clinical Oncology Vol.26, No.8, (March 2008), pp. 1338–1345,ISSN: 1527-7755

Stadlbauer, A., Moser, E., Gruber, S., Buslei, R., Nimscki, C., Fahlbusch, R. & Ganslandt, O. (2004) Improved delination of brain tumors: an automated method for segmentation based on pathologic changes of 1HMRSI metabolites in gliomas. *Neuroimage*, Vol.23, No.2, (October 2004), pp. 454-461, ISSN 1053-8119

Stadlbauer, A., Gruber, S., Nimscki, C. et al. (2006) Preoperative grading of gliomas using metabolite quantification with high-spatial-resolution proton MR spectrospic imaging. *Radiology*, Vol.238, No.3, (March 2006) pp. 958-969, ISSN 0033-8419

Stummer, W., Pichlmeier, U., Meinel, T., Wiestler, O.D., Zanella, F. & Reulen, H-J. for the ALA-Glioma Study Group (2006) Fluorescence-guided surgery with 5-aminolevulinic acid for resection of malignant glioma: a randomised controlled multicentre phase III trial. *The Lancet Oncology*, Vol.7, No.5, (April 2006), pp.392-401, ISSN: 1470-2045

Talacchi, A., Turazzi, S., Locatelli, F., Sala, F., Beltramello, A., Alessandrini, F., Manganotti, P., Lanteri, P., Gambin, R., Ganau, M., Tramontano, V., Santini, B. & Gerosa, M. (2010) Surgical treatment of high-grade gliomas in motor areas. The impact of different supportive technologies: a 171-patient series. *Journal of Neuro-Oncology*, (April 2010), DOI 10.1007/s11060-010-0193-x

Talacchi, A., Santini, B., Savazzi, S. & Gerosa M. (2010) Cognitive effects of tumour and surgical treatment in glioma patients. *Journal of Neuro-Oncology*, (September 2010), DOI 10.1007/s11060-010-0417-0

Talos, I.F., Zou, K.H., Kikinis, R. & Jolesz, F.A. (2007) Volumetric assessment of tumor infiltration of adjacent white matter based on anatomic MRI and diffusion tensor tractography. *Academic Radiology*, Vol.14, No.4, (April 2007), pp. 431–436, ISSN 1076-6332

Taphoorn, M.J.B., Heimans, J.J., Snoek, F.J., Lindeboom, J., Oosterink, B., Wolbers, J.G. & Karim, A.B.M. (1992) Assessment of quality of life in patients treated for low-grade glioma: a preliminary report. *Journal of Neurology, Neurosurgery and Psychiatry*, Vol.55, No.5, (May 1992), pp. 372- 376, ISSN 0022-3050

Taphoorn, M.J.B. & Klein, M. (2004) Cognitive Status in adult patients with brain tumours. *The Lancet Neurology*, Vol.3, No.3, (March 2004), pp. 159-168, ISSN 1474-4422

Taphoorn, M.J.B., Stupp, R., Coens, C., Osaba, D., Kortmann, R., Van den Bent, M.J., Mason, W. et al. (2005) Health-related qualità of life in patients with glioblastoma: a randomised controlled trial. *The Lancet Oncology*, Vol.6, No.12, (December 2005), pp. 934-944, ISSN: 1470-2045

Taylor, M.D. & Bernstein, M. (1999) Awake craniotomy with brain mapping as the routine surgical approach to treating patients with supratentorial intaaxial tumors: a prospective trial of 200 cases. *Journal of Neurosurgery*, Vol.90, No.1, (January 1999), pp. 35-41, ISSN 0022-3085

Taylor, W.A., Thomas, N.W., Wellings, J.A. & Bell, BA. (1995) Timing of postoperative intracranial hematoma development and implications for the best use of neurosurgical intensive care. *Journal of neurosurgery*, Vol.82, No.1, (January 1995), pp. 48-50, ISSN 0022-3085

Thiebaut de Schotten, M., Urbanski, M., Duffau, H., Volle, E., Lévy, R., Dubois, B. & Bartolomeo, P. (2005) Direct evidence for a parietal pathway subserving spatial awareness in humans. *Science*, Vol.309, No.5744, (September 2005), pp. 2226- 2228, ISSN 0036-8075

Toms, S.A., Ferson, D.Z. & Sawaya, R. (1999) Basic surgical techniques in the resection of malignant gliomas. *Journal of Neuro-Oncology*, Vol.42, No.3, (May 1999), pp. 215-226, ISSN 0167-594X

Tucha, O., Smeley, C., Preier, M. & Lange, K,W. Cognitive Deficits Before and After with Brain Tumours. *Neurosurgery*, 2000; Vol.47, No.2, (August 2000), pp. 324- 334, ISSN 0148-396X

Van Buren, J.M., Fedio, P. & Frederick, G.C. (1978) Mechanisms and localization of speech in the parietotemporal cortex. *Neurosurgery*, Vol.2, No.3, (May-June 1978), pp. 233-239, ISSN 0148-396X

Vives, K.P. & Piepmeier, J.M. (1999) Complications and expected outcome of glioma surgery. *Journal of Neuro-Oncology*, Vol.42, No.3, (May 1999), pp. 289-302, ISSN 0167-594X

Waydo, S., Kraskov, A., Quian Quiroga, R., Fried, I. & Koch, C. (2006) Sparse Representation in the Human Medial Temporal Lobe. *The Journal of Neuroscience*, Vol.26, No.40, (Ottobre 2006), pp. 10232-10234, ISSN: 0888-0395

Weitzner, M.A., Meyers, C.A. & Byrne, K. (1996) Psychosocial functioning and quality of life in patients with primary brain tumours. *Journal of Neurosurgery*, Vol.84, No.1, (January 1996), pp. 29-34, ISSN 0022-3085

Weitzner, M.A. & Meyers, C.A. (1997) Cognitive Functioning and quality of life in malignant glioma patients: a review of literature. *Psycho-Oncology*, Vol.6, No.3, (September 1997), pp. 169-177, ISSN 1057-9249

Whittle, I.R., Borthwick et al (2003) Brain dysfunction following 'awake' craniotomy, brain mapping and resection of glioma. *British Journal of Neurosurgery*, April, Vol.17, No.2, (April 2003), pp. 130- 137, ISSN 0007-0912

Whittle, I.R., Midgley, S., Georges, H., Pringle, A.M. & Taylor, R. (2005) Patient perceptions of "awake" brain tumour surgery. *Acta Neurochirurgica (Wien)*, Vol.147, No.3, (March 2005), pp. 275-277, ISSN 0001-6268

Wiedemayer, H., Sandalcioglu, I.E., Armbruster, W., Regel, J., Schaefer, H. & Stolke, D. (2004) False negative findings in intraoperative SEP monitoring: analysis of 658 consecutive neurosurgical cases and review of published reports. *Journal of Neurology, Neurosurgery and Psychiatry*, Vol.75, No.2, (February 2004), pp. 280-286, ISSN 0022-3050

Wu, J.S., Zhou, L.F., Tang, W.J., Mao, Y., Hu, J., Song, Y.Y. et al (2007) Clinical evaluation and follow-up outcome of diffusion tensor imaging-based functional neuronavigation: a prospective, controlled study in patients with gliomas involving pyramidal tracts. *Neurosurgery*, Vol.61, No.5, (November 2007), pp. 935–949, ISSN 0148-396X

Yaşargil, M.G. (1996) Neuropathology, In: *Microneurosurgery, Vol IVA*. Yaşargil MG (Ed), pp. 115-188, Thieme, New York

Yaşargil, M.G. (1996) Surgical approaches, In: *Microneurosurgery, Vol IVB*. Yaşargil MG (Ed), pp. 29-68, Thieme, New York

Yaşargil, M.G. (1996) Strategies, tactics and Techniques, In: *Microneurosurgery, Vol IVB*. Yaşargil MG (Ed), pp. 69-91, Thieme, New York

Yaşargil, M.G., Kadri, P.A. & Yaşargil, D.C. (2004) Microsurgery for malignant gliomas. *Journal of Neuro-Oncology*, Vol.69, No.1, (August-Sptember 2004), pp. 67–81, ISSN 0167-594X

Yoshii, Y., Tominaga, D., Sugimoto, K., Tsuchida, Y., Hyodo, A., Yonaha, H. & Kushi, S. (2008) Cognitive function of patients with brain tumor in pre- and postoperative stage. *Surgical Neurology*, Vol.69, No.1, (January 2008) pp. 51-61, ISSN 0090-3019

16

Clinical Study on Modified Boron Neutron Capture Therapy for Newly Diagnosed Glioblastoma

Shinji Kawabata[1,*], Yoko Matsushita[1], Motomasa Furuse[1], Shin-Ichi Miyatake[1], Toshihiko Kuroiwa[1] and Koji Ono[2]
[1]*Department of Neurosurgery, Osaka Medical College, Takatsuki, Osaka*
[2]*Kyoto University Research Reactor Institute, Kumatori, Osaka*
Japan

1. Introduction

Boron neutron capture therapy (BNCT) is based on the nuclear capture and fission reactions that occur when non-radioactive boron-10 (^{10}B) is irradiated with neutrons of the appropriate energy to yield high energy alpha particles (^{4}He) and recoiling lithium-7 (^{7}Li) nuclei. Since these particles have pathlengths of approximately one cell diameter, their lethality primarily is limited to boron containing cells. BNCT, therefore, can be regarded as both a biologically and a physically targeted type of radiation therapy (Fig. 1). Its success is dependent upon the selective delivery of sufficient amounts of ^{10}B to cancer cells with only small amounts localized in the surrounding normal tissues. A wide variety of boron delivery agents have

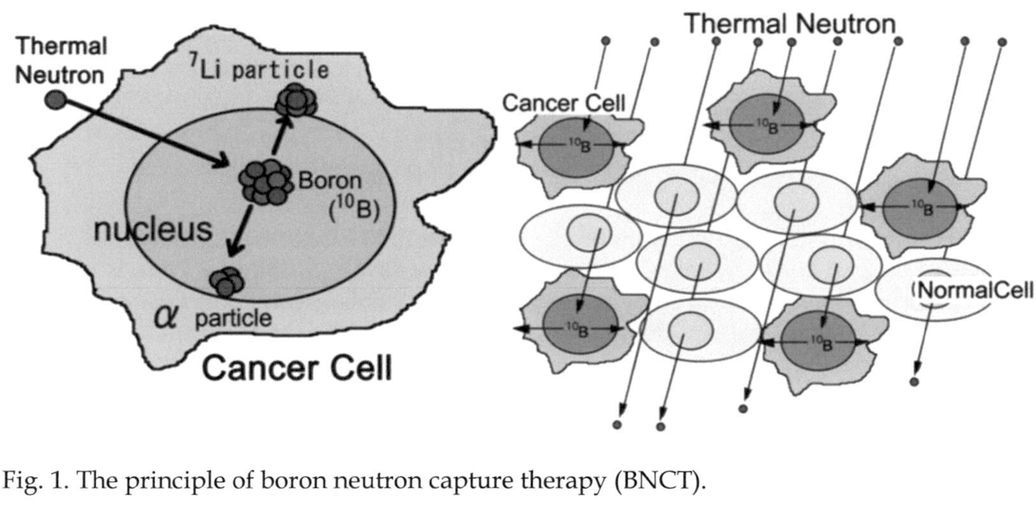

Fig. 1. The principle of boron neutron capture therapy (BNCT).

been synthesized (Hiramatsu *et al.* 2011, Miyata *et al.* 2011, Wu *et al.* 2007, Yang *et al.* 2006), but only two of these currently are being used in clinically. The first, which has been used primarily in Japan, is sodium borocaptate or BSH, and the second is a dihydroxyboryl derivative of phenylalanine referred to as boronophenylalanine or BPA (Barth *et al.* 2005). The latter has been used in clinical trials in Japan, Europe and the United States, primarily for the treatment of high grade gliomas, and more recently for recurrent tumors of the head and neck region (Ariyoshi *et al.* 2007, Haginomori *et al.* 2009, Kimura *et al.* 2009). Following i.v. administration of either BPA or BSH by i.v. infusion, the tumor site is irradiated with neutrons, the source of which is a nuclear reactor.

Recently, BNCT studies carried out by us at Osaka Medical College (OMC) and Kyoto University Research Reactor Institute (KURRI), in which BPA and BSH were administered in combination (Kawabata *et al.* 2003, Miyatake *et al.* 2005, Miyatake *et al.* 2009) for the patients with recurrent tumor after irradiation, or BNCT followed by an X-ray boost showed favorable responses in patients with newly-diagnosed glioblastoma (GB) and especially those in high risk groups (Kawabata *et al.* 2009a).

2. Clinical studies of our modified boron neutron capture therapy

Since the 1950s, BNCT has been used to treat malignant gliomas, although the results have not been satisfactory. We modified the therapy in several ways to resolve problems previously existing, and applied this modified BNCT to malignant gliomas beginning in 2002 by using KURRI (Kawabata et al. 2003). First, we utilized an epithermal rather than a thermal beam to improve the distribution of thermal neutrons in deep sites. Second, we used both of the boron compounds that are currently available worldwide for BNCT: sodium borocaptate (BSH) and boronophenylalanine (BPA). These compounds reach different subpopulations of tumor cells and accumulate in them in a different fashion.

2.1 Survival benefit from modified boron neutron capture therapy in combination with external beam fractionated X-ray treatment

We evaluate the clinical results of a form of tumor selective particle radiation, BNCT in combination with external beam fractionated X-ray treatment (XRT) for newly-diagnosed GB patients. Between 2002 and 2006, we treated 21 patients of newly-diagnosed GB with BNCT utilizing sodium borocaptate and boronophenylalanine simultaneously. The first 10 were treated with only BNCT (protocol 1), and the last 11 were treated with BNCT followed by fractionated XRT of 20 to 30 Gy (protocol 2) to reduce the possibility of local tumor recurrence. No chemotherapy was applied until tumor progression was observed.

2.1.1 Methods and the study design of our modified BNCT with XRT

As mentioned previously, we modified the protocol of BNCT as follows: First, we started using epithermal neutrons instead of thermal neutrons to obtain good penetration for deep-seated lesions. Second, we simultaneously used 2 different boron compounds (BSH and BPA) with different accumulation mechanisms to the tumor cells (Ono *et al.* 1999, Yokoyama *et al.* 2006). Third, we utilized a dose simulation work station, the Simulation Environments for Radiotherapy Applications (SERA; Idaho National Laboratory, Idaho Falls, ID) or the JAERI computational dosimetry system (JCDS). Fourth, ^{18}F-labeled BPA positron emission tomography (^{18}F-BPA-PET) (Fig.2) was applied for the estimation of the boron compound accumulation prior to neutron irradiation (Imahori *et al.* 1998). Fifth, we filled the tumor removed cavity with air to obtain enough neutron flux, especially for the bottom of deep-seated tumors (Sakurai *et al.* 2006). Sixth, we developed a central shielding method with a lithium plate at the center of the irradiation field to obtain uniform neutron distribution and increase the neutron flux relativey at the periphery in the radiation field (Ono 2006, Ono *et al.* 2000). With these modifications, even patients with deep-seated tumors can be treated by BNCT without craniotomy with a short hospital stay. In the present study, the revised protocol was used as a new protocol as follows.

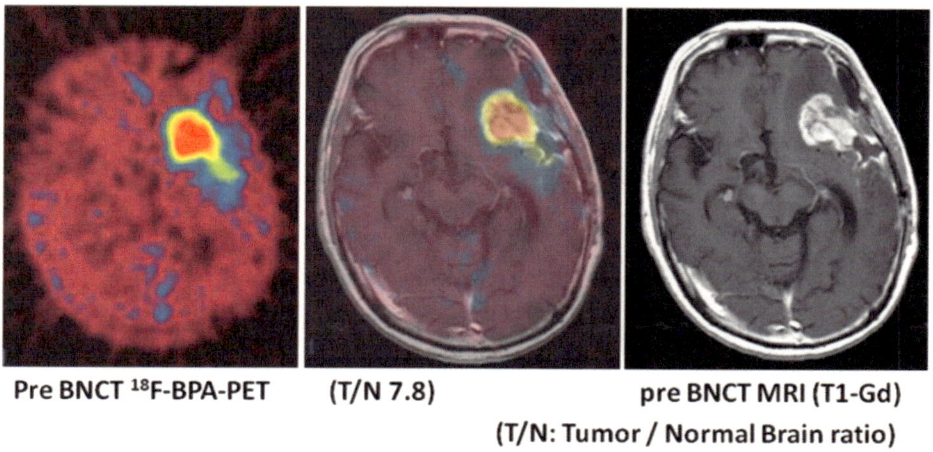

Fig. 2. ^{18}F labeled BPA positron emmision tomography (^{18}F - BPA PET) has been applied for the estimation of the boron compound accumulation prior to BNCT. The tracer is fluororide labelled boron compound. This PET ensures the effectiveness of BNCT. ^{18}F-BPA accumulates well and distributes precisely in the tumor lesion and the infiltrating tumor zone.

Twelve hours before the neutron irradiation, the patients were administered 100mg/kg of BSH intravenously for one hour. 700mg/kg of BPA was infused continuously to the patients for 6 hours before the irradiation, and they were positioned for neutron irradiation in the reactor (KURRI or JRR-4 (Japan Atomic Energy Agency Research Reactor 4)). Just after termination of continuous BPA infusion for 6hrs, neutrons were irradiated. We used the dose-planning workstation to calculate the radiation dose for tumors from the ^{18}F-BPA-PET data and blood ^{10}B concentrations obtained every 2 hours after BSH administration. We used an epithermal neutron beam. Following this, a 2 Gy daily fraction of XRT was applied, for a total of 20 to 30Gy. The total dose of XRT was decided based on the BNCT dose for the normal brain. In Protocol 1, we aimed to apply more than 30 gray-equivalent (Gy-Eq) for gross tumor volume (GTV) and less than 12 Gy-Eq for normal brain, as BNCT. In Protocol 2, we aimed to apply more than 40 Gy-Eq for GTV and less than 15 Gy-Eq for normal brain. No chemotherapy was applied for any of the patients until the tumor progression was confirmed histologically or by ^{18}F-BPA-PET (Miyashita *et al.* 2008).

Survival time from histologically diagnosed as GB was compared with the survival time for the institutional historical controls who were treated by surgical removal followed by XRT and chemotherapy (mainly nitrosourea) from 1990 to 2006 in OMC. In this historical control group, all cases were operated on to aim for the maximum tumor removal, the same as for the cases of the BNCT group. These Kaplan–Meier curves were calculated and the Log-rank test was used for statistical analysis. For the 21 patients who received BNCT, survival time was also compared with the corresponding recursive partitioning analysis (RPA) subclasses by the Radiation Therapy Oncology Group (RTOG) (Curran *et al.* 1993), as the international historical control, and European Organisation for Research and Treatment of Cancer - National Cancer Institute of Canada (EORTC-NCIC) trial (Stupp *et al.* 2009).

2.1.2 Results from our past study

Patients treated with BNCT (n=21) had a median ST of 15.6 months (95% confidence interval (CI): 12.2-23.9) after diagnosis (Fig. 3). Here the date of diagnosis is the initial debulking surgery date. This was significantly longer than the median survival time (MST) for the historical controls at our institute who were treated with surgical removal followed by XRT and chemotherapy (n=27, MST was 10.3 months (95% CI: 7.4-13.2), log-rank test p = 0.0035). The survival time from the date of diagnosis was calculated using the Kaplan-Meier method. The MST of the protocol 2 was 23.5 months (95% CI: 10.2 - undetermined) after diagnosis (n=11), and that of the protocol 1 patients (n=10) was 14.1 months (95% CI: 9.9-18.5), although the difference was not statistically significant (Fig. 4).

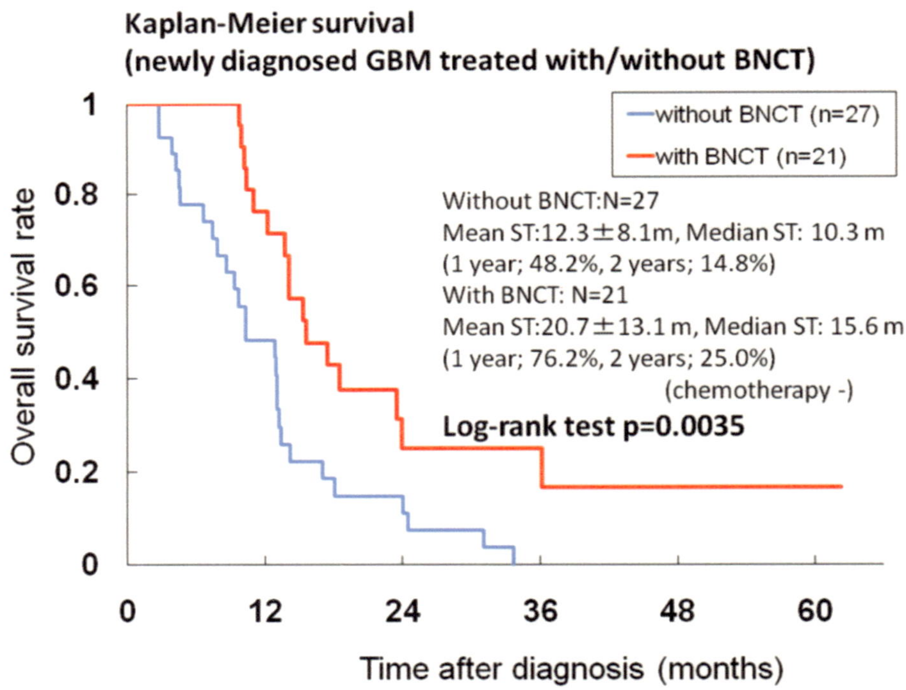

Fig. 3. Cumulative survival data for all newly diagnosed glioblastoma (WHO grade 4, n=21). Blue line is our recent historical control treated by external beam X-ray irradiation. The median survival time (ST) of boron neutron capture therapy (BNCT) group (red line) is 15.6 months. There is statistical significance between both group in Log-rank test (p=0.0035).

The RPA class distribution of 21 patients treated with BNCT at the initial diagnosis was as follows: Class III = 6 (29%); Class IV = 6 (29%); Class V = 8 (38%); Class VI = 1 (5%). The MSTs of the patients in classes III, IV, V, and VI were 23.5, 16.9, 13.2, and 9.8 months, respectively (Table 1). In historical control, the RPA class distribution was as follows: Class III = 3 (11%); Class IV = 14 (52%); Class V = 8 (30%); Class VI = 2 (7%). The distributions of each RPA class in BNCT group and institutional historical control group are a little bit different. We compare the survival of both groups in low risk RPA (class III and IV) and in high risk RPA (class V and IV) separately. The MST of BNCT group in low risk group was 18.5 months (n=12, 95% CI: 13.7-36.1) and that of historical control was 13.0 months (n=17, 95% CI: 8.6-18.0). There is statistical significance in log-rank test (p=0.028). The MST of BNCT group in high risk group was 12.2 months (n=9, 95% CI: 9.8-undetermined) and that of historical control was 7.4 months (n=10, 95% CI: 2.7-10.3). There is also statistical significance in log-rank test (p=0.0083). Therefore, it can be concluded that BNCT group shows the long survival in comparison with historical control not mainly by the difference of distribution of each RPA class in both groups. Our BNCT results for survival among the newly-diagnosed GB cases were favorable in comparison with those obtained from the corresponding RTOG - RPA subclasses.

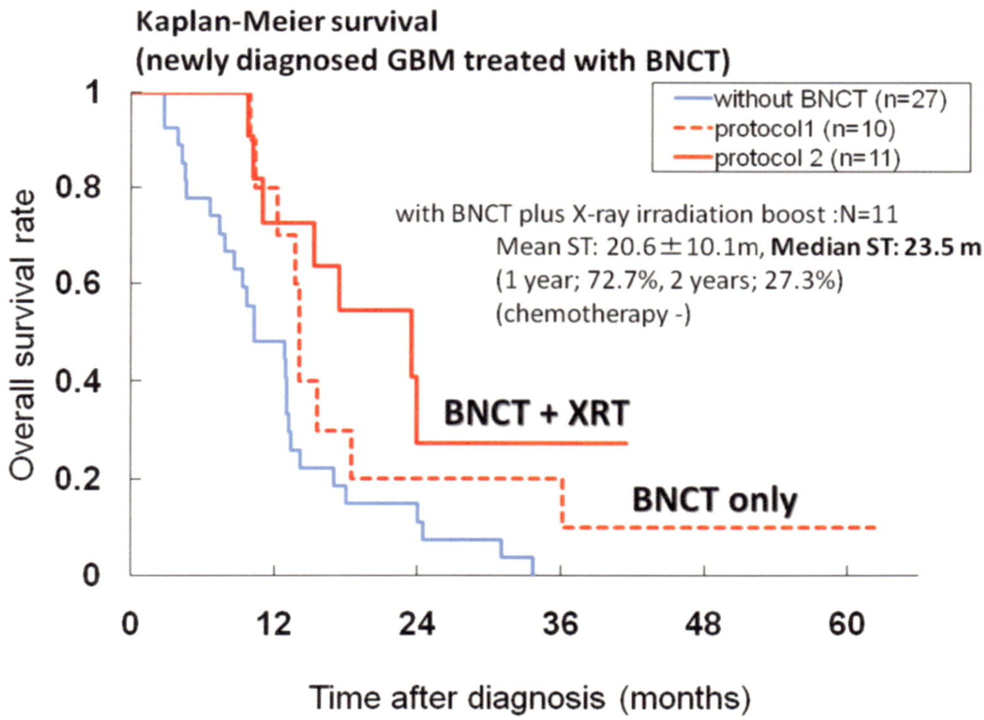

Fig. 4. Cumulative survival data for all newly diagnosed glioblastoma (protocol 1 and 2). External beam X-ray irradiation boost after boron neutron capture therapy (BNCT) (protocol 2, red line) was indicated for later 11 cases. This improve the median survival time as 23.5 months (vs 14.1 months for BNCT only (protocol 1, dotted red line)).

RTOG RPA class	RTOG original	EORTC-NCIC (XRT/TMZ)		BNCT	
	XRT	XRT	TMZ/XRT	XRT	BNCT
III	17.9	14.8	18.7	13.4	23.5
IV	11.1	13.3	16.3	12.8	16.9
V	8.9	9.1	10.7	7.4	13.2
VI	4.6	Not reported		3.6	9.8

*Median survival time (months). RTOG: radiation therapy oncology group, EORTC: european organisation for research and treatment of cancer, NCIC: National Cancer Institute of Canada Clinical Trials, RPA: recursive partitioning analysis, XRT: X-ray radiation therapy, TMZ: Temozolomide, BNCT: boron neutron capture therapy.

Table 1. Comparison of survival data among RPA class in the RTOG database, EORTC-NCIC (XRT/TMZ) trial, and in our cases treated with BNCT.

2.2 Representative case treated by modified boron neutron capture therapy combination with fractionated X-ray irradiation

A 63-year old female had a left parietal tumor removed partially in a hospital in November 2004. The histopathological diagnosis was GB. She was introduced to our hospital for BNCT for the remaining lesion. While she waited for the BNCT, rapid growth of the tumor caused aggravations of right hemiparesis, total aphasia and consciousness disturbance, all of which caused us to remove the tumor again in our hospital prior to BNCT. The tumor was gross totally removed, and the patient received BNCT with air instillation in tumor removed cavity, followed by XRT. At the time of BNCT, the workstation calculates two different estimated doses, one is for the tumor and the other is for the normal brain (Fig. 5).

Dose calculation shows estimated gray-equivalent (Gy-Eq) isodose lines from BNCT. This is mainly based on the decay of the irradiated neutron, boron concentration and biological effectiveness of each tissue. The deepest part of the tumor was 7.5 cm from the scalp in this case. The irradiated minimum tumor dose by BNCT was improved by the air-instilation (star in the Fig. 5) methods from 18.9 Gy-Eq (without air) to 26.9 Gy-Eq (with air). The maximum irradiated point of the normal brain was 2 cm from the scalp and was 12.7 Gy-Eq and scalp surface was 9.0 Gy-Eq. An additional 20 Gy was applied by XRT (daily fraction of 2 Gy x 10 days) aimed for the deep part of the mass but included surface of the tumor and the normal brain.

No tumor recurrence on MRI and no neurological deficit were seen for 13 months after BNCT (Fig. 6). BNCT followed by fractionated XRT could control the tumor for 12 months (Fig. 6B). However, 14 months after BNCT, the patient suffered from right hemiparesis and MRI revealed a Gd-enhanced lesion from the surface area of the tumor removed cavity which was irradiated by BNCT with enough dose and also included into the boost XRT (Fig. 6C). Radiation necrosis was suspected as the pathological condition based on L/N ratio in BPA-PET, but we could not neglect the possibility of a recurrence of the GB. We performed a re-craniotomy to remove this lesion. The pathological diagnosis was radiation necrosis; no apparent tumor cells were found by pathologists. After the surgery, the right hemiparesis was improved, while no tumor progression was observed on MRI in the follow-up for more than 5 years (Fig. 6D). The patient received best medical treatment (anti-coagulants and vitamin E) for a year to prevent a further radiation necrosis.

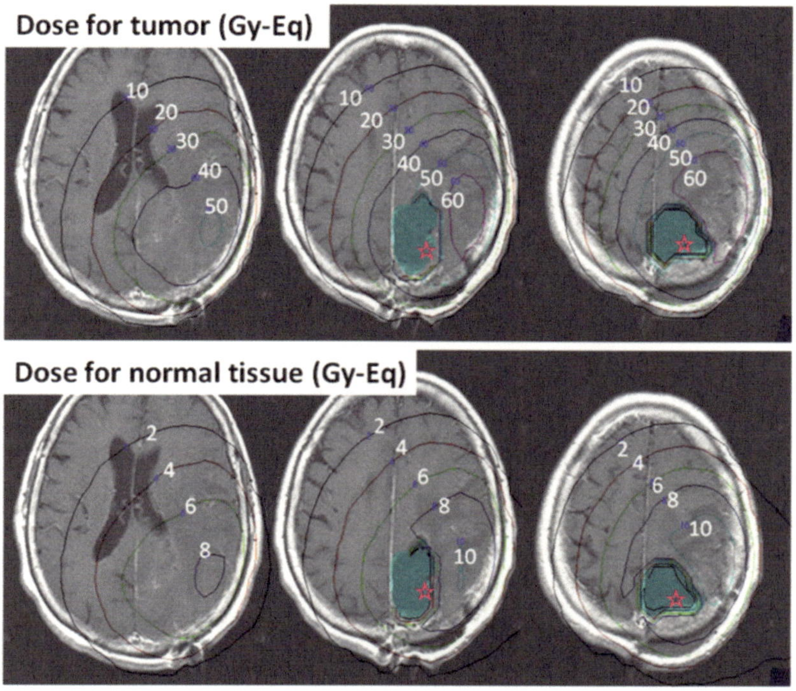

Fig. 5. Dose planning of neutron capture therapy for the tumor (upper) and for the normal brain (lower). (Gy-Eq: gray equivalent, star: air instillation to the tumor removed cavity)

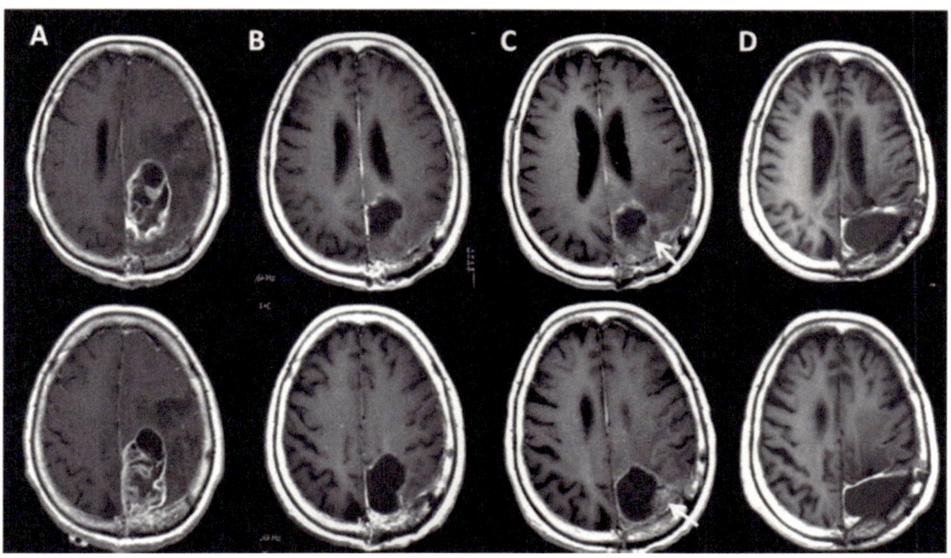

Fig. 6. Serial MRI images (T1-weighted with Gd enhancement) of the patient treated by boron neutron capture therapy combined with fractionated external beam X-ray irradiation. (A: prior to surgical removal and BNCT, B: 12 months, C: 14 months and D: 5 years after BNCT).

2.3 Phase II clinical study of boron neutron capture therapy combined with X-ray radiotherapy / Temozolomide in patients with newly diagnosed glioblastoma multiforme

Results of our clinical study showed the efficacy of combination therapy with external beam XRT and BNCT. For our future study, we planned the Multi-centric Phase II clinical study named "*Boron Neutron Capture Therapy, Radiation Therapy, and Temozolomide in Treating Patients with Newly Diagnosed Glioblastoma Multiforme*" in Japan (OSAKA-TRIBRAIN0902, NCT00974987). The major differences of our protocol from the other past BNCT studies were simultaneous use of both BSH and BPA, and combination with XRT.

2.3.1 Back ground of our recently up-dated protocol using BNCT

Prior to design of new version of the protocol for multi-centric study, we analyzed our previous clinical results of all the patients with malignant glioma treated by BNCT. Main part of the retrospective analysis was as follows. 1. Efficacy of additional fractionated X-ray irradiation, 2. Administration of the boron compouns, 3. Toxicity of our previous study. The median ST of the patients treated with BNCT followed by XRT boost was 23.5 months (95% CI: 10. 2 - undetermined, HR (*vs* control) = 0.32) after diagnosis (n = 11), and that of the patients treated with BNCT only (n = 10) was 14.1 months (95% CI: 9.9–18.5), although the difference was not statistically significant among these two groups.

In our previous study for all of the patients with malignant brain tumor included several doses of boron compounds especially for BPA, 250, 500, 700mg/kg body weight. Blood boron concentration was increased by escalation of the BPA dose. The continuous infusion with reduced BPA dose during irradiation (400mg/kg for 2h + 100mg/kg for 1h, previously used for head and neck cancer in KURRI) was also used and this was useful for dose estimation of BNCT because the blood boron concentration similar as 700mg BPA/kg was kept during irradiation whereas a decline of the blood level was remarkable when we terminated BPA just before neutron irradiation. Adverse events were assessed by common terminology criteria for adverse events (CTCAE) v3.0. Grade 3/4 blood/bone marrow toxicity (hemoglobin, leukocytes, neutrophils, and platelets) were 11% in 250mg/kg, 17% in 500mg/kg, and 28% in 700mg/kg. Other Grade 3/4 adverse events (seizure, AST, ALT, amylase, creatinine) were 64% in 250mg/kg, 25% in 500mg/kg, and 73% in 700mg/kg. All of these adverse events were reversible and transient. Radiation induced edema and/or necrosis occurred mainly in the area that was available for high-dose irradiation by BNCT nearly the surface of the brain of the patients treated with BNCT+XRT. Based on this retrospective analysis, the Multi-centric Phase II clinical study was planned and now on-going.

2.3.2 On-going protocol using BNCT for the newly diagnosed glioblastoma

Based on our former BNCT clinical experience, we included the following points in a new protocol using the two boron compounds, BSH and BPA, in combination (Ono et al. 1999, Yokoyama et al. 2006). The schedule of the administration of boron compounds is settled as follows; 13 hours before the neutron irradiation, 100 mg/kg of BSH will be intravenously infused for one hour, and 500 mg/kg of BPA will be infused continuously 200 mg/kg/h for 2 hours before the irradiation and reduced for 100 mg/kg/h during irradiation to the patients. During continuous BPA infusion of reduced dose as 100 mg/kg, neutrons irradiation is performed. Protocol treatments consist of BNCT, additional 24Gy XRT and chemotherapy with TMZ. Prescription dose by BNCT is regulated as not to be more than 13Gy-Eq for normal brain. Additional XRT is given with 3 gradient such as 8, 16, 24Gy from the surface of scalp to the bottom of tumor infiltrated zone (Fig. 7). Chemotherapy with TMZ is applied concomitantly during XRT treatments and adjuvant chemotherapy with the same agent is repeated in outpatient clinic (Fig. 8) (Stupp *et al.* 2005).

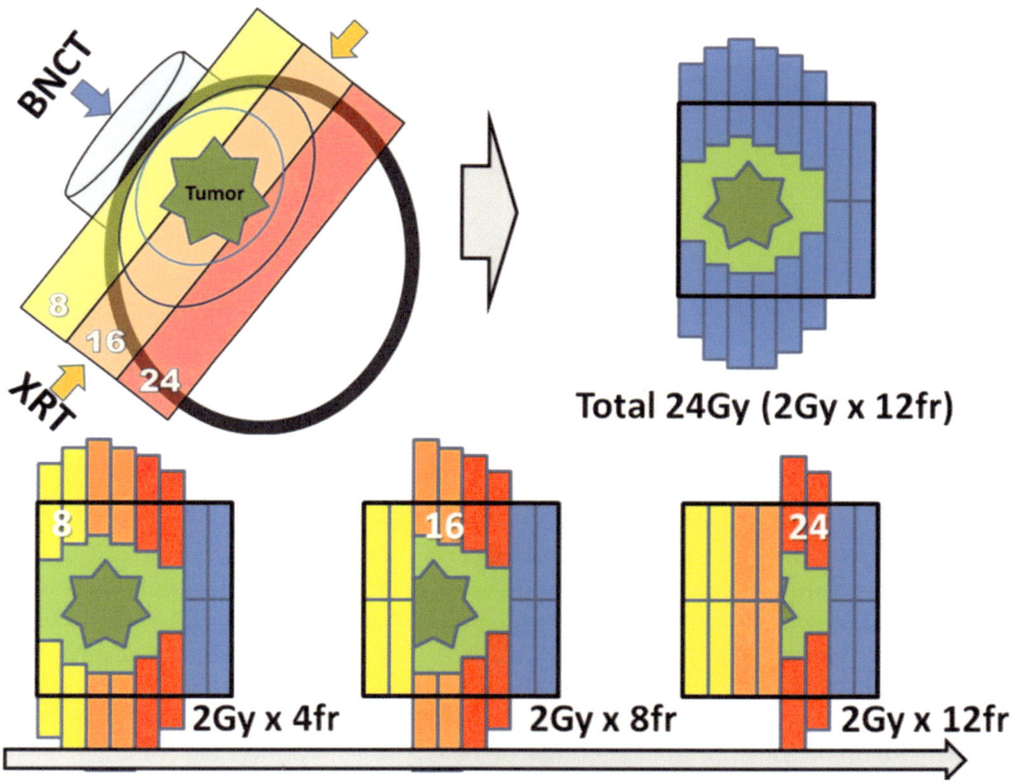

Fig. 7. Illustrated image of the protocol combined with boron neutron capture therapy (BNCT) and 3 gradient fractionated X-ray irradiation (XRT). Gy: gray, fr: fraction.

Based on our previous clinical study, the Hazard ratio of BNCT vs. XRT was simulated as 0.4, so the total estimated number of the patients who should be included in our new study become 45 totally. Primary end point is overall survival and these patients will be followed up for 2 years after the last patient treatment. The most important point in our protocol is diagnosis and treatment of radiation effects such as swelling, radiation induced edema, transient expansion of the tumor, pseudo- progression / response, and radiation necrosis. ^{18}F-BPA-PET study is included for the diagnosis of these pathologies.

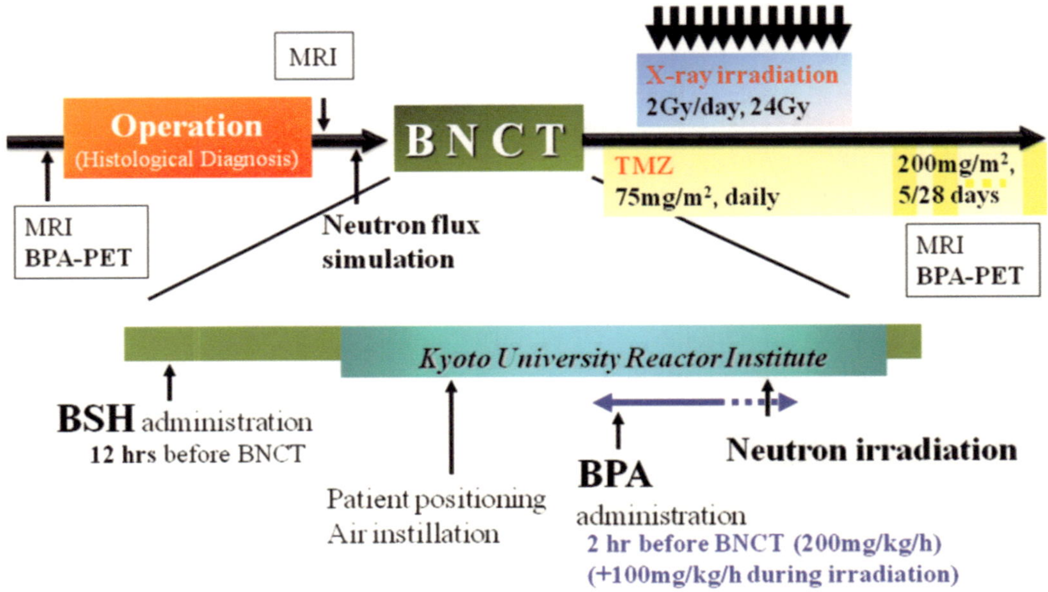

Fig. 8. Treatment protocol of BNCT combination with EBRT/TMZ for Newly diagnosed Malignant Glioma

3. Conclusion

Glioblastoma is currently not curable and the prognosis of it is very poor. A world-wide standard care of newly-diagnosed GB is postoperative XRT with concomitant and adjuvant chemotherapy with new alkylating agent TMZ(Stupp et al. 2005). This standard treatment for newly diagnosed GB prolonged the median ST of patients from 12.1 months to 14.6 months in comparison with XRT alone, which is still pessimistic clinical result of this disease. Therefore an alternative promising treatment should be developed for the improvement of the prognosis of newly diagnosed GB. Several recent clinical studies on the treatment of patients with GB by means of BNCT have reported encouraging results. Careful analysis of survival data from a study, carried out in Sweden (Skold *et al.*) in which BPA was administered at a higher dose over a longer period of time (Skold *et al.*), suggested that a subset of patients had survival times that were at least as good as those obtained with conventional therapy consisting of X-irradiation in combination with TMZ (Stupp et al. 2005).

On the other hand, BNCT is tumor-selective particle radiation. Tumor-seeking boron compounds boronophenylalanine (BPA) and sodium borocapate (BSH) can be delivered selectively in GB tissue with high contrast of accumulation in comparison with normal brain tissue. This tumor selective accumulation of boron compounds is followed by neutron irradiation, which produced high linear energy transfer particles (alpha particle and re-coiled Li nucleus). Thereafter these particles can destroy tumor cells selectively with high efficiency (Barth et al. 2005). The principal investigator of this clinical trial published the excellent survival data of 21 cases of newly diagnosed GB treated by BNCT with the MST of

15.6 months without TMZ. Moreover additional 20 to 30Gy XRT prolonged the MST up to 23.5 months in 11 cases without TMZ (Kawabata *et al.* 2009b). These strategies were also confirmed by pre-clinical bench works (Barth *et al.* 2004). These are the background of our on-going clinical trial. Thereafter in this trial, the protocol is composed of BNCT, followed by 24Gy XRT with concomitant and adjuvant chemotherapy with TMZ for newly diagnosed GB patients.

4. Acknowledgment

This project was supported by the grant-in-aid for Scientific Research from the Ministry of Health, Labor and Welfare of Japan to S-I. Miyatake. This work was also supported in part by the Takeda Science Foundation for S. Kawabata (PI; H. Matsui, Okayama University).
This work was also partly supported by Scientific Research from the Japanese Ministry of Education, Science, and Culture to S. Kawabata, M. Furuse (Scientific Research C), and Y. Matsushita (Grant-in-Aid for Young Scientist B).
This project was approved by the Ethical Committee of Osaka Medical College and by the BNCT Committee of Kyoto University Research Reactor Institute or Japan Atomic Energy Agency. Individual cases were discussed and selected by the latter committee and the signing of the informed consent by each patient.

5. References

Ariyoshi, Y., Miyatake, S., Kimura, Y., Shimahara, T., Kawabata, S., Nagata, K., Suzuki, M., Maruhashi, A., Ono, K. & Shimahara, M. (2007). Boron neuron capture therapy using epithermal neutrons for recurrent cancer in the oral cavity and cervical lymph node metastasis. *Oncol Rep,* Vol. 18, No. 4 pp. (861-866), ISSN. 1021-335X

Barth, R. F., Coderre, J. A., Vicente, M. G. & Blue, T. E. (2005). Boron neutron capture therapy of cancer: current status and future prospects. *Clin Cancer Res,* Vol. 11, No. 11 pp. (3987-4002), ISSN. 1078-0432

Barth, R. F., Grecula, J. C., Yang, W., Rotaru, J. H., Nawrocky, M., Gupta, N., Albertson, B. J., Ferketich, A. K., Moeschberger, M. L., Coderre, J. A. & Rofstad, E. K. (2004). Combination of boron neutron capture therapy and external beam radiotherapy for brain tumors. *Int J Radiat Oncol Biol Phys,* Vol. 58, No. 1 pp. (267-277), ISSN. 0360-3016

Curran, W. J., Jr., Scott, C. B., Horton, J., Nelson, J. S., Weinstein, A. S., Fischbach, A. J., Chang, C. H., Rotman, M., Asbell, S. O., Krisch, R. E. & et al. (1993). Recursive partitioning analysis of prognostic factors in three Radiation Therapy Oncology Group malignant glioma trials. *J Natl Cancer Inst,* Vol. 85, No. 9 pp. (704-710), ISSN. 0027-8874

Haginomori, S., Miyatake, S., Inui, T., Araki, M., Kawabata, S., Takamaki, A., Lee, K., Takenaka, H., Kuroiwa, T., Uesugi, Y., Kumada, H. & Ono, K. (2009). Planned fractionated boron neutron capture therapy using epithermal neutrons for a patient with recurrent squamous cell carcinoma in the temporal bone: a case report. *Head Neck,* Vol. 31, No. 3 pp. (412-418), ISSN. 1097-0347 (Electronic), 1043-3074 (Linking)

Hiramatsu, R., Kawabata, S., Miyatake, S., Kuroiwa, T., Easson, M. W. & Vicente, M. G. (2011). Application of a novel boronated porphyrin (HOCP) as a dual sensitizer for both PDT and BNCT. *Lasers Surg Med,* Vol. 43, No. 1 pp. (52-58), ISSN. 1096-9101 (Electronic), 0196-8092 (Linking)

Imahori, Y., Ueda, S., Ohmori, Y., Sakae, K., Kusuki, T., Kobayashi, T., Takagaki, M., Ono, K., Ido, T. & Fujii, R. (1998). Positron emission tomography-based boron neutron capture therapy using boronophenylalanine for high-grade gliomas: part II. *Clin Cancer Res,* Vol. 4, No. 8 pp. (1833-1841), ISSN. 1078-0432

Kawabata, S., Miyatake, S., Kajimoto, Y., Kuroda, Y., Kuroiwa, T., Imahori, Y., Kirihata, M., Sakurai, Y., Kobayashi, T. & Ono, K. (2003). The early successful treatment of glioblastoma patients with modified boron neutron capture therapy. Report of two cases. *J Neurooncol,* Vol. 65, No. 2 pp. (159-165), ISSN. 0167-594X

Kawabata, S., Miyatake, S., Kuroiwa, T., Yokoyama, K., Doi, A., Iida, K., Miyata, S., Nonoguchi, N., Michiue, H., Takahashi, M., Inomata, T., Imahori, Y., Kirihata, M., Sakurai, Y., Maruhashi, A., Kumada, H. & Ono, K. (2009a). Boron neutron capture therapy for newly diagnosed glioblastoma. *J Radiat Res (Tokyo),* Vol. 50, No. 1 pp. (51-60), ISSN. 0449-3060

Kawabata, S., Miyatake, S., Nonoguchi, N., Hiramatsu, R., Iida, K., Miyata, S., Yokoyama, K., Doi, A., Kuroda, Y., Kuroiwa, T., Michiue, H., Kumada, H., Kirihata, M., Imahori, Y., Maruhashi, A., Sakurai, Y., Suzuki, M., Masunaga, S. & Ono, K. (2009b). Survival benefit from boron neutron capture therapy for the newly diagnosed glioblastoma patients. *Appl Radiat Isot,* Vol. 67, No. 7-8 Suppl pp. (S15-18), ISSN. 1872-9800 (Electronic), 0969-8043 (Linking)

Kimura, Y., Ariyoshi, Y., Miyatake, S., Shimahara, M., Kawabata, S. & Ono, K. (2009). Boron neutron capture therapy for papillary cystadenocarcinoma in the upper lip: a case report. *Int J Oral Maxillofac Surg,* Vol. 38, No. 3 pp. (293-295), ISSN. 1399-0020 (Electronic), 901-5027 (Linking)

Miyashita, M., Miyatake, S., Imahori, Y., Yokoyama, K., Kawabata, S., Kajimoto, Y., Shibata, M. A., Otsuki, Y., Kirihata, M., Ono, K. & Kuroiwa, T. (2008). Evaluation of fluoride-labeled boronophenylalanine-PET imaging for the study of radiation effects in patients with glioblastomas. *J Neurooncol,* Vol. 89, No. 2 pp. (239-246), ISSN. 0167-594X

Miyata, S., Kawabata, S., Hiramatsu, R., Doi, A., Ikeda, N., Yamashita, T., Kuroiwa, T., Kasaoka, S., Maruyama, K. & Miyatake, S. I. (2011). CT imaging of transferrin targeting liposomes encapsulating both boron and iodine contrast agent by CED to F98 rat glioma for boron neutron capture therapy. *Neurosurgery,* Vol., No., ISSN. 1524-4040 (Electronic), 0148-396X (Linking)

Miyatake, S., Kawabata, S., Kajimoto, Y., Aoki, A., Yokoyama, K., Yamada, M., Kuroiwa, T., Tsuji, M., Imahori, Y., Kirihata, M., Sakurai, Y., Masunaga, S., Nagata, K., Maruhashi, A. & Ono, K. (2005). Modified boron neutron capture therapy for malignant gliomas performed using epithermal neutron and two boron compounds with different accumulation mechanisms: an efficacy study based on findings on neuroimages. *J Neurosurg,* Vol. 103, No. 6 pp. (1000-1009), ISSN. 0022-3085

Miyatake, S., Kawabata, S., Yokoyama, K., Kuroiwa, T., Michiue, H., Sakurai, Y., Kumada, H., Suzuki, M., Maruhashi, A., Kirihata, M. & Ono, K. (2009). Survival benefit of

Boron neutron capture therapy for recurrent malignant gliomas. *J Neurooncol,* Vol. 91, No. 2 pp. (199-206), ISSN. 0167-594X

Ono, K. (2006). central shielding. In Y. Nakagawa, T. Kobayashi & H. Fukuda (Eds.), *Advances in Neutron Capture Therapy 2006: "From the past to the future", Proceedings of 12th International Congress on Neutron Capture Therapy.* Kagawa, Japan.

Ono, K., Masunaga, S., Suzuki, M., Kinashi, Y., Takagaki, M. & Akaboshi, M. (1999). The combined effect of boronophenylalanine and borocaptate in boron neutron capture therapy for SCCVII tumors in mice. *Int J Radiat Oncol Biol Phys,* Vol. 43, No. 2 pp. (431-436), ISSN. 0360-3016

Ono, K., Sakurai, Y., Masunaga, S., Kinashi, Y., Takagaki, M. & Kobayashi, T. (2000). Improvement of B-10 dose distribution in water phantom irradiated with epithermal neutron beam and its assessment by colonyformation assay. *Program & Abstracts of the Ninth International Symposium on Neutron Capture Therapy for Cancer (Kyoto University Research Reactor Institute).* Kyoto University Research Reactor Institute: Osaka, Japan.

Sakurai, Y., Ono, K., Miyatake, S. & Maruhashi, A. (2006). Improvement effect on the depth-dose distribution by CSF drainage and air infusion of a tumour-removed cavity in boron neutron capture therapy for malignant brain tumours. *Phys Med Biol,* Vol. 51, No. 5 pp. (1173-1183), ISSN. 0031-9155

Skold, K., B, H. S., Diaz, A. Z., Giusti, V., Pellettieri, L. & Hopewell, J. W. (2010a). Boron Neutron Capture Therapy for glioblastoma multiforme: advantage of prolonged infusion of BPA-f. *Acta Neurol Scand,* Vol. 122, No. 1 pp. (58-62), ISSN. 1600-0404 (Electronic), 0001-6314 (Linking)

Skold, K., Gorlia, T., Pellettieri, L., Giusti, V., B, H. S. & Hopewell, J. W. (2010b). Boron neutron capture therapy for newly diagnosed glioblastoma multiforme: an assessment of clinical potential. *Br J Radiol,* Vol. 83, No. 991 pp. (596-603), ISSN. 1748-880X (Electronic), 0007-1285 (Linking)

Stupp, R., Hegi, M. E., Mason, W. P., van den Bent, M. J., Taphoorn, M. J., Janzer, R. C., Ludwin, S. K., Allgeier, A., Fisher, B., Belanger, K., Hau, P., Brandes, A. A., Gijtenbeek, J., Marosi, C., Vecht, C. J., Mokhtari, K., Wesseling, P., Villa, S., Eisenhauer, E., Gorlia, T., Weller, M., Lacombe, D., Cairncross, J. G. & Mirimanoff, R. O. (2009). Effects of radiotherapy with concomitant and adjuvant temozolomide versus radiotherapy alone on survival in glioblastoma in a randomised phase III study: 5-year analysis of the EORTC-NCIC trial. *Lancet Oncol,* Vol. 10, No. 5 pp. (459-466), ISSN. 1474-5488 (Electronic), 1470-2045 (Linking)

Stupp, R., Mason, W. P., van den Bent, M. J., Weller, M., Fisher, B., Taphoorn, M. J., Belanger, K., Brandes, A. A., Marosi, C., Bogdahn, U., Curschmann, J., Janzer, R. C., Ludwin, S. K., Gorlia, T., Allgeier, A., Lacombe, D., Cairncross, J. G., Eisenhauer, E. & Mirimanoff, R. O. (2005). Radiotherapy plus concomitant and adjuvant temozolomide for glioblastoma. *N Engl J Med,* Vol. 352, No. 10 pp. (987-996), ISSN. 1533-4406 (Electronic), 0028-4793 (Linking)

Wu, G., Yang, W., Barth, R. F., Kawabata, S., Swindall, M., Bandyopadhyaya, A. K., Tjarks, W., Khorsandi, B., Blue, T. E., Ferketich, A. K., Yang, M., Christoforidis, G. A., Sferra, T. J., Binns, P. J., Riley, K. J., Ciesielski, M. J. & Fenstermaker, R. A. (2007).

Molecular targeting and treatment of an epidermal growth factor receptor-positive glioma using boronated cetuximab. *Clin Cancer Res,* Vol. 13, No. 4 pp. (1260-1268), ISSN. 1078-0432

Yang, W., Barth, R. F., Wu, G., Kawabata, S., Sferra, T. J., Bandyopadhyaya, A. K., Tjarks, W., Ferketich, A. K., Moeschberger, M. L., Binns, P. J., Riley, K. J., Coderre, J. A., Ciesielski, M. J., Fenstermaker, R. A. & Wikstrand, C. J. (2006). Molecular targeting and treatment of EGFRvIII-positive gliomas using boronated monoclonal antibody L8A4. *Clin Cancer Res,* Vol. 12, No. 12 pp. (3792-3802), ISSN. 1078-0432

Yokoyama, K., Miyatake, S., Kajimoto, Y., Kawabata, S., Doi, A., Yoshida, T., Asano, T., Kirihata, M., Ono, K. & Kuroiwa, T. (2006). Pharmacokinetic study of BSH and BPA in simultaneous use for BNCT. *J Neurooncol,* Vol. 78, No. 3 pp. (227-232), ISSN. 0167-594X

Multimodal Approach to the Surgical Removal of Gliomas in Eloquent Brain Regions

Giannantonio Spena[1], Antonio Pepoli[2], Marcella Bruno[2], Federico D'Agata[3], Franco Cauda[3], Katiuscia Sacco[3], Sergio Duca[3] and Pietro Versari[1]
[1]*Division of Neurosurgery, Civil Hospital, Alessandria*
[2]*Division of Neurology and Neuropsychology, Civil Hospital, Alessandria,*
[3]*CCS fMRI, Koelliker Hospital and Department of Psychology, University of Turin, Turin*
Italy

1. Introduction

Supratentorial glial neoplasms are the most common primary brain tumor in adults and one of the leading causes of cancer-related death in the general population. Glioblastomas carry the worst prognosis, while low-grade gliomas have the best chance for survival. It has been demonstrated, however, that low-grade gliomas represent a precancerous state, as they have the potential to evolve into higher-grade malignancies. Although management algorithms vary among different types of tumors, surgery remains the mainstay of treatment for several reasons. Surgical resection allows the opportunity to obtain a sufficient amount of tumor for histological identification. This point is of utmost importance, as the best predictors of survival are the World Health Organization (WHO) grade and other immunohistological characteristics of the tumor. Additionally, it has been demonstrated that radical or subtotal resection correlates positively with prolongation of survival and longer time to progression. Given this information, neurosurgeons aim to achieve maximal surgical resection of these tumors whenever feasible. Unfortunately, gliomas are often located in regions of the brain defined as "eloquent" or "critical," meaning that physical damage to these areas can create permanent neurological deficits. A careful evaluation of surgical strategy is mandatory in light of this fact, with the goal being to maximize tumor resection while respecting the highly functional cortical and subcortical regions of the brain.

Different techniques are available that allow the neurosurgeon to study the brain function topography both preoperatively and intraoperatively. These methods of preoperative and intraoperative brain mapping are used to gain essential information about functional and topographic organization in a specific patient. Functional magnetic resonance imaging (fMR) is the most commonly used tool for preoperative visualization of the motor, sensory, language, and visual functional organization of a patient's brain. Since gliomas typically invade white matter, the extent of resection is additionally limited by the degree of infiltration, particularly when critical bundles are involved (e.g., the pyramidal tract). As with the eloquent cortical areas, the relationship of the tumor to the subcortical pathways should be defined in order to avoid permanent deficits. Diffusion tensor imaging (DTI), the

latest MR imaging advancement, allows reconstruction of the anatomy of the main white matter tracts. Using this imaging modality, further information can be gathered on the status of these tracts (e.g., infiltration, displacement, interruption).
It is crucial that contemporary neurosurgeons understand how to properly use these technological advancements to improve postoperative neurological results. It is also vital that critical analysis and discussion of the limits and appropriate use of these devices is part of the neurosurgical routine.
In this chapter, we will focus on some fundamental aspects of brain mapping, particularly regarding the surgical resection of gliomas. First, we will review the concept of eloquent brain regions and the evolution of the concept of critical areas. Then, we will deal with state-of-the-art functional imaging and diffusion tensor imaging, underlining their conceptual and technical limitations and explaining how to use them in surgical planning. Direct brain mapping by CSES will also be examined from a practical point of view, focusing on basic technique, anesthesia, equipment, patient selection, limitations, and future directions. Finally, we will discuss how to integrate these different mapping modalities while highlighting clinical evidence from our experience and that of other authors.
We hope that this chapter will help those who are approaching brain mapping in a clinical and neurosurgical setting not only by showing mechanisms and usefulness but also in posing questions and criticisms.

2. The evolution of the concept of eloquent brain regions

When dealing with brain functions it is quite strange to consider a part of the brain "eloquent" and some other part not, since the brain as a whole is considered the most eloquent organ of the body. Actually, in the routine practice of a neurosurgeon this riddle very often arises, particularly when a tumor is located in an area usually considered "eloquent" (i.e. central region, Broca's area, Wernicke's area). The concept of brain function organization into well defined and localized areas is the legacy of pioneering studies of the 19th and 20th centuries (D'Aubigné 1980; Mohr 2004). The basic method of these revolutionary inquiries rested on the connection between neurological deficits and post-mortem anatomical observations. Consequently, every area of the brain cortex was associated with a specific neurological function and a lesion in that region would have led to a well-defined neurological impairment. This anatomo-functional correlation gave rise to the assertion that some cortical gyri were "eloquent," for example, the triangular gyrus of the frontal operculum (Broca's area), the supramarginal gyrus (Wernicke's area), the angular gyrus, the precentral gyrus (motor area), and so on, while others were not. This tight coupling between anatomy and function has deeply influenced the practice of neurosurgery, making some patients with brain tumors in specific areas aprioristically not suitable for surgery. Even today in clinical practice, neurosurgeons very often rely mainly on standard anatomical cortical references as the initial basis for which resection of a tumor is considered potentially critical or at high risk of causing neurological damage. The excellent anatomical definition produced by MR imaging has made the process of investigation of the cerebral gyri even easier. The Rolandic region, for example, has been extensively portrayed as a model of cerebral landmarks for specific functions (sensory-motor area), but there has also been evidence that reliability is not always absolute. Intrinsic neuroanatomical variability accounts for a distinct challenge to strict anatomo-functional coupling. There are multiple factors that affect neuroanatomical variability, including sex, handedness, aging, and neurological diseases (Annet 1992; Thompson et al. 1998; Toga et al. 2001; Ballmaier et al. 2004; Luders et al. 2005; Narr et al. 2007). In the complex relationship between neuroanatomy and function, the significance of neuroanatomical variability is evidenced by its association with and probable contribution to distinct patterns of functional organization. For example, interhemispheric anatomical asymmetries (especially with respect to the planum temporale) have repeatedly been shown to be related to language lateralization (Josse et al. 2003; Steinmets et al. 1991). A trustworthy functional representation of a defined anatomical landmark is typically feasible for the hand motor area, showing as a correlate a characteristic dorsally oriented convexity in the precentral gyrus (the so-called "hand-knob") (Yousry et al. 1997; Boling et al. 2008). However, motor activity can also be detected outside of the typical landmarks, and the pattern of motor cortex activation is modulated by different physiological factors (Yousry et al. 2001; Mattay & Weinberger 1999). The discrepancy between anatomical references and functions becomes even more complex when dealing with higher cognitive functions, such as language, which have multiple and extensively distributed epicenters. It is nowadays accepted that the classical language model (Lichtheim 1885; Geschwind 1971) is not sufficient to reflect the complexity of cortical language representations (Gabrieli et al. 1998; Grabowski 2000; Bookheimer 2002). The view that there are no well-defined language areas is strongly supported by many fMR studies, as well as cortical and subcortical electrical stimulation (CSES) studies, that have identified widespread and overlapping networks for phonological, semantic, orthographic, and syntactic processing (Ojeman et al. 1989; Herolz et al. 1996; Tzourio-Mazoyer et al. 2004). In an extensive analysis performed on more than 200 patients operated on for intrinsic brain tumor through an awake craniotomy and CSES, Berger et al. (Sanai et al. 2008) showed that sites associated with speech function are variably located along the cortex and can go well beyond the classic anatomical boundaries.

In the neurosurgical population, additional inter-patient anatomical variability arises from the presence of intracranial pathology. Brain tumors can alter the understanding of neuroanatomy and function localization through two mechanisms. The first is related to the deformity created by the space-occupying lesion on adjacent sulci such that normal anatomical and imaging landmarks are more difficult or impossible to identify. The second is related to the reorganization and redistribution that occur in the cortical functional maps as a consequence of the presence of the brain tumor. Post-lesional recovery and the pattern of brain reorganization involved in functional compensations have been well documented in stroke patients (Rijntes & Weiller 2002; Rossini et al. 2003; Ward 2004). These studies have elucidated the concept of cerebral plasticity: the natural capacity of the brain to remodel itself as a consequence of learning and developmental strategy. Cerebral plasticity defines a continuous process that allows reshaping of the neuronosynaptic maps to optimize the functioning of brain networks. It is also the way to recover from lesions of different origin. Gliomas, especially low-grade gliomas, have in the very recent years increasingly attracted researchers because of their tendency to reach large volumes in eloquent areas, frequently without causing neurological symptoms. Functional MR studies have shown how these slow growing tumors can induce functional reshaping by displacing critical epicenters either around the tumor or even to the contralateral hemisphere (Mueller et al., 1996; Carpentier et al. 2001; Baciu et al. 2003). Moreover, several authors have reported series of patients who have undergone awake craniotomy and CSES in whom tumors in critical areas were safely and efficiently removed without permanent morbidity. In these series authors have documented different types and mechanisms of tumor-induced functional reorganization (Duffau 2005; Duffau 2006). In addition, in some cases functional tissue is located within the tumor nidus, and it is now understood that the standard surgical principle of debulking tumor from within to avoid neurological deficits is not always safe (Duffau et al. 2005; Berger et al. 2010; Spena et al. 2010).

The concept of the eloquent area is not limited to cortical functional maps. It is also applied to the bundles of axons connecting a cortical area to secondary neurons and to other areas of a specific cortical network. Hence, the most thorough examination of a tumor requires a careful consideration of its relationship with subcortical white matter. In particular, gliomas are well known to invade white matter tracts through which they can reach the contralateral hemisphere. Accumulating evidence has demonstrated that postsurgical or post-stroke damage to subcortical critical pathways can result in irreversible deficits. There is no documented plasticity in the white matter, and recovery after interruption of a subcortical functional bundle is difficult. Hence, presurgical planning should determine whether tumor invades or simply displaces subcortical pathways. In the very recent years a new application of MR diffusion sequences imaging called Diffusion Tensor Imaging (DTI) has created the opportunity to reconstruct the anatomy of the main white matter tracts. A virtual in vivo dissection of white matter, very similar to those coming from cadaver studies, has been produced, adding new insights into the relationship between tumors and white matter bundles (Catani 2002, Ozawa 2009, Nimsky 2007). The availability of this new tool marks a period in which neuroscientists have given great resonance to connectionism to explain brain functions and neurosurgeons have focused their efforts on gaining preoperative information about subcortical pathways.

This brief overview of advances in understanding of the brain function has given us the opportunity to point out that the modern-era neurosurgeon should be able to preoperatively collect a large amount of information on the distinctive functional and anatomical organization of each patient's brain in order to individualize surgical strategy.

3. Preoperative brain mapping

3.1 Functional MR

Functional MRI is a non-invasive technique that visualizes brain activity indirectly by detection of local hemodynamic changes in cortical capillaries and draining veins (Frahm et al. 1994; Menon et al. 1995). This blood-oxygen level-dependent (BOLD) technique makes use of blood as an intrinsic contrast agent (Ogawa et al. 1993). A BOLD signal is based upon the increase of oxygen consumption by neuronal cells inducing a relative increase in the local perfusion (Heeger 2002; Toronov 2003). The activation spots have been shown to reflect actual neuronal activity with high spatial accuracy (typically between 1 and 5 mm) (Logothetis 2003; Logothetis & Pfeuffer 2004; Logothetis & Wandell 2004). Functional MR imaging maps reflect task-related local changes in the vascular response of brain tissue, and they are therefore an indirect measure of neural activity. Temporal resolution is generally lower than EEG (Gevins, Leong et al. 1995) or MEG (Hämäläinen M 1993) because the hemodynamic BOLD response lags behind the neural response by several seconds. There are other imaging tools that indirectly detect brain activity, such as positron emission tomography (PET) (Fox et al. 1986) (Mazziotta et al. 1982; Raichle 1983) and single-photon emission computer tomography (SPECT) (Holman and Devous 1992), but their description is beyond the scope of this chapter, except to note that they have lower spatial/temporal resolution and are less available for use in clinical scanning. At present, functional magnetic resonance imaging (fMRI) is the most widely used method of functional neuroimaging in both the clinical and research environments. For the latter purpose, and unlike more invasive mapping methods, fMR allows for the study of subjects who are free from neurological illness and enables the modeling of brain processes and of individual differences in brain organization. These are the principal factors that account for the enormous advancements brought by fMR to the understanding brain functional organization.

The two predominant diagnostic aims of presurgical fMR are the localization of eloquent brain areas and their relationships with the tumor, and the determination of the dominant hemisphere for language. As a clinical research tool, fMR can be performed longitudinally pre- and postoperatively to identify neuroplastic changes in brain activity.

Any clinical application of fMRI involves a "paradigm," a defined functional measurement including stimulation, and a task that is presumed to activate the cortical area to be studied. For motor function, the patient is scanned while performing an active blocked motor task. The task consists of 12 seconds of foot plantarflexion/dorsiflexion, hand opening/closing, or tongue movement, with a frequency of 0.5 Hz, followed by 12 seconds of rest for a total acquisition time of 5 minutes. The sensory cortex test is similar, with an active condition of 0.5-Hz brushing of the foot or hand. Language is investigated as follows: in the active condition, the patient listens to a list of nouns and generates associated verbs for 21 seconds; in the rest condition, the patient counts from 1 to 10 for 15 seconds. These paradigms are those usually performed in our routine. For further technical details refer to the bibliography (Moritz & Haughton 2003; Gaillard 2004).

Due to its good spatial resolution and direct correlation to surface anatomy BOLD-fMRI has been used since shortly after its first description (Bandettini et al. 1992) (Kwong et al. 1992; Ogawa et al. 1992) for presurgical localization of the primary sensorimotor cortex in patients with rolandic brain tumors (Jack et al. 1994), for determination of the language dominant hemisphere in patients with left frontal or temporo-parietal tumors (Desmond 1995), and for the localization of Broca and Wernicke language areas (FitzGerald et al. 1997; Stippich et al. 2003; Stippich et al. 2007).

The most relevant concern in presurgical visualization of eloquent areas is the reliability of the spatial position and the extent of the spot of activation as depicted on the fMR. It is important to clarify that the spots of activation are strictly related to the statistical threshold chosen for data evaluation. Even with the use of one or more fixed statistical thresholds, BOLD signal intensities and cluster sizes differ significantly from one patient to another and between different paradigms (e.g. foot movement, hand movement), even when examinations are carried out in a standardized way. This has a direct impact on the planning of the neurosurgeons, who may, based on an fMR map, consider a determined eloquent area to be wider or narrower than it actually is. To address this matter, comparisons of presurgical fMRI data with a reference procedure such as CSES have been performed. In patients with lesions around the central sulcus (Dymarkowski et al. 1998; Achten et al. 1999; Roux et al. 1999), many studies have reported highly concordant data of presurgical fMRI and CSES, with correlation ranging from 83% to 92% (Majos et al. 2005; Lehericy et al. 2000; Spena et al. 2010). However, for language areas, the utility of fMRI to predict the presence of language epicenters in or around the tumor surface is diminished. This is seen in our results (42.8%) as well as in previous works that have indicated variable sensitivities and specificities ranging from 59% to 100% and from 0% to 97%, respectively

(Petrovich et al. 2005, Rutten et al. 2002). Aside from methodological issues, language areas are organized in a large-scale network that is widely variable. Functional MRI maps the entire cortical network involved in a specific task, and it is normally not able to differentiate between essential and substitutable epicenters. These studies mainly addressed the reliability of the position of the focus of an activation spot but no data were produced regarding the extent of those spots (Fig. 1). Furthermore, since a BOLD signal is generated by an increase in blood flow, the presence of infiltration by vascularized tumor can completely alter the local microvascular organization and potentially hamper the reliability of the BOLD signal (Holodny et al. 1999; Ulmer et al. 2004). Therefore, the use of presurgical BOLD activations on fMR to predict resection margins and surgical risks of neurological damage is not routinely indicated. The data available to quantify a safe distance between functional activation and resection borders (Hall et al. 2005; Krishnan et al. 2004) with respect to surgically induced neurological deficits are still very limited and do not justify any general conclusion or recommendation. Moreover, since fMR imaging is only intended to visualize cortical activity, no information is gained about subcortical white matter bundles and connections.

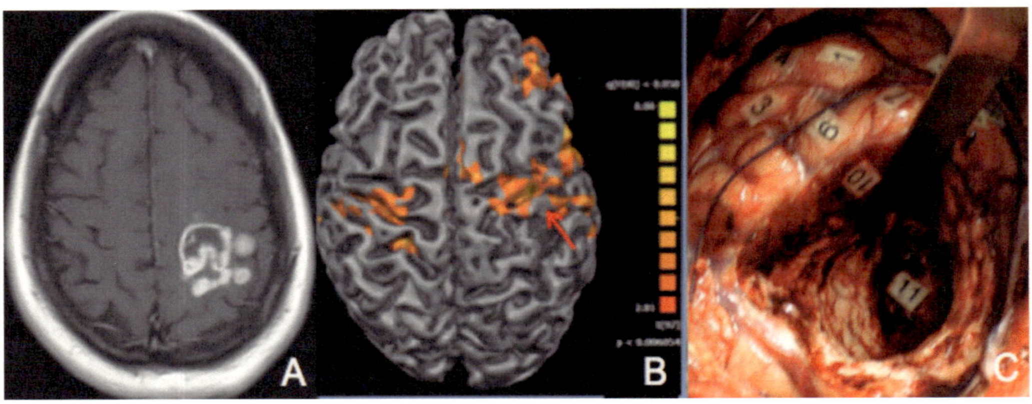

Fig. 1. (A) Preoperative MR showing a retrocentral glioblastoma invading the central gyri. (B). Preoperative fMR showing that the area of the hand seems to be infiltrated by the tumor, and the activation spot seems to be interrupted (red arrow; q< 0.05 FDR corrected, minimum cluster size K>5 voxels in the native resolution). (C) Intraoperative stimulation demonstrated that the infiltrated postcentral gyrus was still functional (hand sensibility: 6, 7, 10) and so was not removed.

Nonetheless, functional MRI is still an important source of non-invasive diagnostic information that can reduce the number of invasive diagnostic procedures, such as the Wada test. We use fMRI in preoperative planning mainly to understand the activation pattern, the location of the pre- or postcentral gyrus, and the approximate distance to the tumor. If the distance from the activation spot is greater than one gyrus or the subcortical infiltration is minimal, we may even choose not to perform an awake surgery with CSES. For tumors in language areas, we calculate the lateralization index that, together with neuropsychological testing, gives an indication about the dominant hemisphere. We strongly recommend precise intraoperative control of functional structures in every situation where there is suspected tumor invasion of an eloquent area.

3.2 Diffusion tensor imaging and fiber tracking

The "eloquence" of a brain region is not only determined by importance of neuron functions. In order to maintain correct functioning of a neural network it is crucial that all the groups of neurons are connected. Consequently, neurosurgeons must try to spare subcortical functional bundles (at least the largest and more essential), otherwise connections between cortical epicenters will be damaged. The seminal works by Kringler, through post-mortem dissections (Agrawal et al. 2011), demonstrated the complex organization of the white matter into bundles of different length and thickness that connect either one gyrus to another or to very distant parts of the brain. Unfortunately these observations are hardly applicable during surgery, when white matter appears as a uniform tissue that can be infiltrated by the tumor. In recent years a new, non-invasive pre-operative technique of white matter signal analysis has been introduced: diffusion tensor imaging (DTI). This is a modification of diffusion weighted imaging (DWI) that is sensitive to the preferential diffusion of brain water along white matter fibers and can detect subtle changes in white matter tracts in disease (Nucifora et al. 2007). The random, diffusion-driven displacements in diffusion magnetic resonance imaging allow microscopic-scale resolution of tissue structure. As diffusion is a three-dimensional process, molecular mobility in tissues can be anisotropic, as in brain white matter. With DTI, diffusion anisotropy effects can be fully extracted, characterized, and exploited, providing even more exquisite detail of tissue microstructure.

DTI has been applied to patients with brain tumors for different purposes. First, measures of mean diffusivity and fractional anisotropy have been used to differentiate normal white matter, edematous brain, and enhancing tumor margins (Sinha 2002, Lu 2003). Anisotropy is reduced in cerebral lesions due to the loss of structural organization (Wieshmann et al. 1999; Mascalchi et al. 2005). It seems that the abnormalities on DTI are more significant than those seen on T2-weighted images in high grade gliomas, but not in metastatic tumors (Beppu et al. 2003; Price et al. 2003). Second, DTI may distinguish if the white matter fibers are displaced (Wieshmann et al. 2000; Gossl et al. 2002), infiltrated, or disrupted by the tumor (Wittwer et al. 2002). Finally, the most fascinating application of DTI is the fiber-tracking technique (DTI-FT) that is able to identify and reconstruct the main white matter connections. This information is very useful for presurgical planning, delineating the spatial relationships of eloquent structures and tumors in order to preserve the functional pathways intraoperatively (Holodny et al. 2002; Tummala et al. 2003; Henry et al. 2004). Since the images generated by DTI-fiber tracking are the result of complex mathematical modeling aimed at resolving the hypercomplex structure of white matter, several authors have worked to answer some practical problems. For instance, what degree of correspondence do the images have to the actual anatomy of the bundles? What is the relationship of the bundle(s) to the tumor (displaced, infiltrated, interrupted)? And, most importantly, what is the function of the bundle(s)? Must it be spared or can it be sacrificed? DTI-FT is currently intended to virtually reconstruct white matter tracts, but it is not able to investigate the function related to a tract. CSES is the gold standard to map subcortical pathways, and DTI-FT findings can be integrated with intraoperative CSES with or without the implementation of intraoperative navigation devices (Henry et al. 2004; Kinoshita et al. 2005; Bello et al. 2008; Ozawa et al. 2009, Leclercq et al. 2010; Spena et al. 2010). The fundamental observation that preoperative DTI-FT cannot itself account for the determination of the presence or absence of functional subcortical tracts in or in the vicinity of the tumor is clearly demonstrated by cases of cystic tumors in which, because of the absence of infiltration and edema, the white matter tract reconstructions are very reliable (fig. 2). DTI-FT underestimates the presence of functional tracts in the context of the tumor, as demonstrated by our finding of 60.4% of infiltrated functional white matter predicted by

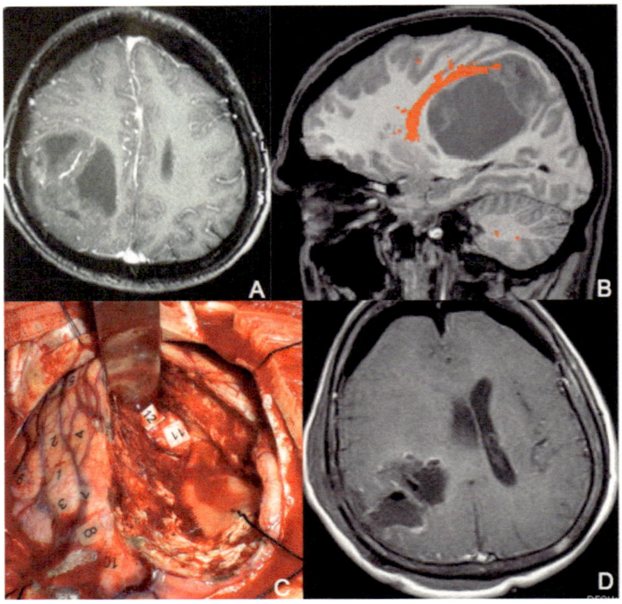

Fig. 2. (A) Male, 43 years old. Preoperative MR showing a large and partly cystic oligodendroglioma (WHO III) in the central area. (B) DTI-FT demonstrates the displacement of the pyramidal tract anteriorly and the close contact to the cystic portion of the tumor. (C) Intraoperative image demonstrating the presence of talamo-cortical fibers at the subcortical level in the anterior aspect of the surgical cavity (11, 12 paraesthesia of the shoulder and neck). (D) On immediate postoperative MRI there was no residual tumor and the patient had no postoperative deficit confirming the DTI-ft hypothesis that the tract was neither damaged nor infiltrated.

DTI compared to the postoperative MRI and intraoperative stimulation results (fig. 3). A typical image featured a white matter bundle in close vicinity to the tumor without any information on how much of the pathway or pathway function was invaded. The tracking of fibers in the vicinity of or within lesions is complicated due to changes in diseased tissue, such as elevated water content (edema), tissue compression, and degeneration. These changes deform the architecture of the white matter, and, in some cases, prevent selection of the seed region of interest (ROI) from which to begin fiber tracking. To overcome this problem, some investigators have suggested posing a seed ROI in the white matter area subjacent to the maximal fMRI activity (i.e., for the pyramidal tract, in the precentral cortex) with the target ROI in the cerebral peduncle (Schomberg et al. 2006; Smits et al. 2007; Staempfli et al. 2007). Also notable is that in language areas, DTI might emphasize the presence of white matter tracts when subcortical stimulation did not show a zone of positive response, favoring an unnecessarily conservative surgery, whereas direct stimulation would have indicated removal of the entire portion of non-eloquent tissue. More recent advances in calculation and characterization of fractional anisotropy have allowed for a more precise reconstruction of the white matter bundles by depicting complex distributions of intravoxel fiber orientation. This new algorithm, called diffusion spectrum imaging (DSI), is a very promising technological advancement (Kuo et al. 2008; Wedeen et al. 2008, Canales-Rodríguez et al. 2010), but unfortunately these methods require very long sessions (up to 60 minutes) of MR scanning that are sometimes unsuitable for patients.

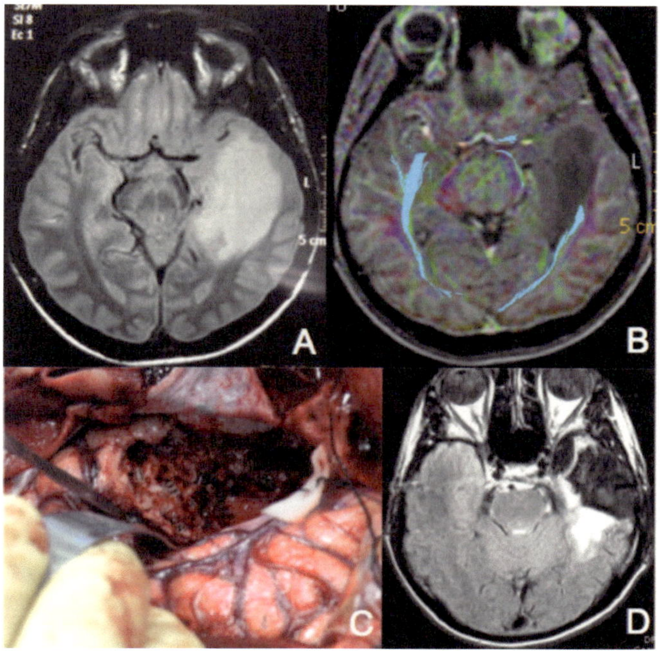

Fig. 3. Man, 42 years old. Three episodes of absence. A) On preoperative MR a temporal mass is demonstrated. B) DTI showed a fascicle just beside the mass that seemed interrupted. No other tract was visualized inside the tumor. By looking at the position and direction, this bundle was referred to the inferior longitudinal fasciculus (ILF). C) CSES confirmed at the subcortical level of naming disturbances (8, 9, 10, 11); consequently resection was arrested, and no language deficit was diagnosed at follow-up. (D) Postoperative MRI confirmed the subtotal resection as well as the functionality of the infiltrated white matter although DTI-FT showed absence of fibers.

4. Intraoperative brain mapping: Awake surgery and cortical and subcortical electrical stimulation (CSES)

4.1 Introduction and indications

Direct electrical stimulation of the brain surface is a technique that has regained greater interest worldwide in the past decade than it has had since its introduction by Foerster, Penfield and Rasmussen in 1930 (Foerster 1931, Penfield & Boldrey 1937, Penfield & Erickson 1941, Penfield & Rasmussen 1950). More recently Berger introduced the technique of subcortical stimulation to spare functional white matter bundles that are very often infiltrated by gliomas (Berger 1994). Indeed, refinement of technical equipment and, mostly, the availability of ultra-short acting anesthetics and new analgesics, have given a strong impetus to the revival of awake surgery and CSES. The goal of CSES is to detect the areas of the brain that are necessary to a given function. The stimulation of neurons provokes either a positive effect (i.e. movement on contralateral muscles or dysaesthesias) or a suppressive effect (speech arrest, anomia, anarthria). In both cases the aim is to define the effect of the resection of that part of brain in order to avoid deficits. The main use of CSES is for intrinsic brain tumors because cortical and mostly subcortical boundaries are very often impossible to define. Moreover, it has been demonstrated that gliomas are frequently located in eloquent areas, thus they are sometimes treated with only a biopsy or a very limited resection. The availability of the direct control of functional topography during surgical tumor resection not only gives the opportunity to avoid permanent neurological impairment, it can also facilitate a larger extirpation. During resection of a tumor, the surgeon does not have to follow anatomical limits, but will follow functional boundaries (Fig. 4). CSES makes it possible to continuously check the integrity of a circuitry at both the cortical and the subcortical level. The ability to maximize resection while preserving a satisfying functional outcome is of particular interest in brain gliomas for two reasons: first, gliomas mostly affect young adults in full social and working activity, so functional outcome is of the utmost relevance. Second, many different studies (Berger 1994; Keles et al. 2001; Sanai & Berger 2009; Stendel 2009) have by now demonstrated that total or subtotal resection has a clear impact on survival and, for LGG (low grade glioma), on malignant transformation, and that the extent of resection is strongly affected by eloquence of the tumor location (Chang et al. 2008).

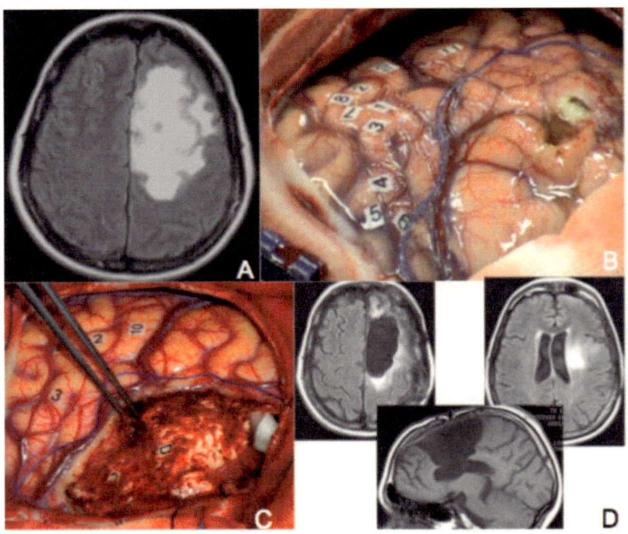

Fig. 4. Female, 38 years old suffering from seizures. (A) Preoperative FLAIR MR showing a left large premotor low grade glioma invading also the supplementary motor area. B) Intraoperative picture: the blue line surrounds the tumor cortical margins. 1, 2, 3, 7, 8: motor area of the face; 10: anartria with face contraction; 4, 5, 6: motor area of the hand. 11: speech arrest). No functional site (neither motor nor language) was detected on the surface of the tumor. C) At subcortical level, resection was stopped when descending motor pathway were stimulated (D and C). D) Postoperative MR showing a residue of tumor on the posterior part of the cavity infiltrating descending motor pathways.

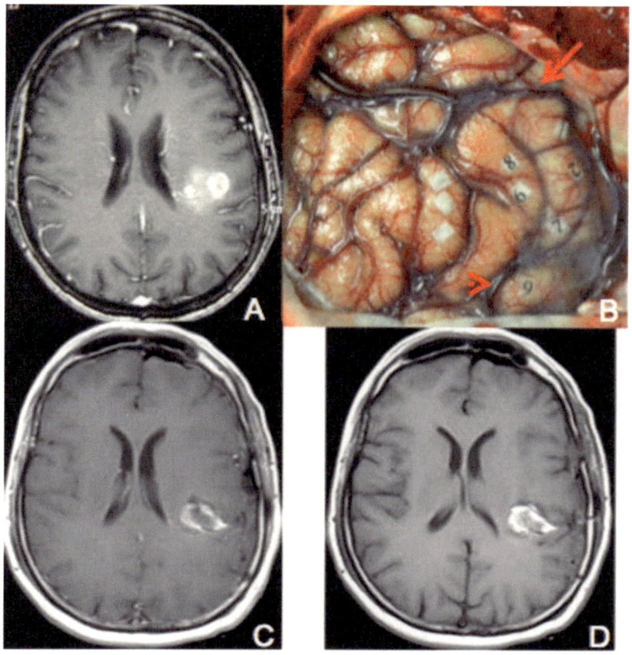

Fig. 5. 63 y.o. woman, transient speech disturbance. A) Preoperative contrast enhanced MR showing an inhomogeneous mass in the white matter of the left fronto-parietal passage. B) Intraoperative picture after cortical mapping (1, 2 speech arrest; 7 anartria; 6 motor area of the mouth; 8, 9 anartria). *Red arrow*: sylvian fissure; *red arrow-head*: central sulcus. The white tags show an area of negative mapping that was chosen to reach the subcortical tumor. Postoperative MR (C with gadolinium and D without) showing complete removal of the tumor. The patient did not present speech disturbance.

In some cases, CSES can also guide in the detection of the safest route for removing purely subcortical tumors. In these circumstances, the surgeon will choose a non-responsive cortical area to perform cortectomy and then will follow a subcortical corridor by alternating stimulation and dissection until the tumor is exposed. Then resection continues, together with the stimulation and monitoring of neurological function of the patient even during stages of non-stimulation (see fig. 5).

From a practical point of view, indication for an awake surgery and CSES is primarily based on the localization of the tumor on an anatomical MR followed by confirmation of the activation pattern on fMR. Typical regions that should be considered for intraoperative mapping are the central regions (sensory-motor areas) on both the dominant and non-dominant hemispheres. Preoperative neurological evaluation is fundamental to detect any sensory, coordination or muscles strength disturbance. For non-dominant hemisphere tumors in the occipito-temporo-parietal junction we also perform a global neuropsychological evaluation of the visuo-spatial abilities (Rey's tangled figures test, copying, spontaneous drawing, clock drawing test, apraxia tasks, line cancellation test, line bisection test, Diller's letter cancellation test, line completion test). It has been established that awake surgery is mandatory since the patient will experience subjective dysaesthesias and will interact with the surgeon, for motor areas there is still debate. In many centers worldwide, neurosurgeons prefer not to operate on awake patients for tumors in motor areas. They argue that the motor responses such as the contraction of muscles do not require a conscious patient. For motor stimulation in an anesthetized patient either the motor evoked potentials (MEPs) method (Kombos et al. 2001; Fujiki et al. 2006; Yoshikawa et al. 2006) or CSES can be chosen. For the former it must be noted that only the action potentials of selected muscles can be controlled, which may hamper both the detection and the avoidance of motor deficits in non-monitored muscles. Furthermore, no information is obtained on the function of cortex adjacent to the central region, and intraoperative evoked potentials presently cannot be used to perform mapping of language or other higher functions. Concerning CSES and the sleeping patient, higher currents are normally required for stimulation, leading to a higher number of intraoperative seizures that can reduce the reliability of mapping. In our experience (Spena et al. 2010) mapping of the motor cortex in an awake patient guarantees more precise cortical and subcortical mapping with a very low risk of intraoperative seizures.

When the tumor is located in the so-called "language areas" (dominant perisylvian, posterior part of F1 and F2, premotor cortex, inferior parietal, posterior temporal, and insular lobes) the first step is to document the hemispheric dominance. A neuropsychological assessment (handedness tests by Edinburgh inventory) and the fMR are sufficient to establish dominance (Stippich et al. 2007). In addition, a detailed and extensive language assessment (Aachen Aphasia Test; WAISS) is necessary to highlight possible subclinical language deficit and to prepare the patients for the intraoperative tests (reading, pictures naming, famous faces naming, counting). At our institution patients with severe motor deficit or language impairments that do not improve after one week of steroid therapy are not considered for awake surgery. This is particularly true for high grade gliomas (HGG) in eloquent areas that more often present with some kind of clinical symptom. These cases merit special consideration because of their natural history and very low survival. In these patients we prefer not to attempt extirpation in cases of low performance status (<70 KPS or >3 Rankin score) unresponsive to steroid drugs; however, we may decide to perform a biopsy. Operating on delicate brain regions often produces a transient deterioration in postoperative status related mostly to manipulation and inflammation, and the presence of rapidly evolving tumors can further impede recovery. Therefore, we can anticipate that a more careful selection of patients with high-grade gliomas located in very delicate regions is the best way to prevent unsatisfying results.

Neurological and neuropsychological tests have a prominent role when treating eloquent area tumor because of different reasons. In general, accumulating information about preoperative neurological and neuropsychological status of the patient gives a great opportunity not only to better document the clinical course and improvements, but also to study the biological behavior of the tumor. In fact, the relapse of a tumor or the passage to a higher grade of malignancies is sometimes predicted by even subtle changes in neuropsychological performance. Moreover, it's fundamental to correlate intraoperative findings with postoperative tests in order to create robust outcome measurements and to document that the resection of a "negative" site has no actual negative effect. That's why tests must be repeated in the early postoperative period (7-10 days) and at least after 3 and 6 months.

Once the surgeon has established the indication for awake surgery, it is very important to consider the patient's general status as well as the psychological profile. In Table 1, some general and anaesthesiological factors that can contraindicate awake surgery are summarized. The idea of undergoing an awake surgery is a source of anxiety for psychologically intact patients. It is essential that a thorough and clear relationship between medical staff and the patient is established and that the patient is correctly informed about every event that he or she is going to experience. Different authors have demonstrated that good preoperative communication is even more effective in alleviating anxiety than preoperative sedative drugs (Egbert 1963; Aglio 2001).

Severe cardio-pulmonary dysfunction (>ASA 3)
Factors predicting difficult intubation
Prior difficult intubation
Claustrophobia
Generalized anxiety disease
Severe obesity
Sleep apnea

Table 1. General and anesthesiology factors contraindicating awake surgery.

4.2 Anesthesia and surgical techniques

The goal of anesthesia is to obtain an easily reversible sedation while maintaining spontaneous respiration. We do not use tracheal masks or other intubation devices. Two large bore venous accesses are sufficient and intra-arterial pressure monitoring is required. Positioning on the operating table is very important and the patient must feel comfortable in order to avoid pain or the need to continuously move. We usually prefer lateral decubitus with the contralateral arm and leg free from drapes so that reaction during stimulation can be easily detected. In men, a urethral catheter is avoided and a condom-like urine reservoir ("Texas catheter") is applied instead. Scalp anesthesia is achieved through nerve block by infiltration of levobupivacaine (0.75%) and mepivacaine (1%). During craniotomy, we sedate spontaneously breathing patients with intravenous remifentanil (0.01 to 0.08 mg/Kg/min) and propofol (0.3 to 1 mg/Kg/h), continuously throughout the procedure. Lidocaine filled cotton paddies are used to locally anesthetize the dura. Before opening the dura, drugs are arrested and the patient is completely awakened. At this time a rapid check of responsiveness and collaboration as well as control of comfort and pain is very important. In case of pain and depending on the site of pain, local anesthetics or intravenous low dose remifentanil is administered.

The craniotomy is targeted to expose the area of the tumor and the motor and/or sensory strips upon which current intensity will be determined by establishing the minimum current required to generate a movement or a dysaesthesia. If the tumor is not visible at the cortical surface, it is important to delineate the superficial projection of its boundaries by using a neuronavigation system or an ultrasound. A bipolar fork, measuring 6 mm in distance between the electrodes (Nimbus, Newmedic, Labege, France), is used to deliver a non-deleterious, biphasic square-wave current in 4-second trains at 60 Hz. We start stimulation at 1 mA and increase by increments of 0.30 mA until the initiation of contralateral face or upper limb movements and paresthesias. Normally no more than 4 mA are necessary to have a positive response. In our experience, factors necessitating higher current intensity are large or deep-seated tumors and the presence of edema. Every positive site is restimulated

to confirm reproducibility of the response. Once the proper current intensity is set, the entire surface of the tumor is thoroughly examined in order to exclude the presence of functional sites. When tumors are located in language areas, a neuropsychologist administers tests on a laptop screen (a series of slides with black and white pictures preceded by the words "this is a....") and describes the type of language disturbance observed (speech arrest, anarthria, anomia, or reading errors). These same tests are administered the day before surgery in order to detect baseline errors or hesitations that could be misinterpreted during intraoperative stimulation. Intraoperatively, the patient is unaware of the timing of stimulation, and the current is delivered just before presentation of the slide. After disruption of a language area, the patient rests for a while, then spontaneous speech and slide reading are tested, and stimulation starts again. Every time a positive response is encountered, a numbered tag is left in place and the function associated to the stimulation of that point is recorded. If the tumor is separated from a functional gyrus by a sulcus, maximal attention is paid in order to respect the arachnoid plane and the vasculature of the sulcus. If the tumor invades functional gyri or subcortical functional tracts, the resection must to be very careful since no anatomical limit is present between the infiltrated parenchyma and the normal functioning cortex. In these situations as well as for subcortical tumors, we test language or motor function throughout the resection even when no stimulation is applied, stopping whenever anomalies appear. Many authors have for a long time postulated a need to maintain a safe distance of at least 1 cm from a functional site (Haglund et al. 1994; Carrabba et al. 2007; Sanai & Berger 2008). More recently, this concept has been evolving because accumulated experiences have clearly demonstrated that continuous cortical and subcortical stimulations can enable the surgeon to identify and preserve eloquent cortex and the white matter bundles. Abandoning the idea of leaving a "safe margin" in favor of reaching functional boundaries yields an increase of the extent of resection, and thus, it is believed, has an increased impact on the natural history of the tumor. This more aggressive strategy is related to a higher percentage of transient postoperative neurological deficits, but it has also led to very satisfying long-term neurological outcomes (Gil-Robles & Duffau 2010).
In order to collect the largest amount of information about the unique functional organization of each individual patient, it is very important to record all the possible data from pre-, intra- and postoperative observations, including intraoperative photographs or films and, in cases of language area tumors, recordings of patients' voices. It also is important to register parameters such as current intensity, reproducibility of stimuli, and seizure occurrence, as well as the degree of pain control (at minimum a visual analog scale should be checked) and other anesthesiology concerns, such as nausea, vomiting, and need for respiratory support or for switching to general anesthesia.

5. Brain mapping in neurosurgery: Criticisms and future perspectives

Ideally, neurosurgeons could detect and locate the exact position of brain functions before performing tumor resection, allowing them to recommend surgery only in those patients with the prospect of radical or grossly subtotal resection. Moreover, technological support would serve as a guide during surgery in order to spare critical areas. Such complete and reliable technology is not yet available, but major advances have been made since the days when neurosurgeons performed brain surgery only via anatomical references.

Undoubtedly, CSES has gained a prominent role in neurosurgery above all because a large number of studies worldwide have shown a clear advantage in terms of usefulness, safety, and neurological and oncological outcomes (Berger 1994; Duffau et al. 2005; Duffau 2006; Kim et al. 2009; Sanai & Berger 2009; De Benedictis et al. 2010; Spena et al. 2010). The spatial accuracy and the ability to perform functional resection (that is, a resection in which limits are represented by spared functions) have met the approval of many neurosurgeons, who now use CSES routinely. However, there are some technical and methodological drawbacks of CSES that have yet to be addressed. First, the application of an electric current on the brain can have effects that are more complex than anticipated. For example, the excitation of the stimulated cortex can diffuse to near or far cortex by short or long-range white matter tracts. Consequently, the observed effect of the stimulation may not be related (or not only) to that portion of a gyrus. In this case the tumor resection might be prematurely arrested. At the same time, at which point is the surgeon sure that a functional area is essential and cannot be substituted by other epicenters? The concept of plasticity can explain recovery after various brain injuries, but the stimulation of a functional site intraoperatively cannot give information about the brain's potential to substitute that site. Another highly debated issue in CSES is the technique of negative stimulation, which means pursuing resection where no positive site is detected. Although results of such strategy have been encouraging (Sanai & Berger 2008; Kim et al. 2009), the question arises concerning the possibility of missing a positive site because of a false negative result during the intraoperative tests. This is especially true for cognitive functions, given that an awake patient has a limited time span for testing before fatigue arrives (normally no more than 90 minutes in our experience). Further, intraoperative cognitive tests (language, calculation, writing, visuo-spatial abilities) are limited to very simple tasks that cannot account for more complex functions. From this point of view, fMR allows a more comprehensive analysis of brain function because all the epicenters involved during a specific task are visualized and a real-time mapping is generated. If this represents a limitation of the spatial accuracy of fMR for surgical planning, at the same time it offers a means to non-invasively study a patient pre- and postoperatively, which is undoubtedly a unique opportunity to gain precious insights into functional organization and post-lesional adaptation at the individual level.

Direct mapping methods such as CSES are, at the moment, the safest procedures to achieve the most extensive resections with controllable risks. Preoperative brain mapping is useful when planning awake surgery to estimate the relationship between the tumor and functional brain regions. However, these techniques cannot directly lead the surgeon during resection. Intraoperative brain mapping is necessary to safely guide maximal resection and to guarantee a satisfying neurological outcome. It is unlikely that the study of functional connectivity and the longitudinal modification of brain maps will leave behind the integration of repeated fMR. This multimodal approach is more aggressive, leads to better outcomes, and should be used routinely for resection of lesions in eloquent brain regions.

It is probably no longer necessary to compare different methods of brain mapping because of their intrinsically different functioning; rather, we propose that now it would be most desirable to share preoperative (fMR, DTI, and neuropsychology) and postoperative protocols in order to accumulate a major cohort of patients in multicenter studies. At the same time, results of intraoperative stimulations should be well documented and standardized to create a common comprehensive database of intraoperative brain mapping results.

6. References

Achten E., Jackson, G.D., Cameron, J.A., Abbott, D.F., Stella, D.L. & Fabinyi, G.C. (1999). Presurgical evaluation of the motor hand area with functional MR imaging in patients with tumors and dysplastic lesions. *Radiology* Vol. 210(No.2):529–538.

Aglio, L.S. & Gugino, L.D. (2001). Conscious sedation for Intraoperative Neurosurgical Procedures Techniques in Neurosurgery, Vol. 7, No. 1, March.

Agrawal, A., Kapfhammer, J.P., Kress, A., Wichers, H., Deep, A., Feindel, W., Sonntag, V.K., Spetzler, R.F., & Preul, M.C. (2011). Josef Klingler's Models of White Matter Tracts: Influences on Neuroanatomy, Neurosurgery, and Neuroimaging. *Neurosurgery* Vol. 26 Epub ahead of print.

Annett, M. (1992). Parallels between asymmetries of planum temporale and of hand skill. *Neuropsychologia* Vol. 30:951–962.

Baciu, M., Le Bas, J.F., Segebarth C. & Benabid A.L. (2003). Presurgical fMRI evaluation of cerebral reorganization and motor deficit in patients with tumors and vascular malformations. *European Journal of Radiology*. Vol. 46(No. 2):139-46.

Ballmaier, M., Sowell, E.R., Thompson, P.M., Kumar, A., Narr, K.L. & Lavretsky H. (2004). Mapping brain size and cortical gray matter changes in elderly depression. *Biological Psychiatry* Vol. 55:382–389.

Bandettini, P.A., Wong, E.C., Hinks, R.S., Tikofsky, R.S. & Hyde J.S. (1992). Time course EPI of human brain function during task activation. *Magnetic Resonance in Medicine* Vol. 25(No. 2):390–397.

Bello L., Gambini, A., Castellano, A., Carrabba, G., Acerbi, F., Fava, E., Giussani, C., Cadioli, M., Blasi, V., Casarotti, A., Papagno, C., Gupta, A.K., Gaini, S., Scotti, G. & Falini A. (2008). Motor and language DTI Fiber Tracking combined with intraoperative subcortical mapping for surgical removal of gliomas. *Neuroimage* Vol. 39(1):369–382.

Beppu, T., Inoue, T., Shibata, Y., Kurose, A., Arai, H., Ogasawara, K., Ogawa, A., Nakamura, S. & Kabasawa, H. (2003). Measurement of fractional anisotropy using diffusion tensor MRI in supratentorial astrocytic tumors. *Journal of Neurooncology* Vol. 63: 109-16.

Berger, M.S. (1994). Lesions in functional ("eloquent") cortex and subcortical white matter. *Clinical Neurosurgery*. Vol. 41:444-63.

Berger, M.S., Deliganis, A.V., Dobbins, J.D. & Keles, G.E. (1994): The effect of extent of resection on recurrence in patients with low-grade cerebral hemisphere gliomas. *Cancer* Vol. 74: 1784-1791.

Boling, W., Parsons, M., Kraszpulski, M., Cantrell, C. & Puce A. (2008). Whole-hand sensorimotor area: cortical stimulation localization and correlation with functional magnetic resonance imaging. *Journal of Neurosurgery* Vol. 108(No.3):491-500.

Bookheimer, S. (2002). Functional MRI of language: new approaches to understanding the cortical organization of semantic processing. *Annual Review of Neuroscience* Vol. 25:151–188.

Canales-Rodríguez, E.J., Iturria-Medina, Y., Alemán-Gómez, Y. & Melie-García, L. (2010). Deconvolution in diffusion spectrum imaging. *Neuroimage* Vol. 50(No.1):136-49.

Carpentier, A.C., Constable, R.T., Schlosser, M.J., de Lotbinière, A., Piepmeier, J.M., Spencer, D.D. & Awad, I.A. (2001). Patterns of functional magnetic resonance imaging activation in association with structural lesions in the rolandic region: a classification system. *Journal of Neurosurgery* Vol. 94(No. 6):946-54.

Carrabba, G., Fava, E., Giussani, C., Acerbi, F., Portaluri, F., Songa, V., Stocchetti, N., Branca, V., Gaini, S.M. & Bello, L. (2007). Cortical and subcortical motor mapping in rolandic and perirolandic glioma surgery: impact on postoperative morbidity and extent of resection. *Journal of Neurosurgical Science* Vol. 51:45–51.

Catani, M., Howard, R.J., Pajevic, S. & Jones, D.K. (2002). Virtual in vivo interactive dissection of white matter fasciculi in the human brain. *Neuroimage* Vol. 17:77–94.

Chang, E.F., Smith, J.S., Chang, S.M., Lamborn, K.R., Prados, M.D., Butowski, N., Barbaro, N.M., Parsa, A.T., Berger, M.S. & McDermott, M.M. (2008). Preoperative prognostic classification system for hemispheric low-grade gliomas in adults. *Journal of Neurosurgery* Vol. 109:817–824.

D'Aubigné, R.M. (1980). Paul Broca and surgery of the motor system. *Chirurgie* Vol. 106(10):791-3.

De Benedictis, A., Moritz-Gasser, S. & Duffau, H. (2010). Awake mapping optimizes the extent of resection for low-grade gliomas in eloquent areas. *Neurosurgery*. Vol. 66(No.6):1074-84.

Desmond, J.E., Sum, J.M., Wagner, A.D., Demb, J.B., Shear, P.K., Glover, G.H., Gabrieli, J.D. & Morrell, M.J. (1995). Functional MRI measurement of language lateralization in Wada-tested patients. *Brain* Vol. 118 (No. 6):1411–1419.

Duffau, H., Lopes, M., Arthuis, F., Bitar, A., Sichez, J.P., Van Effenterre, R. & Capelle, L. (2005). Contribution of intraoperative electrical stimulations in surgery of low grade gliomas: a comparative study between two series without (1985-96) and with (1996-2003) functional mapping in the same institution. *Journal of Neurology, Neurosurgery and Psychiatry* Vol. 76:845–851.

Duffau, H. (2005). Lessons from brain mapping in surgery for lowgrade glioma: insights into associations between tumour and brain plasticity. *Lancet Neurology* Vol. 4:476–486.

Duffau, H. (2006). New concepts in surgery of WHO grade II gliomas: functional brain mapping, connectionism and plasticity—a review. *Journal of Neurooncology* Vol. 79:77–115.

Dymarkowski, S., Sunaert, S., Van Oostende, S., Van Hecke, P., Wilms, G., Demaerel, P., Nuttin, B., Plets, C.& Marchal, G. (1998). Functional MRI of the brain: localisation of eloquent cortex in focal brain lesion therapy. *European Radiology* Vol. 8(No. 9):1573–1580.

Egbert, L.D., Battit, G., Turndorf, H. & Beecher, H.K. (1963). The value of the preoperative visit by an anesthetist. *Journal of the American Medical Association* Vol.185:553–5.

FitzGerald, D.B., Cosgrove, G.R., Ronner, S., Jiang, H., Buchbinder, B.R., Belliveau, J.W., Rosen, B.R. & Benson, R.R. (1997). Location of language in the cortex: a comparison between functional MR imaging and electrocortical stimulation. *American Journal of Neuroradiology* Vol. 18(No. 8):1529–1539.

Foerster, O. (1931). The cerebral cortex in man. *Lancet* Vol. 2:309–312.

Fox, P.T., Mintun, M.A., Raichle, M.E., Miezin, F.M., Allman, J.M. & Van Essen, D.C. (1986). Mapping human visual cortex with positron emission tomography. *Nature* Vol. 323(No. 6091):806–809.

Frahm, J., Merboldt, K.D., Hänicke, W., Kleinschmidt, A. & Boecker, H. (1994). Brain or vein - oxygenation or flow? On signal physiology in functional MRI of human brain activation. *NMR in Biomedicine* Vol. 7(No.1-2):45–53.

Fujiki, M., Furukawa, Y., Kamida, T., Anan, M., Inoue, R., Abe, T. & Kobayashi, H. (2006). Intraoperative corticomuscular motor evoked potentials for evaluation of motor function: a comparison with corticospinal D and I waves. *Journal of Neurosurgery* Vol. 104(No.1):85–92.

Gabrieli, J.D., Poldrack, R.A. & Desmond, J.E. (1998). The role of left prefrontal cortex in language and memory. *Proceedings of Natural Academic Science* Vol. 95(3):906–913.

Gaillard, W.D. (2004). Functional MR imaging of language, memory, and sensorimotor cortex. *Neuroimaging Clinics of North America* Vol. 14 (No. 3):471-85.

Geschwind, N. (1971). Current concepts: aphasia. *New England Journal of Medicine* Vol. 284(No. 12):654–656.

Gevins, A., Leong, H., Smith, M.E., Le, J. & Du, R. (1995). Mapping cognitive brain function with modern high-resolution electroencephalography. *Trends in Neuroscience* Vol. 18(No. 10):429–436.

Gil-Robles, S. & Duffau, H. (2010). Surgical management of World Health Organization Grade II gliomas in eloquent areas: the necessity of preserving a margin around functional structures. *Neurosurgical Focus* Vol. 28(2):E8

Gossl, C., Fahrmeir, L., Putz, B., Auer, L.M. & Auer, D.P. (2002). Fiber tracking from DTI using linear state space models: detectability of the pyramidal tract. *Neuroimage* Vol. 16: 378-88.

Grabowski, T.J. (2000). Investigating language with functional neuroimaging, *in* MJ Toga AW, *Brain mapping: the systems*, Academic Press, San Diego, San Francisco, New York, Boston, London, Sydney, Tokio, 425–461.

Haglund, M., Berger, M., Shamseldin, M., Lettich, E. & Ojemann, G. (1994). Cortical localization of temporal lobe language sites in patients with gliomas. *Neurosurgery* Vol. 34: 567–576

Hämäläinen, M., Ilmoniemi, R.J., Knuutila, J. & Lounasmaa, O.V. (1993). Magnetoencephalography -theory, instrumentatation and applications to noninvasive studies of the working human brain. *Review of modern physics* Vol. 65:413–487.

Hall, W.A., Liu, H. & Truwit, C.L. (2005). Functional magnetic resonance imaging-guided resection of low-grade gliomas. *Surgical Neurology* Vol. 64(No.1):20–27.

Heeger, D.J. & Ress, D. (2002). What does fMRI tell us about neuronal activity? *Nature Reviews Neuroscience* Vol. 3: 142-51.

Hendler, T., Pianka, P., Sigal, M., Kafri, M., Ben-Bashat, D., Constantini, S., Graif, M., Fried, I. & Assaf, Y. (2003). Delineating gray and white matter involvement in brain lesions: three-dimensional alignment of functional magnetic resonance and diffusion-tensor imaging. *Journal of Neurosurgery* Vol. 99: 1018-27.

Henry, R.G., Berman, J.I., Nagarajan, S., Mukherjee, P. & Berger, M.S. (2004). Subcortical pathways serving cortical language sites: initial experience with diffusion tensor imaging fiber tracking combined with intraoperative language mapping. *Neuroimage* Vol. 21:616–622.

Herholz, K., Thiel, A., Wienhard, K., Pietrzyk, U., von Stockhausen, H.M., Karbe, H., Kessler, J., Bruckbauer, T., Halber, M. & Heiss, W.D. (1996). Individual functional anatomy of verb generation. *Neuroimage* Vol. 3:185–194.

Holman, B.L. & Devous, M.D. (1992). Functional brain SPECT: the emergence of a powerful clinical method. *Journal of Nuclear Medicine* Vol. 33(No. 10):1888–1904.

Holodny, A.I. & Ollenschleger, M. (2002). Diffusion imaging in brain tumors. *Neuroimaging Clinic of North America* Vol. 12: 107-24.

Holodny, A.I., Schulder, W.C., Liu, J.A., Maldjian, J.A. & Kalnin, A.J. (1999). Decreased BOLD functional MR activation of the motor and sensory cortices adjacent to a glioblastoma multiforme: implications for image-guided neurosurgery. *American Journal of Neuroradiology* Vol. 20:609–612.

Jack, C.R., Thompson, P.M., Butts, R.K., Sharbrough, F.W., Kelly, P.J., Hanson, D.P., Riederer, S.J., Ehman, R.L., Hangiandreou, N.J. & Cascino, G.D. (1994). Sensory motor cortex: correlation of presurgical mapping with functional MR imaging and invasive cortical mapping. *Radiology* Vol. 190(No.1): 85–92.

Josse, G., Mazoyer, B., Crivello, F. & Tzourio-Mazoyer, N. (2003). Left planum temporale: an anatomical marker of left hemispheric specialization for language comprehension. *Cognitive Brain Research* Vol. 18:1–14.

Keles, G.E., Lamborn, K.R. & Berger, M.S. (2001). Low-grade hemispheric gliomas in adults: a critical review of extent of resection as a factor influencing outcome. *Journal of Neurosurgery* Vol. 95: 735-745.

Kim, S.S., McCutcheon, I.E., Suki, D., Weinberg, J.S., Sawaya, R., Lang, F.F., Ferson, D., Heimberger, A.B., DeMonte, F. & Prabhu. S.S. (2009). Awake craniotomy for brain tumors near eloquent cortex: correlation of intraoperative cortical mapping with neurological outcomes in 309 consecutive patients. *Neurosurgery* Vol. 64(No.5):836–845.

Kinoshita, M., Yamada, K., Hashimoto, N., Kato, A., Izumoto, S. & Baba T. (2005). Fiber-tracking does not accurately estimate size of fiber bundle in pathological condition: initial neurosurgical experience using neuronavigation and subcortical white matter stimulation. *Neuroimage* Vol. 25:424–429.

Kombos, T., Suess, O., Ciklatekerlio, O. & Brock, M. (2001). Monitoring of intraoperative motor evoked potentials to increase the safety of surgery in and around the motor cortex. *Journal of Neurosurgery* Vol. 95(No.4):608- 614

Krings ,T., Reinges, M.H., Thiex, R., Gilsbach, J.M. & Thron, A. (2001). Functional and diffusion-weighted magnetic resonance images of space-occupying lesions affecting the motor system: imaging the motor cortex and pyramidal tracts. *Journal of Neurosurgery* Vol. 95: 816-24.

Krishnan, R., Raabe, A., Hattingen, E., Szelényi, A., Yahya, H., Hermann, E., Zimmermann, M. & Seifert V. (2004). Functional magnetic resonance imaging-integrated neuronavigation: correlation between lesion-to-motor cortex distance and outcome. *Neurosurgery* Vol. 55 (No.4):904–914.

Kuo, L.W., Chen, J.H., Wedeen, V.J. & Tseng, W.Y. (2008). Optimization of diffusion spectrum imaging and q-ball imaging on clinical MRI system. *Neuroimage*. Vol. 41(No.1):7-18.

Leclercq, D., Duffau, H., Delmaire, C., Capelle, L,, Gatignol, P., Ducros, M., Chiras, J. & Lehéricy, S. (2010). Comparison of diffusion tensor imaging tractography of language tracts and intraoperative subcortical stimulations. *Journal of Neurosurgery* Vol. 112(No.3):503-11.

Lehéricy, S., Duffau, H., Cornu, P., Capelle, L., Pidoux, B., Carpentier, A., Auliac, S., Clemenceau, S., Sichez, J.P., Bitar, A., Valery, C.A., Van Effenterre, R., Faillot, T., Srour, A., Fohanno, D., Philippon, J., Le Bihan, D. & Marsault, C. (2000). Correspondence between functional magnetic resonance imaging somatotopy and individual brain anatomy of the central region: comparison with intraoperative stimulation in patients with brain tumors. *Journal of Neurosurgery* Vol. 92(4):589–598.

Lichtheim, L. (1885). On aphasia. *Brain* Vol. 7:433–484.

Logothetis, N.K. (2003) The underpinnings of the BOLD functional magnetic resonance imaging signal. *Journal of Neuroscience* Vol. 23(10):3963–3971.

Logothetis, N.K. & Pfeuffer, J. (2004). On the nature of the BOLD fMRI contrast mechanism. *Magnetic Resonance Imaging* Vol. 22(10):1517–1531.

Logothetis, N.K. & Wandell, B.A. (2004). Interpreting the BOLD signal. *Annual Review of Physiology* Vol. 66:735–769.

Lu, S., Ann, D., Johnson, G. & Cha, S. (2003). Peritumoral diffusion tensor imaging of high-grade gliomas and metastatic brain tumors. *American Journal of Neuroradiology* Vol. 24: 937-41.

Luders, E., Narr, K.L., Thompson, P.M., Woods, R.P., Rex, D.E., Jancke, L., Steinmetz, H. & Toga, A.W. (2005). Mapping cortical gray matter in the young adult brain: effects of gender. *Neuroimage* Vol. 26:493–501.

Majos, A., Tybor, K., Stefańczyk, L. & Góraj, B. (2005). Cortical mapping by functional magnetic resonance imaging in patients with brain tumors. European Radiology Vol. 15(No. 6):1148-58.

Mascalchi, M., Filippi, M., Floris, R., Fonda, C., Gasparotti, R. & Villari, N. (2005). Diffusion-weighted MR of the brain: methodology and clinical application. *Radiologia Medica* Vol. 109(3):155-97.

Mattay, V.S. & Weinberger, D.R. (1999). Organization of the human motor system as studied by functional magnetic resonance imaging. *European Journal of Radiology* Vol. 30(No.2):105-14.

Mazziotta, J.C., Phelps, M.E. & Carson, R.E. (1982). Tomographic mapping of human cerebral metabolism: auditory stimulation. *Neurology* Vol. 32(No. 9):921–937.

Menon, R.S., Ogawa, S., Hu, X., Strupp, J.P., Anderson, P. & Uğurbil, K. (1995). BOLD based functional MRI at 4 Tesla includes a capillary bed contribution: echoplanar imaging correlates with previous optical imaging using intrinsic signals. *Magnetic Resonance in Medicine* Vol. 33(No.3):453–459

Mohr, J.P. (2004). Historical observations on functional reorganization. *Cerebrovascular Disease* Vol. 18(No.3):258-9

Moritz, C. & Haughton, V. (2003). Functional MR imaging: paradigms for clinical preoperative mapping. Magnetic Resonance Imaging *Clinics of North America* Vol. 11(No. 4):529-42.

Mueller, W.M., Yetkin, F.Z., Hammeke, T.A., Morris, G.L. 3rd, Swanson, S.J., Reichert, K., Cox, R. & Haughton, V.M. (1996). *Neurosurgery* Vol. 39(No.3):515-20

Narr, K.L., Bilder, R.M., Luders, E., Thompson, P.M., Woods, R.P., Robinson, D., Szeszko, P.R., Dimtcheva, T., Gurbani, M. & Toga, A.W. (2007). Asymmetries of cortical shape: effects of handedness, sex and schizophrenia. *Neuroimage* Vol. 34:939–948.

Nimsky, C., Ganslandt, O., Hastreiter, P., Wang, R., Benner, T., Sorensen, A.G. & Fahlbusch, R. (2007). Preoperative and intraoperative diffusion tensor imaging-based fiber tracking in glioma surgery. *Neurosurgery* Vol. 61(1 Suppl):178-85.

Nucifora, P.G., Verma, R., Lee, S.K. & Melhem, E.R. (2007). Diffusion-Tensor MR Imaging and Tractography: Exploring Brain Microstructure and Connectivity. *Radiology* Vol. 245(No.2): 367-384.

Ogawa, S., Menon, R.S., Tank, D.W., Kim, S.G., Merkle, H., Ellermann, J.M. & Ugurbil, K. (1993). Functional brain mapping by blood oxygenation level-dependent contrast magnetic resonance imaging. A comparison of signal characteristics with a biophysical model. *Biophysical Journal* Vol. 64(No.3):803–812.

Ogawa, S., Tank, D.W., Menon, R., Ellermann, J.M., Kim, S.G., Merkle, H. & Ugurbil, K. (1992). Intrinsic signal changes accompanying sensory stimulation:functional brain mapping with magnetic resonance imaging. *Proceedings of the National Academy of Science* Vol. 89(No.13):5951–5955.

Ojemann, G., Ojemann, J., Lettich, E. & Berger, M. (1989). Cortical language localization in left, dominant hemisphere. An electrical stimulation mapping investigation in 117 patients. *Journal of Neurosurgery* Vol. 71:316–326.

Ozawa, N., Muragaki, Y., Nakamura, R. & Iseki, H. (2009). Identification of the pyramidal tract by neuronavigation based on intraoperative diffusion-weighted imaging combined with subcortical stimulation. *Stereotactic Functional Neurosurgery* Vol. 87(1):18–24.

Penfield, W. (1950). The cerebral cortex of man. New York, MacMillan.

Penfield, W. & Boldrey, E. (1937). Somatic motor and sensory representation in the cerebral cortex of man as studied by electrical stimulation. *Brain* Vol. 60:389–443

Penfield,W. & Erickson, T.C. (1941). Epilepsy and Cerebral Localization. A Study of the Mechanism, Treatment, and Prevention of Epileptic Seizures. Springfield, IL: Charles C Thomas.

Penfield, W. & Rasmussen, T. (1950). Secondary Sensory and Motor Representation. New York, Macmillan.

Petrovich, N., Holodny, A.I., Tabar, V., Correa, D.D., Hirsch, J., Gutin, P.H. & Brennan. C.W. (2005). Discordance between functional magnetic resonance imaging during silent speech tasks and intraoperative speech arrest. *Journal of Neurosurgery* Vol. 103:267–274

Price, S.J., Burnet, N.G., Donovan, T., Green, H.A., Peña, A., Antoun, N.M,, Pickard, J.D., Carpenter, T.A. & Gillard. J.H. (2003).Diffusion tensor imaging of brain tumors at 3 T : a potential tool for assessing white matter tract invasion? *Clinical Radiology* Vol. 58: 455-62.

Raichle, M.E. (1983). Positron emission tomography. *Annual Review of Neuroscience* Vol. 6:249–267.

Rijntjes, M. & Weiller, C. (2002). Recovery of motor and language abilities after stroke: the contribution of functional imaging *Progress in Neurobiology* Vol. 66:109–22.

Rossini, P.M., Calautti, C., Pauri, F. & Baron, J.C. (2003). Post-stroke plastic reorganisation in the adult brain. *Lancet Neurology* Vol. 2: 493–502.

Roux, F.E., Boulanouar, K., Ranjeva, J.P., Manelfe, C., Tremoulet, M., Sabatier, J. & Berry, I. (1999). Cortical intraoperative stimulation in brain tumors as a tool to evaluate spatial data from motor functional MRI. *Investigative Radiology* Vol. 34(No.3):225–229.

Rutten, G.J., Ramsey, N.F., van Rijen, P.C., Noordmans, H.J. & van Veelen, C.W. (2002). Development of a functional magnetic resonance imaging protocol for intraoperative localization of critical temporo-parietal language areas. *Annals of Neurology* Vol. 51:350–360.

Rutten, G.J. & Ramsey, N.F. (2010). The role of functional magnetic resonance imaging in surgery. *Neurosurgical Focus* Vol. 28(No.2):E4.

Sanai, N. & Berger, M.S. (2008). Mapping the horizon: techniques to optimize tumor resection before and during surgery. *Clinical Neurosurgery* Vol. 55:14–19.

Sanai, N., Mirzadeh, Z. & Berger, M.S. (2008). Functional outcome after language mapping for glioma resection. *New England Journal of Medicine* Vol. 358:18–27.

Sanai, N. & Berger, M.S. (2009). Operative techniques for gliomas and the value of extent of resection. *Neurotherapeutics* Vol. 6(3):478-86.

Sanai, N. & Berger, M.S. (2010). Intraoperative stimulation techniques for functional pathway preservation and glioma resection.. *Neurosurgical Focus* Vol. 28(No.2): E1

Schonberg, T., Pianka, P., Hendler, T., Pasternak, O. & Assaf, Y. (2006). Characterization of displaced white matter by brain tumors using combined DTI and fMRI. *Neuroimage* Vol. 30(No.4):1100–1111.

Sinha, S., Bastin, M.E., Whittle, I.R. & Wardlaw, J.M. (2002). Diffusion tensor MR Imaging of high-grade cerebral gliomas. *American Journal of Neuroradiology* Vol. 23: 520-7.

Smits, M., Vernooij, M.W., Wielopolski, P.A., Vincent, A.J., Houston, G.C. &van der Lugt, A. (2007). Incorporating functional MR imaging into diffusion tensor tractography in the preoperative assessment of the corticospinal tract in patients with brain tumors. *American Journal of Neuroradiology* Vol. 28(No.7):1354–1361.

Spena, G., Nava, A., Cassini, F., Pepoli, A., Bruno, M., D'Agata, F., Cauda, F., Sacco, K., Duca, S., Barletta, L. & Versari P. (2010). Preoperative and intraoperative brain mapping for the resection of eloquent-area tumors. A prospective analysis of methodology, correlation, and usefulness based on clinical outcomes.
Acta Neurochirurgica(Wien) Vol. 152(No.11):1835-46.

Staempfli, P., Reischauer, C., Jaermann, T., Valavanis, A., Kollias, S. & Boesiger, P. (2007). Combining fMRI and DTI: a framework for exploring the limits of fMRI-guided DTI fiber tracking and for verifying DTI-based fiber tractography results. *Neuroimage* Vol. 39 (No. 1):119–126.

Steinmetz, H., Volkmann, J., Jäncke, L. & Freund, H.J. (1991). Anatomical left-right asymmetry of language-related temporal cortex is different in left- and right-handers. *Annals of Neurology* Vol. 29:315–319

Stendel R. (2009). Extent of resection and survival in glioblastoma multiforme: identification of and adjustment for bias. *Neurosurgery* Vol. 64(No. 6) E1206.

Stippich, C., Rapps, N., Dreyhaupt, J., Durst, A., Kress, B., Nennig, E., Tronnier, V.M. & Sartor, K. (2007). Localizing and lateralizing language in patients with brain tumors: feasibility of routine preoperative functional MR imaging in 81 consecutive patients. *Radiology* Vol. 243(3):828-36.

Stippich, C., Mohammed, J., Kress, B., Hähnel, S., Günther, J., Konrad, F. & Sartor, K. (2003). Robust localization and lateralization of human language function: an optimized clinical functional magnetic resonance imaging protocol. *Neuroscience Letters* Vol. 31;346(No. 1-2):109-13

Thompson, P.M., Moussai, J., Zohoori, S., Goldkorn, A., Khan, A.A., Mega, M.S., Small, G.W., Cummings, J.L. & Toga, A.W. (1998). Cortical variability and asymmetry in normal aging and Alzheimer's disease. *Cerebral Cortex* Vol. 8:492–509.

Toga, A.W., Thompson, P.M., Mega, M.S., Narr, K.L. & Blanton, R.E. (2001). Probabilistic approaches for atlasing normal and disease-specific brain variability. *Anatomy and Embryology* Vol. 204:267–282.

Toh, C.H., Castillo, M., Wong, A.M., Wei, K.C., Wong, H.F., Ng, S.H. & Wan, Y.L. (2008). Primary Cerebral Lymphoma and Glioblastoma Multiforme: Differences in Diffusion Characteristics Evaluated with Diffusion Tensor Imaging. *American Journal of Neuroradiology* Vol. 29: 471-75.

Toronov, V., Walker, S., Gupta, R., Choi, J.H., Gratton, E., Hueber, D. & Webb, A. (2003). The roles of changes in deoxy-hemoglobin concentration and regional cerebral blood volume in the fMRI BOLD signal. *Neuroimage* Vol. 19: 1521-31.

Tummala, R.P., Chu, R.M., Liu, H. & Hall, W.A. (2003). Application of duffusion tensor imaging to magnetic-resonance-guided brain tumor resection. *Paediatric Neurosurgery* Vol. 39: 39-43.

Tzourio-Mazoyer, N., Josse, G., Crivello, F. & Mazoyer, B. (2004). Interindividual variability in the hemispheric organization for speech. *Neuroimage* Vol. 21(No.1):422-35.

Ulmer, J.L., Hacein-Bey, L., Mathews, V.P., Mueller, W.M., DeYoe, E.A., Prost, R.W., Meyer, G.A., Krouwer, H.G. & Schmainda, K.M. (2004). Lesion-induced pseudo-dominance at functional magnetic resonance imaging: implications for preoperative assessments. *Neurosurgery* Vol. 55:569–579.

Ward NS. (2004). Functional reorganization of the cerebral motor system after stroke. *Current Opinion in Neurology* Vol. 17(No.6):725-30.

Wedeen, V.J., Wang, R.P., Schmahmann, J.D., Benner, T., Tseng, W.Y., Dai, G., Pandya, D.N., Hagmann, P., D'Arceuil, H., de Crespigny, A.J. (2008). Diffusion spectrum magnetic resonance imaging (DSI) tractography of crossing fibers. *American Journal of Neuroimage* Vol. 41(No. 4):1267-77.

Wieshmann, U.C., Clark, C.A., Symms, M.R., Franconi, F., Barker, G.J. & Shorvon, S.D. (1999). Reduced anisotropy of water diffusion in structural cerebral abnormalities demonstrated with diffusion tensor imaging. *Magnetic Resonance Imaging* Vol. 17: 1269-74.

Wieshmann UC, Symms MR, Parker, G.J., Clark, C.A., Lemieux, L., Barker, G.J. & Shorvon, S.D. (2000). Diffusion tensor imaging demonstrates deviation of fibres in normal appearing white matter adjacent to a brain tumour. *Journal of Neurology, Neurosurgery and Psychiatry* Vol. 68: 501-3.

Witwer, B.P., Moftakhar, R., Hasan, K.M., Deshmukh, P., Haughton, V., Field, A., Arfanakis, K., Noyes, J., Moritz, C.H., Meyerand, M.E., Rowley, H.A., Alexander, A.L. & Badie, B. (2002). Diffusion-tensor imaging of white matter tracts in patients with cerebral neoplasm. *Journal of Neurosurgery* Vol. 97: 568-75.

Yoshikawa, K., Kajiwara, K., Morioka, J., Fujii, M., Tanaka, N., Fujisawa, H., Kato, S., Nomura, S. & Suzuki, M. (2006). Improvement of functional outcome after radical surgery in glioblastoma patients: the efficacy of a navigation-guided fence-post procedure and neurophysiological monitoring. *Journal of Neurooncology* Vol. 78(No.1):91–97.

Yousry, I., Naidich, T.P. & Yousry, T.A. (2001). Functional magnetic resonance imaging: factors odulating the corticalactivation pattern of the motor system. *Neuroimaging Clinic of North America* Vol. 11(No. 2):195–202.

Yousry, T.A., Schmid, U.D., Alkadhi, H., Schmidt, D., Peraud, A., Buettner, A. & Winkler, P. (1997). Localization of the motor hand area to a knob on the precentral gyrus. A new landmark. *Brain* Vol. 120 (No. 1): 141–57.

18

Radiation Immune Modulation Therapy of Glioma

Bertil R.R. Persson
Lund University
Sweden

1. Introduction

Since Roentgens discovery of the X-rays 1895, radiation therapy (RT) has been one of the most successful modalities used to treat cancer (Rontgen 1995). The experimental radiation treatment of glioma, however, took place first in 1938 (Bailey & Brunschwig 1938). Since then advances in radiation technology have expanded the role and value of using ionizing radiation in diagnosis, imaging and therapy of glioma. But despite substantial technical improvements in the current treatment modalities the survival rate for glioma patients is still very low (Barnholtz-Sloan, et al. 2007). Although the recently addition of temozolomide to conventional fractionated radiotherapy for newly diagnosed glioblastoma has resulted in an increased time of survival (Stupp, et al. 2005).

Immunotherapy utilizes the fact that the immune system has a potential to react against tumour antigens and that this can result in immunological control of the tumour. There is an increasing body of evidence that the activation of cytotoxic T-lymphocytes (CTL) has a positive effect on the long-term survival of cancer patients receiving traditional therapies such as surgery, chemo- or radiation-therapy (Nakano 2001; Prall 2004; L. Zhang, et al. 2003). It has been clearly demonstrated that tumour immune reactivity is of importance in treatment of several types of tumours (Shankar & Salgaller 2000). The immune response to glioma is primarily a result of the cell-killing function by the activated cytotoxic T cells (CTL). The aim of vaccination regimes is to enhance the effectors functions of CTL and the number of lymphoid cells within the glioma. But even if immune therapy cause large populations of lymphocytes to enter CNS tumours, total eradication of the glioma do not occur. This is partly due to the immunosuppressive factors produced by the glioma, which result in non-functioning CTL (Roszman, et al. 1991).

Traditional fractionated radiation therapy decrease the number of radiation sensitive T cells and damping the immune response of immunotherapy. Thus the interest in combining radiation therapy and immunotherapy has so far been very sparse. The use of sterotactic techniques with single radiation exposure or hypo-fractionated radiation therapy, however, does modulate the immune response and increases the therapeutic outcome (Lee, et al. 2009; Wersäll, et al. 2006). This radioimmuno modulatory effect of radiation opens for a new approach in glioma therapy by the combination of radiation- and immune-therapy.

Currently, there is a growing interest in combining radiation with other kinds of therapy, of which some are immunotherapy, to treat a broad range of malignancies (Chakraborty, et al.

2004; Gulley, et al. 2005; Sharp, et al. 2007). There is also an ongoing pre-clinical search for methods to enhance the therapeutic response of malignant glioma by combining immunotherapy with single fraction or hypo-fractionated radiation therapy (Demaria, et al. 2005a; Graf, et al. 2002; Lumniczky, et al. 2002; Newcomb, et al. 2006; B. R. R. Persson, et al. 2002; B. R. R. Persson, et al. 2003; B. R. R. Persson, et al. 2010; B. R. R. Persson, et al. 2008). The clinical trials using this approach, however, are still very sparse.

This chapter will summarize the aspects of the interaction of ionizing radiation with the immune system and its immunomodulatory effects and its implications for glioma therapy (Friedman 2002). Preclinical studies of the combinational approaches of radiation and immune therapies, which results in high fractions complete remissions of glioma in animal models, is reviewed. Various clinical studies towards combination of radiation- and immune-therapy for treatment of glioma are summarized in a final section.

2. Immune response of glioma

2.1 T cell infiltration in tumours and prognosis

Many tumours are potentially immunogenic and exhibit tumour-specific immune responses in vivo (Curiel 2008; Curiel, et al. 2004). Tumour-specific antigens are released from the tumour cells and then captured by antigen presenting dendritic cells (Huang, et al. 2010). Dendritic cell migration brings tumour antigen to the lymphoid organ where the antigen presentation stimulates immature T cells to become either "cytotoxic" CD8(+) T-cells (CTL), "helper" CD4(+) T-cells or memory T-cells (Fig. 1). Lymphocytes and some innate immune cells (macrophages, natural killer cells) migrate to the tumour in order to kill and eliminate tumour cells. Patients with high infiltration of lymphocytes in their tumours have usually found to have a better prognosis of survival.

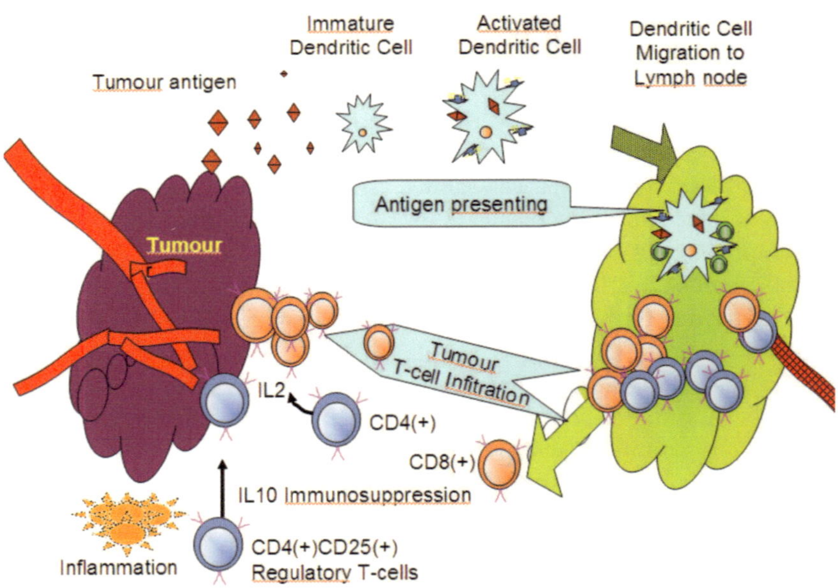

Fig. 1. Tumour immune response

Tumour infiltrating lymphocytes (TILs) of various subtypes represent the host-to-tumour reaction. Anti-tumour immune response is mediated by infiltrating CD8(+) T cells which have been shown to lyses tumour cells directly via recognition of the major histocompatibility complex class I (MHC-I) present on most tumour cells. But some tumours, which have low or none expression of MHC-I, are not affected by the CTL. Tumour infiltrating CD4(+) helper T cells seems to play a role in regulating and amplifying tumours response by priming tumour-specific cytotoxic CD8(+) T cells, as well as macrophages involved in clearance of dead tumour cells (Toes, et al. 1999; Vesalainen, et al. 1994).

In Fig. 1 is shown how tumour antigens are captured by antigen presenting cells such as dendritic cells, which migrate to regional lymph nodes. There they present the antigen to T-cells which differentiate into CD8(+) cytotoxic T-cells, CD4(+) helper T-cells, and memory T-cells. The cytotoxic CD8(+) T-cells (CTL) are transferred to the tumour in order to kill the tumour cells. The CD4(+) release IL2 which help the CD8(+) T-Cells to proliferate. But the CD4(+) can also form CD4(+)CD25(+) regulatory T-cells which excrete IL10 to suppress the activity of the CD8(+) cytotoxic T-cells.

The number of tumour infiltrating lymphocytes can be used as prognostic factor for several types of cancer (Cho, et al. 2003; Rauser, et al. 2010; Schumacher, et al. 2001; Zingg, et al. 2010). But in malignant glioma the use of tumour infiltrating lymphocytes as a prognostic factor seems to be more complex. The overall reports on tumour-infiltrating CD8(+), CD4(+) T-cells and major histocompatibility complex class I (MHC-I) expression in malignant glioma do not yield consistent correlation with clinical outcome (Dunn, et al. 2007). There seems to be factors present in patients with glioma that suppress the action of tumour infiltrated lymphocytes, and it has been demonstrated that glioma cells can actively paralyze T cell migration by the expression of Tenascin-C (Huang, et al. 2010).

Regulatory CD4(+)CD25(+)FoxP3(+) T cells (Treg) have been shown to play a major role in suppression of the immune response to malignant glioma. In human CNS tumor samples both CD4(+) and Treg infiltration have found to be significantly increased throughout the time of metastatic tumor progression. Thus immunotherapeutic strategies for treating metastatic CNS tumors must fight against Treg (Sugihara, et al. 2009). In an experimental GL261 intracranial tumor model, it was shown that depletion of CD25(+) regulatory T-cells (Treg) using anti-CD25 antibodies enhance the efficacy of DC immunotherapy (Maes, et al. 2009).

Infiltration of myeloid suppressor cells (MSC) is another factor inhibiting the function of the CD8(+) T cells, which results in tumour progression (Graf, et al. 2005). Other studies indicate that glioma seems to secrete factors such as TGF_{β} and prostaglandins (PGE2) that depress the cell-mediated immunity by down regulating the function of infiltrated CD8(+) T-cells and monocytes (Dix, et al. 1999; Farmer, et al. 1989). This might be one of the reasons why anti-tumour response of the immune system is decreased in patients with primary glioma (Brooks, et al. 1972).

2.2 Radio-immune-modulating effects by local irradiation

Recent studies have shown that local single fraction radiotherapy stimulates the immune response by enhancing the antigen presentation of MHC class I (Liao, et al. 2004). The mechanism underlying these effects is probably at the level of the proteasome in the cytoplasm of the tumour cell, which are essential for production of antigenic peptides for loading onto MHC class I molecules. The proteasome in tumour cells is a sensitive target for radiation, resulting in decreased processing of endogenous self antigens. The processing of tumour antigens is, however, increased by radiation, which enhance the accumulation of antigen/MHC class I complexes on the cell surface (Pajonk &Mcbride 2001).

Radiation therapy also causes an increase in production of the cytokine IFNγ in the target region which up-regulates low levels of MHC class I, creating a tumour microenvironment conducive for CD8(+) T cell infiltration and their recognition of tumour cells (Lugade, et al. 2008).

It has been demonstrated that antigen presentation by MHC class I is increased for many days by single fraction radiation therapy. The most pronounced effect was recorded at 7 days after irradiation with an absorbed dose of 8 Gy. This might be one of the reasons why the efficacy of tumour immunotherapy is most effective in combination with single fraction radiation therapy (Reits, et al. 2006). Maximum loading of the tumour micro-environment with cancer antigen occurred 2 days after radiation therapy and coincided with the optimal time for CD8(+) T cell transfer (Bin Zhang, et al. 2007).

2.3 Radiation effecting dendritic cells DC function

It has been demonstrated that the radiation modulation of MHC-I mediated antitumor immunity also depends on the antigen presenting pathways of the dendritic cells (Liao, et al. 2004). The dendritic cells either initiate an effective cytotoxic response against antigen-bearing cells, or produce tolerance, depending on the context in which those antigens are presented (Zou 2005). It has been shown that cell death caused by radiation therapy release tumour antigen, which facilitates an effective cytotoxic response of the dendritic cells (Hatfield, et al. 2005). Radiation therapy activation of dendritic cells (DC), induce secretion of interleukin-1 beta ($IL\text{-}1_{\beta}$), which is required for the adequate polarization of IFN_{γ} producing CD8(+) T-cells (Aymeric, et al. 2010).

3. Preclinical experience of glioma-radio-immune-modulatory therapy

In the Lund clinical study, named "Brain-Immuno-Gene-Tumour-Therapy" (BRIGTT), patients were immunized with their own tumour cells, cultivated from their surgical specimens and transfected with human IFNγ gene (Salford, et al. 2002). The cells taken from the surgically removed tumour were grown in culture. The day before immunization the karyotyped tumour cells were infected with an Adenovirus expressing human IFNγ. At the day after transfection, the immunization of the patient takes place soon after the cells have been irradiated with Cs-137 gamma radiations to an absorbed dose of 100 Gy (Baureus-Koch, et al. 2004). By subcutaneous (s.c.) implantation of these cells in the arm of the patient it is expected that the host immune system is activated against the tumour. The activated CD8(+) T-cells will pass the BBB and attack the cancer cells present at the primary tumour site as well as the distant metastases "*guerrilla cells*" (Salford, et al. 2006; Salford, et al. 2001; Salford, et al. 2002; Salford, et al. 2004; Siesjö, et al. 1993; Visse, et al. 1999). Results from the first eight human treatments in the phase 1−2 BRIGTT study show that immunization with transfected tumour cells is safe for the patients and improves survival (A. Persson, et al. 2005; Salford, et al. 2005; Salford, et al. 2011; Salford, et al. 2004).

In order to further enhance the effect of this immunotherapy we investigated the effect of combining it with a single fraction radiation therapy in an animal model. The results of these preclinical experiments, which were performed already 2001, showed that a single fraction of RT combined with immunotherapy resulted in a significantly increased survival time of rats with intra-cranially implanted N29 or N32 glioblastoma. Further there were significant numbers of complete remissions of the most infiltrative N29 tumour implanted in Fischer-344 rats (B.R.R. Persson, et al. 2010). Other researchers have also reported substantial tumour regression by single fraction radiation therapy combined with various regimes of immune therapy (Bradley 1999; Chakraborty, et al. 2003; Demaria, et al. 2005a; Friedman 2002; Garnett, et al. 2004; Graf, et al. 2002; Lumniczky, et al. 2002).

3.1 The Lund experience of combined single fraction RT and Immunization with IFN-γ secreting tumour cells

3.1.1 Animals and tumour cell lines

Fischer-344 rats were maintained by continuous, single-line brother to sister mating in the laboratory at Lund. During the experiments rats of both sexes, females weighing around 190 g and males 370 g respectively, were housed in a climate controlled cabinet. Otherwise they were kept in Macralon cages provided with food pellets and water *ad libitum*. All experimental animal procedures were approved by the Animal Ethical Committee in Malmö/Lund (Lunds tingsrätt, Box 75, 22100 Lund Sweden).
All cells were maintained in culture flasks (Nunc, Denmark) and harvested by treatment with trypsin/EDTA. The culture medium was antibiotic-free RPMI-1640 medium supplemented with 5-10% foetal calf serum, L-glutamine (2 mM), HEPES (10 mM), pyruvate (0.5 mM) and $NaHCO_3$ (11 mM). The cell-cultures were regularly checked for contaminating microbes by staining with the fluorescent dye Hoechst 32 258 and examined with fluorescent microscopy. If *Mycoplasma* infection was indicated the cultures were discharged or treated with *Mycoplasma Removal Agent* (Hoechst, Germany) twice with 7 days interval, and repeatedly confirmed free of infection.
The tumour cells (N29 or N32) used for immunization were interferon-gamma (IFN-γ) gene modified to enhance secretion of IFN_{γ}. The cells were cultured for one week, washed twice, and suspended in serum free medium (IMDM-0) to a cell density of $2{\cdot}10^4$ cells/ml. Just before immunization the cells were transferred from the culture flasks to 15 ml centrifuge test tubes (Nanclon) and stored on melting ice to prevent the cells to grow during the procedure. Irradiation of the cells was performed during 20 minutes at room temperature to an absorbed dose of 70 Gy by using a ^{137}Cs gamma-ray source (*Gammacell 2000;* Mølsgaard Medical, Risø, Denmark) (Siesjö, et al. 1996; Sjögren, et al. 1996; Visse, et al. 1999).

3.1.2 Inoculation and treatment of intracerebrally tumours

Inoculation was performed by injecting 5 000 tumour cells in 5 μl nutrient solution into the head of Fischer 344 rats, using a stereotactic technique with a Hamilton syringe. To avoid extra-cranial tumour growth, the injection site was cleaned with 70% ethanol after injection and the borehole was sealed with wax. The animals were arranged into 6 groups, which included: controls, RT with either 5 or 15 Gy, immunization with IFN-γ gene modified tumour cell, and RT with either 5 or 15 Gy combined with immunization (Table 1).
Animals were given a single radiation treatment using a ^{60}Co radiotherapy unit (Siemens Gammatron S) with a source-skin distance (SSD) of 50 cm and the maximum absorbed dose rate 0.65-0.70 Gy/min. The radiation field size was collimated to cover the brain. The adsorbed dose of either 5 or 15 Gy was measured both by an dose-meter diode and TLD

dose meter. A sheet of tissue equivalent bolus, 5 mm thick, was placed over the head for radiation build up.

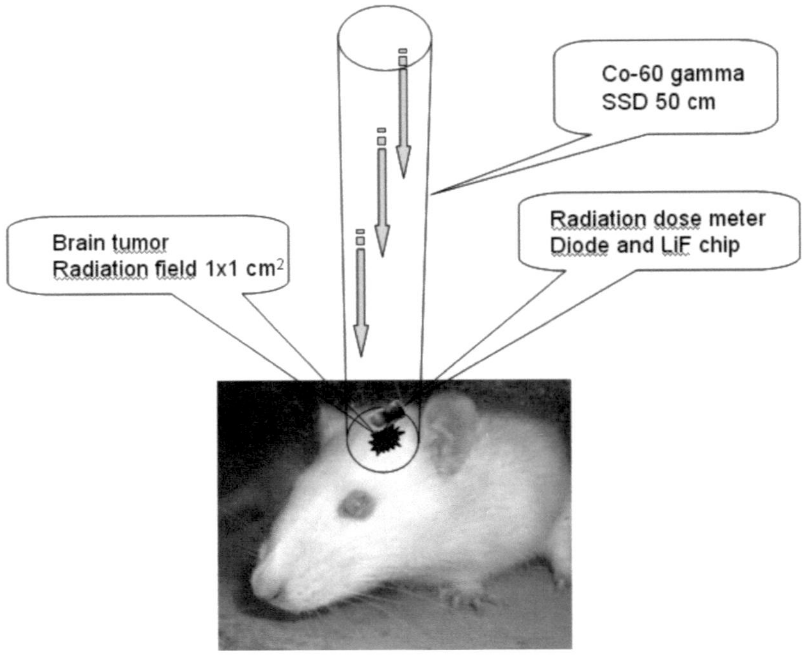

Fig. 2. Radiation therapy was performed at day 7 after inoculation with the animals anesthetized with 5% chloral hydrate given intraperitoneally (i.p.) or Ketalar®/Rompun®, 0.55 ml per 100g. The animals were given a single radiation exposure using a ^{60}Co radiotherapy unit (Siemens Gammatron S) at a source-skin distance (SSD) of 50 cm with a maximum absorbed dose rate of 0.70 Gy/min. The radiation field (1 cm^2) was collimated to cover the brain (Fig. 2). The delivered adsorbed dose of either 5 or 15 Gy was measured both by an dose-meter diode and a Lithium fluoride (LiF) TLD chip placed next to the tumour in the field under the bolus.

The animals were immunized by intraperitoneally administration of 3 x 10^6 IFN-γ gene modified N29 or N32 tumour cells, which immediately before had been irradiated with 70 Gy ^{134}Cs gamma-radiation. The first immunization was performed within one hour after the radiotherapy session at day 7. In the rats still alive it was repeated at least two more times at days 21 and 35.

Group No.	Treatment	Number of N29 Animals Experiment A	Number of N32 Animals Experiment B	Number of N32 Animals Experiment C
1	Controls with no treatment	6	9	3
2	Radiation 5 Gy	8	7	
3	Radiation 15 Gy	8	6	6
4	Immunization	6	7	6
5	Radiation 5 Gy + Immunization	8	7	
6	Radiation 15 Gy + Immunization	8	7	6

Table 1. Number of animals in the groups of various treatments used in the experiments with either N29 or N32 tumours. The various experiments A, B and C respectively, were performed at different occasions

Following symptoms of the rats were used as signs of progressing tumour growth:

- keeping their heads turned to one side,
- rotating or losing weight,
- unwillingness to move,
- shaggy fur and
- reddening of the eyes and nose.

The rats were examined daily and when the animals developed symptoms, they were euthanatized and the brains were stained for histopathological examination.
None of the rats, which were inoculated with N32 tumour cells, survived longer than 30 days. But in the group inoculated with N29 tumour cells, surviving animals could be observed for more than 170 days. In this group of animals with N29 tumours, re-challenge was performed with $2 \cdot 10^5$ N29 glioma cells in 200 µl, administered just under the skin in the thigh of the hind leg. Fourteen out of the originally 46 rats, and 4 extra control rats with no previous treatment were inoculated.

3.1.3 Survival of rats with intracerebrally implanted N29 tumours

In Table 2 are given the fractions of animals intracerebrally implanted with N29 tumour cells, which were surviving more than 170 days: Controls; IFNγ cell immunization (IMU IFNγ), single fraction radiation therapy (RT with either 5 or 15 Gy), and their combinations (IMU IFNγ + RT with either 5 or 15 Gy). RT and first immunization was performed at 7 days after inoculation. Immunizations were then repeated for at least two more times at days 21 and 35. In the 2nd column of Table 2 are given the numbers of animals survived more than 170 days, versus the number in each group of animals with intra cerebral N29 tumour. In the 3rd column is given the number of tumours appeared, relative to the number of animals that were re- challenged, including the 4 extra controls.
In the last column of Table 2 is given the number of re-challenged animals without tumour versus the original number in each group. Those animals, which resisted re-challenge, seem to have been cured from their primary glioma.

Type of treatment	Fraction of Animals Survived >170 d	Fraction of animals with tumour in the re challenged survivors	Fraction of Cured animals
Controls	1/6	5/(1+4+)	0
IMU IFNγ 3x	2/6	1/2	1/6
RT 5 Gy	0/8	-	0
RT 15 Gy	2/8	2/2	0
IMU IFNγ 3x + RT 5 Gy	**6/8*)**	**4/6**	**2/8**
IMU IFNγ 3x + RT 15 Gy	3/8	2/3	1/8

*) p=0.03; +) extra controls

Table 2. The fraction of living rats in the various groups with different treatments, followed during 170 days after inoculation of N29 tumour cells in their brain, number of tumours after re-challenge, and fraction of cure.

By using Fisher exact probability test the results show that treatment with 5 Gy radiation therapy combined with immunization resulted in significantly increased number of survivals versus controls (p = 0.03). But neither immunization alone nor radiation therapy alone with single fractions of 5 or 15 Gy resulted in any significant therapeutic effect versus the controls. The combination of radiation therapy with immunization compared with radiotherapy alone, however, resulted in significant survival fraction at both 5 Gy and 15 Gy, with p-values <0.01** and p <0.05* respectively.
The number of living rats in the various groups with different treatments, followed during 170 days after inoculation of N29 tumour cells in their brain, is displayed in Fig. 3 for each group respectively.
In Table 3 is given the median survival time and the p-values of two-sided non-parametric Mann-Whitney test versus the control. Immunization with N29 cells significantly increased

Type of treatment	Num. Rats	Median survival time (days)		Mann-Whitney 2-tailed versus Control	Tumour weight g	
Control	6	82	± 46		0.39	± 0.22
IMU IFNγ	6	132	± 44	P=0.04 *	0	
RT 5 Gy	8	46	± 14	NS	0.25	± 0.25
RT 15 Gy	8	93	± 35	NS	0,24	± 0.14
IMU IFNγ + RT 5 Gy	**8**	**153**	**± 31**	**P=0.003 ****	**0**	
IMU IFNγ + RT 15 Gy	8	119	± 35	P=0.03 *	0.01	± 0.01

Table 3. Number of rats; mean survival time and tumour weight at time of death of rats with intra cerebrally implanted N29 tumours treated one week after inoculation, with IFNγ cell immunization, radiation therapy (RT) and their combination. Immunization (IMU-IFNγ) was repeated for at least two more times at days 21 and 35. The rats were observed during up to 170 days after inoculation.

the survival time by 60% (p=0.04). Radiation therapy alone with 5 Gy, however, did not significantly increased the survival time. But immunization combined with 5 Gy radiation therapy resulted in a significantly increased survival time with 87% (p=0.003). Radiation therapy alone with 15 Gy did not significantly increased the survival time. But 15 Gy RT combined with immunization increased the survival time with 45% (p=0.03).

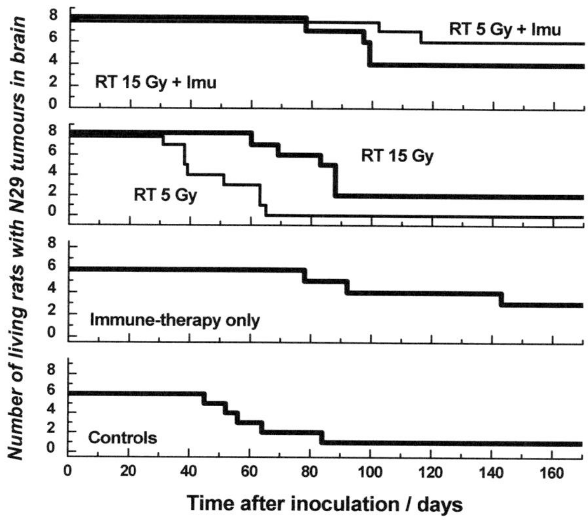

Fig. 3. Survival plot of intra cerebral implanted N29 tumours: Controls (Lower panel), immunization with syngeneic N29 tumour cells (2nd panel); radiation therapy (3rd panel) and combinations of radiation therapy and immunization (upper panel).

3.1.4 Survival of rats with intracerebrally implanted N32 tumours

The pooled results of the two experimental series (B and C in Table 1) with rats implanted with N32 tumours are displayed in Table 4. The results are given in terms of the mean survival time and weight of tumour at the time of death for each group animals. None of the rats with N32 tumours survived more than 30 days and thus no re-challenging could be done.

The survival of all rats with implanted N32 tumours were followed during 30 days and the results in the various groups of rats with different treatments are displayed in Fig. 4.

For the N32 tumours given a single fraction radiation therapy with 15 Gy resulted in significant increase of survival time with about 20% (p<0.001). The combination of 15 Gy single fraction radiation therapy with immunization of IFN-γ secreting syngeneic cells resulted in increased survival time by about 40% (p<0.001), although there were no complete remissions. But neither immunization with IFN-γ secreting syngeneic cells alone, nor radiation therapy with a single fraction of 5 Gy alone, or in combination with immunization, resulted in any increase in survival time of the N32 tumours in rats.

There is no significant difference in the weight of tumours in the different groups. Although the average growth rate of the N32 tumours treated with 5 Gy radiation therapies combined with immunization was decreased by 30% compared with the controls.

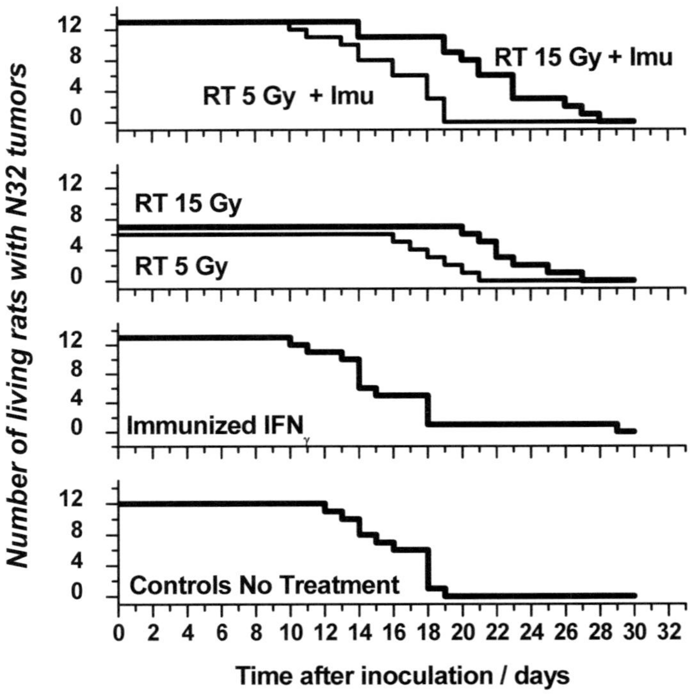

Fig. 4. Survival plot of intra-cerebral implanted N32 tumours: Controls (Lower panel); Immunization with syngeneic N32 tumours cells (2nd panel); radiation therapy (3rd panel), and a combination of radiation therapy and immunization (upper panel).

Type of treatment	Num. Rats	Median Survival time days		Mann-Whitney 2-tailed test versus Control	Tumour weight g	
Control	12	19	± 3		0.19	± 0.16
IMU IFNγ	13	19	± 6	NS	0.25	± 0.23
RT 5 Gy	6	19.5	± 2	NS	0.18	± 0.10
RT 15 Gy	13	23	± 2	P<0.001***	0.16	± 0.13
RT 5 Gy +IMU IFNγ	7	19	± 2	NS	0.14	± 0.09
RT 15 Gy + IMU IFNγ	**13**	**27**	**± 3**	**P<0.0001*** **	**0.30**	**± 0.28**

Table 4. Number of rats, mean survival time, and the significance of Mann-Whitney 2-tailed test versus control is shown in columns 2-4. In the last column is given the tumour weight at time of death of intra cerebral N32 tumours treated with syngeneic IFNγ transfected tumour cells (IMU IFNγ), radiation therapy (RT) and their combination (RT + IMU IFNγ).

3.1.5 Summary of the LUND experiment

The results of the Lund experiments reveal that a single fraction radiotherapy session of 5 or 15 Gy combined with immunization by i.p. injection of irradiated syngeneic tumour cells induces a significant anti-tumour response to intra cranial implanted glioblastoma tumours in Fischer-344 rats. In the rats, which were inoculated with N32 tumour cells, the combination of 15 Gy single fraction radiation therapy with immunization of IFN-γ secreting syngeneic cells resulted in increased survival time by about 40% ($p<0.001$). But none of these rats survived longer than 30 days. In the group inoculated with N29 tumour cells and treated with 5 Gy RT combined with immunization the survival time was significantly increased by 87% ($p=0.003$), and 75% of the animals survived for more than 170 days. The difference in response of N29 and N32 cell lines indicate that there is difference in immune response in different clones of glioma.

3.2 The Hungarian experience of single fraction RT and Immunization with (GM-CSF, IL-4, IL-12) in a mouse glioma (Gl261) brain tumour model

In Hungary a study was performed in a mouse glioma (Gl261) brain tumour model with single fraction radiotherapy combined with administration of cytokine-producing cancer cell vaccines (Lumniczky, et al. 2002). Their brain tumour bearing mice were treated with various cytokine producing vaccines made by in vitro transduction of Gl261 tumour cells with different genes such as: IL-4, IL-6, IL-7, GM-CSF, TNF_{α}. Immunotherapy alone with vaccines producing either IL-4 or GM-CSF resulted in complete remission in 20–40% of the mice. By combining immunotherapy using (GM-CSF, IL-4, IL-12) producing vaccines with local tumour radiotherapy (single fraction 6 Gy X-ray radiations) about 80–100% of the glioma-bearing mice were cured. The high efficiency of the combined treatment was maintained even under suboptimal conditions when neither of the individual modalities alone cured any of the mice (Lumniczky, et al. 2002). Their results are in good agreement the survival rate of 75% ($p<0.05$) achieved in the Lund study of N29 tumours in rats treated with IFN-γ secreting vaccine combined with 5 Gy single fraction RT (B. R. R. Persson, et al. 2010).

3.3 The U.S. experience of radiation therapy combined with vaccination of mice with Glioma or mammary carcinoma

3.3.1 Combining radiation therapy with blockade of the CTLA-4 pathway

The cytotoxic T lymphocyte-associated protein CTLA-4 is involved in the immune regulatory mechanisms that control the early stage of the T cell response. It has previously been demonstrated that blockade of the CTLA-4 protein enhance anti-tumour responses both in experimental systems and in clinical trials (Chambers, et al. 2001; Egen, et al. 2002).
In a mouse model of the poorly immunogenic metastatic mouse mammary carcinoma 4T1, however, neither anti-tumour response nor survival-time was affected by using an anti-CTLA-4 monoclonal antibody for blocking the CTLA-4 protein. But anti-CTLA-4 monoclonal antibody administration combined with one 12 Gy fraction of radiation therapy, inhibited the growth of the primary irradiated tumour. Also the survival-time of the mice was significantly increased by this combined treatment (Demaria, et al. 2004; Demaria, et al. 2003; Demaria, et al. 2005b).
Another investigation of the effects of systemic CTLA-4 blockade with monoclonal antibody (9H10) to CTLA-4 employed in a mice model with well-established glioma, showed that CTLA-4 blockade confers long-term survival in 80% of treated mice (Fecci, et al. 2007). Thus the combination of local RT with CTLA-4 blockade might be applied as radio-immune-modulating therapeutic strategy also against glioma.

3.3.2 Combination of radiation therapy and vaccination of mice with glioma

In a study of combining radiation therapy and vaccination, mice with intracerebrally established invasive GL261 glioma were treated with two fraction of radiation therapy (2x4 Gy) to the whole brain, peripheral vaccination with cells transfected to secrete granulocyte-macrophage colony-stimulating factor GM-CSF and their combination (Newcomb, et al. 2006).

Less than 10% increase in survival time was observed in mice given radiation therapy or vaccination alone. But by combining radiation therapy and vaccination a highly significant increase in the survival time, with about 40-80%, was observed. The surviving animals showed acquired antitumor immunity by rejecting challenge tumours (Newcomb, et al. 2006). These results are in good agreement with the results of (75 %) long term survivals and acquired antitumor immunity in N29 rats treated with the combination of radiation and immune therapy with cells secreting IFN_{γ} (B. R. R. Persson, et al. 2010).

3.3.3 Combination of radiation therapy and anti-CD137 antibodies in treatment of mice with glioma

The immune response induced by CD137 monoclonal antibodies (BMS-469492, Bristol-Meyer Squibb) directed to the co-stimulatory molecule CD137 has shown to generate effective antitumor responses in several animal models and in clinical trials (Ascierto, et al. 2010; Mazzolini, et al. 2007; Nam, et al. 2005).

Treatment of murine lung (M109) and breast (EMT6) carcinoma with CD137 monoclonal antibodies BMS-469492 generate tumour growth retardation of 3 days in M109 tumours and of 12.5 days in EMT6 tumours. In combination with radiation therapy, however, the tumour responses were enhanced in both tumour models (Shi & Siemann 2006).

A recent study in mice with intracerebrally established invasive GL261glioma applied the combination of radiotherapy with anti-CD137 antibody directed to the co-stimulatory molecule CD137 (Newcomb, et al. 2010). The mice were treated with two fractions (2x4 Gy) radiation therapy to the whole brain. Non-specific rat IgG or anti-CD137 mAb was administered either alone or in combinations with RT.

Type of treatment	Median survival time days	Number of > 120 days survivals out of 9 rats
IgG	31	0
anti-CD137	42	0
RT (4Gy×2) alone	No data	No data
IgG + RT (4Gy×2)	37	2
anti-CD137 + RT (4Gy×2)	114	6

Table 5. Median survival time of rats, with 9 animals in each group, after the different types of treatments (Newcomb, et al. 2010).

The results summarized in Table 5 show that the combination of radiation (4 Gy×2) with anti-CD137 therapy resulted in complete tumour eradication and prolonged survival in six of nine (67%) mice with established brain tumours ($p < 0.001$). Five of the six long-term survivors in the combination group demonstrated acquired antitumor immunity by rejecting challenge tumours. Antitumor immunity was associated with an increased number of tumour-infiltrating lymphocytes (TILs) in brain tumours and increased tumour-specific production of IFNγ. Since anti-CD137 therapy is already used in clinical trials it was suggested to be studied further in combination with local hypo-fractionated (2x4 Gy) radiation therapy for clinical translation (Newcomb, et al. 2010).

4. Clinical studies of combining radiation and immune therapy

The expression profiles of CD4(+) and CD8(+) T cells and T_{reg} from patients with newly diagnosed *glioblastoma multiforme* are quite different when compared with normal healthy volunteers (Learn, et al. 2006). But how various absorbed dose or various fractionation pattern or methods of radiation delivery can affect T-cell populations and alternative regulatory molecules in glioma patients is still under debate (Chiba, et al. 2010; Teitz-Tennenbaum, et al. 2008; Verastegui, et al. 2003).

4.1 Effects of concomitant temozolomide and radiation therapies on WT1-specific T-cells in malignant glioma

Like many other solid tumours, glioma have been found to express a protein characteristic for Wilms' tumour 1 (WT1) (Hashiba, et al. 2007). A peptide based immunotherapy targeting the WT1 gene has successfully been used in patients with recurrent glioma. The clinical response indicates that CD8(+) cytotoxic T lymphocytes (CTLs) are the main effectors of this WT1 vaccination (Oka, et al. 2004). A phase II clinical trial of the WT1 vaccination for patients with recurrent malignant glioma resulted in a partial response rate of 9.5% but none complete response. The median length of period with progression-free survival was 20 weeks (Izumoto, et al. 2008).

In planning for a clinical trial of WT1 vaccination involving patients with newly diagnosed malignant glioma, it is also aimed to combine concurrent radiation /TMZ therapy with WT1 immunotherapy. The critical question is, however, if the depletion of lymphocytes caused by the current standard radiation/TMZ treatment is a drawback for a combination with WT1 immunotherapy. Therefore a clinical study was performed in order to determine how the concomitant radiation/TMZ therapy affects the WT1-specific T-cells and other T-cells in terms of their frequencies and total numbers. This study concluded that, even after the decrease of the absolute numbers of lymphocytes, the fraction of WT1 specific T-cells was stable. They concluded that it may the possible to apply WT1 immunotherapy after the end of 6 weeks of radiation/TMZ therapy (Chiba, et al. 2010).

In another clinical study of 8 patients with primary glioma it was found that concomitant radiation/TMZ therapy integrated with autologous dendritic cell-based immunotherapy was feasible and well tolerated. The median progression-free survival (PFS) was 75% and at 6 months and 50% at 18 months. The median time of survival for all patients is 24 months. One patient was still free from progression or recurrence at 34 months (Ardon, et al. 2010).

4.2 Treatment recurrent malignant glioma with hypo-fractionated radiotherapy combined with immune therapy

A single fraction of high dose radiation therapy has been demonstrated to dramatically increase the priming of T-cell in draining lymphoid tissues, which increased the action of the CD8(+) T cells and lead to reduction and eradication of the primary tumour or distant metastasis. This immune response, however, is abrogated by conventional fractionated RT or adjuvant chemotherapy (Lee, et al. 2009). So far only preclinical studies of hypo-fractionated radiation therapy in combination with immune therapy have been performed. The results are however encouraging and clinical trials using this therapeutic regime is urgently needed for both primary and recurrent glioma (Newcomb, et al. 2006; B. R. R. Persson, et al. 2002; B. R. R. Persson, et al. 2010; B. R. R. Persson, et al. 2008).

Henke et al. (2010) found that retreatment of recurrent high-grade glioma with hypo-fractionated radiation therapy with 20 Gy given over 1 week seems to be feasible even after a previous complete course of radiotherapy (Henke, et al. 2009). Thus it should be feasible to consider hypo-fractionated radiotherapy with about 8 Gy in one or two fractions to recurrent glioma in combination with immune therapy.

4.3 Treatment of newly diagnosed glioma with fractionated radiotherapy combined with vaccination therapy

An autologous formalin-fixed tumor vaccine (AFTV) has been prepared from formalin-fixed and/or paraffin-embedded glioma tumor tissue obtained upon surgery and premixed with original adjuvant materials. In a clinical pilot study, AFTV inoculations of 12 patients took place at least 4 weeks after prior primary conventional glioma treatments were concluded. Of these 12 patients, four responded to the AFTV therapy: one showed a complete response, one showed a partial response, two showed minor responses, and one had stabilization of disease. The median survival period was about 11 months from the initiation of the AFTV treatment. But three of these patients survived for 20 months or more after AFTV inoculation (Ishikawa, et al. 2007). In a subsequent phase I/IIa clinical trial, the AFTV was inoculated in 24 patients with newly diagnosed glioblastoma multiforme, in combination with conventional fractionated radiotherapy. The treatment protocol in that study included aggressive tumor resection, fractionated radiotherapy, 2 Gy per fraction, up to a total dose of 60 Gy, and 3 concomitant courses of AFTV administered with an interval of one week during the last 3 weeks of irradiation. The median duration of overall survival was 21.4 months (95% CI 13.8–31.3 months). The actuarial 2-year survival rate was 40%. These results demonstrate that vaccine treatment in combination with fractionated radiotherapy may be effective in patients with newly diagnosed glioblastoma (Muragaki, et al. 2011). Since the previous pilot study with AFTV therapy only, also has shown a good response, the outcome of the phase I/IIa clinical trial might have been even better if it has been combined with hypo-fractionated radiation therapy as described in the previous paragraph 4.3.

5. Summary and conclusion

Many pre-clinical models have proven that one or two radiotherapy fractions with a total absorbed dose in the range of 5 - 16 Gy in combination with immune therapy result in enhanced therapeutic response to glioma. This finding opens for the possibility of clinical testing of new challenging therapeutic regimes for glioma, based on a combination of immune-therapy and hypo-fractionated radiotherapy. A regime of one or two radiation sessions with a total radiation target dose in the order of 8 Gy in combination with clinically proven immunotherapy seem so be adequate (De Vleeschouwer, et al. 2008; Gulley, et al. 2005; J. Nemunaitis, et al. 2006a; J. J. Nemunaitis, et al. 2006b; Newcomb, et al. 2010; B. R. R. Persson, et al. 2010; Salford, et al. 2006; Salford, et al. 2004).

Although the total lymphocyte count decrease as a consequence of the current radiation/temozolomide therapy, it seems not affect the frequency of antigen specific T-cells, which suggest that combination with immunotherapy might be successful (Ardon, et al. 2010; Chiba, et al. 2010).

6. Acknowledgement

This chapter is dedicated to emeritus professor Leif G. Salford who spent his career as neuro-surgeon to fight against the "*guerrilla cells*" of glioma. He initiated the Brain Immuno Gene Tumour Therapy project "BRIGTT" with support of Märit and Hans Rausing Charitable Foundation. Berta Kamprad's foundation of cancer and the Faculty of Medicine at Lund University are gratefully acknowledged for their support in publishing this chapter.

7. References

Ardon H., Van Gool, S., Lopes, I. S., Maes, W., Sciot, R., Wilms, G., Demaerel, P., Bijttebier, P., Claes, L., Goffin, J., Van Calenbergh, F., and De Vleeschouwer, S., (2010). Integration of autologous dendritic cell-based immunotherapy in the primary treatment for patients with newly diagnosed glioblastoma multiforme: a pilot study, *Journal of Neuro-Oncology*, Vol. 99, No. 2, pp. 261-272, ISSN 0167-594X

Ascierto P. A., Simeone, E., Sznol, M., Fu, Y. X., and Melero, I., (2010). Clinical Experiences With Anti-CD137 and Anti-PD1 Therapeutic Antibodies, *Seminars in Oncology*, Vol. 37, No. 5, pp. 508-516, ISSN 0093-7754

Aymeric L., Apetoh, L., Ghiringhelli, F., Tesniere, A., Martins, I., Kroemer, G., Smyth, M. J., and Zitvogel, L., (2010). Tumor Cell Death and ATP Release Prime Dendritic Cells and Efficient Anticancer Immunity, *Cancer Research*, Vol. 70, No. 3, pp. 855-858, ISSN 0008-5472

Bailey P., and Brunschwig, A., (1938). Experiments with x-ray treatment of neural glioma, *Zeitschrift Fur Die Gesamte Neurologie Und Psychiatrie*, Vol. 161, No., pp. 214-221, ISSN 0303-4194

Barnholtz-Sloan J. S., Sloan, A. E., and Schwartz, A. G., (2007). *Cancer of the Brain and Other Central Nervous System*(National Cancer Institute, SEER Program, Bethesda, MD,).

Baureus-Koch C., Nyberg, G., Widegren, B., Salford, L. G., and Persson, B. R. R., (2004). Radiation sterilisation of cultured human brain tumour cells for clinical immune tumour therapy, *British Journal of Cancer*, Vol. 90, No. 1, pp. 48-54, ISSN 0007-0920

Bradley J. D., Kataoka, Y., Advani, S., Chung, S. M., Arani, R. B., Gillespie, G. Y., Whitley, R. J., Markert, J. M., Roizman, B., Weichselbaum, R. M. , (1999). Ionizing radiation improves survival in mice bearing intracranial highgrade gliomas injected with genetically modified herpes simplex virus, *Clinical Cancer Research*, Vol. 5, No. June, pp. 1517-1522, ISSN

Brooks W. H., Netsky, M. G., Normanse.De, and Horwitz, D. A., (1972). Depressed cell-mediated immunity in patients with primary intracranial tumors - Characterization of a humoral immunosuppressive factor., *Journal of Experimental Medicine*, Vol. 136, No. 6, pp. 1631-&, ISSN 0022-1007

Chakraborty M., Abrams, S. I., Camphausen, K., Liu, K. B., Scott, T., Coleman, C. N., and Hodge, J. W., (2003). Irradiation of tumor cells up-regulates Fas and enhances CTL lytic activity and CTL adoptive immunotherapy, *Journal of Immunology*, Vol. 170, No. 12, pp. 6338-6347, ISSN 0022-1767

Chakraborty M., Abrams, S. I., Coleman, C. N., Camphausen, K., Schlom, J., and Hodge, J. W., (2004). External beam radiation of tumors alters phenotype of tumor cells to render them susceptible to vaccine-mediated T-cell killing, *Cancer Research*, Vol. 64, No. 12, pp. 4328-4337, ISSN 0008-5472

Chambers C. A., Kuhns, M. S., Egen, J. G., and Allison, J. P., (2001). CTLA-4-mediated inhibition in regulation of T cell responses: Mechanisms and manipulation in tumor immunotherapy, *Annual Review of Immunology*, Vol. 19, No., pp. 565-594, ISSN 0732-0582

Chiba Y., Hashimoto, N., Tsuboi, A., Oka, Y., Murao, A., Kinoshita, M., Kagawa, N., Oji, Y., Hosen, N., Nishida, S., Sugiyama, H., and Yoshimine, T., (2010). Effects of Concomitant Temozolomide and Radiation Therapies on WT1-specific T-cells in Malignant Glioma, *Japanese Journal of Clinical Oncology*, Vol. 40, No. 5, pp. 395-403, ISSN 0368-2811

Cho Y., Miyamoto, M., Kato, K., Fukunaga, A., Shichinohe, T., Kawarada, Y., Hida, Y., Oshikiri, T., Kurokawa, T., Suzuoki, M., Nakakubo, Y., Hiraoka, K., Murakami, S., Shinohara, T., Itoh, T., Okushiba, S., Kondo, S., and Katoh, H., (2003). CD4(+) and CD8(+) T cells cooperate to improve prognosis of patients with esophageal squamous cell carcinoma, *Cancer Research*, Vol. 63, No. 7, pp. 1555-1559, ISSN 0008-5472

Curiel T. J., (2008). Regulatory T cells and treatment of cancer, *Current Opinion in Immunology*, Vol. 20, No. 2, pp. 241-246, ISSN 0952-7915

Curiel T. J., Coukos, G., Zou, L. H., Alvarez, X., Cheng, P., Mottram, P., Evdemon-Hogan, M., Conejo-Garcia, J. R., Zhang, L., Burow, M., Zhu, Y., Wei, S., Kryczek, I., Daniel, B., Gordon, A., Myers, L., Lackner, A., Disis, M. L., Knutson, K. L., Chen, L. P., and Zou, W. P., (2004). Specific recruitment of regulatory T cells in ovarian carcinoma fosters immune privilege and predicts reduced survival, *Nat Med*, Vol. 10, No. 9, pp. 942-949, ISSN 1078-8956

De Vleeschouwer S., Fieuws, S., Rutkowski, S., Van Calenbergh, F., Van Loon, J., Goffin, J., Sciot, R., Wilms, G., Demaerel, P., Warmuth-Metz, M., Soerensen, N., Wolff, J. E. A., Wagner, S., Kaempgen, E., and Van Gool, S. W., (2008). Postoperative adjuvant dendritic cell-based immunotherapy in patients with relapsed glioblastoma multiforme, *Clinical Cancer Research*, Vol. 14, No. 10, pp. 3098-3104, ISSN 1078-0432

Demaria S., Bhardwaj, N., Mcbride, W. H., and Formenti, S. C., (2005a). Combining radiotherapy and immunotherapy: A revived partnership, *International Journal of Radiation Oncology Biology Physics*, Vol. 63, No. 3, pp. 655-666, ISSN 0360-3016

Demaria S., Kawashima, N., Yang, A. M., Devitt, M. L., Babb, J. S., Allison, J. P., and Formenti, S. C., (2003). Immune-mediated inhibition of metastases after treatment with local radiation and CTLA-4 blockade in a mouse model of breast cancer, *45th Annual Meeting of the American-Society-for-Therapeutic-Radiology-and-Oncology*, Vol., No., pp. 728-734, ISSN

Demaria S., Kawashima, N., Yang, A., Devitt, M., Babb, J., Allison, J. P., and Formenti, S. C., (2004). Reduction of immature myeloid cells by treatment with all-trans-retinoic acid (ATRA) improves the immunotherapeutic effect of the combination of local radiation with CTLA-4 blockade, *International Journal of Radiation Oncology Biology Physics*, Vol. 60, No. 1, pp. 76, ISSN 0360-3016

Demaria S., Newcomb, E. W., Zagzag, D., Lukyanov, E., Schnee, T., Kawashima, N., Devitt, M., and Formenti, S. C., (2005b). The combination of ionizing radiation and peripheral vaccination produces long-term survival of mice bearing invasive GL261 glioma, *International Journal of Radiation Oncology Biology Physics*, Vol. 63, No. 2, pp. 1044, ISSN 0360-3016

Dix A. R., Brooks, W. H., Roszman, T. L., and Morford, L. A., (1999). Immune defects observed in patients with primary malignant brain tumors, *Journal of Neuroimmunology*, Vol. 100, No. 1-2, pp. 216-232, ISSN 0165-5728

Dunn G. P., Dunn, I., P.,, and William T. Curry, W. T., (2007). Focus on TILs: Prognostic significance of tumor infiltrating lymphocytes in human glioma, *Cancer Immunity*, Vol. 7, No., pp. 16, ISSN

Egen J. G., Kuhns, M. S., and Allison, J. P., (2002). CTLA-4: new insights into its biological function and use in tumor immunotherapy, *Nature Immunology*, Vol. 3, No. 7, pp. 611-618, ISSN 1529-2908

Farmer J. P., Antel, J. P., Freedman, M., Cashman, N. R., Rode, H., and Villemure, J. G., (1989). Characterization of lymphoid-cells isolated from human gliomas, *Journal of Neurosurgery*, Vol. 71, No. 4, pp. 528-533, ISSN 0022-3085

Fecci P. E., Ochiai, H., Mitchell, D. A., Grossi, P. M., Sweeney, A. E., Archer, G. E., Cummings, T., Allison, J. P., Bigner, D. D., and Sampson, J. H., (2007). Systemic CTLA-4 blockade ameliorates glioma-induced changes to the CD4(+) T cell compartment without affecting regulatory T-cell function, *Clinical Cancer Research*, Vol. 13, No. 7, pp. 2158-2167, ISSN 1078-0432

Friedman E. J., (2002). Immune modulation by ionizing radiation and its implications for cancer immunotherapy, *Current Pharmaceutical Design*, Vol. 8, No. 19, pp. 1765-1780, ISSN 1381-6128

Garnett C. T., Palena, C., Chakarborty, M., Tsang, K. Y., Schlom, J., and Hodge, J. W., (2004). Sublethal irradiation of human tumor cells modulates phenotype resulting in enhanced killing by cytotoxic T lymphocytes, *Cancer Research*, Vol. 64, No. 21, pp. 7985-7994, ISSN 0008-5472

Graf M. R., Prins, R. M., Hawkins, W. T., and Merchant, R. E., (2002). Irradiated tumor cell vaccine for treatment of an established glioma. I. Successful treatment with combined radiotherapy and cellular vaccination, *Cancer Immunology Immunotherapy*, Vol. 51, No. 4, pp. 179-189, ISSN

Graf M. R., Sauer, J. T., and Merchant, R. E., (2005). Tumor infiltration by myeloid suppressor cells in response to T cell activation in rat gliomas, *Journal of Neuro-Oncology*, Vol. 73, No. 1, pp. 29-36, ISSN 0167-594X

Gulley J. L., Arlen, P. M., Bastian, A., Morin, S., Marte, J., Beetham, P., Tsang, K. Y., Yokokawa, J., Hodge, J. W., Menard, C., Camphausen, K., Coleman, C. N., Sullivan, F., Steinberg, S. M., Schlom, J., and Dahut, W., (2005). Combining a recombinant cancer vaccine with standard definitive radiotherapy in patients with localized prostate cancer, *Clinical Cancer Research*, Vol. 11, No. 9, pp. 3353-3362, ISSN 1078-0432

Hashiba T., Izumoto, S., Kagawa, N., Suzuki, T., Hashimoto, N., Maruno, M., and Yoshimine, T., (2007). Expression of WT1 protein and correlation with cellular proliferation in glial tumors, *Neurologia Medico-Chirurgica*, Vol. 47, No. 4, pp. 165-170, ISSN 0470-8105

Hatfield P., Merrick, A., Harrington, K., Vile, R., Bateman, A., Selby, P., and Melcher, A., (2005). Radiation-induced cell death and dendritic cells: Potential for cancer immunotherapy?, *Clinical Oncology*, Vol. 17, No. 1, pp. 1-11, ISSN 0936-6555

Henke G., Paulsen, F., Steinbach, J. P., Ganswindt, U., Isijanov, H., Kortmann, R. D., Bamberg, M., and Belka, C., (2009). Hypofraktionierte Rebestrahlung bei rezidivierten malignen Gliomen, *Strahlentherapie Und Onkologie*, Vol. 185, No. 2, pp. 113-119, ISSN 0179-7158

Huang J. Y., Cheng, Y. J., Lin, Y. P., Lin, H. C., Su, C. C., Juliano, R., and Yang, B. C., (2010). Extracellular Matrix of Glioblastoma Inhibits Polarization and Transmigration of T Cells: The Role of Tenascin-C in Immune Suppression, *Journal of Immunology*, Vol. 185, No. 3, pp. 1450-1459, ISSN 0022-1767

Ishikawa E., Tsuboi, K., Yamamoto, T., Muroi, A., Takano, S., Enomoto, T., Matsumura, A., and Ohno, T., (2007). Clinical trial of autologous formalin-fixed tumor vaccine for glioblastoma multiforme patients, *Cancer Science*, Vol. 98, No. 8, pp. 1226-1233, ISSN 1347-9032

Izumoto S., Tsuboi, A., Oka, Y., Suzuki, T., Hashiba, T., Kagawa, N., Hashimoto, N., Maruno, M., Elisseeva, O. A., Shirakata, T., Kawakami, M., Oji, Y., Nishida, S., Ohno, S., Kawase, I., Hatazawa, J., Nakatsuka, S., Aozasa, K., Morita, S., Sakamoto, J., Sugiyama, H., and Yosihmine, T., (2008). Phase II clinical trial of Wilms tumor 1 peptide vaccination for patients with recurrent glioblastoma multiforme, *Journal of Neurosurgery*, Vol. 108, No. 5, pp. 963-971, ISSN 0022-3085

Learn C. A., Fecci, P. E., Schmittling, R. J., Xie, W. H., Karikari, I., Mitchell, D. A., Archer, G. E., Wei, Z. Z., Dressman, H., and Sampson, J. H., (2006). Profiling of CD4(+), CD8(+), and CD4(+) CD25(+) CD45RO(+) FoxP3(+) T cells in patients with malignant glioma reveals differential expression of the immunologic transcriptome compared with T cells from healthy volunteers, *Clinical Cancer Research*, Vol. 12, No. 24, pp. 7306-7315, ISSN 1078-0432

Lee Y. J., Auh, S. L., Wang, Y. G., Burnette, B., Wang, Y., Meng, Y. R., Beckett, M., Sharma, R., Chin, R., Tu, T., Weichselbaum, R. R., and Fu, Y. X., (2009). Therapeutic effects of ablative radiation on local tumor require CD8(+) T cells: changing strategies for cancer treatment, *Blood*, Vol. 114, No. 3, pp. 589-595, ISSN 0006-4971

Liao Y. P., Wang, C. C., Butterfield, L. H., Economou, J. S., Ribas, A., Meng, W. S., Iwamoto, K. S., and Mcbride, W. H., (2004). Ionizing radiation affects human MART-1 melanoma antigen processing and presentation by dendritic cells, *Journal of Immunology*, Vol. 173, No. 4, pp. 2462-2469, ISSN 0022-1767

Lugade A. A., Sorensen, E. W., Gerber, S. A., Moran, J. P., Frelinger, J. G., and Lord, E. M., (2008). Radiation-induced IFN-gamma production within the tumor microenvironment influences antitumor immunity, *Journal of Immunology*, Vol. 180, No. 5, pp. 3132-3139, ISSN 0022-1767

Lumniczky K., Desaknai, S., Mangel, L., Szende, B., Hamada, H., Hidvegi, E. J., and Safrany, G., (2002). Local tumor irradiation augments the antitumor effect of cytokine-producing autologous cancer cell vaccines in a murine glioma model, *Cancer Gene Therapy*, Vol. 9, No. 1, pp. 44-52, ISSN

Maes W., Rosas, G. G., Verbinnen, B., Boon, L., De Vleeschouwer, S., Ceuppens, J. L., and Van Gool, S. W., (2009). DC vaccination with anti-CD25 treatment leads to long-term immunity against experimental glioma, *Neuro-Oncology*, Vol. 11, No. 5, pp. 529-542, ISSN 1522-8517

Mazzolini G., Murillo, O., Atorrasagasti, C., Dubrot, J., Tirapu, I., Rizzo, M., Arina, A., Alfaro, C., Azpilicueta, A., Berasain, C., Perez-Gracia, J. L., Gonzalez, A., and Melero, I., (2007). Immunotherapy and immunoescape in colorectal cancer, *World Journal of Gastroenterology*, Vol. 13, No. 44, pp. 5822-5831, ISSN 1007-9327

Muragaki Y., Maruyama, T., Iseki, H., Tanaka, M., Shinohara, C., Takakura, K., Tsuboi, K., Yamamoto, T., Matsumura, A., Matsutani, M., Karasawa, K., Shimada, K., Yamaguchi, N., Nakazato, Y., Sato, K., Uemae, Y., Ohno, T., Okada, Y., and Hori, T., (2011). Phase I/IIa trial of autologous formalin-fixed tumor vaccine concomitant with fractionated radiotherapy for newly diagnosed glioblastoma Clinical article, *Journal of Neurosurgery*, Vol. 115, No. 2, pp. 248-255, ISSN 0022-3085

Nakano O., Sato M, Naito Y, Suzuki K, Orikasa S, Aizawa M, Suzuki Y, Shintaku I, Nagura H, Ohtani H, (2001). Proliferative activity of intratumoral CD8(+) T-lymphocytes as a prognostic factor in human renal cell carcinoma: clinicopathologic demonstration of antitumor immunity, *Cancer Research*, Vol. 61, No. 13, pp. 5132-5136, ISSN

Nam K. O., Kang, W. J., Kwon, B. S., Kim, S. J., and Lee, H. W., (2005). The therapeutic potential of 4-1BB (CD137) in cancer, *Current Cancer Drug Targets*, Vol. 5, No. 5, pp. 357-363, ISSN 1568-0096

Nemunaitis J. J., Dillman, R. O., Schwarzenberger, P., Senzer, N., Tong, A., Devol, E., Chamberlin, T., Shawler, D., and Fakhrai, H., (2006b). Phase II study of a TGF-beta 2 antisense gene modified allogeneic tumor cell vaccine (Lucanix) in advanced NSCLC, *Journal of Clinical Oncology*, Vol. 24, No. 18, pp. 368S-368S, ISSN 0732-183X

Nemunaitis J., Dillman, R. O., Schwarzenberger, P. O., Senzer, N., Cunningham, C., Cutler, J., Tong, A., Kumar, P., Pappen, B., Hamilton, C., Devol, E., Maples, P. B., Liu, L. L., Chamberlin, T., Shawler, D. L., and Fakhrai, H., (2006a). Phase II study of belagenpumatucel-L, a transforming growth factor beta-2 antisense gene-modified allogeneic tumor cell vaccine in non-small-cell lung cancer, *Journal of Clinical Oncology*, Vol. 24, No. 29, pp. 4721-4730, ISSN 0732-183X

Newcomb E. W., Demaria, S., Lukyanov, Y., Shao, Y. Z., Schnee, T., Kawashima, N., Lan, L., Dewyngaert, J. K., Zagzag, D., Mcbride, W. H., and Formenti, S. C., (2006). The combination of ionizing radiation and peripheral vaccination produces long-term survival of mice bearing established invasive GL261 gliomas, *Clinical Cancer Research*, Vol. 12, No. 15, pp. 4730-4737, ISSN 1078-0432

Newcomb E. W., Lukyanov, Y., Kawashima, N., Alonso-Basanta, M., Wang, S. C., Liu, M. L., Jure-Kunkel, M., Zagzag, D., Demaria, S., and Formenti, S. C., (2010). Radiotherapy Enhances Antitumor Effect of Anti-CD137 Therapy in a Mouse Glioma Model, *Radiation Research*, Vol. 173, No. 4, pp. 426-432, ISSN 0033-7587

Oka Y., Tsuboi, A., Taguchi, T., Osaki, T., Kyo, T., Nakajima, H., Elisseeva, O. A., Oji, Y., Kawakami, M., Ikegame, K., Hosen, N., Yoshihara, S., Wu, F., Fujiki, F., Murakami, M., Masuda, T., Nishida, S., Shirakata, T., Nakatsuka, S., Sasaki, A., Udaka, K., Dohy, H., Aozasa, K., Noguchi, S., Kawase, L., and Sugiyama, H., (2004). Induction of WT1 (Wilms' tumor gene)-specific cytotoxic T lymphocytes by WT1 peptide vaccine and the resultant cancer regression, *Proceedings of the National Academy of Sciences of the United States of America*, Vol. 101, No. 38, pp. 13885-13890, ISSN 0027-8424

Pajonk F., and Mcbride, W. H., (2001). Ionizing radiation affects 26s proteasome function and associated molecular responses, even at low doses, *Radiotherapy and Oncology*, Vol. 59, No. 2, pp. 203-212, ISSN 0167-8140

Persson A., Skagerberg, G., Salford, L. G., Englund, E., and Brain Immuno Gene Tumour Therapy, (2005). Immunotreatment in patients with glioblastoma multiforme - a histopathological evaluation of reactive and inflammatory changes, *Clinical Neuropathology*, Vol. 24, No. 5, pp. 201-208, ISSN 0722-5091

Persson B. R. R., Bauréus Koch, C., Grafström, G., Engström, P. E., and Salford, L. G., (2003). A model for evaluating therapeutic response of combined cancer treatment modalities: Applied to treatment of subcutaneously implanted brain tumors (N32 and N29) in Fischer rats with pulsed electric fields (PEF) and (CO)-C-60-gamma radiation (RT), *Technology in Cancer Research & Treatment*, Vol. 2, No. 5, pp. 459-470, ISSN 1533-0346

Persson B. R. R., Bauréus Koch, C., Grafström, G., Engström, P., Brun, A., Widegren, B., and Salford, L. G., (2002). Tumor Treatment by using Pulsed Electric Fields Combined with Radiation Therapy and Immunization with syngeneic Interferon-gamma secreting tumor cells, *Neuro-Oncology*, Vol. 4, No. Supplement 2, pp. 68 ISSN

Persson B. R. R., Koch, C. B., Grafström, G., Ceberg, C., af Rosenschöld, P. M., Nittby, H., Widegren, B., and Salford, L. G., (2010). Radiation Immunomodulatory Gene Tumor Therapy of Rats with Intracerebral Glioma Tumors, *Radiation Research*, Vol. 173, No. 4, pp. 433-440, ISSN 0033-7587

Persson B. R. R., Koch, C. B., Grafström, G., Ceberg, C., af Rosenschöld, P. M., Widegren, B., and Salford, L. G., (2008). Survival of rats with N29 brain tumours after irradiation with 5 or 15 Gy and immunization with IFN-gamma secreting tumour cells., *Bmei 2008: Proceedings of the International Conference on Biomedical Engineering and Informatics, Vol 2*, Vol., No., pp. 243-247, ISSN

Prall F., Dührkop, T., Weirich, V., Ostwald, C., Lenz, P., Nizze, H., and Barten, M., (2004). Prognostic Role of CD8 Tumor-Infiltrating Lymphocytes in Stage III Colorectal Cancer With and Without Microsatellite Instability., *Human Pathology* Vol. 35, No. 7, pp. 808 - 816, ISSN

Rauser S., Langer, R., Tschernitz, S., Gais, P., Jutting, U., Feith, M., Hofler, H., and Walch, A., (2010). High number of CD45RO+tumor infiltrating lymphocytes is an independent prognostic factor in non-metastasized (stage I-IIA) esophageal adenocarcinoma, *Bmc Cancer*, Vol. 10, No., ISSN 1471-2407

Reits E. A., Hodge, J. W., Herberts, C. A., Groothuis, T. A., Chakraborty, M., Wansley, E. K., Camphausen, K., Luiten, R. M., De Ru, A. H., Neijssen, J., Griekspoor, A., Mesman, E., Verreck, F. A., Spits, H., Schlom, J., Van Veelen, P., and Neefjes, J. J., (2006). Radiation modulates the peptide repertoire, enhances MHC class I expression, and induces successful antitumor immunotherapy, *Journal of Experimental Medicine*, Vol. 203, No. 5, pp. 1259-1271, ISSN 0022-1007

Rontgen W. C., (1995). December 28, 1895 - On a new kind of rays (Reprinted), *Veterinary Radiology & Ultrasound*, Vol. 36, No. 5, pp. 371-374, ISSN 1058-8183

Roszman T., Elliot, L., and Brooks, W., (1991). Modulation of T-cell function by gliomas, *Immunol Today*, Vol., No. 12, pp. 370, ISSN

Salford L. G., Ask, E., Siesjö, P., Skagerberg, G., Baureus-Koch, C., Blennow, C., Darabi, A., Elfgren, C., Englund, E., Janelidze, S., Larsson, E. M., Lilja, A., Persson, B. R. R., Rydelius, A., Stromblad, S., Visse, E., and Widegren, B., (2005). Immunization with autologous glioma cells transfected with IFN-g gene significantly prolongs survival in GBM-patients older than 50 years, *Neuro-Oncology*, Vol. 7, No. 3, pp. 370-370, ISSN 1522-8517

Salford L. G., Rydelius, A., Skagerberg, G., Siesjö, P., Darabi, A., Persson, B., Visse, E., and Widegren, B., (2006). Immune therapy significantly prolongs survival of GBM patients, *Neuro-Oncology*, Vol. 8, No. 4, pp. 351-351, ISSN 1522-8517

Salford L. G., Siesjö, P., Skagerberg, G., Persson, B. R. R., Larsson, E. M., Lindvall, M., Visse, E., and Widegren, B., (2001). Search for effective therapy against glioblastoma multiforme - clinical immunisation with autologous glioma cells transduced with the human Interferon-γ gene, *The 2nd International Mt. BANDAI Symposium for Neuroscience 2001*, Vol., No., pp. 143-149, ISSN

Salford L. G., Siesjö, P., Skagerberg, G., Persson, B. R. R., Visse, E., Larsson, E. M., Englund, E., and Widegren, B., (2002). A-32 Clinical Immunizatrion with autologous glioma cells transduced with human interferon-γ gene, *Neuro-Oncology*, Vol. 4, No. Supplement 2, ISSN

Salford L. G., Siesjö, P., Skagerberg, G., Rydelius, A., Blennow, C., Lilja, Å., Persson, B. R. R., Strömblad, S., Visse, E., and Widegren, B., (2011). Immunization with autologous IFN-γ secreting glioma cells in patients with Glioblastoma Multiforme - a phase 1-2 clinical trial, *To be published*, Vol., No., ISSN

Salford L. G., Siesjö, P., Skagerberg, G., Visse, E., Darabi, A., Lilja, A., Blennow, C., Strömblad, S., Ask, E., Rydelius, A., Persson, B. R. R., Koch, C. B., Englund, E., Larsson, E. M., Mandahl, N., and Widegren, B., (2004). Brain immuno gene tumour therapy (BRIGTT), *Neuro-Oncology*, Vol. 6, No. 4, pp. 344-344, ISSN 1522-8517

Schumacher K., Haensch, W., Roefzaad, C., and Schlag, P. M., (2001). Prognostic significance of activated CD8(+) T cell infiltrations within esophageal carcinomas, *Cancer Research*, Vol. 61, No. 10, pp. 3932-3936, ISSN 0008-5472

Shankar G., and Salgaller, M. L., (2000). Immune monitoring of cancer patients undergoing experimental immunotherapy, *Current Opinion in Molecular Therapeutics*, Vol. 2, No. 1, pp. 66-73, ISSN

Sharp H. J., Wansley, E. K., Garnett, C. T., Chakraborty, M., Camphausen, K., Schlom, J., and Hodge, J. W., (2007). Synergistic antitumor activity of immune strategies combined with radiation, *Frontiers in Bioscience*, Vol. 12, No., pp. 4900-4910, ISSN 1093-9946

Shi W. Y., and Siemann, D. W., (2006). Augmented antitumor effects of radiation therapy by 4-1BB antibody (BMS-469492) treatment, *Anticancer Research*, Vol. 26, No. 5A, pp. 3445-3453, ISSN 0250-7005

Siesjö P., Visse, E., and Sjögren, H. O., (1996). Cure of established, intracerebral rat gliomas induced by therapeutic immunizations with tumor cells and purified APC or adjuvant IFN-gamma treatment, *Journal of Immunotherapy*, Vol. 19, No. 5, pp. 334-345, ISSN 1053-8550

Siesjö P., Visse, E., Lindvall, M., Salford, L., and Sjögren, H. O., (1993). Immunization with mutagen-treated (tum-) cells causes rejection of nonimmunogenic rat glioma isografts, *Cancer Immunology Immunotherapy*, Vol. 37, No. 1, pp. 67-74, ISSN 0340-7004

Sjögren H. O., Visse, E., Siesjö, P., and Widegren, B., (1996). Regression of intracerebral isografts of malignant rat glioma by therapeutic subcutaneous immunization with tumor cells transduced with IFN-gamma, IL-7 or B7-1, *Cancer Gene Therapy*, Vol. 3, No. 6, pp. O8-O8, ISSN 0929-1903

Stupp R., Mason, W. P., Van Den Bent, M. J., Weller, M., Fisher, B., Taphoorn, M. J. B., Belanger, K., Brandes, A. A., Marosi, C., Bogdahn, U., Curschmann, J., Janzer, R. C., Ludwin, S. K., Gorlia, T., Allgeier, A., Lacombe, D., Cairncross, J. G., Eisenhauer, E., Mirimanoff, R. O., Van Den Weyngaert, D., Kaendler, S., Krauseneck, P., Vinolas, N., Villa, S., Wurm, R. E., Maillot, M. H. B., Spagnolli, F., Kantor, G., Malhaire, J. P., Renard, L., De Witte, O., Scandolaro, L., Vecht, C. J., Maingon, P., Lutterbach, J., Kobierska, A., Bolla, M., Souchon, R., Mitine, C., Tzuk-Shina, T., Kuten, A., Haferkamp, G., De Greve, J., Priou, F., Menten, J., Rutten, I., Clavere, P., Malmstrom, A., Jancar, B., Newlands, E., Pigott, K., Twijnstra, A., Chinot, O., Reni, M., Boiardi, A., Fabbro, M., Campone, M., Bozzino, J., Frenay, M., Gijtenbeek, J., Brandes, A. A., Delattre, J. Y., Bogdahn, U., De Paula, U., Van Den Bent, M. J., Hanzen, C., Pavanato, G., Schraub, S., Pfeffer, R., Soffietti, R., Weller, M., Kortmann, R. D., Taphoorn, M., Torrecilla, J. L., Marosi, C., Grisold, W., Huget, P., Forsyth, P., Fulton, D., Kirby, S., Wong, R., Fenton, D., Fisher, B., Cairncross, G., Whitlock, P., Belanger, K., Burdette-Radoux, S., Gertler, S., Saunders, S., Laing, K., Siddiqui, J., Martin, L. A., Gulavita, S., Perry, J., Mason, W., Thiessen, B., Pai, H., Alam, Z. Y., Eisenstat, D., Mingrone, W., Hofer, S., Pesce, G., Curschmann, J.,

Dietrich, P. Y., Stupp, R., Mirimanoff, R. O., Thum, P., Baumert, B., and Ryan, G., (2005). Radiotherapy plus concomitant and adjuvant temozolomide for glioblastoma, *New England Journal of Medicine*, Vol. 352, No. 10, pp. 987-996, ISSN 0028-4793

Sugihara A. Q., Rolle, C. E., and Lesniak, M. S., (2009). Regulatory T cells actively infiltrate metastatic brain tumors, *International Journal of Oncology*, Vol. 34, No. 6, pp. 1533-1540, ISSN 1019-6439

Teitz-Tennenbaum S., Li, Q., Okuyama, R., Davis, M. A., Sun, R., Whitfield, J., Knibbs, R. N., Stoolman, L. M., and Chang, A. E., (2008). Mechanisms involved in radiation enhancement of intratumoral dendritic cell therapy, *Journal of Immunotherapy*, Vol. 31, No. 4, pp. 345-358, ISSN 1524-9557

Toes R. E. M., Ossendorp, F., Offringa, R., and Melief, C. J. M., (1999). CD4 T cells and their role in antitumor immune responses, *Journal of Experimental Medicine*, Vol. 189, No. 5, pp. 753-756, ISSN 0022-1007

Verastegui E. L., Morales, R. B., Barrera-Franco, J. L., Poitevin, A. C., and Hadden, J., (2003). Long-term immune dysfunction after radiotherapy to the head and neck area, *International Immunopharmacology*, Vol. 3, No. 8, pp. 1093-1104, ISSN 1567-5769

Vesalainen S., Lipponen, P., Talja, M., and Syrjanen, K., (1994). Histological grade, Perineural infiltration, Tumor-Infiltrating Lymphocytes and Apoptosis as Determinants of long-term Prognosis In Prostatic Adenocarcinoma, *European Journal of Cancer*, Vol. 30A, No. 12, pp. 1797-1803, ISSN 0959-8049

Visse E., Siesjö, P., Widegren, B., and Sjögren, H. O., (1999). Regression of intracerebral rat glioma isografts by therapeutic subcutaneous immunization with interferon-gamma, interleukin-7, or B7-1-transfected tumor cells, *Cancer Gene Therapy*, Vol. 6, No. 1, pp. 37-44, ISSN 0929-1903

Wersäll P. J., Blomgren, H., Pisa, P., Lax, I., Kalkner, K. M., and Svedman, C., (2006). Regression of non-irradiated metastases after extracranial stereotactic radiotherapy in metastatic renal cell carcinoma, *Acta Oncologica*, Vol. 45, No. 4, pp. 493-497, ISSN 0284-186X

Zhang B., Bowerman Natalie, A., Salama Joseph, K., Schmidt, H., Spiotto Michael, T., Schietinger, A., Yu, P., Fu, Y.-X., Weichselbaum Ralph, R., Rowley Donald, A., Kranz David, M., and Schreiber, H., (2007). Induced sensitization of tumor stroma leads to eradication of established cancer by T cells, *Journal of Experimental Medicine*, Vol. 204, No. 1, pp. 49-55, ISSN 00221007

Zhang L., Conejo-Garcia, J. R., Katsaros, D., Gimotty, P. A., Massobrio, M., Regnani, G., Makrigiannakis, A., Gray, H., Schlienger, K., Liebman, M. N., Rubin, S. C., and Coukos, G., (2003). Intratumoral T cells, recurrence, and survival in epithelial ovarian cancer, *New England Journal of Medicine*, Vol. 348, No. 3, pp. 203-213, ISSN 0028-4793

Zingg U., Montani, M., Frey, D. M., Dirnhofer, S., Esterman, A. J., Went, P., and Oertli, D., (2010). Tumour-infiltrating lymphocytes and survival in patients with adenocarcinoma of the oesophagus, *Ejso*, Vol. 36, No. 7, pp. 670-677, ISSN 0748-7983

Zou W. P., (2005). Immunosuppressive networks in the tumour environment and their therapeutic relevance, *Nature Reviews Cancer*, Vol. 5, No. 4, pp. 263-274, ISSN 1474-175X

19

Confocal Neurolasermicroscopy - Modern Perspectives for Glioma Resection on a Cellular Level

Hans-Georg Schlosser[1] and Christian Bojarski[2]
[1]*Universitätsmedizin Berlin, Charité – Campus Virchow Klinikum, Department of Neurosurgery, Berlin*
[2]*Universitätsmedizin Berlin, Charité – Campus Benjamin Franklin Department of Gastroenterology, Berlin*
Germany

1. Introduction

Confocal neurolasermicroscopy (NLM)(Schlosser et al., 2009 (Epub)) is the current front end of the innovative process in neurosurgery for optimizing the operative results. Hence NLM is the continuance of a protracted development. Microscopic imaging technologies in neurosurgery invented 50 years ago revealed new strategies and possibilities for surgeons. These techniques were first used with magnifying lenses in research for introducing blood into the subarachnoid space in the region of circle of Willis in dog (Lougheed and Tom, 1961). It was further used in cerebrovascular diseases (Jacobson et al., 1962) (Chou, 1963), graft interposition (Woringer and Kunlin, 1963) (Lougheed et al., 1971) and aneurysm surgery (Pool and Colton, 1966) (Rand and Jannetta, 1967). From studies assessing radical surgery in the excision of fluorescence labelled tumours (Stummer et al., 2006) (Stummer et al., 1998) the necessity for a high-resolution imaging technique was clearly evident. Intravital fluorescence microscopy was used in animal studies to investigate tumorangiogenesis and microcirculation (Read et al., 2001) (Vajkoczy et al., 2000).
In the following section our pilot study using NLM in the neurosurgical operating condition is introduced (Schlosser et al., 2009 (Epub)). We aimed to demonstrate a technique with the potential to be adapted intraoperatively to define cellular and subcellular structures during ongoing neurosurgery. Here we show our results of miniaturized confocal lasermicroscopy in normal brain and brain tumor tissue which we termed NLM. Our pilot study was initiated to test the feasibility of this new technique and to open the door for high resolution imaging during ongoing neurosurgery.

2. Technical background

We used a miniaturized confocal laser microscope (Optiscan, Australia, Fig. 1) for tissue examination as described earlier (Schlosser et al., 2009 (Epub)). This technique was first described as confocal laser endoscopy in gastrointestinal endoscopy and was used for high-resolution in-vivo imaging while endoscopy of the upper or lower gastrointestinal tract was performed (Kiesslich et al., 2004). The ability to detect or exclude premalignant conditions and/or other pathologies which were normally not visible created a complete new field of gastrointestinal diagnosis followed by specific treatment before classical histology was accessible (Bojarski et al., 2009). For the use in humans intravenous applied fluorescein sodium distributes throughout the mucosa, however, most of the serum albumin bound fraction of fluorescein highlights the blood vessels and the capillaries.

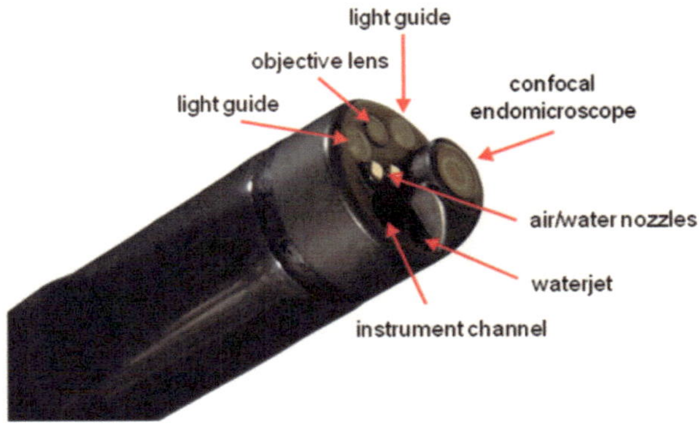

Fig. 1. Distal tip of the confocal endomicroscope EC-3870CIFK (Pentax, Europe) used in gastrointestinal endoscopy. As a protrusion on the end of a conventional endoscope a microscopic lens is mounted (diameter of the lens is 5 mm). All other features of the distal tip are standard in routine endoscopy.

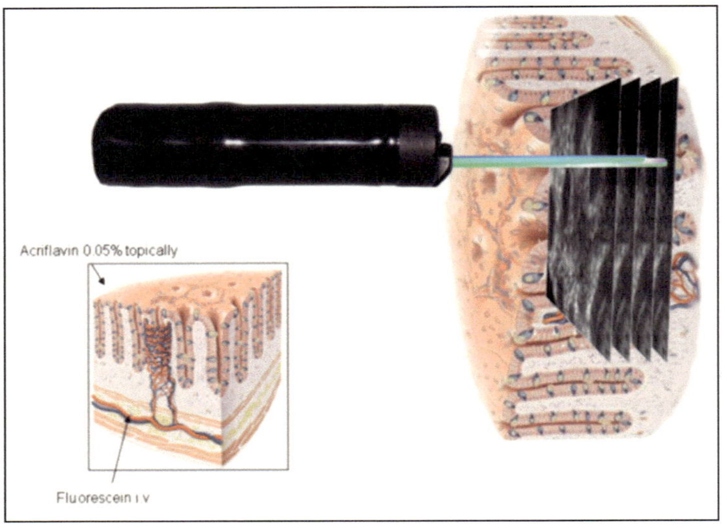

Fig. 2. (With kind permission of Peter Delaney, Optiscan, Australia and Ralf Kiesslich, University Medicine Mainz, Germany). The use of confocal endomicroscopy in human gastrointestinal tract. When the confocal lens was hold in gentle contact with the gastrointestinal mucosa, blue laser light generated a series of images every 7μm up to an imaging depth of 250μm. Typical contrast dyes were fluorescein and acriflavine as indicated.

Topically applied acriflavine hydrochloride (0.05% in saline, Sigma Aldrich, Germany) accentuates the superficial cell borders and their nuclei (Hoffman et al., 2006). Acriflavine is not approved for the use in humans due to a low but theoretical risk of inducing mutagenesis as described in cell culture systems (Ferenc et al., 1999). However, in special clinical indications there are several studies in which this substance was used safely (Leong et al., 2008) (Günther et al., 2010).

3. Pilot study

In our pilot study NLM was performed in an ex vivo approach on small tissue samples of patients suspicious to suffer from GBM (WHO IV, n=9) or meningeoma (grade I n=2, grade II n=1) after diagnostic radiology. Open tumor resection was performed in the neurosurgical OR in all patients. No prior histological diagnosis was available before neurosurgery. One sample of tumor tissue was used for direct comparison of NLM and histopathology of the same area. After the examination with NLM the specimen was transferred to neuropathology for conventional tissue examination. Additional fragments of the tumor center and border were analysed by NLM. Different additional fragments were sent for conventional pathological diagnosis. These were not marked as study material and therefore assessment and diagnosis was blinded.

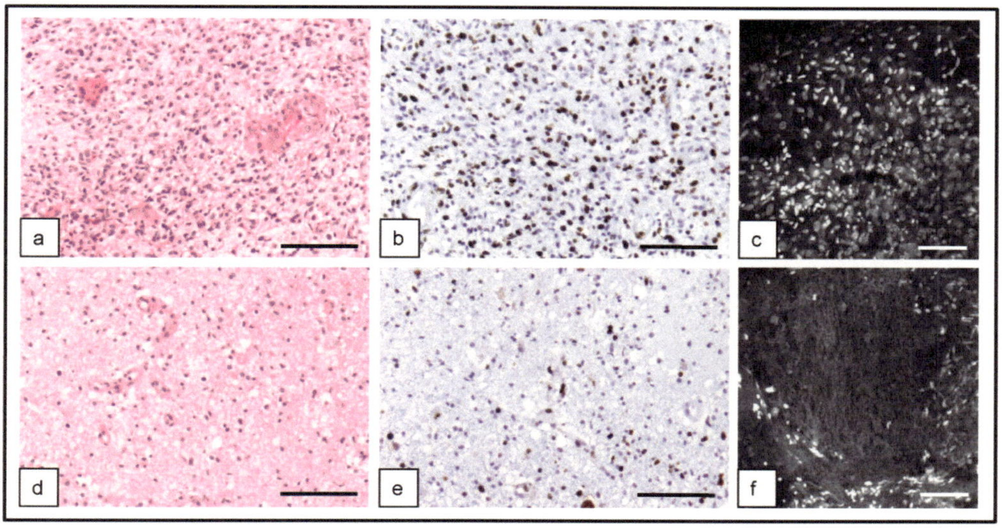

Fig. 3. (Removed with approval Schlosser, Cen Eur Neurosurg, 2010, 71(1):13-9) Histopathology and Neurolasermicroscopy (NLM) of a GBM (a-f same patient, a-c center; d-f infiltration zone, bar = 100 µm). a, d: H&E staining of tumor border (a) and infiltration zone (d). H&E staining of tumor center shows a high density of tumor cells; b, e: immunohistochemical staining with MIB-1antibody to assess proliferation in tumor center (b) and infiltration zone (e). c, f: NLM of tumor center (c) and infiltration zone (f) with detection of a high density of tumor cells in the center and markedly reduced cell density in the infiltration zone. The margin of the tumor appears similar to a parabolic curve.

Frozen sections were done in 4 out of the 9 patients with GBM and all patients with meningeoma (n=3). It was beyond the scope of the present study to directly compare the diagnostic outcome of frozen sections, conventional histology and NLM even because all patients had a final histological confirmation of glioblastoma or meningeoma. However, we see some future indications for NLM to contribute to a rapid diagnosis intraoperatively and to reduce the proportion of frozen sections reasonably.

After the tissue sample was coated with acriflavine 0.05% the NLM device was hold in gentle contact with the surface of the tumor and confocal scanning process was initiated. Histological processing included staining with hematoxylin and eosin (HE), periodic acidic Schiff (PAS), silver-impregnation for reticulin or immunohistochemical staining.

Histopathology was performed according to the criteria for GBM of the recent WHO classification respecting the exceptions and subtypes (Louis et al., 2007). In nine patients with histologically proven GBM, in which no case of "small cell glioblastoma" or glioblastoma with oligodendroglial component" occurred, the presence of the following WHO criteria for GBM were analysed in the NLM obtained images: a) cell number and density, b) cell pleomorphy, c) mitotic figures and rate of mitosis (high, moderate, low), d) microvascular proliferation and e) pseudopalisading necrosis. Diagnosis and specific findings of NLM images and conventional histopathology were compared when all data were available. In three patients with histologically proven meningeoma typical features were visible with NLM including pleomorphy, onion-skin shaped appearance of tumor cells and single apoptotic cells.

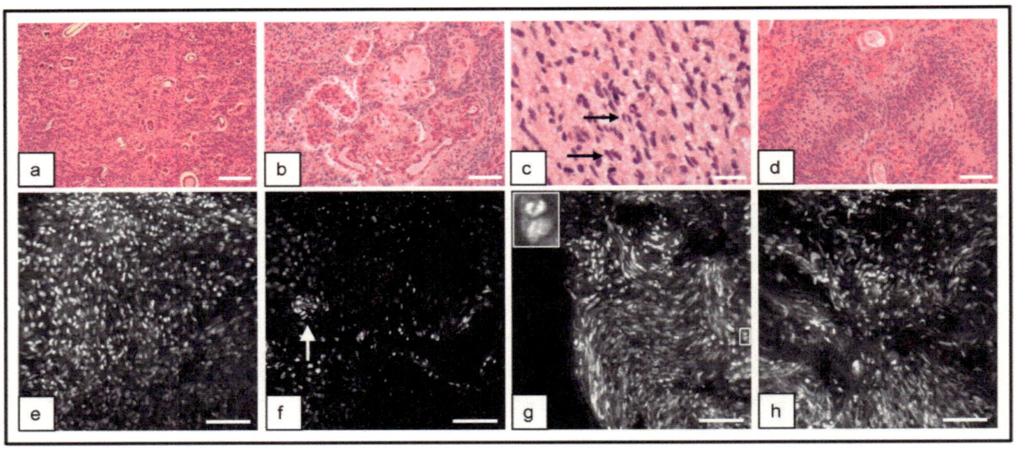

Fig. 4. (Removed with approval Schlosser, Cen Eur Neurosurg, 2010, 71(1):13-9) Histology (H&E; a-d, bar = 100 µm; c, bar = 50 µm) and NLM (e-h, bar = 100 µm) of WHO criteria for the diagnosis of GBM. a, e: tumor center with a high density of pleomorphic tumor cells. b, f: microvascular proliferation within the tumor formation (arrow). c, g: mitotic figures (arrows in c, square in g), higher magnification in g shows the mitosis within the nucleus (inset). d, h: pseudopalisading necrosis.

NLM was an easy to handle tool and revealed in all nine patients with GBM and three patients with meningeoma typical characteristics of tumor architecture. This unique technique provided evaluable scans for all patients with GBM from the center and from the border depicting the differences of both areas. The overall image quality was good. In one patient with GBM the scanning images directly correspond to conventional histopathology in all five diagnostic aspects. The WHO criteria for the diagnosis of GBM - cell density, cell pleomorphy, mitoses, microvascular proliferation and pseudopalisading or ischemic necrosis - were all detectable by NLM.

Identification of the infiltration zone or the center of the tumor was possible in any patient by determination of the cell density comparing center and border resection bloc (Fig 3). Further WHO criteria for tumor classification to identify GBM were compared to histology in the same resection bloc and were identified in some but not all patients (Fig. 4).

The NLM images of nine patients with histologically proven GBM were analysed for the presence of WHO criteria of GBM. In all 9 patients cell density and cell pleomorphy were clearly visible with NLM. In 44% of the patients (4/9) microvascular proliferation was visible and in 22% of the patients (2/9) mitosis and stroke like necrosis was identified.

Additional aspects, e.g. apoptotic figures in perinecrotic palisading tumor cells, and important histological structures such as giant cells, fibrillary tumor matrix and blood vessels were also visible with NLM (Fig. 5). Typical features of NLM in patients with histologically proven meningeoma are shown in Fig. 6.

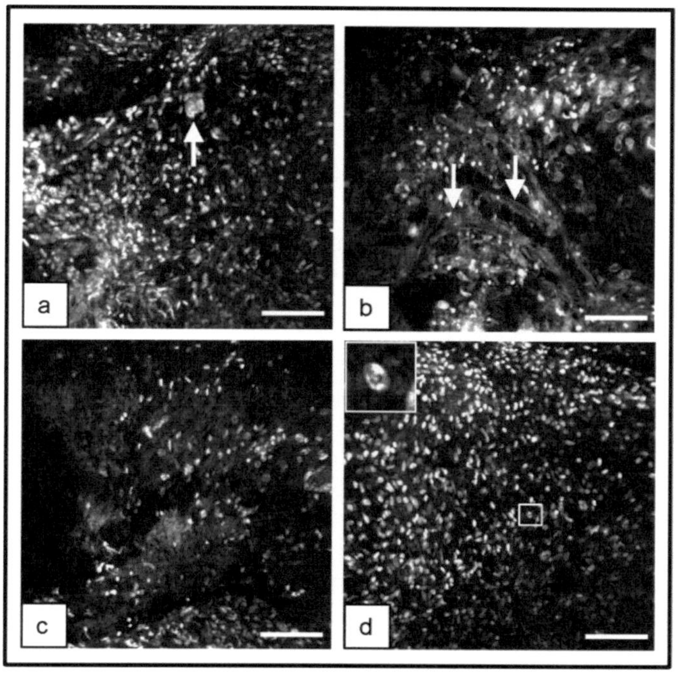

Fig. 5. (Removed with approval Schlosser, Cen Eur Neurosurg, 2010, 71(1):13-9) Additional findings of GBM with NLM (bar = 100 µm). a: giant cell within the tumor formation. b: pathological blood vessel, the thickened wall of the vessel is clearly visible (arrows). c: necrosis formation in the near of tumor cells. d: apoptotic figure within the tumor center (square), magnification shows characteristic chromatin fragments at the inner side of the nuclear membrane (inset).

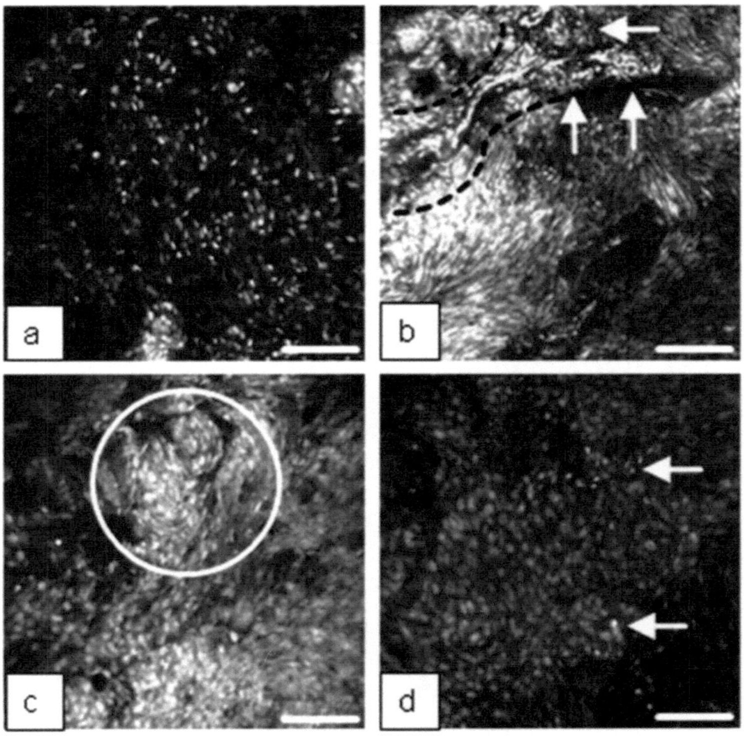

Fig. 6. Representative NLM images from patients with histologically proven meningeoma (n=3, bar = 100 µm). a: tumor center with a high density of pleomorphic tumor cells in grade II meningeoma, b: undirected tumor cells with a pathological blood vessel (in between the spotted line) and neoangiogenesis (arrows) in the same patient; c: typical onion-shaped tumor cell configuration in grade I meningeoma (circle), d: single apoptotic cells (arrows) in the tumor border in the same patient.

4. Discussion

Neurolasermicroscopy (NLM) was shown to recognize malignant brain tumor characteristics in patients with histologically proven GBM in our pilot feasibility study (Schlosser et al., 2009 (Epub)). There was a good accordance of the NLM images compared to the histopathological findings with respect to the WHO classification (Louis et al., 2007). The differentiation of more specific tumor entities by NLM should be performed after this promising technique is transferred into the intraoperative situation. Our ex vivo approach opened the door for a neurosurgical in vivo diagnosis on a cellular and subcellular level. Moreover, the combination of confocal laser microscopy and flexible video systems may promote a variety of potential developments eligible for neurosurgical procedures. This ranges from process optimization in the operating room (OR) to new ways to corroborate regenerative therapy (Wessels et al., 2007). Current research data showed the same technique we use in our pilot study to be useful in patients during neurosurgery (Sanai et al., 2011 (Epub), Schlosser, H.G., Bojarski, C. (2011 (Epub)). Confocal Neurolasermicroscopy (NLM). Neurosurgery, Epub,).

5. Definition of histological borders

Realizing in vivo histology during neurosurgery would contribute to a better definition of the histological borders of the tumor. This would improve the definition of the resection margins significantly. However, due to the infiltrative growth of many primary brain tumours it is not possible to clearly define the exact margins of a tumor mass in all cases, neither by conventional histology nor by NLM. The in vivo look on these areas from tumor to intact brain tissue (probably by using a histopathological NLM classification) could provide new insights towards a standardized diagnosis during neurosurgery.
On a cellular basis the excision could be performed as much as necessary but as little as possible which could be beneficial for patients suffering from a brain tumor (Lacroix et al., 2001) (Ammirati et al., 1987). The amount of residual tumor mass after surgery is one of the most important prognostic factors (Burger and Green, 1987) (Wood et al., 1988). NLM scans on a cellular and subcellular level could be more accurate than performing the whole investment of brain navigation even with shift correction (Asthagiri et al., 2007).
Regarding those aspects one has to focus on the appearance of the NLM scans depicting tumor pathologies. Cell types, cell division, neovascularisation and boarder zones have to become acquainted to the observer as well as th possibility for dynamic investigation. This histology is different from the appearance in classical histopathology. So neurosurgeon and pathologist have to share their insight and practically an atlas for defining all pathologies seen in NLM with regard for the process in the theatre has to be developed in the near future.

6. Targeted biopsies

Compared to conventional "random" brain tissue biopsies with the possibility of sampling errors NLM allowed "targeted" biopsies which could increase the reliability of the diagnosis when multiple cell types contribute to a tumor.

7. Potential indications

By using NLM the process of frozen sections could be influenced considerably. On the one hand thee cellular findings could be discussed between surgeon and pathologist demonstrating different areas and shifting the focus depending on the microscopic results which can affect the further direction of the procedure, on the other hand the NLM scans could be transferred directly to the pathologist via a network with marked reduction of the processing time for serial-cuts. This would also eliminate transfer time of the tissue bloc from the OR to the laboratory.

8. Molecular imaging

The presented scans show also vascular and important subcellular aspects contributing to the final diagnosis by predicting typical disease features. The options for biochemical or immunologic in vivo imaging by using antibodies or cell surface markers can be evaluated in the future after establishing NLM as an in vivo tool for neurosurgery providing a cellular and subcellular view. This subcellular view already enabled physiologic investigations in skin (Lademann et al., 2007) (Suihko et al., 2005).

9. Further developments

The next step in evaluating NLM for a diagnostic approach in humans during ongoing neurosurgery would be to utilize an adapted miniaturized confocal instrument specially designed for neurosurgery applications. The technical settings for the laser system can be directly transferred from the system used in this study. However, one important problem should be addressed concerning the reprocessing of the microscopic device. The way of reprocessing will be an essential step to use the microscope in a sterile condition within routine neurosurgical procedures. The first data in humans during ongoing neurosurgery are meanwhile available (Sanai et al., 2011 (Epub), Schlosser, H.G., Bojarski, C. (2011 (Epub)). Neurosurgery, however the problem of reprocessing is not completely fixed. The confocal laser technique for the reusable equipment has been licensed by Zeiss, Germany, for neurosurgery from its initial developer in Australia. Here the integration of NLM into a conventional microscope system is advanced including the option of navigation and matching image-guidance data. A hand-held device has been designed and used in animal research (Sankar et al., 2010) and in humans (Schlosser, H.G., Bojarski, C. 2011 (Epub)). For the reusable system used in endoscopy in the last years a setrilizablility has not been achieved. So the application in routine neurosurgical procedures is severely limited. One has to think to introduce a disposable system which is already in clinical use for different applications. An adaptation of a reusable system could be the step to provide a confocal neurolasermicroscope for routine clinical use in neurosurgery.

Furthermore, the use of contrast agents has to be adapted to the in vivo situation. We would prefer using intravenously injected fluorescein (Makale, 2007) instead of topically applied acriflavine. Fluorescein is used for decades in ophthalmology and is permitted as a medical investigational drug with a very low rate of side effects (Lipson and Yannuzzi, 1989). Moreover, fluorescein is an established contrast agent in confocal endomicroscopy in gastroenterology where it distributes the entire gastrointestinal tissue up to 250 µm in depth (Hoffman et al., 2006). When fluorescein is applied in neurosurgery one has to consider the effect of passing the blood brain barrier (BBB), presumably only a small amount of serum albumin unbound fraction of fluorescein will pass BBB and the dye mainly stay intravascular. The amount of cellular staining has to be explored in further studies. In the neoplastic tissue the vessels probably will show a different pattern compared to healthy brain. We would expect abnormal branching and looping of the vasculature as well as abrupt changes in diameter contributing to stricture-like structures. The extravascular distribution of fluorescein, however, in a disturbed BBB as in neoplastic conditions may show the pathologic vascularisation in combination with a cellular staining.

The next step after defining the pathologies in an NLM atlas and after ascertain the affiliated operative proceeding clinical studies have to proof the benefit for the patients depending on the disease.

10. References

[1] Schlosser, H. G., Suess, O., Vajkoczy, P., van Landeghem, F. K., Zeitz, M. & Bojarski, C. (2009 (Epub)). Confocal neurolasermicroscopy in human brain - perspectives for neurosurgery on a cellular level (including additional comments to this article). *Cen Eur Neurosurg*, 71, 1, 13-19

[2] Lougheed, W. M. & Tom, M. (1961). A method of introducing blood into the subarachnoid space in the region of the circle of Willis in dogs. *Can J Surg.*, 4, 1, 329-37.

[3] Jacobson, J. H., 2nd, Wallman, L. J., Schumacher, G. A., Flanagan, M., Suarez, E. L. & Donaghy, R. M. (1962). Microsurgery as an aid to middle cerebral artery endarterectomy. *J Neurosurg*, 19, 108-15

[4] Chou, S. N. (1963). Embolectomy of Middle Cerebral Artery: Report of a Case. *J Neurosurg*, 20, 161-3

[5] Woringer, E. & Kunlin, J. (1963). [Anastomosis between the Common Carotid and the Intracranial Carotid or the Sylvian Artery by a Graft, Using the Suspended Suture Technic.]. *Neurochirurgie*, 200, 181-8

[6] Lougheed, W. M., Marshall, B. M., Hunter, M., Michel, E. R. & Sandwith-Smyth, H. (1971). Common carotid to intracranial internal carotid bypass venous graft. Technical note. *J Neurosurg*, 34, 1, 114-8

[7] Pool, J. L. & Colton, R. P. (1966). The dissecting microscope for intracranial vascular surgery. *J Neurosurg*, 25, 3, 315-8

[8] Rand, R. W. & Jannetta, P. J. (1967). Micro-neurosurgery for aneurysms of the vertebral-basilar artery system. *J Neurosurg*, 27, 4, 330-5

[9] Stummer, W., Pichlmeier, U., Meinel, T., Wiestler, O. D., Zanella, F. & Reulen, H. J. (2006). Fluorescence-guided surgery with 5-aminolevulinic acid for resection of malignant glioma: a randomised controlled multicentre phase III trial. *Lancet Oncol*, 7, 5, 392-401

[10] Stummer, W., Stocker, S., Wagner, S., Stepp, H., Fritsch, C., Goetz, C., Goetz, A. E., Kiefmann, R. & Reulen, H. J. (1998). Intraoperative detection of malignant gliomas by 5-aminolevulinic acid-induced porphyrin fluorescence. *Neurosurgery*, 42, 3, 518-25; discussion 525-6

[11] Read, T. A., Farhadi, M., Bjerkvig, R., Olsen, B. R., Rokstad, A. M., Huszthy, P. C. & Vajkoczy, P. (2001). Intravital microscopy reveals novel antivascular and antitumor effects of endostatin delivered locally by alginate-encapsulated cells. *Cancer Res*, 61, 18, 6830-7

[12] Vajkoczy, P., Ullrich, A. & Menger, M. D. (2000). Intravital fluorescence videomicroscopy to study tumor angiogenesis and microcirculation. *Neoplasia*, 2, 1-2, 53-61

[13] Kiesslich, R., Burg, J., Vieth, M., Gnaendiger, J., Enders, M., Delaney, P., Polglase, A., McLaren, W., Janell, D., Thomas, S., Nafe, B., Galle, P. & Neurath, M. (2004). Confocal laser endoscopy for diagnosing intraepithelial neoplasias and colorectal cancer in vivo. *Gastroenterology*, 127, 706-713

[14] Bojarski, C., Günther, U., Rieger, K., Heller, F., Loddenkemper, C., Grünbaum, M., Uharek, L., Zeitz, M. & Hoffmann, J. (2009). In vivo diagnosis of acute intestinal graft-versus-host disease by confocal endomicroscopy. *Endoscopy*, 41, 433-438

[15] Hoffman, A., Goetz, M., Vieth, M., Galle, P. R., Neurath, M. F. & Kiesslich, R. (2006). Confocal laser endomicroscopy: technical status and current indications. *Endoscopy*, 38, 12, 1275-83

[16] Ferenc, T., Janik-Spiechowicz, E., Bratkowska, W. & Denys, A. (1999). Mutagenic activity of 3,6-diamino-10-methyl-9,10-dihydroacridine in Salmonella typhimurium cells. *Int J Occup Med Environ Health*, 12, 67-72

[17] Leong, R., Nguyen, N., Meredith, C., Al-Sohaily, S., Kukic, D., Delaney, P., Murr, E., Yong, J., Merrett, N. & Biankin, A. (2008). In vivo confocal endomicroscopy in the diagnosis and evaluation of celiac disease. *Gastroenterology,* 135, 1870-1876

[18] Günther, U., Daum, S., Heller, F., Schumann, M., Loddenkemper, C., Grünbaum, M., Zeitz, M. & Bojarski, C. (2010). Diagnostic value of confocal endomicroscopy in celiac disease. *Endoscopy,* 42, 3, 197-202

[19] Louis, D. N., Ohgaki, H., Wiestler, O. D., Cavenee, W. K., Burger, P. C., Jouvet, A., Scheithauer, B. W. & Kleihues, P. (2007). The 2007 WHO classification of tumours of the central nervous system. *Acta Neuropathol,* 114, 2, 97-109

[20] Wessels, J. T., Busse, A. C., Mahrt, J., Dullin, C., Grabbe, E. & Mueller, G. A. (2007). In vivo imaging in experimental preclinical tumor research--a review. *Cytometry A,* 71, 8, 542-9

[21] Sanai, N., Eschbacher, J., Hattendorf , G., Coons, S. W., Preul, M. C., Smith, K. A., Nakaji, P. & Spetzler, R. F. (2011 (Epub)). Intraoperative Confocal Microscopy for Brain Tumors: A Feasibility Analysis in Humans. *Neurosurgery,* Epub,

[22] Schlosser, H.G., Bojarski, C. (2011 (Epub)). Confocal Neurolasermicroscopy (NLM). Neurosurgery, Epub

[23] Lacroix, M., Abi-Said, D., Fourney, D. R., Gokaslan, Z. L., Shi, W., DeMonte, F., Lang, F. F., McCutcheon, I. E., Hassenbusch, S. J., Holland, E., Hess, K., Michael, C., Miller, D. & Sawaya, R. (2001). A multivariate analysis of 416 patients with glioblastoma multiforme: prognosis, extent of resection, and survival. *J Neurosurg,* 95, 2, 190-8

[24] Ammirati, M., Vick, N., Liao, Y. L., Ciric, I. & Mikhael, M. (1987). Effect of the extent of surgical resection on survival and quality of life in patients with supratentorial glioblastomas and anaplastic astrocytomas. *Neurosurgery,* 21, 2, 201-6

[25] Burger, P. C. & Green, S. B. (1987). Patient age, histologic features, and length of survival in patients with glioblastoma multiforme. *Cancer,* 59, 9, 1617-25

[26] Wood, J. R., Green, S. B. & Shapiro, W. R. (1988). The prognostic importance of tumor size in malignant gliomas: a computed tomographic scan study by the Brain Tumor Cooperative Group. *J Clin Oncol,* 6, 2, 338-43

[27] Asthagiri, A. R., Pouratian, N., Sherman, J., Ahmed, G. & Shaffrey, M. E. (2007). Advances in brain tumor surgery. *Neurol Clin,* 25, 4, 975-1003, viii-ix

[28] Lademann, J., Otberg, N., Richter, H., Meyer, L., Audring, H., Teichmann, A., Thomas, S., Knuttel, A. & Sterry, W. (2007). Application of optical non-invasive methods in skin physiology: a comparison of laser scanning microscopy and optical coherent tomography with histological analysis. *Skin Res Technol,* 13, 2, 119-32

[29] Suihko, C., Swindle, L. D., Thomas, S. G. & Serup, J. (2005). Fluorescence fibre-optic confocal microscopy of skin in vivo: microscope and fluorophores. *Skin Res Technol,* 11, 4, 254-67

[30] Sankar, T., Delaney, P. M., Ryan, R. W., Eschbacher, J., Abdelwahab, M., Nakaji, P., Coons, S. W., Scheck, A. C., Smith, K. A., Spetzler, R. F. & Preul, M. C. (2010). Miniaturized handheld confocal microscopy for neurosurgery: results in an experimental glioblastoma model. *Neurosurgery,* 66, 2, 410-417

[31] Makale, M. (2007). Intravital imaging and cell invasion. *Methods Enzymol,* 426, 375-401

[32] Lipson, B. K. & Yannuzzi, L. A. (1989). Complications of intravenous fluorescein injections. *Int Ophthalmol Clin,* 29, 3, 200-5

20

Ultrafractionated Radiation Therapy (3 Daily Doses of 0.75 Gy) - A New and Promising Radiotherapy Schedule for Glioblastoma Patients

Patrick Beauchesne
Neuro-Oncology Department,
CHU de NANCY
France

1. Introduction

Malignant glioma is one of the most radio-resistant tumor types and accounts for approximately 60% of all primary brain tumors in adults (Behin et al., 2003; Black, 1991a, 1991b; DeAngelis, 2001). There are three distinct histological types: anaplastic astrocytoma (AA), anaplastic oligodendroglioma (AO), and glioblastoma multiforme (GBM). The prognosis of malignant glioma patients remains dismal (Behin et al., 2003; Black, 1991a, 1991b; De Angelis, 2001). The median survival for patients with newly diagnosed GBM is 8 to 15 months, prognosis is slightly better for newly diagnosed AA with a median survival of 24 to 36 months, and the prognosis for AO gives a median survival of 60 months (Behin et al., 2003; Black, 1991a, 1991b; De Angelis, 2001). For AA and GBM, the standard of care consists of surgical resection of as much of the tumor as is considered to be safe, followed by radiation and chemotherapy and has been so for many decades (Behin et al., 2003; Black, 1991a, 1991b; DeAngelis, 2001, Fine et al., 1993; Stewart, 2002; Walker et al., 1978, 1980). A new standard procedure for GBM has recently been defined by the EORTC phase III trial which randomized patients in two groups, receiving either temozolomide (TMZ) concomitant and adjuvant to radiation therapy or radiation therapy alone (Stupp et al., 2005). A significant increase in overall survival (OS) was seen in the radiation therapy plus TMZ group compared to the radiation therapy alone group. Survival rates were respectively 14.6 and 12.1 months. For AO, the standard treatment is surgical resection followed by radiation therapy (Stupp et al., 2005). Adjuvant chemotherapy does not provide significant benefits in OS (Van den Bent et al., 2006).

Radiation therapy remains the backbone of care for glioblastomas, even in patients who have undergone a prior presumed complete resection. The infiltrative nature of these tumors makes a truly complete resection nearly impossible in most cases (Behin et al., 2003; Black, 1991a, 1991b; DeAngelis, 2001, Fine et al., 1993; Hall, 1978; Stewart, 2002; Walker et al., 1978, 1980). Standard fractionated radiation therapy delivers a total radiation dose of 60 Gy given in 30 fractions over 6 weeks. The target is usually the tumor bulk as visualized on CT or MRI, with a wide margin of 2-3 cm (Behin et al., 2003; Black, 1991a, 1991b; DeAngelis,

2001, Fine et al., 1993; Hall, 1978; Stewart, 2002; Walker et al., 1978, 1980). Although radiation therapy is not a curative treatment for glioblastomas, it results in prolongation of life with optimized quality (Behin et al., 2003; Black, 1991a, 1991b; DeAngelis, 2001, Fine et al., 1993; Stewart, 2002; Walker et al., 1978, 1980). Whether the clinical radioresistance of GBM is due solely to inherent radioresistance at the cellular level is unclear. Overall, malignant glioma cell lines exhibit SF2 (SF - 2 Gy) values at the upper end of the range compared with other human tumor cell lines, though studies have failed to link clinical response with SF2 (Taghian, 1992, 1993). Defining the molecular basis of radioresistance is, therefore, important. Disruption of cell-cycle arrest or apoptotic pathways by *INK4a* loss or by *p53* mutations or inactivation (approx. 40–60% of malignant gliomas have *p53* mutations) associated with *CDK4* amplification or *Rb* loss may be significant factors in determining the response of these tumors to irradiation and treatment outcome (James & Olson, 1986; Kleihues & Ohgaki, 1999, Watanabe et al., 1996).

The radiation survival response of mammalian cells is more complicated than once believed. A few studies indicate that some human cell lines are sensitive to killing by low radiation doses (1 Gy). This has been termed *low-dose hyper-radiosensitivity* (HRS) (Joiner et al., 1986; Lambin et al., 1994b, 1996; Marples et al., 1997; Short et al., 1999b; Turesson & Joiner, 1996). This phenomenon is more apparent in radioresistant cell lines such as glioma cells, and is substantially underestimated by the linear-quadratic (LQ) model (Joiner et al., 1986; Lambin et al., 1994b, 1996; Marples et al., 1997; Short et al., 1999b, 2001; Turesson & Joiner, 1996; Wouters et al., 1996). It may reflect differential triggering or induction of repair mechanisms. Cells may be sensitive to low doses because repair mechanisms are not induced, whereas higher doses may cause enough damage to induce or trigger repair mechanisms and, therefore, exhibit increased radioresistance (Joiner et al., 1986; Lambin et al., 1994b, 1996; Marples et al., 1997; Short et al., 1999b, 2001; Turesson & Joiner, 1996; Wouters et al., 1996). Still, new modalities of radiation therapy are urgently needed.

2. *In Vitro* studies

2.1 Cell lines experiments

The GRAY laboratory first demonstrated an increased X-ray sensitivity in murine skin and kidney after very low doses per fraction (Joiner & Denekamp, 1986; Joiner et al., 1986; Joiner & Johns, 1988). They irradiated the V79 murine fibroblast cell line with 250kVp X-rays and measured cell survival with a Dynamic Microscopic Imaging Processing Scanner (DMIPS) cell analyzer (Joiner et al., 1993a; Marples et al., 1994). Briefly, 3000-5000 cells were plated into 25 cm^2 tissue culture flasks and left to incubate for 4 to 6 hours at 37° C. The flasks were removed from the incubator halfway through the initial 4-6 hour incubation period, the medium removed, and the flasks were then immediately completely refilled with fresh medium before being sealed. Following irradiation, the DMIPS cell analyser was used to locate and record the positions of 300-400 isolated cells within 10 cm^2 in the centre of each flask. After 6-7 days of incubation at 37°C, all the originally recorded cell locations were revisited to assay for colony formation using a criterion for survival of 50 cells or more per colony as determined by manual microscopic examination of each selected location in the flask (Marples et al., 1994). The results displayed an increased X-ray sensitivity (hypersensitivity) after very small doses (< 0.3 Gy), followed by an increase in survival after the doses increased from 0.3 – 1 Gy (Joiner et al., 1993a; Marples et al., 1994). The first phenomenon was defined and termed "low-dose hyper-radiosensitivity" (HRS), and the second phenomenon "increased radio-resistance" (IRR) (Joiner et al., 1986; Lambin et al., 1994b, 1996; Marples et al., 1997; Short et al., 1999b, 2001; Turesson & Joiner, 1996; Wouters et al., 1996). While the LQ model underestimates the HRS phenomenon, it correlates to the data at doses ranging from 2 - 5 Gy. HRS was represented as an undeniable downward "kink" on survival curve for doses below 1 Gy (Fig. 1). This was demonstrated by Wouters et al using the flow cytometry survival (FACS) method thus showing that it was not merely an artifact associated with the DMIPS assay (Wouters & Skarsgard, 1994). HRS has also been triggered in the human lung epithelial cell line, L132, after exposition to very low-doses of X-rays (Singh et al., 19974), and found with Chinese Hamster cells (Joiner et al., 1993a; Marples et al., 1994).

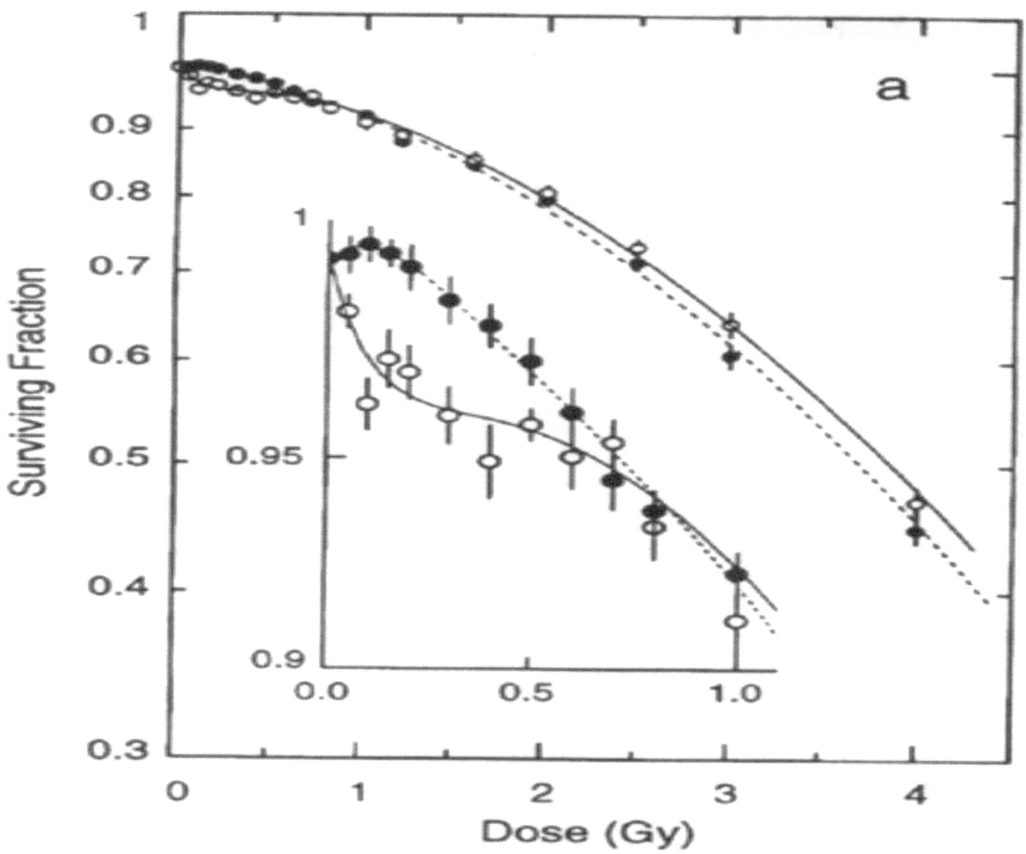

Fig. 1. Low-dose hypersensitivity was represented as an undeniable downward "kink" on survival curve for doses below 1 Gy, followed for doses superior to 2 Gy by "IRR" or "increased radio-resistance" phenomenon.

Lambin et al irradiated the HT 29 cell line, derived from a human colorectal tumor and considered as a radio-resistant tumor at usual X-ray doses, with single-doses of X-rays from 0.05 to 5 Gy. They focused on cell survival at doses of less than 1 Gy, using the DMIPS cell analyzer (Lambin et al., 1993a, 1993b). At doses < 0.5 Gy, an increased X-ray sensitivity was observed. The HT 29 cell line was also irradiated with neutrons [d(4)-Be], obtained by a Van de Graaff accelerator bombarding a thick beryllium target with 4 MeV deuterons, at a dose rate of 0-20 Gy/min, but no HRS was observed (Lambin et al., 1993a, 1993b). In another study, Lambin et al studied an RT 112 cell line derived from a bladder carcinoma (Lambin et al., 1994a, 1994b). At a survival fraction of 60 % at 2 Gy (SF 2 Gy) this tumor was considered to be as radio-resistant (Lambin et al., 1994a, 1994b). The cell line was irradiated with low doses X-ray, and the HRS phenomenon observed at doses of < 0.5 Gy using the DMIPS method (Lambin et al., 1994a, 1994b).

The cell lines Be 11 and MeWo derived from melanoma, SW 48 from a colorectal tumor, and HX 142 from a neuroblastoma were irradiated with low doses X-ray as described above (Lambin et al., 1996). The cell line Be 11 was considered as radio-resistant - the SF 2 Gy ranged from 60 to 70 % - but the cell lines MeWo, SW 48 and HX 142 were radio-sensitive tumors with an SF 2 Gy ranging from 3 to 29 % (Lambin et al., 1996). The response obtained for doses ranging from 2 – 5 Gy for all cell lines fit with the LQ model, but HRS at doses < 0.5 Gy was not observed for the cell lines MeWo, SW 48 and HX 142 (Lambin et al., 1996). This absence of HRS in radiosensitive cell lines could be explained by the decreased inducible response of these cell lines (Lambin et al., 1996).

Human glioblastoma is considered to be one of the most radio-resistant tumors. Short et al studied five human glioblastoma cell lines, T98G – A7 – U87MG – U138 – HGL21, and one cell line derived from an anaplastic astrocytoma, U373 (Short et al., 1999a, 1999b). All the cell lines were irradiated with low doses of X-ray (Short et al., 1999a, 1999b). Survival time was calculated for the T98G – A7 – U373T9 lines using the DMIPS method. Survival time for U87MG – U138 – HGL21 which are not suitable for the DMIPS methods, were obtained from the cell shorter (CS) protocol as modified by Wouters et al (Wouters et al., 1996). HRS was noted at very low doses of X-rays in all five of the human glioblastoma cell lines, and most markedly in the A7 – U138 – TG98 cell lines (Short et al., 1999a, 1999b). The grade III cell line, U373, did not express HRS, though no clear explanation for this was put forward; possibly limitations of the CS methods or because this cell line could expresses HRS at much lower doses than is technically possible to test (Short et al., 1999a, 1999b).

To date, the low-dose responses have been reported by several laboratories in more than 26 different human cell lines, and survival times obtained using both DMIPS and the colony assay formation (CFA) (Beauchesne et al., 2003; Joiner et al., 1986, 1993a, 1993b; Lambin et al., 1993a, 1993b, 1994a, 1994b, 1994c, 1996; Marples et al., 1994, 1997; Short et al., 1999a, 1999b, 2001; Singh et al., 1994; Turesson & Joiner, 1996; Wouters et al., 1994, 1996). These include cell lines from colorectal carcinoma, bladder carcinoma, melanoma, prostate carcinoma, cervical squamous carcinoma, lung adenocarcinoma, neuroblastoma, gliomas, one non-malignant lung epithelial line, and one primary human fibroblast line.

Beauchesne et al also studied the HRS phenomenon in a French laboratory, using a linear accelerator to deliver the daily the radiation therapy for hospitalized patients (Beauchesne et al., 2003; Pedeux et al., 2003). The following human malignant cell lines established in this laboratory and previously described were tested; G5 – CL35 (a clone derived from G5) – G111 – G142 – G152. Cell survival was calculated from the CFA technique. Three hours after plating, cells were exposed to X-rays delivered by a linear accelerator (X photons of 10 MeV, dose rate of 2.43 Gy/min) with the irradiator placed at a distance of 1 m from the target, and an irradiation field of 40 X 40 cm (Beauchesne et al., 2003; Pedeux et al., 2003). The irradiation doses ranged from 0.2 to 2 Gy. HRS was once more reported at doses lower than 1 Gy for the glioma cell lines G5-G111-G142-G152, though, CL35, a regular sub-clone of G5, failed to express this HRS phenomenon (Fig. 2) (Beauchesne et al., 2003; Pedeux et al., 2003).

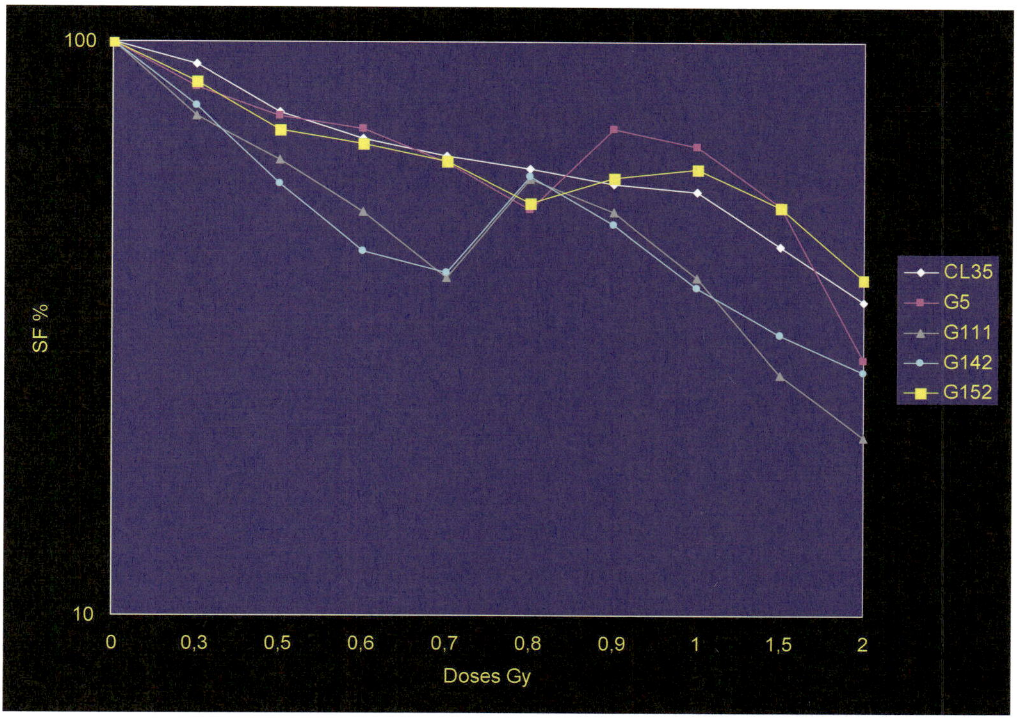

Fig. 2. Survival of human glioma cells following irradiation. Cells were irradiated with 0–2 Gy. G111, G142 and G152 glioma cell lines display HRS at doses below 1 Gy. HRS was observed only with G5 cells, whereas its clone, CL35, displayed conventional sensitivity to radiation therapy.

The authors demonstrated HRS in four human melanoma tumor cell lines, M4Be - A375P - MeWo - SKMe12, at doses below 1 Gy, and in the MRC5 human fibroblast cell strain (Beauchesne et al., 2003; Pedeux et al., 2003). HRS was not expressed in two radio-sensitive cell lines, H460 (from a lung cancer) and MCF7 (from breast cancer) (Beauchesne et al., 2003; Pedeux et al., 2003).
The same team (Beauchesne et al) also tested the chemotherapy combination etoposide - temozolomide concomitantly with low-doses fractions on the human glioblastoma cell lines, G5 - G142 - G152 (Beauchesne et al., 2003; Pedeux et al., 2003). Cells were incubated immediately after an ultrafractionated irradiation regimen with etoposide and temozolomide at determined doses for 24 hours. A marked radio-sensizitation effect was observed with the CL35 line, and an enhancement of the HRS phenomenon was reported for G142 and G152 (Beauchesne et al., 2003; Pedeux et al., 2003). Thus, the combination of chemotherapy and radiotherapy enhances the effects of the therapies, thus further improving the effect of repeated low-radiation doses on malignant glioma cells (Beauchesne et al., 2003; Pedeux et al., 2003).

2.2 Repeated irradiations

Short et al in another set of experiments using the T98G human cell line (derived from a human glioblastoma), tested low-doses irradiations given at < 0.5 Gy once or more daily

(Short et al., 1994a, 2001). Cell survival was calculated by DMIPS cell assay after 15 fractions of 0.4 Gy, given three times a day and compared to the same total dose given as once-daily 1.2 Gy. The low-doses were administered at 4-hours intervals (09.00 - 13.00 - 17.00 hours) each day for 5 consecutive days, and the single dose of 1.2 Gy was also given for 5 consecutive days (Short et al., 1994a, 2001). The repeated low-doses produced a significantly increased tumor cell kill; cell survival after three consecutive 0.4 Gy fractions was lower than after the same total dose given as a single fraction (1.2 Gy), the difference was significant ($p<0.0002$) (Short et al., 1994a, 2001). Cell survival after 2 Gy single doses was not different to that obtained after three consecutive 0.4 Gy fractions (Short et al., 1994a, 2001).Two other human glioblastoma cell lines, A7 - U87, were also tested: the lowest cell survival occurred with doses administered at 4 and 6 hours intervals for A7 and at 1 and 5 hours intervals for U87 (Short et al., 1994a, 2001). The cell line U373 (obtained from a human astrocytoma grade III) did not express HRS phenomenon, repeated low-doses did not enhance cell killing (Short et al., 1994a, 2001). The conclusions of this work were that multiple low-doses (< 1 Gy) per day spaced at appropriate intervals (4 hours) could increase cell killing by the enhancing he HRS phenomenon (Short et al., 1994a, 2001). The authors termed this multiple low-doses per fraction per day as an "ultrafractionated regimen" (Short et al., 1994a, 2001).

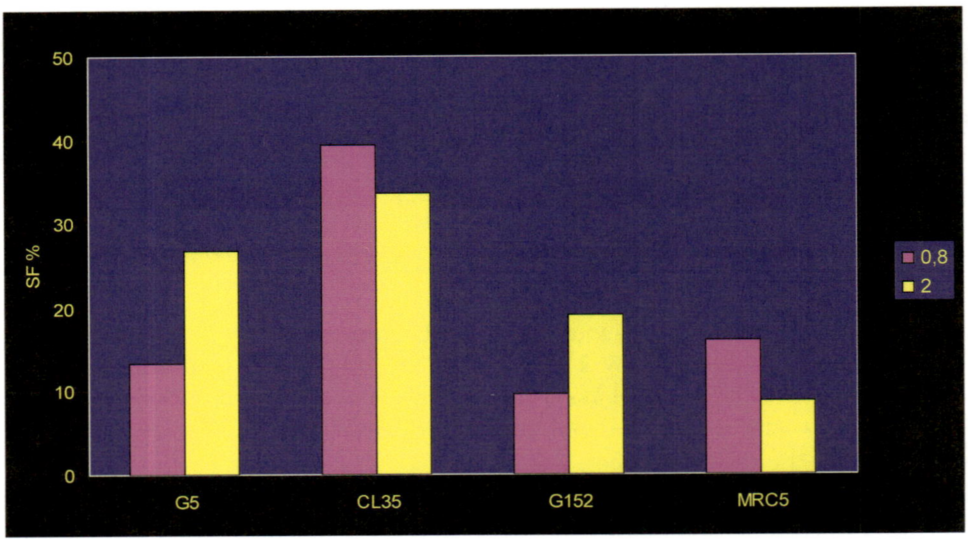

Fig. 3. Survival of human glioma cells following repeated irradiations. G5, CL35, G152 or MRC5 cells were exposed to 0.8 Gy 3 times/day spaced by 4 hr for 2 consecutive days or to 2 Gy once/day for 2 consecutive days. Cell survival was assessed by a clonogenic assay.

Beauchesne et al also tested the cumulative effect of low radiation doses on cell survival on the following human glioblastoma cell lines; G5 - CL35 - G152 (Beauchesne et al., 2003; Pedeux et al., 2003). Three fractions of 0.8 Gy spaced at 4 hour intervals were compared to a biologically equivalent single dose of 2 Gy. Irradiations were given for 2 consecutive days. A marked increase in cell killing was reported with the ultrafractionated regimen (repeated low-doses) in the G5 and G152 cell lines, but not in the CL35 cell line (Fig. 3) (Beauchesne et al., 2003; Pedeux et al., 2003). The experiments were repeated with a linear accelerator used daily for clinical therapies for patients. G5 and CL35 cell lines were exposed to 0.8 Gy, three times per day, spaced at 4 hour intervals for 2 consecutive days and to 2.4 Gy once a day for

2 days. Again, a marked and significant increase in cell killing occurred after the repeated low-doses for G5 but not the CL35 cell line (Beauchesne et al., 2003; Pedeux et al., 2003). It was postulated that te HRS phenomenon was responsible for the lower cell survival obtained after ultrafractionated regimen (Beauchesne et al., 2003; Pedeux et al., 2003).

3. *In Vivo* experiments

The first study which tested ultrafractionated irradiation on an animal model was reported by Beck-Bornholdt; the rat rhabdomyosarcoma R1H was irradiated with 126 fractions over 6 weeks. Top-up irradiations were not given (different doses per fraction between 0.43 and 0.71 Gy were applied) (Beck-Bornholdt et al., 1989). The results were compared to "historical control", and the authors demonstrated that the ultrafractionated regimen was slight more effective than the conventional approach (Beck-Bornholdt et al., 1989).

With a view to demonstrating a potential therapeutic benefit of the ultrafractionated irradiation schedule for malignant glioma patients, Beauchesne et al tested the fractionated low-dose irradiation in a glioma animal model, previously developed by the same team, on the G152 cell line (Beauchesne et al., 2003; Pedeux et al., 2003). Briefly the model was developed as follows; G152 malignant glioma cells (2 x10^6) suspended in 0.1 ml of PBS were subcutaneously injected into the inter-scapular region of 4-week-old mice (female nude mice, Swiss *nu/nu*). Drinking water was supplemented with estrone (0.1 ml/100 ml of water) until death of the animal. Two perpendicular diameters (D1 and D2) of the tumors were measured once a week and tumor volume calculated from the following equation: $(D1 + D2/2)^3 X (\pi/6)$ (Beauchesne et al., 2003; Pedeux et al., 2003). G152 xenograft tumors were grown for 17 days, and the mice were then exposed to either 0.8 Gy per fraction (3 times per day, spaced at 4 hour intervals, 4 days per week, for 2 consecutive weeks) or to a single dose of 2 Gy (once per day, 4 days per week, for 2 consecutive weeks). Another arm of tumor-bearing mice were not treated. The ultrafractionated irradiation was delivered by a clinical linear accelerator, with the mice immobilized in plastic tubes, and only the tumor exposed to the irradiation (Beauchesne et al., 2003; Pedeux et al., 2003).

Tumors grew faster in the untreated mice with an average tumor volume at week 12 of 1223 mm^3. As expected, radiation therapy had a therapeutic effect on the tumor growth resulting in an inhibition of tumor growth of 80-90 % (Beauchesne et al., 2003; Pedeux et al., 2003). At week 12, tumor volume of the mice in the ultrafractionated arm (repeated low-doses) was half that of the mice in the standard treatment arm (single dose, each day) representing a highly significant difference (p=0.0022) (Beauchesne et al., 2003; Pedeux et al., 2003). A second experiment gave similar results with neuropathology analysis revealed that the grafted tumor had the same characteristics as the initial human primary glioma tumor from which the G152 was obtained.

To further assert the therapeutic efficiency of ultrafractionated regimen, a third experiment was performed to compare the irradiation regimens for the same total doses (Beauchesne et al., 2003; Pedeux et al., 2003). Seventeen days after grafting, the mice were exposed to either 0.8 Gy, 3 times/day spaced at 4 hour intervals 5 days/week for 2 consecutive weeks (total dose = 24 Gy) or to 2.4 Gy once/day 5 days/week for 2 consecutive weeks (total dose = 24 Gy). Another group of mice was left untreated. Tumor size was measured once a week. As previously demonstrated, the ultrafractionated regimen led to a dramatic inhibition of tumor growth, and in the group of mice irradiated with fractions of 2.4 Gy, the tumor growth was not very different from mice irradiated with 2 Gy per fractions (Fig. 4)

(Beauchesne et al., 2003; Pedeux et al., 2003). These experiments show that ultrafractionated irradiation provides a marked benefit compared to a more classical irradiation regimen. It is worth noting that the use of a clinical linear accelerator is more feasible and the ultrafractionated regimen could thus be suitable for clinical treatment (Beauchesne et al., 2003; Pedeux et al., 2003).

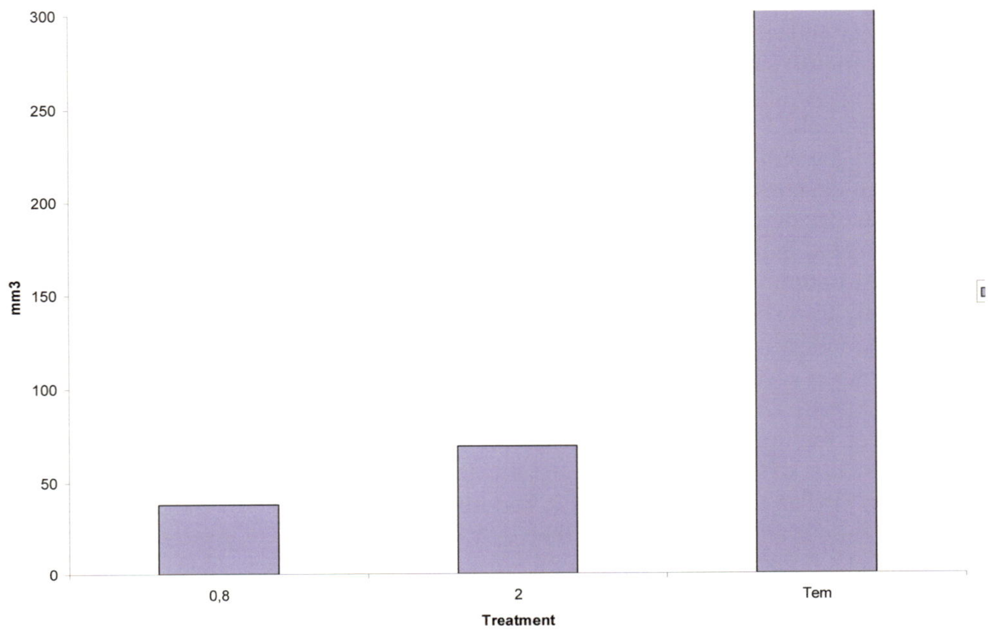

Fig. 4. Inhibition of glioma tumor growth following repeated irradiation with low doses. G152 glioma cells injected into the interscapular region of 4-week-old female nude mice (Swiss *nu/nu*). Seventeen days after grafting, mice were exposed either to 0.8 Gy 3 times/day spaced by 4 hr 5 days/week for 2 consecutive weeks or to 2.4 Gy once/day 5 days/week for 2 consecutive weeks. Tumor size was measured once a week.

Krause et al tested the ultrafractionated regimen in an animal model grafted with cells derived from the A7 human cell line which expressed the HRS phenomenon (Krause et al., 2003). Cryoprereserved tumor tissue was transplanted subcutaneously onto the backs of five mice. The tumor with the median volume doubling time was transplanted onto the back of another eight to 12 mice. 1-2 mm pieces of tissue from the median tumor were then transplanted subcutaneously into the right hind leg of the experimental animals (Krause et al., 2003). Irradiation protocols were started daily when the tumours reached a mean diameter of 5 mm, corresponding to a volume of 57 mm^3; the ultrafractionated regimen consisted of 26 fractions over 6 weeks (0.4 Gy per fraction, 3 fractions per day, 21 fractions per week, spaced at 6 hour intervals), and conventional treatment consisted of 30 fractions over 6 weeks (1.68 Gy per fraction, once daily, 5 fractions per week) (Krause et al., 2003). A local irradiator was used. Endpoints were tumor growth delay and local tumor control 180 days after the end of the treatment, and for the first 60 days after the end of irradiation. The tumors were measured twice weekly and once weekly thereafter (Krause et al., 2003). The authors were unable to demonstrate a therapeutic benefit of the ultrafractionated regimen; growth delay in the ultrafractionated arm was significantly shorter than after conventional treatment (Krause et al., 2003).The top-up TCD_{50} values were 28.3 Gy for conventional irradiation and 40 Gy for the ultrafractionated regimen (p=0.047) (Krause et al., 2003). The use of a local irradiator with a dose rate 0.2 - 0.4 Gy/min could alter the molecular mechanisms and perhaps modify the mechanisms responsible for the HRS phenomenon (Krause et al., 2003).

4. Clinical trials

The ultrafractionated radiation therapy regimen

To translate these *in vitro* and *in vivo* observations into a clinical setting, Beauchesne et al initiated a phase I/II clinical trial using an ultrafractionated radiation therapy protocol (3 times 0.75 Gy for a total of 67.5 Gy) (Beauchesne et al., 2010). The main purpose of this study was to assess the toxicity of the ultrafractionated regimen. This protocol was initiated before concomitant radio-chemotherapy became standard of care. For this pilot trial, the authors purposely selected patients with unfavourable clinical prognostic factors: newly unresectable glioblastoma (Beauchesne et al., 2010).

4.1 The population

This phase I/II study was conducted in seven French centres. Patients (> 18 years and who were able to give informed consent) with newly diagnosed, supratentorial, unresectable but histologically confirmed glioblastoma (astrocytoma grade IV according to the WHO classification), with a WHO performance status of 0-2 were eligible (Beauchesne et al., 2010). Patients were included based on local pathology. Patients with an estimated survival of less than 3 months, who had undergone partial or complete tumor resection, or who had previously received prior radiation therapy were not eligible. The primary end-points of the study were the treatment-related toxicity and tolerability (Beauchesne et al., 2010). Secondary end-points were progression-free survival (PFS) and overall survival (OS) of glioblastoma patients (Beauchesne et al., 2010).

4.2 Treatment

The radiation therapy regimen consisted of ultrafractionated focal irradiation with three daily doses of 0.75 Gy delivered at least four hours apart five days a week (Monday through Friday), for 6-7 consecutive weeks. A total dose of 67.5 Gy was delivered in 90 fractions (Beauchesne et al., 2010). Irradiation was delivered to the gross tumor volume with a 2.5 cm margin for the clinical target volume. Radiation therapy was planned with dedicated computed tomography (CT) or magnetic resonance imaging (MRI), and three-dimensional planning systems; conformal ultrafractionated radiotherapy was delivered with linear accelerators with a nominal energy of 6 MeV or more (Beauchesne et al., 2010). The patients were treated with thermoplastic immobilization masks to ensure adequate immobilization and reproducibility.

4.3 Patient evaluation

The patients were assessed weekly for tolerability and toxicity during the radiation therapy. The baseline examination included cranial MRI (with and without contrast), physical and neurological examination and included Mini-Mental-Status score (MMS) and a quality-of-life questionnaire (EORTC - QLQ-C30, Brain Cancer Module BN-20) (Beauchesne et al., 2010). Baseline examination was performed at the end of radiation therapy regimen (within the first 10 days after completion of ultrafractionated irradiation) and then every 2 months until death. The first MRI (at the end of radiation therapy) constituted the baseline imaging to evaluate tumor response keeping in mind that radiation therapy artifacts if present should be taken into account when interpreting the images (Beauchesne et al., 2010). Tumor progression was defined according to the modified WHO criteria (Macdonald criteria) as an increase in tumor size by 25 percent (size of the product of the largest perpendicular diameters of contrast-enhancing tumor), the appearance of new lesions, or an increased need for corticosteroids (MacDonald et al., 1990). When there was tumor progression, patients were treated at the investigator's discretion, and the type of subsequent therapy (usually chemotherapy) was recorded (Beauchesne et al., 2010).

4.4 Patient characteristics

From September 2003 until June 2006, 31 patients were enrolled in this phase II study (16 males and 15 females). Median patient was 58 years (range 37 to 76). Median Karnofsky Performance Status (KPS) was 80, ranging from 60 to 100 (Beauchesne et al., 2010). The median time from diagnosis to the beginning of ultrafractionated radiation therapy was 6 weeks (ranging from 2 to 10 weeks) (Beauchesne et al., 2010). Four patients died before the beginning of irradiation and two decided to revert to the standard radiation therapy regimen after starting (Beauchesne et al., 2010). The radiation course was completed in 22 patients. Multi-focal glioblastoma was diagnosed in seven patients, four of whom received and completed the ultrafractionated regimen (Beauchesne et al., 2010). Neuropathology was review reviewed by a central laboratory and all but one case was diagnosed as glioblastoma as WHO classification, and one case was secondary and classified as anaplastic oligodendroglioma.

4.5 Safety and tolerability

No toxic death occurred during the ultrafactionated irradiation and no radiation therapy regimen was discontinued. All but three patients (25 patients) received the ultrafractionated irradiation, and 22 completed the course of the treatment (Beauchesne et al., 2010). Two patients with a very large tumor progressed during the radiation therapy, and radiation therapy leading to premature discontinuation after 48 and 56 Gy. The most common adverse event was fatigue, as is frequently observed in standard cranial radiation therapy (Beauchesne et al., 2010). Although the ultrafractionation regimen was a constraint to patients, it was well accepted; only one out of 25 changed his mind during the course of the treatment, and was withdrawn. Overall, the ultrafractionated regimen was well tolerated.

4.6 Survival

After a median follow-up of 4 years, two of the 31 initial patients were alive (6.5 %). The median survival was 9.53 months (Beauchesne et al., 2010). The OS at 6, 12, 18 and 24 months was respectively 74.19 %, 29.03 %, 19.35 % and 15.48 %. The median PFS was 5.09 months. The PFS at 6, 12, 18, and 24 months was respectively 45.16 %, 12.90 %, 6.45 % and 6.45 % (Beauchesne et al., 2010). No difference was found in the median survival for age and sex: 8.4 months for males vs. 8.9 months for females, 8.4 months for < 55 years vs. 9.5

months for > 55 years (Beauchesne et al., 2010). The trial design allowed the use of fotemustine, a nitrosourea component, as first line of chemotherapy at tumor progression, but patients were treated at the physician's discretion. At the cut-off date, 16 patients had received chemotherapy; fotemustine was given in 14 cases, and temozolomide in 2 (Beauchesne et al., 2010). One patient underwent surgery, and radio-surgery was performed in one case. The response to salvage chemotherapy was not recorded as part of our study.

4.7 Response to treatment

Tumor response was analyzed (at the end of the ultrafractionated regimen and then 2 months later) using the WHO criteria. Eight stabilizations (corresponding to a decrease of less than 25 % of perpendicular transversal diameters - no cerebral edema and mass effect) were observed among the patients who had received the ultrafractionated radiation therapy (Fig. 5) (Beauchesne et al., 2010). In addition, the doses of corticosteroids were stable or decreased for these patients. Stabilization of tumor responses was observed either at the end of radiation therapy or in the following months. In the remaining cases, the tumor was non-progressive (Beauchesne et al., 2010). In most cases, corticosteroids were decreased and stopped for several weeks. Half of the long term survivors did not receive a chemotherapy line.

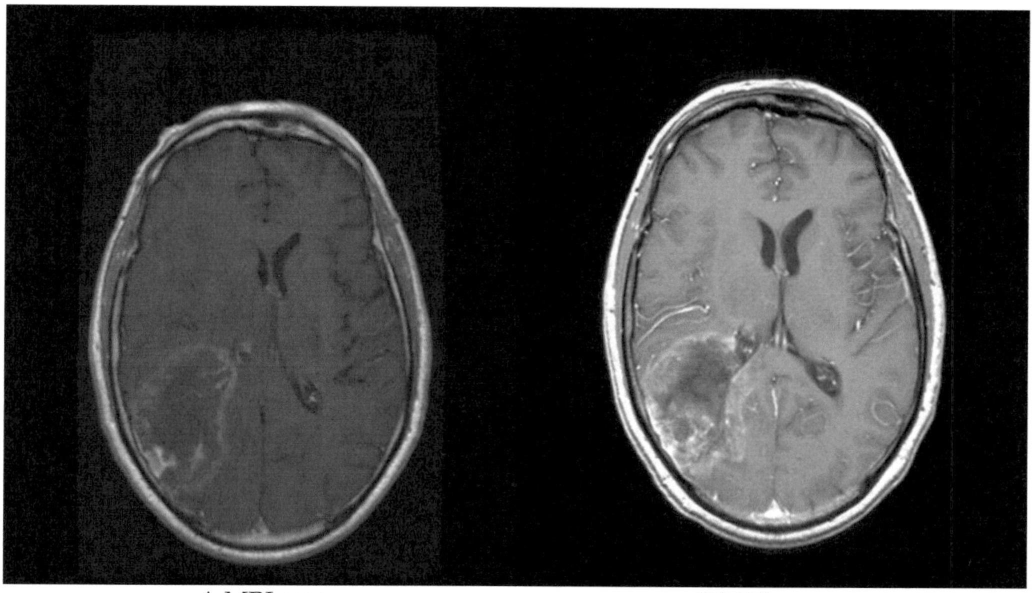

A MRI scan B MRI scan.

Fig. 5. A stabilisation response was seen on a cranial MRI. A- At the beginning of treatment. B- At the end of radiotherapy.

4.8 Commentaries

Before this study was conducted, the safety and tolerability of this new regimen of radiation therapy, three doses per day administered at intervals at least 4 hours, were unknown. This was the first time that such an ultrafractionated radiation therapy regimen was clinically performed (Beauchesne et al., 2010). The study showed that the regimen is safe, well tolerated and well accepted by the patients. No toxic death occurred and no neurological symptoms evoking a post-radiation therapy leuco-encephalopathy were recorded (Beauchesne et al., 2010). Neither were any abnormal radiological findings suggesting a potential toxic effect of ultrafractionated irradiation noted on cranial MRI. Fatigue, as is usually observed with the standard cranial irradiation, was the main adverse event recorded.

The median survival compares favorably with the best outcomes observed in the recent large randomized studies (Athanassiou et al., 2005; Westphal et al., 2003). Moreover, these studies had included a high percentage of patients with better prognosis (good WHO performance status - young age - resection of tumor - a single tumor), and the adjuvant chemotherapy was systematically administered (Athanassiou et al., 2005; Westphal et al., 2003). The EORTC-NCIC study reported a median survival of 7.85 and 9.4 months respectively for radiation therapy alone and temozolomide/radiotherapy together administered to patients with inoperable glioblastomas (Stupp et al., 2005).

Beauchesne et al's study resulted in both a longer median survival time and higher OS at 24 months (9.53 months - 15.38 % and 7.4 months - 8 % respectively) than the RTOG 90-06 trial (7.4 months and 8 % respectively) (Beauchesne et al., 2010; Scott et al., 1998). Furthermore, there were an unexpectedly high number of long survivors; 19.35 % and 15.48 % at 18 and 24 months. This compares favorably with the 24 months survival in the EORTC-NCIC study which stands at 4.59 % for the radiation therapy alone arm and 10.42 % for the temozolomide/radiation therapy arm (Beauchesne et al., 2010; Stupp et al., 2005). Furthermore half of the patients in the Beauchesne et al trial did not receive a chemotherapy line or other therapy (Beauchesne et al., 2010). It seems reasonable therefore to claim an ultrafractionated radiation therapy regimen may result in better long survival and OS compared with the best results reported in the literature.

These encouraging results support the development of a randomized phase II study to test the efficacy of a concomitant combination of ultrafractionated radiation therapy and temozolomide in no-operable glioblastomas. Beauchesne et al initiated such a study in February 2008 in France to test this new combination of ultrafractionated irradiation and temozolomide. Patients over 18 years of age who are able to give informed consent and have histologically proven, newly diagnosed inoperable and supratentorial glioblastoma are eligible. Three doses of 0.75 Gy are delivered daily at a minimum of 4 hour intervals, 5 days a week for 6 consecutive weeks (67.5Gy). Concomitant chemotherapy consisting of temozolomide is given 7 days per week during the ultrafractionated radiation therapy. After a 4-week break, chemotherapy is resumed with up to 6 cycles of adjuvant temozolomide every 28 days. Tolerability and toxicity are the primary endpoints and survival and PFS the secondary endpoints.

To date 36 patients have been enrolled in this study, 24 men and 12 women with a median age of 62, years and median KPS of 80. The ultrafractionated radiation therapy - temozolomide combination has been well tolerated; no acute grade 3 and/or 4 CNS toxicity has been observed and only one grade 4 hematological toxicity has been reported. Two patients progressed during the radiation therapy, and two patients died of pulmonary embolism. Median survival has not yet been reached. Half of the patients have survived for more than one year.

5. Conclusions

The "Low Dose Hypersensitivity" phenomenon has been demonstrated *in vitro* in a number of various human malignant glioma cell lines, when cells were irradiated with single-doses of X-rays from 0.05 to 5 Gy, and focusing on cell survival at doses less than 1 Gy. Interestingly, daily repeated irradiation of cells with low doses compared to irradiation with a single biologically equivalent dose resulted in significantly higher cell kill (as measured with a clonogenic assay).

Experiments conducted on glioma xenografts went on to demonstrate that repeated irradiation with low doses (0.8 Gy, 3 times a day) is more effective than a single dose (2 or 2.4 Gy, once a day) to inhibit tumor growth.

Clinical trials on ultrafractionated radiation regimens confirm these experimental results and have proved to be safe and well tolerated. No acute grade 3 and/or 4 CNS toxicity has been observed in such trials. Median progression-free and survival from initial diagnosis have been found to be 5.1 and 9.5 months. When compared with the EORTC/NCIC trial in both PFS and OS multivariate analysis, ultrafractionation showed superiority over radiation therapy alone but not over radiation therapy and temozolomide. Nevertheless, the treatment regimen has proved feasible, well tolerated and deserves to be further evaluated in combination with the current standard concomitant chemotherapy agents.

6. References

Athanassiou H, Synodinou M, Maragoudakis E, et al. (2005). Randomized phase II study of temozolomide and radiotherapy compared with radiotherapy alone in newly diagnosed glioblastoma multiforme. *J Clin Oncol*, 23, 2372-2377.

Beauchesne PD, Bertrand S, Branche R, et al. (2003). Human malignant glioma cell lines are sensitive to low radiation doses. *Int J Cancer*; 105, 33-40.

Beauchesne PD, Bernier V, Carnin C, et al. (2010). Prolonged survival for patients with newly diagnosed, inoperable glioblastoma with 3-times daily ultrafractionated radiation therapy. *Neuro Oncol*, 12, 595-602.

Beck-Bornholdt HP, Maurer T, Becker S, et al. (1989). Radiotherapy of the rhabdomyosarcoma R1H of the rat: hyperfractionation–126 fractions applied within 6 weeks. *Int J Radiation Oncology Biol Phys*, 16, 701–705.

Behin A, Hoang-Xuan K, Carpentier AF, et al. (2003). Primary brain tumours in adults. *Lancet*; 36, 323-31.

Black PM. (1991a). Brain tumor. Part 2. *N Engl J Med*, 324, 1555-1564.

Black PM. (1991b). Brain tumors. Part 1. *N Engl J Med*, 324, 1471-1476.

DeAngelis LM. (2001). Brain tumors. *N Engl J Med*, 344, 114-123.

Fine HA, Dear KB, Loeffler JS, et al. (1993). Meta-analysis of radiation therapy with and without adjuvant chemotherapy for malignant gliomas in adults. *Cancer*, 71, 2585-2597.

Hall EJ. (1978). Radiobiology for the radiologist, 2nd ed. Hargestown ; Harper and Row.

James CD, Olson JJ. (1996). Molecular genetics and molecular biology advances in brain tumors. *Curr Opin Oncol*, 8, 188 –195.

Joiner MC, Denekamp J. (1986). The effect of small radiation doses on mouse skin. *British J Cancer*, 7, 63–66.

Joiner MC, Denekamp J, Maughan RL. (1986). The use of 'top-up' experiments to investigate the effect of very small doses per fraction in mouse skin. *Int J Radiat Biol Relat Stud Phys Chem Med*, 49, 565-580.

Joiner MC, Johns H. (1988). Renal damage in the mouse: the response to very small doses per fraction. *Radiat Res*, 114, 385–398.

Joiner MC, Marples B, Johns H. (1993a). The response of tissues to very low doses per fraction: a reflection of induced repair? *Cancer Res*, 130, 27–40.

Joiner MC, Marples B, Johns H. (1993b). The limitation of the linear–quadratic model at low doses per fraction. In H. P. Beck-Bornholdt (ed.), Current Topics in Clinical Radiobiology of Tumors (Berlin: Springer), 51–66.

Joiner MC, Lambin P, Malaise EP, et al. (1996). Hypersensitivity to very-low single radiation doses: its relationship to the adaptive response and induced radioresistance. *Mutation Res*, 358, 171–183.

Joiner MC, Marples B, Lambin P, et al. (2001). Low-dose hypersensitivity: current status and possible mechanisms. *Int J Radiat Oncol Biol Phys*, 49, 379-89.

Kleihues P, Ohgaki H. (1999). Primary and secondary glioblastoms: from concept to clinical diagnosis. *Neuro-Oncol*, 1, 44 –51.

Krause M, Hessel F, Wohlfarth J, et al. (2003). Ultrafractionation in A7 human malignant glioma in nude mice. *Int J Cancer*, 79, 377-383.

Lambin P, Marples B, Fertil B, et al. (1993a). Hypersensitivity of a human tumour cell line to very low radiation doses. *Int J Radiat Biol*, 63, 639-650.

Lambin P, Malaise EP, Joiner MC. (1993b). Megafractionnement: une methode pour agir sur les tumeurs intrinsequement radioresistantes? *Bull Cancer Radiother*, 80, 417–423.

Lambin P, Coco-Martin J, Legal JD, et al. (1994a) Intrinsic radiosensitivity and chromosome aberration analysis using fluorescence in situ hybridization in cells of two human tumor cell lines. *Radiat Res*, 138, S40–43.

Lambin P, Malaise EP, Joiner MC. (1994b). The effect of very low radiation doses on the human bladder carcinoma cell line RT112. *Radiother Oncol*, 32, 63-72.

Lambin P, Fertil B, Malaise EP, et al. (1994c). Multiphasic survival curves for cells of human tumor cell lines: induced repair or hypersensitive subpopulation? *Radiat Res*, 138, S32–36.

Lambin P, Malaise EP, Joiner MC. (1996). Might intrinsic radioresistance of human tumour cells be induced by radiation? *Int J Radiat Biol*, 69, 279-290.

McDonald DR, Cascino TL, Schold SC, et al. (1990). Response criteria for phase II studies of supratentorial malignant glioma. *J Clin Oncol*, 8, 1277–1280.

Marples B, Lam GK, Zhou H, et al. (1994). The response of Chinese hamster V79-379A cells exposed to negative pi-mesons: evidence that increased radioresistance is dependent on linear energy transfer. *Radiat Res*, 138, S81-4.

Marples B, Lambin P, Skov KA, et al. (1997). Low dose hyper-radiosensitivity and increased radioresistance in mammalian cells. *Int J Radiat Biol*, 71, 721-735.

Pedeux R, Boniol M, Dore JF, et al. (2003). Ultrafractionation radiation therapy of human gliomas ; a pre-clinical model. *Int J Cancer*, 107, 334.

Scott CB, Scarantino C, Urtasun R, et al. (1998). Validation and predictive power of Radiation Therapy Oncology Group (RTOG) recursive partitioning analysis classes for malignant glioma patients: a report using RTOG 90-06. *Int J Radiat Oncol Biol Phys*, 40, 51–55.

Short SC, Mayes CR, Woodcock M, et al. (1999a). Low dose hypersensitivity in the T98G human glioblastoma cell line. *Int J Radiat Biol*, 75, 847–855.

Short SC, Mitchell SA, Boulton P, et al. (1999b). The response of human glioma cell lines to low-dose radiation exposure. *Int J Radiat Biol*, 75, 1341-1348.

Short SC, Kelly J, Mayes CR, et al. (2001). Low-dose hypersensitivity after fractionated low-dose irradiation in vitro. *Int J Radiat Biol*, 77, 655-664.

Singh, B, Arrand JE, Joiner MC. (1994). Hypersensitive response of normal human lung epithelial cells at low radiation doses. *Int J Radiat Biol*, 65, 457-464.

Stewart LA. (2002). Chemotherapy in adult high-grade glioma: a systematic review and meta-analysis of individual patient data from 12 randomised trials. *Lancet*; 359, 1011-1018.

Stupp R, Mason WP, van den Bent MJ, et al. (2005). Radiotherapy plus concomitant and adjuvant temozolomide for glioblastoma. *N Engl J Med*, 352, 987-996.

Taghian A, Suit H, Pardo F, et al. (1992). In vitro intrinsic radiation sensitivity of glioblastoma multiforme. *Int J Radiat Oncol Biol Phys*, 3, 55- 62.

Taghian A, Ramsay J, Allalunis-Turner J, et al. (1993). Intrinsic radiation sensitivity may not be the major determinant of the poor clinical outcome of glioblastoma multiforme. *Int J Radiat Oncol Biol Phys*, 25, 243–249.

Turesson I, Joiner MC. (1996). Clinical evidence of hypersensitivity to low doses in radiotherapy. *Radiother Oncol*, 40, 1–3.

Walker MD, Alexander E, Jr, Hunt WE, et al. (1978). Evaluation of BCNU and/ or radiotherapy in the treatment of anaplastic gliomas. A cooperative clinical trial. *J Neurosurg*, 49, 333–343.

Walker MD, Green SB, Byar DP, et al. (1980). Randomized comparisons of radiotherapy and nitrosoureas for the treatment of malignant glioma after surgery. *N Engl J Med*, 303, 1323–1329

Van den Bent MJ, Carpentier AF, Brandes AA, et al. (2006). Adjuvant procarbazine, lomustine, and vincristine improves progression-free survival but not overall survival in newly diagnosed anaplastic oligodendrogliomas and oligoastrocytomas: a randomized European organisation for research and treatment of cancer phase III trial. *J Clin Oncol*, 24, 2715-2722.

Watanabe K, Tachibana O, Sata K, et al. (1996). Overexpression of the EGF receptor and *p53* mutations are mutually exclusive in the evolution of primary and secondary glioblastomas. *Brain Pathol*, 6, 217–223.

Westphal M, Hilt DC, Bortey E, et al. (2003). A phase 3 trial of local chemotherapy with biodegradable carmustine (BCNU) wafers (Gliadel wafers) in patients with primary malignant glioma. *Neuro-Oncol*, 5, 79-88.

Wouters BG, Skarsgard LD. (1994). The response of a human tumor cell line to low radiation doses: evidence of enhanced sensitivity. *Radiat Res*, 138, S76–80.

Wouters BG, Sky AM, Skarsgard LD. (1996). Low dose hypersensitivity and increased radioresistance in a panel of human tumor cell lines with different radiosensitivity. *Radiat Res*, 146, 399–413.

21

Immunotherapy for Malignant Gliomas: A Roadmap for the Future

S. De Vleeschouwer and SW. Van Gool
Catholic University Leuven
Belgium

1. Introduction

Since many decades, medical doctors and researchers have been intrigued by the possible beneficial contribution of the immune system in the long-lasting combat against cancer. Both in the cellular and humoral immunity arms, powerful tools are available to target the cancer cell. Moreover, the gradual shift of a focus on aspecific reinforcement of the innate immune system towards a specifically activated adaptive immunity in order to reject cancer cells has dominated the field of the last 10 to 20 years(1). Restorative immunotherapy in which cytokine balances are restored or reset and aspecific adoptive immunotherapy using e.g. natural killer (NK) cells or lymphokine-activated killer (LAK) cells are classical representations of the first wave. Specific adoptive immunotherapy using ex vivo activated antitumor cytotoxic T cells and especially active specific immunotherapy ('cancer vaccines') are representative for the second wave. Thorough changes in the underlying basic immunology mechanism guide these novel approaches. To date, only the different variants of cancer vaccines are able to induce an immunological memory, as such being the only approach potentially protecting the patients for future cancer re-challenges(2). A perceived low rate of classical objective responses, restricted to volume changes of a measurable tumor burden, has been the principal body of criticism against these therapies.

Several new insights however, especially focusing on changes in the micro-environment of the tumors, are only starting to be unraveled. Without any doubt, they're already now revealing much more than the previous tips of the curtains. Nowadays, converging evidence is being gained in a rapid way, for the need to move towards a third wave of immunotherapy approaches, those of the multimodal integrated immunotherapy paradigms, considering all the relevant players in the complex field of tumor immunology.

2. Proof of the principle: A solid body of preclinical evidence

The idea to actively prime cytotoxic T cells to specifically kill a tumor target cell has become a well established scientific fact. Several approaches all aiming to induce specifically activated, tumor-rejecting effector T cells have been investigated and found to be reproducible and reliable technologies. Genetically engineered tumor cells but especially autologous dendritic cells charged with tumor associated antigens have become the most potent and popular immunological adjuvants to install an active anti-tumoral immunity(3;4). An additional advantage of the latter is the activation of both the innate and adaptive immunity arms of the patient. The mechanisms underlying this antitumoral priming capacity of dendritic cells seem to be fully consistent with the established paradigms of antigen uptake, processing and presentation. The exclusive potential of DC to present and cross-present exogenous antigens in the same antigen presenting cell is the critical characteristic for a successful antigen presentation to cytotoxic and helper T cells. DC pick up tumor-associated antigens from diverse sources, process them and present them in both an Major Histocompatibility Complex (MHC) class I and II context to cytotoxic and helper T cells respectively. This has been clearly shown, also for glioma associated antigens from a whole-tumor-cell lysate(5). To date, efficient priming of the patient by dendritic cells implies four sequences of interaction between the dendritic cell and the T cell. Upon binding of the T cell receptor with the MHC complex on the antigen presenting cell displaying the appropriate epitope, a specific activation of the antitumor T cells with high enough avidity for the epitope takes place. Expansion of this T cell clones requires co-stimulatory molecules on the DC. A polarized immune response, preferentially with a Th-1 cytokine profile, should result from the previous interactions. Finally, some indication about the target location should be transferred to the T cells leading to the appropriate T cell homing properties(6-8).

Many rodent models have demonstrated that prophylactic vaccination of mice with tumor-antigen loaded DC can protect immune competent animals from tumor challenge and outgrow. The most relevant experiments are being performed with syngeneic mice-tumor models, to prove the efficacy of the vaccination in an autologous setting underscoring the possibility to break tolerance for self-derived antigens. Moreover, one can raise an anti-tumor immunological memory to make mice survive a re-challenge of cancer cells. More elaborated manipulations of the immune system like e.g. regulatory T cell depletion before vaccination even yield a much stronger protective effect in up to 100% of the exposed animals(9;10). The step towards therapeutic vaccination models, being more relevant for the clinical reality of all day can be made if the crucial timing of inoculation and vaccination is being respected. Probably also due to the aggressive nature of the investigated models, where all mice are dead within 3 weeks after tumor inoculation, it appears crucial to vaccinate the animals not later than one week after the tumor inoculations. After that period, the course of the disease can hardly be influenced, presumably because of the establishment of an efficient immune suppressive, pro-tumor micro-environment around the tumor inocula. This should be understood as the first evidence to use DC vaccinations as an adjuvant therapy in minimal residual disease settings, resembling most the prophylactic setting in which anti-tumor vaccines are so efficient.

3. From proof of the principle to proof of efficacy

Tumor vaccination therapy, even in its more basic form did yield some interesting results in terms of benefit in overall survival in several fields of oncology e.g. renal cell carcinoma, prostate carcinoma, non-small cell lung cancer, colon carcinoma and others(11). Historically, most attention has been paid to so called immunogenic tumors like melanomas. Although proof of the principle has been extensively demonstrated in these tumors using different vaccine approaches and the clinical results obtained until now are equivalent to standard of care chemotherapy regimens, the final results of immunotherapy in these entities are still modest. Malignant gliomas, the most common primary brain tumors have always been considered to be not suitable for immunotherapy because of their location in the immune privileged central nervous system. To date however, we know that all the obstacles like the blood brain barrier, the lack of lymphatic vessels, the lack of residing antigen presenting cells in the brain, the low MHC expression on the tumor target cells are quite relative. They don't seem to hamper the documented immune responses in patients harboring such tumors(12). To the current understanding the real hurdles in glioma vaccination strategies are the multiple immunosuppressive pathways orchestrated by this type of cancer cells and the lack of universally expressed glioma associated antigens that are really crucial for tumor cell survival. Surprisingly, preliminary data might be pointing to an exploitable lack of spontaneous immunogenicity of malignant gliomas. As such, they develop in a micro-environment protecting them from too extensive immune editing: especially that characteristic could be of major help to try to reset the patients' immunity resulting in a much better immune rejection or control since the original immune-sensitive tumor clones have not yet been eliminated by the natural immune surveillance mechanisms(13).

Immune responses in the brain always elicit some fear for potentially disastrous consequences of an auto-immune attack by the patient's immunity. Unlike vitiligo or even destruction of normal prostate tissue, an auto-immune encephalomyelitis could result in devastating neurological symptoms and deficits. Until now however, no preclinical –other than in a heavily manipulated immune environment- and no clinical data have been published showing any suspicion of serious auto-immunity in the central nervous system, using tumor vaccination strategies. Moreover, numerous phase I and small phase II trials have been published showing the safety and the very attractive low toxicity profile of dendritic cell vaccines in brain cancer. As we're still dealing with a palliative treatment thus far, this perfect patient tolerance profile is highly valuable to build upon for upcoming vaccination strategies. Although today's technology to produce autologous dendritic cell vaccines is still very labour-intensive, it proved to be perfectly feasible to implement it in the daily clinical practice, both in the case of relapsed or newly diagnosed high grade gliomas.

The main criticism against tumor vaccine approaches, often raised till today, comprises the presumed low rate of objective tumor responses. Objective, radiological responses as defined according to RECIST(14) or McDonalds(15) criteria have indeed been developed for radio-and especially chemotherapy regimens during which one aims to reduce the measurable tumor load in the patient. Although they provide valuable information in terms of proof of the principle of the investigated chemotherapy, they should not be considered a synonym for clinically relevant efficacy: in only a few cases, one was really able to demonstrate a clear correlation between objective responses and overall survival benefits(16). More intriguing even is the existence of the so-called 'pseudo-progression' since radiochemotherapy with temozolomid became the standard of care(17). In up to 25% (or even 40%) of cases, one might see an initial increase in radiological tumor volume, rather early after the concomitant radiochemotherapy: strikingly, often especially these patients seem to have a better overall survival chance than the group not displaying these types of misleading radiological changes. Dendritic cell vaccination is known to cause similar radiological images in which transient contrast-enhancements on magnetic resonance imaging (MRI) might represent inflammatory, vaccine-induced radiological changes that can easily be mistaken for disease progression(18). Although the available literature mentions objective responses in about 13% of vaccinated patients with high grade gliomas, objective responses are not the most appropriate outcome measure for this therapy nor for other experimental therapies. Especially the growing consensus that immunotherapy should be used as an adjuvant treatment for minimal residual disease settings, implies that in many cases there will be no measurable tumor volume at the start of the treatment. Indeed, not all patients today are good candidates to possibly benefit from DC-based immunotherapy. Only tumors amenable to meaningful surgical resections should be considered candidates for adjuvant DC vaccination(19). Several reasons exist for that restriction: first of all one need enough tumor specimen to obtain tumor associated antigens. Secondly, one should be able to stably wean the patient from peri-operative steroids, which might dampen an efficient immune response in case of vaccinations under steroids. Thirdly, by reducing the bulky tumor load, one partially corrects the immune suppressive environment, both locally and systemically, that results from the presence of an organized tumor. In that context, one should mention that modern resection techniques like the use of 5-ALA induced fluorescence guided resections, leading to more extensive glioma resections, can be a complement to the postoperative DC vaccination.

In the past, many researchers have focused on the measurable immune responses in the blood of vaccinated patients as a surrogate endpoint and even as a surrogate of the desired objective clinical responses. The many immunological assays like delayed type hypersensitivity (DTH) reactions - even with skin biopsies of the test sites - , ELISA, ELISPOT, tetramer analysis and diverse in vitro cytotoxicity assays have provided us with valuable insights in relevant immunological mechanisms contributing to the proof of the principle and to our understanding of the complex interaction of the immune system and cancer cells. Regardless the assay used, there seem to be a fairly constant rate of about 50% immune responders in vaccinated cancer patients with malignant gliomas. Apart from a rare exception, most assays failed to correlate with clinical results. We should realize that we have to leave the former linear paradigm stating that cancer vaccines induce a detectable immune response that results in a detectable clinical response (tumor rejection), finally leading to improved overall survival. It did teach us however the important lesson that to date, dendritic cells indeed seem to be the best adjuvants available for clinical use to elicit measurable immune responses in cancer patients, even if almost all of them had been heavily pretreated with radio-and chemotherapy. It has to be mentioned that a rational combination of preferentially, non-myelo-ablative chemotherapy leading to 'pro-inflammatory' immunogenic apoptosis of cancer cells rather synergizes than antagonizes with modern vaccine approaches. Several excellent reviews are dealing with that particular finding(20-22).

Indeed, since recent years a growing consensus on the way to proceed with clinical research in cancer vaccine strategies has arisen. The Cancer Vaccine Clinical Trial Working Group already suggested two parallel tracts of investigation: trials focusing on proof of principle and efficacy trials(23). The former should aim to demonstrate immunological activity, the latter should be designed to show clinical benefit for the patients.

The clinical outcome measures that really do have an impact on the patients' perspectives are overall survival and quality of life. The well tolerated vaccinations often result in a minimal interference with a good quality of life, that is actually only being threatened by disease progression but not substantially by the therapy itself(24). The ambulatory nature of the vaccination schedules further contribute to this low impact on the treatment burden for the individual patient. Especially this low toxicity profile adds to the merits of this therapy in the subgroup of long-term surviving brain cancer patients. Indeed, even more than the possible statistically important impact on median survival data, the substantial group of patients with malignant glioma, both WHO grade III and IV lesions, surviving for many years after vaccination, is the best advocate of this therapeutic approach. Both newly diagnosed, but even more strikingly, relapsed and multi-relapsed patients with high grade gliomas display survival periods of more than 4 to 9 years (manuscript submitted). Considering the classical definition of long-term survivor in the malignant glioma literature, being patients surviving 24 or more months after diagnosis (of primary disease or relapse), substantial numbers of patients, including up to 25% of the relapsed HGG patients undergoing DC vaccination are actually benefitting this opportunity. These long-term survivors are not only an encouragement for this –even not fully mature - immunotherapy approach, but also a source of scientificly important translational knowledge to learn more about the factors predicting this type of outcome after immunotherapy. Final scientific proof of efficacy can of course only be delivered by well-designed, sound randomized controlled trials, several of which are currently running throughout the world.

4. Lack of standards: Disadvantage or opportunity for further improvement?

The 'dendritic cell therapy for cancer'-world today is still characterized by a large variety of similar but not identical approaches. Even the definition of dendritic cell can slightly vary according to their progenitors with different resulting markers on their surface. Although direct harvesting from the peripheral blood is possible, some DC are differentiated out of stem cells or cord blood, but for the vast majority of clinical grade DC today, monocytes are harvested out of the peripheral blood and differentiated into DC. Different culture protocols and conditions result in different phenotypes, but the minimal criteria should be respected before one can claim the cells to be dendritic cells for clinical use: they should display clear cytoplasmic veils, have a high expression of MHC class II molecules as well as co-stimulatory molecules like CD86 and have lost their 'monocyte' markers like CD14. Growing consensus is being reached about the mature DC being the preferred state of the cells to re-inject into the patients, rather than immature cells being able to tolerize rather than immunize the patient. Several maturation cocktails are being used, none of them however have been proven to be superior to the other variants in clinical use, although some evidence exists for the critical involvement of TNFα in the cocktail(25). As the serum of cancer patients might contain identified and unidentified immune suppressive agents inhibiting a good DC differentiation in ex vivo cultures, some favor the use of serum free culture conditions.

Dendritic cells should be loaded with relevant glioma-associated antigens. The sources of these antigens differ widely from well-defined, possibly acid-eluted peptides, proteins, whole tumor cell lysates and homogenates, total tumor RNA, vector constructs, apoptotic and necrotic bodies. The same lack of data about which source of antigen leads to the most effective vaccine construct is blurring a uniformal approach today. However, many theoretical considerations, could rather support the use of whole tumor cell antigens rather than well-defined single peptides. The most important argument against the exclusive use of a single peptide is the well-established phenomenon of selecting antigen-loss variants of the tumor, leading to an inevitable tumor escape of probably less immune susceptible tumor clones after vaccination. Moreover, the broad repertoire of whole tumor cell derived tumor associated antigens, will lead to presentation of the relevant processed antigens in any type of HLA constitution of the patient, both in an MCH class I and II context. An efficient immunization in these cases is more prone to result in a comprehensive polyclonal T and B cell activation able to provide a better coverage of different tumor clones of the intrinsic heterogenous malignant glioma cells. Nevertheless, further improvements might be expected if a more immunogenic apoptosis pathway could be used to create the source of tumor antigens. Nanoparticles could maybe improve uptake and processing efficiency in the DC and justify further investigation.

Even harder to estimate today, is the optimal use of the appropriate danger signals (PAMP's or pathogen associated molecular patterns or DAMP's being danger associated molecular patterns) to further increase the potency of the vaccine preparation(26). Several candidates, most of them being Toll-like receptor agonists, could substantially potentiate the clinical impact of the dendritic cell-based vaccine. To date, only preliminary data exist to support the use of e.g. imiquimod , poly I:C or clinical grade LPS in the clinical applications of DC vaccines. Several others like ssRNA even have to start being explored for this application. It is evident that with so many parameters being undecided in terms of the most clinically potent DC-based vaccination approach, that a large spectrum of DC-based vaccines result, going from the crude 'dirty' vaccines to the highly elaborated, often genetically engineered cell constructs.

The lack of standards is not only to be found in the vaccine production arm, but even in the target population of patients to treat with DC-based vaccines. Most immunotherapy trials, not only those in brain cancer patients, have been performed in end-stage patients, often heavily pre-treated. Anergic states, either induced by myelo-ablative regimens or by the advanced state of the cancer itself, compromise the theoretical potential of tumor vaccines. Mounting evidence exists nowadays, that DC-based cancer vaccines should be applied to patients with a minimal residual disease status rather than in end-stage cancer patients. Some researchers even advocate the use of cancer vaccines in pre-cancerous lesions, as such referring to the historical prophylactic nature of vaccines and the abundant evidence of the prophylactic efficacy of tumor vaccines in rodent models. In terms of glioma patients, this would imply a shift of the focus to patients with low grade gliomas, as these tumors tend to dedifferentiate over time to secondary high grade gliomas. It would however be very hard, if possible at all in this state of knowledge, to show any survival benefit of this approach in low grade gliomas as the natural course of this condition is so variable that one would need very extensive patient numbers to reach an adequate statistical power in any trial design. Malignant gliomas on the other hand, have the disputable statistical advantage of being rapidly progressive lesions with an almost invariable fatal outcome: a substantial deviation from this natural evolution in vaccinated patients will rapidly result in a broad clinical awareness and possible recognition of the value of cancer vaccines in this setting.

Not only the state of the disease, but also the patient's age and possible timing of vaccination in the course of the treatment are relevant items to consider in the global treatment paradigm using DC-based vaccinations. Indeed, like in many types of oncological treatments, younger age seems to be correlated to a better response and survival after tumor vaccination. This can easily be understood as basic immunological features like thymic involution over time are very likely to influence the potential of active specific immunotherapy approaches in general. As for timing of the implementation of immunotherapy, the question remains whether an upfront integration of the DC-based vaccines in the standard postoperative radiochemotherapy regimen(27) will result in a netto benefit over the alternative approach to apply DC-based tumor vaccination after re-operation for recurrent disease as a single postoperative adjuvant treatment modality without interference of e.g. chemotherapy. Even more basic questions like the best frequency, dose, administration route and boost vaccine frequency and content are unanswered as yet. We do know that in DC-based tumor vaccination, no dose-response, nor dose-toxicity phenomenon is involved, but the optimal 'pharmacological' vaccine characteristics can only be concluded after further comparative clinical data.

Although clinical trials with the current standards of tumor vaccines are mandatory to define the presumed position of cancer immunotherapy in the global oncological treatment regimens, we should realize ourselves that further improvements of the products itself will continue to be made in the next decade. This is of utmost importance to estimate the future potentials of the therapy without losing credits for further innovations of the technology itself.

5. How to learn more? A difficult interplay between the technique, the tumor and the patient

Three main areas of elucidation arise at the moment. First of all, intrinsic improvements of the vaccine details itself are to be monitored by advanced immune monitoring techniques(28). Apart from the classical monitoring assays aimed at detecting a specific anti-tumoral immune response, we should move towards a more global appreciation of the immune system and changes under therapy, both conventional and vaccination therapy. Indeed, preliminary evidence is emerging about the importance of the global immune status of the patient at time of diagnosis and treatment steps. Radiochemotherapy leads to a 're-setting' of the patient's immune system, possibly already then priming it towards a favorable or unfavorable starting position for subsequent immunotherapy. The vaccine itself might cause quantitative and qualitative shifts in immune cell subtypes, not only regulatory or effector T cells, but also natural killer cells or natural killer T cells. We should start to include monitoring of local immune cells in the target environment, i.e. the brain and brain tumor micro-environment, rather than only in the blood, which is often not (at all) correlating with the local immune conditions in the target organs. Probably coinciding with shifts in cellular compartments of the immune system, cytokine environments might mimic the underlying changes and are good candidates to represent relevant switches in micro-environment facilitating or suppressing an effective tumor rejection by the immune system. Usually, a Th-1 pro-inflammatory environment is believed to be beneficial for tumor rejection, although other types of cytokine profiles, like e.g. a Th-17 mediated immune response are gaining importance in the global picture. Moreover, a TLR-agonist matured, fully Th-1 polarized DC vaccine has not yet been applied in larger clinical trials. A pro-inflammatory environment however is only facilitating a tumor rejection, if there's no evolution to a chronic inflammatory state, like in chronic inflammatory diseases : in this particular situation indeed, the immune system exhibits important signs of immune exhaustion. Even this state can be detected and monitored to date in an increasingly accurate way e.g. by analyzing zeta-chain down regulation in the T cell compartments(29). Many other relevant cell types from tumor infiltrating macrophages (especially those with pro-tumor 'M2' phenotype - called 'alternatively activated macrophages'), or tumor infiltrating myeloid-derived suppressor cells (MDSC), both abundantly present in several glioma models and human glioma specimens are only beginning to be unraveled. Analogue to the regulatory T cell compartment, which has been recognized for years as a relevant player in the balance between tumor rejection and immune tolerance, the first preliminary reports arise about 'regulatory dendritic cells'. It goes without saying that the fast acquisition of growing knowledge on the complex interplay between all these immune cells will influence our future understanding and concept of the current vaccine approaches.

A second important source of contributing insights will come from the molecular analysis of the tumor specimens. The molecular profile of a malignant glioma with the characterization of MGMT promotor methylation status, 1p19q co-deletion, PTEN loss, IDH1 mutation etc is rapidly gaining access to the routine clinical assessment of a common high grade glioma. To the same extent, predictive (or prognostic) markers for immunotherapy will become available as there are already now the reports on tumoral HOX genes relevant for 'immune reactions' (30)or the suggestion of an 'immunotherapy prone' mesenchymal phenotype of the glioblastoma tumor cells(31).

A third emerging field is the 'predictive' radiology field. In era's of pseudo-progression and therapy-induced radiological changes on gadolinium(Gd)-enhanced MRI of the brain tumor patients, distinctive radiological techniques predicting a tumor response or a tumor progression are of utmost importance. Especially its non-invasive character turns MRI into a preferred monitoring tool for malignant glioma follow-up especially for the new therapy classes. Preliminary steps are being made to try to distinguish vaccine-induced radiological changes from tumor progression in Gd-enhancing lesions on the MRI, using perfusion-weighted (regional cerebral blood volume-rCBV) and diffusion-weighted (apparent diffusion coefficient-ADC) images in combination with spectroscopic findings(18). In terms of correct patient counseling, these new monitoring paradigms are considered crucial for the near future.

6. How to proceed?

It is clear that we're at a crucial step in the decision to move on with immunotherapy or not. Therefore we should acknowledge the particular difficulty to find a balance between gaining the appropriate clinical evidence that immunotherapy adds to the favorable outcome of the patients with high grade gliomas on the one hand and creating a stimulating environment for further optimalisation of an as yet immature technology on the other hand.

A too quick global 'dissemination' of today's technologies will probably kill the credits for further development as too many aspects of the tumor vaccine approach itself are rapidly evolving towards a theoretical optimum.

The combination of both objectives can be accomplished by performing further preclinical experiments and small-scale early-clinical trials to optimize the vaccine technology as such and a gradual implementation of solid techniques of DC-based vaccine production and administration in large, randomized trials with the appropriate control arms to stepwise introduce the best available DC vaccine at that moment. The latter element is imperfect in se, but nevertheless highly required, even already at the moment, given the unmet medical need and the promising results for important subgroups of patients thus far.

It is hard to predict the outline of the final, optimal DC-based vaccine for the future. Nevertheless it is clear it will have to integrate all the aspects of the difficult interplay between the technique, the tumor and the patient. Indeed, all of these three elements are highly relevant for a successful immunotherapy approach and probably for any approach at all. As for the anti-glioma DC-based vaccine production itself, preliminary evidence is being reported that whole tumor cell -based preparations are superior to defined epitopes in terms of overall survival data. Which types of other therapies that might synergize the most with cancer vaccines is subject of further investigations. Many candidates from radio-and chemotherapy over anti-angiogenesis, blood-brain barrier disruption techniques or oncolytic virus therapy do exist or are emerging today. Immune modulators and strategies able to modify the tumor micro-environment will play a crucial role in the future cancer vaccines. For anti-glioma vaccines, again many candidates immune modulators are at the edge of a clinical application to improve the overall vaccine efficiency. Substances like galectin-1, transforming growth factor β, interleukin 10, interleukin 6 and vascular endothelial growth factor are known to hamper vaccine efficiency and might even be interconnected, so interference with either of these locally secreted factors could result in a dramaticly increased vaccine efficacy. Finally, the patient itself creates the background that might alter the impact of all the interventions according to pre-existing parameters. In that regard, the notion of inherent immune cycles is an intriguing finding that needs however further clarification. Nevertheless, it might explain the indirect evidence we have for the tremendous importance of the timing of immunotherapy interventions on the final outcome of the patient.

All this implies that we should consequently move into the direction of 'individualized' or 'customized' cancer vaccines rather than mass-produced 'off the shelf' constructs. Therefore , we should not mix up the ideal medical tracts with the desired 'manufacturing profile' of a cancer vaccine. It is highly likely that clinical results in this area of research will proceed the elucidation of all the underlying mechanisms rather than vice versa. Also for regulating agencies of cellular therapies, all the above mentioned aspects hold an enormous challenge but also a 'life-important' responsibility.

7. References

[1] Weller RO, Engelhardt B, Phillips MJ. Lymphocyte targeting of the central nervous system: a review of afferent and efferent CNS-immune pathways. Brain Pathol 1996; 6(3):275-288.

[2] De Vleeschouwer S, Van Gool SW, Van Calenbergh F. Immunotherapy for malignant gliomas: emphasis on strategies of active specific immunotherapy using autologous dendritic cells. Childs Nerv Syst 2005; 21:7-18.
[3] Steinman RM. The dendritic cell system and its role in immunogenicity. Annu Rev Immunol 1991; 9:271-296.
[4] Steinman RM, Mellman I. Immunotherapy: bewitched, bothered, and bewildered no more. Science 2004; 305:197-200.
[5] De Vleeschouwer S, Arredouani M, Ade M, Cadot P, Vermassen E, Ceuppens JL et al. Uptake and presentation of malignant glioma tumor cell lysates by monocyte-derived dendritic cells. Cancer Immunol Immunother 2005; 54:372-382.
[6] Gilboa E. DC-based cancer vaccines. J Clin Invest 2007; 117(5):1195-1203.
[7] Kalinski P, Hilkens CMU, Wierenga EA, Kapsenberg ML. T-cell priming by type-1 and type-2 polarized dendritic cells: the concept of a third signal. Immunol Today 1999; 20:561-567.
[8] Kalinski P, Urban J, Narang R, Berk E, Wieckowski E, Muthuswamy R. Dendritic cell-based therapeutic cancer vaccines: what we have and what we need. Future Oncol 2009; 5(3):379-390.
[9] Maes W, Galicia Rosas G, Verbinnen B, Boon L, De Vleeschouwer S, Ceuppens JL et al. DC vaccination with anti-CD25 treatment leads to long-term immunity against experimental glioma. Neuro-oncol 2009; 11(5):529-542.
[10] Maes W, Van Gool SW. Experimental immunotherapy for malignant glioma: lessons from two decades of research in the GL261 model. Cancer Immunol Immunother 2011; 60(2):153-160.
[11] Mocellin S, Rossi CR, Lise M, Marincola FM. Adjuvant immunotherapy for solid tumors: from promise to clinical application. Cancer Immunol Immunother 2002; 51(11-12):583-595.
[12] Dunn GP, Dunn IF, Curry WT. Focus on TILs: Prognostic significance of tumor infiltrating lymphocytes in human glioma. Cancer Immun 2007; 7:12.
[13] Van Gool SW, Maes W, Ardon H, Verschuere T, Van Cauter S, De Vleeschouwer S. Dendritic cell therapy of high grade gliomas. Brain Pathol 2009; 19:694-712.
[14] Therasse P, Arbuck SG, Eisenhauer EA, Wanders J, Kaplan RS, Rubinstein L et al. New guidelines to evaluate the response to treatment in solid tumors. European Organization for Research and Treatment of Cancer, National Cancer Institute of the United States, National Cancer Institute of Canada. J Natl Cancer Inst 2000; 92(3):205-16.
[15] Macdonald DR, Cascino TL, Schold SC, Jr., Cairncross JG. Response criteria for phase II studies of supratentorial malignant glioma. J Clin Oncol 1990; 8(7):1277-1280.
[16] De Vleeschouwer S, Rapp M, Sorg RV, Steiger HJ, Stummer W, Van Gool S et al. Dendritic cell vaccination in patients with malignant gliomas: current status and future directions. Neurosurgery 2006; 59(5):988-999.
[17] Taal W, Brandsma D, de Bruin HG, Bromberg JE, Swaak-Kragten AT, Smitt PA et al. Incidence of early pseudo-progression in a cohort of malignant glioma patients treated with chemoirradiation with temozolomide.

Cancer 2008; 113(2):405-410.
[18] Vrabec M, Van Cauter S, Himmelreich U, Van Gool SW, Sunaert S, De Vleeschouwer S et al. MR perfusion and diffusion imaging in the follow-up of recurrent glioblastoma treated with dendritic cell immunotherapy: a pilot study. Neuroradiology 2010.
[19] Rutkowski S, De Vleeschouwer S, Kaempgen E, Wolff JEA, Kuhl J, Demaerel P et al. Surgery and adjuvant dendritic cell-based tumour vaccination for patients with relapsed malignant glioma, a feasibility study. Br J Cancer 2004; 91:1656-1662.
[20] Masucci GV, Mansson-Brahme E, Ragnarsson-Olding B, Nilsson B, Wagenius G, Hansson J. Alternating chemo-immunotherapy with temozolomide and low-dose interleukin-2 in patients with metastatic melanoma. Melanoma Res 2006; 16(4):357-363.
[21] Nowak AK, Robinson BW, Lake RA. Synergy between chemotherapy and immunotherapy in the treatment of established murine solid tumors. Cancer Res 2003; 63(15):4490-4496.
[22] van der Most RG, Currie A, Robinson BW, Lake RA. Cranking the immunologic engine with chemotherapy: using context to drive tumor antigen cross-presentation towards useful antitumor immunity. Cancer Res 2006; 66(2):601-604.
[23] Hoos A, Parmiani G, Hege K, Sznol M, Loibner H, Eggermont A et al. A clinical development paradigm for cancer vaccines and related biologics. J Immunother 2007; 30(1):1-15.
[24] De Vleeschouwer S, Fieuws S, Rutkowski S, Van Calenbergh F, Van Loon J, Goffin J et al. Postoperative adjuvant dendritic cell-based immunotherapy in patients with relapsed glioblastoma multiforme. Clin Cancer Res 2008; 14(10): 3098-3104.
[25] McIlroy D, Gregoire M. Optimizing dendritic cell-based anticancer immunotherapy: maturation state does have clinical impact. Cancer Immunol Immunother 2003; 52(10):583-591.
[26] Koski GK, Cohen PA, Roses RE, Xu S, Czerniecki BJ. Reengineering dendritic cell-based anti-cancer vaccines. Immunol Rev 2008; 222:256-76.:256-276.
[27] Ardon H, Van Gool S, Lopes IS, Maes W, Sciot R, Wilms G et al. Integration of autologous dendritic cell-based immunotherapy in the primary treatment for patients with newly diagnosed glioblastoma multiforme: a pilot study. J Neurooncol 2010.
[28] Jian B, Yang I, Parsa AT. Monitoring immune responses after glioma vaccine immunotherapy. Neurosurg Clin N Am 2010; 21(1):195-199.
[29] Baniyash M. Chronic inflammation, immunosuppression and cancer: new insights and outlook. Semin Cancer Biol 2006; 16(1):80-88.
[30] Murat A, Migliavacca E, Gorlia T, Lambiv WL, Shay T, Hamou MF et al. Stem cell-related "self-renewal" signature and high epidermal growth factor receptor expression associated with resistance to concomitant chemoradiotherapy in glioblastoma. J Clin Oncol 2008; %20;26(18):3015-3024.

[31] Prins RM, Soto H, Konkankit V, Odesa SK, Eskin A, Yong WH et al. Gene expression profile correlates with T-cell infiltration and relative survival in glioblastoma patients vaccinated with dendritic cell immunotherapy. Clin Cancer Res 2011; 17(6):1603-1615.